SECOND EDITION

DIABETES MELLITUS IN PREGNANCY

SECOND EDITION
DIABETES MELLITUS IN PREGNANCY

E. ALBERT REECE, M.D.

Abraham Roth Professor and Chairman
Department of Obstetrics, Gynecology, and
Reproductive Sciences
Professor
Department of Internal Medicine
Temple University School of Medicine
Director, Division of Maternal-Fetal Medicine
Department of Obstetrics, Gynecology, and
Reproductive Sciences
Temple University Hospital
Philadelphia, Pennsylvania

DONALD R. COUSTAN, M.D.

Professor and Chairman
Department of Obstetrics and Gynecology
Brown University School of Medicine
Obstetrician and Gynecologist-in-Chief
Department of Obstetrics and Gynecology
Women and Infants' Hospital
Providence, Rhode Island

Churchill Livingstone
New York, Edinburgh, London, Melbourne, Tokyo

Library of Congress Cataloging-in-Publication Data

Diabetes mellitus in pregnancy / [edited by] E. Albert Reece, Donald
    R. Coustan. — 2nd ed.
        p.   cm.
    Includes bibliographical references and index.
    ISBN 0-443-08979-5
    1. Diabetes in pregnancy.   I. Reece, E. Albert. II. Coustan,
Donald R.
    [DNLM: 1. Pregnancy in Diabetes. WQ 248 D5358 1995]
RG580.D5D524 1995
618.3—dc20
DNLM/DLC
for Library of Congress   95-12415
                                                               CIP

Second Edition © Churchill Livingstone Inc. 1995
First Edition © Churchill Livingstone Inc. 1988

Distributed in the United Kingdom by Churchill Livingstone, Robert Stevenson House, 1–3
Baxter's Place, Leith Walk, Edinburgh EH1 3AF, and by associated companies, branches, and
representatives throughout the world.

Accurate indications, adverse reactions, and dosage schedules for drugs are provided in this
book, but it is possible that they may change. The reader is urged to review the package information data of the manufacturers of the medications mentioned.

The Publishers have made every effort to trace the copyright holders for borrowed material. If
they have inadvertently overlooked any, they will be pleased to make the necessary arrange-
ments at the first opportunity.

Acquisitions Editor: *Jennifer Mitchell*
Production Editor: *Bridgett Dickinson and Dorothy J. Birch*
Production Supervisor: *Laura Mosberg-Cohen*
Cover Design: *Jeannette Jacobs*

Printed in the United States of America

First published in 1995   7   6   5   4   3   2   1

To my wife, Sharon,
and our children,
Kelie, Brynne, and Sharon–Andrea,
with love and gratitude for being supportive, patient, and long–suffering.

E. A. R.

To Terri, Becky, Rachel, and David,
who keep me from taking myself too seriously.

D. R. C.

Contributors

Roberta A. Ballard, M.D.

Professor, Department of Pediatrics, University of Pennsylvania School of Medicine; Director, Division of Neonatology, Children's Hospital of Philadelphia and Hospital of the University of Pennsylvania, Philadelphia, Pennsylvania

Peter H. Bennett, M.B., F.R.C.P., F.F.C.M.

Chief, Phoenix Epidemiology and Clinical Research Branch, National Institute of Diabetes and Digestive and Kidney Diseases, Phoenix, Arizona

Walter P. Borg, M.D.

Postdoctoral Fellow and Research Affiliate, Department of Internal Medicine, Yale University School of Medicine, New Haven, Connecticut; Resident, Department of Internal Medicine, John Dempsey Hospital, University of Connecticut Health Center, Farmington, Connecticut

Florence M. Brown, M.D.

Instructor in Medicine, Harvard Medical School; Associate Staff Physician, Joslin Diabetes Center, Boston, Massachusetts

Thomas A. Buchanan, M.D.

Associate Professor, Departments of Medicine and Obstetrics-Gynecology, University of Southern California School of Medicine; Attending Physician, Departments of Medicine and Obstetrics and Gynecology, LAC-USC Medical Center, Los Angeles, California

Marshall W. Carpenter, M.D.

Associate Professor, Department of Obstetrics and Gynecology, Brown University School of Medicine; Director, Maternal-Fetal Medicine, Women and Infants' Hospital, Providence, Rhode Island

Nam H. Cho, Ph.D.

Associate Professor, Department of Preventive Medicine, Ajou University School of Medicine, Suwon, Korea

C. Andrew Combs, M.D., Ph.D.

Associate Director, Department of Maternal-Fetal Medicine, Good Samaritan Health System, San Jose, California

Joshua Copel, M.D.

Professor, Department of Obstetrics and Gynecology, Yale University School of Medicine; Director, Department of Obstetrics, Yale-New Haven Hospital, New Haven, Connecticut

Larry Cousins, M.D.

Director, Maternal-Fetal Medicine, Division of Perinatology, Mary Birch Hospital for Women at Sharp Memorial and Sharp Perinatal Center, San Diego, California

Donald R. Coustan, M.D.

Professor and Chairman, Department of Obstetrics and Gynecology, Brown University School of Medicine; Obstetrician and Gynecologist–in–Chief, Department of Obstetrics and Gynecology, Women and Infants' Hospital, Providence, Rhode Island

Ulf J. Eriksson, M.D.

Associate Professor, Department of Medical Cell Biology, University of Uppsala, Uppsala, Sweden

Ann M. Ferris, Ph.D., R.D.

Professor and Head, Department of Nutritional Sciences, University of Connecticut College of Agriculture and Natural Resources, Storrs, Connecticut

Alan M. Friedman, M.D.
Assistant Professor, Department of Pediatrics, Yale University School of Medicine, New Haven, Connecticut

Steven G. Gabbe, M.D.
Professor and Chairman, Department of Obstetrics and Gynecology, Ohio State University College of Medicine; Attending Perinatologist, Division of Maternal–Fetal Medicine, Ohio State University Hospitals, Columbus, Ohio

Susan H. Guttentag, M.D.
Assistant Professor, Department of Pediatrics, University of Pennsylvania School of Medicine; Attending Neonatologist, Division of Neonatology, Children's Hospital of Philadelphia, Philadelphia, Pennsylvania

John W. Hare, M.D.
Associate Clinical Professor of Medicine, Harvard Medical School; Senior Physician, Joslin Diabetes Center, Consultant (Obstetrics), Brigham and Women's Hospital, Boston, Massachusetts

Carol J. Homko, R.N., M.S.
Diabetes Nurse Specialist, Division of Maternal-Fetal Medicine, Department of Obstetrics, Gynecology, and Reproductive Sciences, Temple University School of Medicine; Coordinator, Diabetes-in-Pregnancy and Research Programs, Division of Maternal-Fetal Medicine, Department of Obstetrics, Gynecology, and Reproductive Sciences, Temple University Hospital, Philadelphia, Pennsylvania

Lois Jovanovic–Peterson, M.D.
Professor, Department of Medicine, University of Southern California School of Medicine, Los Angeles, California; Senior Scientist, Clinical Research Department, Sansum Medical Research Foundation, Santa Barbara, California

John L. Kitzmiller, M.D.
Professor, Department of Obstetrics, Gynecology, and Reproductive Services, University of California, San Francisco, School of Medicine; Director, Maternal-Fetal Medicine, Good Samaritan Health Systems, San Jose, California

Charles S. Kleinman, M.D.
Professor, Departments of Pediatrics and Obstetrics and Gynecology, Yale University School of Medicine, New Haven, Connecticut

Susan Koch, M.S.
Genetic Counselor and Director, Perinatal Genetics, Department of Obstetrics, Gynecology, and Reproductive Services, Temple University School of Medicine, Philadelphia, Pennsylvania

Mark B. Landon, M.D.
Associate Professor, Department of Obstetrics and Gynecology, Ohio State University College of Medicine; Attending Perinatologist, Division of Maternal–Fetal Medicine, Ohio State University Hospitals, Columbus, Ohio

Oded Langer, M.D.
Professor, Division of Obstetrics and Maternal–Fetal Medicine, Department of Obstetrics and Gynecology, University of Texas Medical School at San Antonio; Director, Division of Obstetrics and Maternal–Fetal Medicine, Department of Obstetrics and Gynecology, University Health System, San Antonio, Texas

Barbara Luke, Sc.D., M.P.H., R.D.
Associate Professor and Director, Section of Reproductive and Perinatal Epidemiology, Department of Obstetrics and Gynecology, Rush Medical College of Rush University; Associate Scientist, Department of Obstetrics and Gynecology, Rush–Presbyterian–St. Luke's Medical Center, Chicago, Illinois

Frank Manning, M.Sc., F.R.C.S.(C)
Professor, Department of Obstetrics, Gynecology, and Reproductive Sciences, University of Manitoba Faculty of Medicine; Division Head, Maternal–Fetal Medicine, Department of Obstetrics and Gynecology, Women's Center, Winnipeg, Manitoba, Canada

Jennifer B. Marks, M.D.
Assistant Professor, Department of Medicine, University of Miami School of Medicine, Miami, Florida

Boyd E. Metzger, M.D.

Professor, Department of Medicine, Center for Endocrinology, Metabolism, and Molecular Medicine, Northwestern University Medical School, Attending Physician, Department of Medicine, Northwestern Memorial Hospital, Chicago, Illinois

Maureen A. Murtaugh, Ph.D., R.D.

Assistant Professor, Department of Clinical Nutrition, Rush University College of Health Sciences; Clinical Dietitian, Department of Food and Nutrition Services, Rush–Presbyterian–St. Luke's Medical Center, Chicago, Illinois

William Oh, M.D.

Professor and Chairman, Department of Pediatrics, Brown University School of Medicine; Pediatrician-in-Chief, Department of Pediatrics, Women and Infants' Hospital and Rhode Island Hospital, Providence, Rhode Island

John B. O'Sullivan, M.D.

Medical Director, Diabetes and Arthritis Foundation, Inc., Boston, Massachusetts

Mary Jo O'Sullivan, M.D.

Chief, Division of Perinatology, Professor, Department of Obstetrics and Gynecology, University of Miami School of Medicine, Miami, Florida

Charles M. Peterson, M.D.

Professor, Department of Medicine, University of Southern California School of Medicine, Los Angeles, California; Director, Research Department, Sansum Medical Research Foundation, Santa Barbara, California

David J. Pettitt, M.D.

Assistant Chief, Diabetes and Arthritis Epidemiology Section, Phoenix Epidemiology and Clinical Research Branch, National Institute of Diabetes and Digestive and Kidney Diseases, Phoenix, Arizona

E. Albert Reece, M.D.

Abraham Roth Professor and Chairman, Department of Obstetrics, Gynecology, and Reproductive Services, and Professor, Department of Internal Medicine,

Temple University School of Medicine; Director, Division of Maternal–Fetal Medicine, Department of Obstetrics, Gynecology, and Reproductive Services, Temple University Hospital, Philadelphia, Pennsylvania

Robert S. Sherwin, M.D.

Director, Diabetes Endocrinology Research Center, and Professor, Department of Internal Medicine, Yale University School of Medicine; Attending Endocrinologist, Department of Medicine, Yale–New Haven Hospital, New Haven, Connecticut

Don B. Singer, M.D.

Professor, Department of Pathology and Laboratory Medicine, Brown University School of Medicine; Pathologist–in–Chief, Department of Pathology, Women and Infants' Hospital of Rhode Island and Rhode Island Hospital, Providence, Rhode Island

Jay S. Skyler, M.D.

Professor, Departments of Medicine, Pediatrics, and Psychology, University of Miami School of Medicine, Miami, Florida

Judith M. Steel, M.B., Ch.B. F.R.C.P.Ed.

Honorary Lecturer, Department of Medical Science, University of St. Andrews, St Andrews, Fife, Scotland; Associate Specialist, Department of Diabetes, Victoria Hospital, Kirkcaldy, Fife, Scotland

John B. Susa, Ph.D.

Research Associate Professor, Department of Pediatrics, Brown University School of Medicine; Director, Pediatric Metabolic Research Laboratories, Providence, Rhode Island

William V. Tamborlane, M.D.

Section Chief, Pediatric Endocrinology, Director, Children's Clinical Research Center, and Professor, Department of Pediatrics, Yale University School of Medicine; Attending Pediatric Endocrinologist, Department of Pediatrics, Yale–New Haven Hospital, New Haven, Connecticut

Preface to the Second Edition

The first edition of *Diabetes Mellitus in Pregnancy: Principles and Practice* appeared in 1988. Since that time, management of both diabetes mellitus and diabetes in pregnancy have continued to undergo dramatic developments. The outlook for women with diabetes and their offspring continues to improve. Publication of the results of the Diabetes Control and Complications Trial (DCCT) in June 1994 has again brought to the attention of the scientific community and the lay public the importance of tight metabolic control in the management of diabetes.

The second edition of *Diabetes Mellitus in Pregnancy* has been extensively revised and rewritten to reflect changes in clinical practice. The developments highlighted in this edition include immunotherapeutic strategies for the prevention of type I diabetes in high risk individuals, clinical implications of the DCCT results, and advances in our understanding and prevention of diabetes-associated malformations. Many new figures and tables have been added and some illustrative materials have been replaced to further enhance the information presented.

This edition presents critical discussion of the current and expected state-of-the-art in diabetes in pregnancy. Once again, major authoritative up-to-date reviews and guidance cover the topics of general medical considerations, effects of diabetes on the fetus, management, pregnancy outcomes, counseling, and postpartum care. It remains the editors' intention that this book continues to be authoritative and a useful contribution to an expanding field. We also hope that it will serve practitioners, resident physicians, and other health care providers in the day-to-day care of patients.

We are indebted to the outstanding internationally recognized contributors without whose expertise and efforts this edition would not be possible. For this, we will be forever grateful.

E. Albert Reece, M.D.
Donald R. Coustan, M.D.

Preface to the First Edition

Diabetes mellitus, by virtue of its frequency and severity of its metabolic effects, has long been one of the most common and significant medical conditions complicating pregnancy. During the pre-insulin era, diabetic women found it difficult to become pregnant. When pregnancy occurred, both maternal and fetal mortalities were extremely high. The discovery and availability of insulin during the 1930s brought a rapid decline in maternal mortality, such that by the 1950s health-care providers and researchers could focus their efforts on the prevention of perinatal mortality. Except for deaths related to congenital malformations, perinatal mortality was reduced to background levels in the 1970s, and perinatal morbidity came to the foreground as the largest remaining unsolved problem of the 1980s.

Currently the presence of diabetes during pregnancy raises concerns about the course of fetal growth and development. It is becoming more and more clear that normal metabolic fuels are essential for normal embryogenesis, and that normalization of metabolism is best accomplished prior to conception, rather than after organogenesis has occurred. As pregnancy proceeds, the prevention of maternal complications and perinatal morbidity and mortality requires continued normalization of metabolism and close surveillance of the fetal condition. The achievement of these goals necessitates the cooperation of obstetricians/perinatologists, pediatricians/neonatologists, internists/diabetologists, nutritionists, diabetes educators, social workers, and other health-care practitioners. No other medical complication during pregnancy so strikingly brings into focus recent advances in technology, physiology, clinical care, and the social sciences as does diabetes mellitus.

Because of improvements in the care of diabetes mellitus, women with this disorder are living longer and experiencing more of its long-term complications. Thus, those who care for complicated pregnancies are encountering increasing numbers of diabetic women with vascular involvement of multi-organ systems. In the past, standard textbooks supported termination of such pregnancies. However, with recent improvements in prognosis, recommendations against conception or continuation of pregnancy are seldom warranted. Unfortunately, newer forms of management and technology are unfamiliar to many clinicians, and the counseling of pregnant women with diabetes may be influenced by this lack of up-to-date information.

In creating this book, the editors and authors have sought to provide a comprehensive overview of available information on the pathophysiology of both diabetes and pregnancy, and to describe appropriate methods for management of various aspects of this multifaceted problem. Sections on the epidemiology, genetics, and immunology of diabetes offer insight into issues that are usually of great concern to diabetic individuals planning a family, and thus to physicians and diabetes educators counseling these patients. Discussions of carbohydrate metabolism in normal and diabetic pregnancies provide the background for understanding later recommendations for clinical care. Maternal diabetes is examined for the ways it may be expressed as disorders in the feto-placental unit. Guidelines are presented for the management of gestational diabetes. Recommendations for when and how to deliver infants of diabetic mothers are followed by discussions of perinatal mortality and morbidity, neonatal management, and long-term outcomes for these children.

It is the editors' intention that this evaluation of the effects of diabetes mellitus in pregnancy will be a useful contribution to an expanding field, and that it will serve practitioners, resident physicians, and other health-care providers in the day-to-day care of patients.

We would like to express our gratitude to the contributors, who worked hard with little reward to provide state-of-the-art chapters in their particular fields of expertise. Their contributions are not only scholarly but also comprehensive and highly informative. We would also like to thank our secretaries for the many hours invested in typing, reviewing, and correcting the many versions of the manuscripts, and the editors at Churchill Livingstone, whose patience and forbearance allowed us to complete this book in good spirits and on friendly terms.

E. Albert Reece, M.D.
Donald R. Coustan, M.D.

Acknowledgment

We would also like to express our gratitude to our contributors, who have painstakingly written comprehensive, highly informative, and scholarly chapters. Efforts like these can only be described as labors of love. We truly appreciate as well the efforts invested in this book by Ms. Carol Homko, R.N., M.S., C.D.E., who not only was a contributor to this text, but assisted in coordinating the project. In addition, all our secretaries collectively deserve much praise and commendation for the many hours invested in typing, reviewing, and correcting the many versions of the manuscripts. Finally, we remain indebted to the editors of Churchill Livingstone, especially Ms. Jennifer Mitchell, whose patient yet persistent demeanor permitted the timely publication of this book.

Our lives have been greatly touched as we interacted with everyone who participated in the successful completion of this book—to you all we remain deeply grateful.

A Tribute to
Dr. Priscilla White
(March 17, 1900 to December 16, 1989)

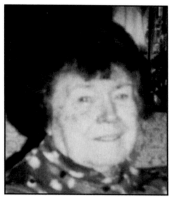
Dr. White in 1987.

The past half century has seen dramatic changes in the management of pregnancy complicated by diabetes, and equally dramatic improvements in outcomes. We of a younger generation of researchers have come late upon the scene, at a time when many of the major advances of the past are taken for granted. For this reason, we feel it appropriate to credit the formative work of early investigators, particularly Dr. Priscilla White, who is acknowledged to be one of the outstanding contributors to the study of diabetes in pregnancy.

In the course of working on the first edition of this book, we were privileged to confer with Dr. White and to hear her personal recollections of 50 years of research and patient care, in which Dr. White captured quite vividly the sadness and gloom, and the dismal reproductive prognosis for diabetic women. As Dr. White remembered:

> Diabetic women were discouraged from becoming pregnant, and termination of pregnancy was often recommended for those who did. Before insulin was available, patients often died during the course of their pregnancy, or their fetuses often died before birth, or as infants. Any successful pregnancy was remarkable, so doctors spent almost the entire pregnancy with their patients. We saw them weekly, practically. When they came in labor, I was notified immediately and stayed with them through the entire labor.

> Delivery was often done prematurely, because if patients were allowed to go to term, the babies would die. We did see, however, fewer mothers die following the introduction of insulin.

Dr. White spent virtually all her distinguished career in Boston, primarily at the Joslin Clinic, caring for pregnant women with diabetes. Her writings have been extensive and have served as mileposts chronicling the advances in management and outcome from the early 1920s through the late 1970s. Her system of classification of diabetes among pregnant women was the international standard by which such patients were described.

Her descriptions of the hardships experienced by diabetic individuals prior to the discovery of insulin underscore the tremendous contribution made by Dr. White and her contemporaries. Dr. White will always be respected and remembered with affection by diabetologists, obstetricians, and others who care for diabetic women during their pregnancies. Without the immense strides made by these forerunners, today's advancements might still be out of reach. We presented a copy of the first edition of this book to Dr. White. She graciously accepted our tribute. In 1989, Dr. White died at the age of 89. Fortunately, her contributions live on!

E. Albert Reece, M.D.
Donald R. Coustan, M.D.

xvii

Contents

xix

1

The History of Diabetes Mellitus

E. ALBERT REECE

The history of diabetes probably dates back to the beginning of humankind, encompassing centuries, generations, and civilizations. An historical review of the events surrounding the evolution of our current knowledge of diabetes mellitus must examine the oldest civilizations, including the Babylonians, Assyrians, Egyptians, Chinese, and Japanese, as well as the contributions of the Greeks, Romans, Europeans, and Americans. This chapter doses not attempt to give credit to all contributors to our present knowledge but rather attempts to develop a cohesive story of the evolution of the field of diabetes mellitus. To place some chronology to events and to put them in the context of the times in which they occurred, it is necessary to describe some societal or political occurrences of those times that had an effect on the development of this field.

EARLY CIVILIZATION AND RECORDS OF DIABETES

Early Egyptian Medicine

Although no consensus exists as to the beginnings of civilization, the period 5000 to 4500 BC is often cited to represent that era. At that time, Babylon was founded by the Sumerians but was later conquered in 3800 BC by the Babylonians and the Assyrians.[1,2] Babylon was a powerful empire encompassing many nations. In modern terms, such growth would be referred to as imperialism and expansionism. In any event, the rulership was theocratic, with religion dominating politics as well as medicine. Disease was considered to be due to evil spirits or demons that influenced the physical and mental well-being of humans. Beliefs or concepts of this nature led to the beginning of medical astrology. Much of early Babylonian and Assyrian medicine was inscribed on some 800 medical tablets, much of which was translated by Morris Jastrow.[1,2]

The Sumerians made inscriptions in clay; the Egyptians used strips of papyrus, reeds fastened together and shaped into rolls, on which they inscribed information. These strips subsequently became permanent records.[3] For our purposes, the most interesting of these papyri is Papyrus Ebers, written about 1500 BC, which records medical knowledge of ancient days. This contains a record of abnormal polyuria, now believed to be related to diabetes.[1,3,4] This probably represents the first recorded reference to the symptoms of diabetes.

Early Greek Medicine

As previously mentioned, the dominant ideology in early civilization was theocracy, with religion dictating every aspect of human life. It was not until about the time of Hippocrates (466–377 BC) that there came about some separation of medicine from religion. In the Hippocratic writings, no direct reference to diabetes exists. This was probably because the disease was rare and incurable, and the Hippocratic philosophy was to pay little attention to such diseases. There is some indirect evidence that Hippocrates was familiar with diabetic conditions. In the writing of the Ermerins edition of Hippocrates (p. 354), a word is used that is translated to mean "to make water much or often." This word was also referred to by Aristotle and may be the condition known to writers of that time as "wasting of the body."[3,5]

Aretaeus of Cappadocia (AD 30–90) was highly respected in his time and was of similar stature in society to Hippocrates. He embraced most of the philosophy of his contemporaries, namely, Hippocrates and Pythagoras, but not totally. At the time, there was a Pythagorean philosophy, described in the works of Plato,[3] that stated:

> He who instead of accepting his destiny endeavors to prolong life by medicine is likely to multiply and magnify his diseases; regimen and not medicine is the true cure when a man has time at his disposal. No attempt should be made to cure a disease system and afford a long and miserable life to the Man himself and to his descendants.

Although Aretaeus did not agree with the above philosophy at the time, he apparently was politically shrewd enough not to disagree with a dominant philosophy yet maintain the respect of his peers. He was known for his dignity and his love of the art of medicine, his sympathy for sick patients, and his unswerving belief that, whenever possible, medicine should be used to prolong life. In addition, he believed that a physician should also feel obliged to attend to incurable cases even though he may be able to do no more than express sympathy.[3,6] One might reflect on such a principle and possibly find it difficult to distinguish that position from those held by most 20th century physicians.

Although diabetes had always been present, it was Aretaeus who is credited for naming this medical illness. The term *diabetes* means to pass through or to siphon. The following quote will demonstrate how severe these patients with diabetes were and the sense of frustration and hopelessness that such a disease generated, not only to the patient but to the physicians as well. Aretaeus[7] describes diabetes as

> a wonderful affliction, not very frequently in men, being a melting down of the flesh and limbs into urine. Its cause is of a cold and humid nature as in dropsy, for the patients never stop making water, but the flow is incessant as if from the opening of aqueducts. The nature of the disease is chronic, but the patient is short lived, for the illness is rapid and the death speedly. Moreover, the life is disgusted and painful, thirst unquenchable, with excessive drinking which, however, is disproportionate to the large quantity of urine. If at times they abstain from drinking, the mouth becomes

parched and the body dry. The viscera seems scorched up. They are affected with nausea, restlessness and burning thirst and at no distant time they expire.

In another quotation, Aretaeus describes further the symptoms of diabetes, particularly the severe polyuria and the progressive nature of this disease. Except for acquired immunodeficiency syndrome, we can hardly comprehend the sense of hopelessness that such a disease evoked in both patients and physicians. Aretaeus[3] recreates the sorrow, pain, and gloom:

> Diabetes is a wasting of the flesh and limbs into urine from a cause similar to dropsy. The patient never ceasing to make water and the discharge is an incessant sluice let off. The patient does not survive long for the marasmus is rapid and death speedy. The thirst is ungovernable. The copious potations are more than equaled by the diffuse urinary discharge, for more urine flows away, how indeed could the making of water be stopped, or what sense of modesty is paramount to pain? The epithet diabetes has been assigned from the disorder being somewhat like passing of water by a siphon.

We can sense the frustrations in the writings of Aretaeus as he describes the fate of patients with diabetes. Medical therapy was not emphasized for more than one reason. As stated before, the Pythagorean philosophy advocated that medicine should not be used to prolong the sufferings of an incurable disease, and no available cure for diabetes existed.

Early Roman Medicine

Celsus (30 BC to AD 50), a Roman translator of Greek medicine, summarized the medical and surgical progress of both the Hippocratic and the Alexandrian periods. Celsus also described individuals with diabetes as "patients with a discharge of urine greater than the amount of fluid taken in by mouth," a definition similar to that of Aretaeus.[8,9]

Early Arabian Medicine

Arabian medicine was highlighted by an acclaimed physician named Avicenna (AD 980–1027). He was not only a meticulous physician but a prolific writer. It is said that he wrote more than 100 articles that were compiled to form a canon. Such scholarship is worthy of congratulations. However, some may argue strongly that the peer review process was entirely different then and, of course, more difficult now. In any event, Avicenna made important observations regarding diabetes. He commented that diabetes may be primary or secondary to another disease. He also observed that diabetic patients have an irregular appetite associated with thirst, mental exhaustion, inability to work, and loss of sexual functions. In essence, Avicenna described many of the features related to diabetes that we are well aware of today. In fact, he observed the carbuncles, furuncles, and the variety of diabetic complications. It is said that Avicenna believed that diabetes affected the liver, probably causing enlargement of the organ.[1,10]

Early Asian Medicine

The Hindus had three leading medical texts, the Charaka, the Susruta, and the Vagbhata. The Susruta was the book of surgery, and the Charaka was the book of medicine. The Hindu medical writings of the sixth century refer to diabetes as honey urine. It describes diabetes[11]:

A disease of the rich and one that is brought about by gluttony or overindulgence in flour and sugar. This disease is ushered in by the appearance of morbid secretions about the teeth, nose, ears and eyes. The hands and feet are very hot and burning. The surface of the skin is shiny as if oil had been applied to it, this accomplished by the thirst and the sweet taste in the mouth. The different varieties of this disease are distinguished from each other by the symptoms and by the color of the urine. If the disease is produced by phlegm, insects approach the urine. The person is languid. His body becomes flat and there is discharge with mucus from the nose and mouth with dyspeptic symptoms and looseness of the skin. He is always sleeping with cough and difficulty breathing.

The ancient Hindus were known for their surgical skills and their many operative procedures. The Susruta described 121 different surgical instruments. They performed lithotomy, cesarean section, excision of tumor, removal of omental hernia, and amputations. Evidently, these surgical procedures remained unimproved by the Greeks and Romans.[8,11]

The earliest of the Chinese medicine texts is based on the works of Huag-ti of 2697 BC. Records were preserved on lacquer on strips of bamboo or palm leaves. These writings represent the counterpart of the Egyptian picture writing. The Chinese must be credited for physical anthropometry. Japanese medicine began much later, with the first medical book dating back to AD 982.

The Chinese and Japanese also recognized the symptoms of diabetes but were even less restrained with their description and wrote "the urine of diabetics was very large in amount and it was so sweet that it attracted dogs."[8] One can imagine the folklore that accompanied this disease. It is unfortunate that such information is not readily available. However, one can imagine that patients afflicted with diabetes were considered demonic and often were ostracized.

European and American Medicine

Observations of patients having diabetes were also made by Italian, Portuguese, Greek, Dutch, and other Europeans, as well as American physicians. In more recent times, many more observations regarding diabetes were made. Physicians went beyond merely describing the hopelessness and the osmotic diuretic effect of severe diabetes but began thinking of possible causes and exploring these ideas. Some conducted experiments to simulate the medical illness in order to apply a scientific approach to the understanding of this disease.

Sylvanus (1478–1555) believed that diabetes was a disease of the blood, whereas Cardano (1505–1576) did not accept the dictum that diabetes was a disease of greater fluid output than intake. Therefore, he compiled a table in which he recorded the intake of liquid and urinary output in diabetic patients. Willis Wyatt (1621–1675) of Oxford University claimed diabetes to be a primary disease of the blood. He explained that the sugar present in the urine of patients with diabetes represented excretion of sugar that was initially in the blood. In fact, he made the best qualitative urinalysis studies possible in that time.[3]

In 1682, Brunner[12] created an animal model to study diabetes by destroying the pancreas of experimental animals, causing polyuria and polydypsia. Other observations were made that continued to refine the understanding and characterization of diabetes. Dobson[13] in 1776 demonstrated that diabetic urine contained sugar that fermented. In 1888, Cawley[14] diagnosed diabetes for the first time by demonstrating the presence of sugar in the urine. He observed that the disease may result from injury to the pancreas, as had already been observed in experimental animals in 1682 by Brunner.[12]

Throughout this time, diabetes had been recognized and many of its symptoms described. As more observations were made, its clinical and diagnostic features were characterized.[15] However, no mention was made of attempts to control the disease. The foundation for systematic treatment of diabetes by restricting the diet should be credited to Rollo[16,17] in 1797. Soon thereafter, Bouchardat (1806–1866) proposed a management of diet and exercise that seems rather contemporary.[18] He advocated the use of fresh fats as a substitute for carbohydrate, the avoidance of milk because of its lactose, and the use of alcohol as a fluid. He also invented gluten bread, stressed the use of green vegetables in the diet, and emphasized the importance of "undernutrition." Bouchardat[18] has been credited for professing a modern viewpoint concerning diabetes. Such a therapeutic approach suggests that physicians were then convinced that the disease was caused by the inability of the body to handle carbohydrates properly. Several physicians and investigators subsequently emphasized dietary management of diabetes. Clearly, the Pythagorean era had ended and was replaced by the philosophy of Aretaeus; a potentially incurable disease was now being treated, and diligent efforts were made to prolong life. In any event, as one reads the literature, one understands diabetes as a curable problem, since much effort was dedicated toward this disease. Both clinicians and investigators focused on potential causes and possible cures.[3,19] Naunyn[19] devoted most of his life to the study of diabetes. He strongly advised dietary management and suggested the following points[3,19]:

1. The alpha and omega care of diabetes is dietetic treatment and not drugs.
2. Diabetic glycosuria increases with time while the weight of the patient decreases.
3. When the diabetic patient is free from sugar, tolerance usually increases; therefore aim to manage the patient sugar-free to prevent glycosuria.
4. Reduction of carbohydrates and proteins is useful for the removal of glycosuria.
5. Sugar-producing foods are carbohydrates and proteins.

6. Determine the exact qualitative and quantitative diet for every diabetic patient who comes under treatment.
7. Patients get along well on 30 to 35 calories/kg body weight.
8. Sugar production from fat does not play such an important role as to influence diabetic glycosuria to a notable extent.
9. For this reason and on account of its high caloric value, fat is the most valuable food for the diabetic.

As we look back at history, we see that the recommendations and observations of Avicenna, Bouchardat, and Naunyn were similar to what we currently recommend for the treatment of diabetes. Progress seems almost episodic, whereby great strides were made rather rapidly, then progress slowed and remained in a steady state for a long while.

EARLY PATHOPHYSIOLOGY

As mentioned, experimental work began as early as 1682 by Brunner,[12] demonstrating that the pancreas was the diseased organ in diabetic individuals. In 1869, Langerhans[20] described little islands within the pancreas, now known as islets of Langerhans. He offered no suggestion as to their physiologic significance. Shaffer in 1895 suggested that these islets, when diseased, produced diabetes.[3] Six years later in the United States, Opie[21,22] elaborated on the idea that diabetes was a disease due to degeneration of the islets of Langerhans in the pancreas and that these islets had an internal secretion that, when altered in form and function, resulted in diabetes.

Minkowski and von Mering became interested in diabetes research tangentially. They were investigating the role and function of the pancreas in digestion and conducted a pancreatectomy in a dog. The dog was house-trained but nevertheless developed an uncontrollable polyuria similar to that seen in diabetic patients. This research subsequently led to the confirmation that removal of the pancreas caused diabetes.[7,23–25] Although Langerhans[20] had previously described the islets of Langerhans, neither he nor any other investigator suggested any physiologic significance to these islets until Opie.[21,22] The work of Minkowski[25] and the observations by Opie[21,22] began to close the link between islet cell disease and diabetes. In fact, Opie in 1901[21,22] observed changes in the structure of the islet tissue that could be demonstrated in the pancreas of patients dying of diabetes.

For the next 18 years, many investigators concentrated on the islet cells.[25,26] Paulesco, a physiologist in Bucharest, had succeeded in making an extract from the pancreas in 1916, which he called pancreine that when injected into a diabetic dog gave temporary relief from the symptoms. The German regime stopped his research, and he was not able to resume his scientific work until 1920. It was not until 1921 that he published his paper. Unfortunately, Paulesco never succeeded in obtaining a pure extract suitable for humans.[7,27] By the early 1900s, the association of diabetes with islet cell pancreatic disease became an established medical fact. At this point, research was directed at replacement therapy. It became clear that the substance secreted by these islet cells was insufficient in diabetic patients. Zuelzer et al. (1906–1909) prepared an extract from the expressed juice of the pancreas, treated it with alcohol, and dissolved the residue with the salt. This extract was tested in pancreatectomized dogs with hyperglycemia and ketonuria, eight diabetic humans, and four cases of humans with ketosis.[3,28] This was clearly the right direction and probably as close as anyone came to the discovery of insulin before Banting and Best. This extract contained a variety of impurities, and after injection, subjects became very ill with chills and fever. The efforts of Zuelzer and colleagues were recognized by MacLeod, in whose laboratory insulin was eventually discovered. MacLeod stated, "Zuelzer in 1908 came very near to isolating what we now call insulin."[7]

DISCOVERY OF INSULIN

A variety of experiments conducted at that time were aimed at further exploring the pathophysiologic bases of diabetes. Barron wrote a comprehensive article of his work on the pancreas. Banting describes how he became impressed with Barron's work but particularly with the analogy he drew between the degenerative changes induced by experimental ligation of the pancreatic duct or blockage of the duct by gallstones.[7,29] As we all know, good science is created in the morning. Such was true with the discovery of insulin. Banting apparently awoke at 2:00 AM and was bothered by an

idea resulting from his late night reading, so he got up and scribbled on a piece of paper, "Ligate pancreatic duct of dogs, wait 6–8 weeks for degeneration, and remove the residue and extract."[7]

At that time (1920), Banting was a young general practitioner in London and a demonstrator in anatomy. MacLeod was a successful investigator at the University of Toronto. Banting wrote MacLeod and submitted a proposal for doing a series of experiments that would cure diabetes. He was rather precise in detailing his needs. He wanted two medical students, a few dogs, laboratory space, and certainly sufficient funding. Such an ambitious proposal by a new investigator submitted to granting agencies of our time would not pass the receptionist's desk. In any event, MacLeod allocated two medical student assistants, Best and Naunyn, but Best started working with Banting first. By the end of the first month, Best had enjoyed the work so much that he decided that he would work a second month. Shortly after the end of the 8-week period, they both were successful in isolating the pancreatic extract that was injected into a pancreatectomized dog. Banting[30] describes how he will never forget:

> the joy of opening the door of the cage and seeing the dog which had been unable to walk previously, jump on the floor and run around the room in a normal fashion following injection of the extract.

The first patient who received the new hormone was Leonard Thompson, a 14-year-old boy, on January 11, 1922.[7,30] He was admitted to the Toronto General Hospital with nocturia of 2.5 years' duration and weighed only 29 kg. Because neither Banting nor Best had practice privileges at Toronto General, Dr. Ed Jeffrey, an intern, administered the first dose of insulin, which consisted of 7.5 ml of pancreatic extract being injected into each of the patient's buttocks. Leonard was discharged from the hospital on May 15, 1922. He lived a relatively normal life, playing sports and working intermittently. Leonard died at the age of 27 years from bronchopneumonia.[31]

DIABETES IN PREGNANCY

Before 1856, there is hardly any report of pregnancy complicating diabetes. Blott wrote that "true diabetes is inconsistent with conception."[7,28] It was not until

1882 that a report by Duncan described 22 pregnancies in the literature, and for the first time, the aforementioned statement of Blott as well as the dominant philosophy at the time was challenged.[32,33] Subsequently, in 1909, Peel collected 66 cases; 27 percent of the mothers died at the time of labor or within 1 to 2 weeks afterward, and during the following 2 years, 22 percent more mothers died. One-eighth of the pregnancies ended in abortion, and in one-third of the cases that went to term, the baby was born dead.[7,34] This trend of high maternal and fetal mortality continued until the discovery of insulin. However, physicians were somewhat consoled in that the diabetic pregnancies were rare. In fact, Jellet,[7] in a 1905 edition of his manual of midwifery, made the following observation: "First of all, the disease is not a common one, and in the second place, the disability by it is usually so great that as a rule sexual functions including menstruation are arrested." One of the earliest descriptions of gesta-

tional diabetes is by Beunewitz. He quotes a series of 19 cases of diabetes in pregnancy, 10 of which resulted in death of the mother during labor or shortly thereafter.[7,28]

As described previously, diabetes was a disease with a dismal prognosis, and reproductive success in these women was not common. Pregnancy worsened the disease and shortened the lives of these patients, many of whom died during or shortly after the pregnancy. In 1920, De Lee[35] wrote that sterility was common among diabetics, probably due to atrophy of the uterus and ovaries, which might also explain the frequent intermittent and premature menopause. He continued by saying that abortion and premature labor occurred in 33 percent of the pregnancies. The children, if pregnancies went to term, often died shortly after birth, with an overall perinatal mortality rate of about 60 to 70 percent. Diabetes was described as becoming progressively worse with each pregnancy. The nervous

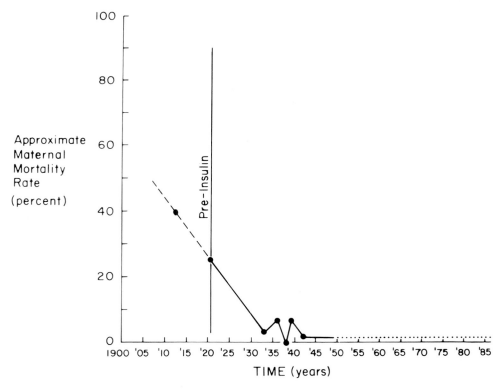

Fig. 1-1. Maternal mortality before and after the discovery of insulin. A precipitous decline in maternal deaths is depicted shortly after the discovery and use of insulin.

system was affected, and about 30 percent of mothers died, primarily because of diabetic ketoacidosis.

The advent of insulin brought about a dramatic change in the overall outlook for diabetic women and their reproductive potential. There was a dramatic fall in the maternal mortality from 45 percent to just over 2 percent shortly after the introduction of insulin (Fig. 1-1). However, the perinatal mortality did not rapidly change but, rather, slowly decreased over time (Fig. 1-2). Other problems not altered by the use of insulin included the very large babies and the associated traumatic injury to these fetuses and their mothers during parturition. Other continuing problems were neonatal hypoglycemia, congenital malformations, toxemia of pregnancy, and infections.[7,36–40]

In view of the lack of significant improvements in perinatal mortality with the advent of insulin therapy, which contrasted with the reduced maternal mortality observed, several attempts were made to reduce the fetal death rate. It was observed that beyond 36 weeks of gestation, there was a significant increase in the stillbirth rate, on the order of 10-fold. It was said that the fetal mortality was about 25 percent if the birth weight of the baby was approximately 7 lb (3.2 kg). However, when supervision was poor or totally absent, there was a 70 percent fetal mortality usually associated with a birth weight of 10 lb (4.5 kg) or more. Because of these concerns, diabetic patients were routinely delivered at or before 36 weeks by cesarean section or by induction of labor if fetal death had not already occurred, or sooner if maternal complications necessitated early delivery.

Diabetes care soon became centralized, and large centers such as King's College in England and the Joslin Clinic in the United States became major referral centers to which patients from all over the world were referred. Various institutional protocols emerged, all aimed at improving fetal outcome. There was a domi-

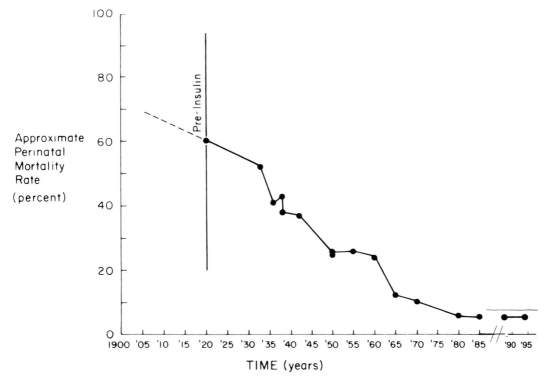

Fig. 1-2. Perinatal mortality before and after the discovery of insulin. Although a decline in perinatal death was observed, this decline was gradual over time.

nant theory originating in Boston that hormone use could improve pregnancy outcome. This later led to White in 1945 claiming a 97 percent fetal survival rate in cases with normal hormone balance and 47 percent survival in the cases with abnormal hormone balance.[41] Subsequent studies, however, showed that the use of estrogens in the doses that were used did not reduce infant mortality in diabetic patients and did not seem to have any beneficial effects on maternal health. In Copenhagen in 1954, Pedersen showed that the fetal mortality rate was significantly lower in patients who were being followed over a long period than in those who were first seen at or about the time of their delivery.[7] So, as early as the 1950s, there was an emerging philosophy that closer surveillance of patients seemed to result in improved fetal outcome. This led to a management policy of long-term or frequent hospitalizations and early delivery of pregnant patients with diabetes.

Other advances included new types of insulin, particularly the long-acting type and, most recently, human insulin with its low antigenic properties. Other adjunctive tools included estriol measurement, human placental lactogen measurement, assessment of fetal growth with ultrasound, antepartum fetal heart rate testing, fetal blood sampling techniques during labor, glucose meters, insulin pumps, neonatal intensive care units, and skilled pediatric care. These "tools" have been used to a lesser or greater extent over the years, and some have been considered to improve perinatal outcome whereas others, such as estriols and human placental lactogen, have been dropped from clinical use as other newer therapies were found to be of greater value. In 1977, Karlsson and Kjellmer[42] showed

in a retrospective study that there was a linear relationship between glycemic control and perinatal mortality. These findings were corroborated by many other studies and subsequently led to a new trend in diabetes care. Ambient glucose was stringently maintained as close to nondiabetic levels as possible, with a fairly rapid decline in perinatal mortality rates. These data were reported both in Europe[43] and the United States[44] (Tables 1-1 and 1-2). At the present time, most centers around the country report an average perinatal rate of less than 5 percent. Patients are living much longer, hence they are experiencing more of the vascular complications of diabetes with its potential effects of pregnancy. In fact, the cause of maternal deaths has shifted from primarily diabetic ketoacidosis to cardiorenal complications[45] (Table 1-3).

As many of these complications appeared, an increased incidence in perinatal mortality was found to be associated with patients having complications of diabetes, and recommendations were made regarding the avoidance of pregnancy or the termination of preg-

Table 1-2. Viable Fetal Survival in 416 Pregnancies with Maternal Vascular Disease at the Joslin Clinic

White Classification	1924–1962		1963–1975	
	No.	Survival Rate (%)	No.	Survival Rate (%)
R	34	74	48	84
F	126	65	59	72
RF	53	54	30	81
H	0	0	4	100
T	0	0	4	75

(From Hare and White,[44] with permission.)

Table 1-1. Perinatal Mortality Among 1,332 Infants of Diabetic Mothers Born at the Rigshospital, 1946–1972

White Classification	Total No. of Infants	Perinatal Mortality (%)
A	181	5.0
B	316	13.9
C	331	18.1
D	425	17.9
F	79	35.4
Total	1,332	16.3

(From Pedersen et al,[43] with permission.)

Table 1-3. Cause of Death in 27,966 Diabetic Patients at the Joslin Clinic 1897–1968

Period	Diabetic Ketoacidosis (%)	Cardiorenal Vascular Disease (%)
1897–1914	64.0	18.0
1914–1922	41.5	25.0
1922–1936	8.3	54.4
1937–1949	2.2	69.0
1950–1965	1.0	77.0
1966–1968	1.0	74.0

(Modified from Marble et al,[45] with permission.)

nancy in patients who had various forms of moderate to severe diabetic vasculopathy. It was also believed that diabetes was worsened by the effects of pregnancy. Evolving data to the present time have shown that, except for coronary artery disease, pregnancy is not contraindicated in diabetic patients with vascular complications. Also, the perinatal outcome among these pregnancies does not appear to be significantly different from other insulin-dependent diabetic patients when metabolic control is stringently maintained.[46]

There is no doubt that very impressive strides have been made with regard to diabetes in pregnancy, so that at the present time the expectation of the diabetic mother regarding pregnancy performance and fetal outcome can be fairly similar to that of a nondiabetic patient. There are, however, some unresolved problems, namely, macrosomia and congenital malformations. The incidence of birth defects has not significantly changed over time, and most series report a rate of 6 to 12 percent. Both clinical and laboratory studies suggest that these malformations are caused by derangement in metabolism during organogenesis.[40,47] Recent work has also shown that by the normalization of metabolism in the preconceptual period, such malformations can be prevented.[48] It is also true, however, that despite encouragement for preconceptional control, patients will become pregnant during unsatisfactory metabolic control. Some studies are now looking at possible therapeutic measures that may either ameliorate or prevent defects caused by hyperglycemia during organogenesis. Recent studies in rodents have demonstrated that fatty acid supplementation can prevent malformations, even in the presence of severe hyperglycemic conditions.[40,47]

As we look over the relatively brief history of pregnancy and diabetes, it is apparent that significant strides have been made. It was only in 1776 that Buchan[7,15] wrote:

> In our matrimonial contracts it is amazing so little regard is given to the health and form of the object. Our sportsmen know that the generous courser cannot be bred out of the foundered jade, nor the sagacious spaniel out of the snarling cur. This is settled upon immutable laws. A man who marries a woman of sickly constitution and descended from unhealthy parents, whatever his views may be, cannot be said to act as a prudent part. A diseased woman may prove fertile. Should this be the case, the family must become

an infirmary. What prospect of happiness a father of such a family has, we shall leave anyone to judge.

Fortunately, we have surpassed that age when people viewed diabetes as a disease of sorrow and unhappiness with little chance for procreation. Today we can look at such quotes with cynicism.

Although diabetes is probably as old as humankind, some problems still remain without solution. A visionary of our time might see history describing our generation as one in which improved techniques were achieved, leading to better glucose monitoring and control; complex problems relating to pathogenesis of diabetes were unraveled; the various effects of diabetes on organ systems were determined; new methods were introduced for the prevention of diabetes; and the various causes of aberrations of fetal growth and the effects of long-term metabolic control on the development of vasculopathy were explored. We hope the future will also bring about a cure for diabetes, technological or insulin pump or islet cell or embryonic pancreas transplantation, or possibly even the microinjection of insulin genes into somatic cells with subsequent autoregulation of insulin production.

REFERENCES

1. Banting FG: The internal secretion of the pancreas. Am J Physiol 59:479, 1922
2. Jastrow M: The medicine of the Babylonians and Assyrians. Proc R Soc Med Lond (Sect Hist Med) 7:109, 1913–1914
3. Barach JH: Historical facts in diabetes. Ann Med Hist 10:387, 1928
4. Ebbell B (trans): The Papyrus Ebers: The Greatest Egyptian Medical Document. Levin and Munksgaard, Copenhagen, 1937
5. Gemmill CL: The Greek concept of diabetes. Bull NY Acad Med 48:1033, 1972
6. Aretaeus of Cappadocia: On diabetes. pp. 338 and 485. In Adams F (ed): The Extant Works. London, 1856
7. Peel J: A historical review of diabetes and pregnancy. J Obstet Gynecol Br Cwlth 79:385, 1972
8. Ballard JF: A descriptive outline of the history of medicine from its earliest days of 600 BC. Ann Med Hist 6:53, 1924
9. Celsus AAC: De Medicina. 3 vols. (English translation by WG Spencer). W. Heinemann, London, 1935–1938
10. Gruner OC: Avicenna Ibn Sina. A treatise on the Canon

of Medicine incorporating a translation of the first book. London, 1930

11. Frank LL: Diabetes mellitus in the texts of old Hindu medicine (Charaka, Susruta, Vagbhata). Am J Gastroenterol 27:76, 1957

12. Brunner JC: Experimenta nova circa pancreas. Amstelaedami, apud. H. Weststenium, 1683

13. Dobson M: Experiments and observations on the urine in diabetes. Med Obs Inq Lond 5:298, 1776

14. Cawley T: A singular case of diabetes, consisting entirely in the quality of the urine; with an inquiry into the different theories of that disease. Lond Med J 9:286, 1888

15. Buchan W: Of the diabetes, and other disorders of the kidneys and bladder. p. A2. In: Domestic Medicine. 10th Ed. London, 1778

16. Rollo J: Cases of the Diabetes Mellitus. 2nd Ed. C. Dilly, London, 1798

17. Rollo J: An Account of Two Cases of the Diabetes Mellitus, with Remarks as They Arose during the Progress of the Cure. C. Dilly, London, 1797

18. Bouchardat A: Du Diabete Sucre ou glycourie; son traitement hygienique. Germer-Bailliere, Paris, 1875

19. Naunyn B: Der Diabetes mellitus. A. Holder, Wien, 1898

20. Langerhans P: Beitrage zur mikroskopichen Anatomie der Bauchspeicheldr use. Inaugural-Dissertation. Berlin, 1869

21. Opie EL: On the relation of chronic interstitial pancreatitis to the islands of Langerhans and to diabetes mellitus. J Exp Med 5:397, 1900–1901

22. Opie EL: The relation of diabetes mellitus to lesions of the pancreas. Hyaline degeneration of the islands of Langerhans. J Exp Med 5:527, 1990–1901

23. Mann RJ: Historical vignette: "honey urine" to pancreatic diabetes: 600 BC–1922. Mayo Clin Proc 46:56, 1971

24. von Mering J, Minkowski O: Diabetes mellitus nach Pankreas-extirpation. Arch Exp Pathol Pharm Leipzig 26:371, 1890

25. Minkowski O: Ueber das Vorkommen von Oxybuttersaure im Harn bei Diabetes mellitus. Arch Exp Pathol Pharm Leipzig 18:35, 1884

26. Nelken L: Chairman's remarks. In Insulin in Retrospect. Isr J Med 8:467, 1972

27. Paulesco NC: Recherches sur le role du pancreas dans l'assimilation nutritive. Arch Int Physiol 17:85, 1921

28. Zuelzer GL: Uber Versuch einer specifischen Fermenttherapie des Diabetes. Z Exp Pathol Ther Berlin 5:307, 1908

29. Barron M: The relation of the islets of Langerhans to diabetes, with special reference to cases of pancreatic lithiasis. Surg Gynecol Obstet 31:437, 1920

30. Banting FG, Best CH: The internal secretion of the pancreas. J Lab Clin Med 7:251, 1922

31. Burrow G, Hazlett B, Phillips MJ: A case of diabetes mellitus. N Engl J Med 306:304, 1982

32. Duncan GG: Diabetes Mellitus: Principles and Treatment. WB Saunders, Philadelphia, 1951

33. Duncan JM: On puerperal diabetes. Trans Obstet Soc Lond 24:256, 1882

34. Williams JW: Obstetrics. 5th Ed. Appleton & Lange, East Norwalk, CT, 1923

35. De Lee JB: The Principles and Practice of Obstetrics. 3rd Ed. WB Saunders, Philadelphia, 1920

36. Joslin EP: Diabetic Manual. 8th Ed. Lea & Febiger, Philadelphia, 1948

37. Joslin EP, Root HF, White P et al: The Treatment of Diabetes Mellitus. 8th Ed. Lea & Febiger, Philadelphia, 1948

38. Papaspyros NS: The History of Diabetes Mellitus. 1st Ed. Thieme, Stuttgart, 1952

39. Papaspyros NS: The History of Diabetes Mellitus. 2nd Ed. Thieme, Stuttgart, 1964

40. Reece EA, Hobbins JC: Diabetic embryopathy: pathogenesis, prenatal diagnosis and prevention. Obstet Gynecol Surv 41:325, 1986

41. White P, Raymond ST, Elliott PJ: Prediction and prevention of late pregnancy accidents in diabetes. Am J Med Sci 198:482, 1939

42. Karlsson K, Kjellmer I: The outcome of diabetic pregnancies in relation to the mother's blood sugar level. Am J Obstet Gynecol 112:213, 1972

43. Pedersen J, Molsted-Pedersen L, Andersen B: Assessors of fetal perinatal mortality in diabetic pregnancy. Diabetes 23:302, 1974

44. Hare JW, White P: Pregnancy and diabetes complicated by vascular disease. Diabetes 26:953, 1977

45. Marble A, White P, Bradley RF, Krall LP (eds): Joslin's Diabetes Mellitus. 11th Ed. Lea & Febiger, Philadelphia, 1971

46. Coustan DR, Berkowitz RL, Hobbins JC: Tight metabolic control of overt diabetes in pregnancy. Am J Med 68:845, 1980

47. Pinter E, Reece EA, Leranth C et al: Yolk sac failure in embryopathy due to hyperglycemia: ultrastructural analysis of yok sac differentiation in rat conceptuses under hyperglycemic culture conditions. Teratology 33:363, 1986

48. Fuhrmann K, Reiher H, Semmler K et al: Prevention of congenital malformations in infants of insulin dependent diabetic mothers. Diabetes Care 6:219, 1983

2

Epidemiology and Genetics

BOYD E. METZGER
NAM H. CHO

Diabetes mellitus is a clinical syndrome characterized by an absolute or relative deficiency of insulin action in responsive organs, thereby exposing all tissues to chronic hyperglycemia. It is estimated that about 12 million persons in the United States have diabetes mellitus (approximately 5 percent of the population). Its economic impact is great, estimated at $92 billion in 1994, approximately 15 percent of the total national expenditures for health care.[1]

In 1979, the National Diabetes Data Group recommended using the terms *insulin-dependent diabetes mellitus (IDDM)* and *non-insulin-dependent diabetes mellitus (NIDDM)* to distinguish the two main categories of idiopathic diabetes mellitus.[2] In common usage, IDDM is synonymous with type I diabetes and NIDDM with type II diabetes. Since the classification of diabetes mellitus has been more standardized and epidemiologic studies of it have become more common, the incidence and prevalence of both type I and type II diabetes mellitus have increased substantially worldwide.[3,4] Several explanations have been offered for this, including more complete and accurate ascertainment and a global increase in the average age of the population. However, other factors are also implicated, and the reasons for this strong secular trend are not fully understood. A similar increase in the prevalence of gestational diabetes mellitus (GDM) has been suggested. However, this issue is further confounded by the fact that the definition of GDM and surveillance for the condition in various populations are not uniform.[5,6] In this chapter, we review the known and postulated epidemiologic and genetic contributions to the incidence and prevalence of the different types of diabetes mellitus, especially as they relate to women of childbearing potential. Comprehensive detailed general reviews of the epidemiology and genetics of diabetes mellitus are available.[7-9]

EPIDEMIOLOGY: WORLDWIDE TRENDS

Insulin-Dependent Diabetes Mellitus

IDDM as it is classically seen in the child and adolescent is abrupt in onset, with a clinical course characterized by polyuria, polydipsia, polyphagia, weight loss, and fatigue. If the diagnosis is not made at this stage, there is eventual progression to diabetic ketoacidosis.[10] Many factors indicate that IDDM is an autoimmune disorder that develops in individuals with specific genetic predisposition. This is reviewed in detail below. There is also much evidence that development of IDDM in susceptible persons involves the participation of secondary factors that may be environmental in nature. Thus, the concordance for IDDM in identical twins is only 40 to 50 percent, rather than much higher as would be expected for a condition that is primarily genetic in origin.[11] In this section, we summarize some of the evidence that supports the contribution of environmental factors in the etiology of IDDM.

In 1984, Keen and Ekoe[12] stated that "insulin-dependent diabetes mellitus (IDDM) [type I]) is characteristic of white people and much less common in, or even absent from, some other ethnic groups." However, several more recent studies from Asia have demonstrated that the frequency of IDDM, although low, appears to be increasing over the past several years.[13,14] The reasons for this phenomenon are not known.

In the United States and western Europe, the current

11

incidence rate for IDDM is second only to that of asthma among severe chronic disease of childhood.[15] An estimated 22,000 children younger than the age of 15 years developed IDDM in the United States during 1978 to 1980. Many population-based reports indicate that there are marked geographic differences in the incidence of IDDM in the world; high risk in Scandinavian countries, moderate risk in Europe and North America, and low risk in Asia.[16–22] Furthermore, there is a strong south-north gradient in incidence, with rates increasing with the latitude away from the equator. In the current literature, the highest nationwide incidence rate has been reported Finland (28.8 per 100,000 person-years) and the lowest in Korea (0.7 per 100,000 person-years).[13,23] This represents a 41-fold difference in incidence rates. Furthermore, major differences in incidence rates have also been reported within the same country. Sevenfold differences have been noted within the midwestern region of Poland,[24] and in Sardinia, Italy, an incidence rate of 38 per 100,000 per year has been observed.[25]

There have been two workshops on IDDM registries, the first in 1983[26] and another in 1985.[27] As a result, data collection and assessment have been standardized, and the international patterns and trends in incidence were validated. These efforts have made a significant contribution to understanding the epidemiology of IDDM and have facilitated direct comparison of the disease across countries.

Despite significant geographic differences in the incidence of IDDM, clinical characteristics and patterns of onset are similar. It has been found consistently that the risk of IDDM in boys is slightly in excess of that in girls.[16,22] In both sexes, the incidence of IDDM in the age groups of 5 to 9 and 10 to 14 years is approximately 2.5 and 3 times higher, respectively, than in the younger age group (0 to 4 years).[16,22] A seasonal pattern of IDDM onset has been observed across continents, with a drop of incidence in summer months and the highest incidence in winter months.[16,22,24] These wide variations in the incidence of the disease have been interpreted as evidence of both environmental and genetic factors in the etiology of IDDM.

Infection with certain viruses, in particular Coxsackie B, at a critical period of vulnerability has been implicated in IDDM.[28,29] Expression of certain antigens or exposure to related antigens has been postulated to increase vulnerability or protect against IDDM (e.g., cow milk versus human breast milk).[30,31]

Non-Insulin-Dependent Diabetes Mellitus

In the United States, NIDDM accounts for 90 to 95 percent of all diabetes mellitus.[4,7,8] Onset and diagnosis of NIDDM are strongly associated with age; however, the patterns vary substantially among different racial/ethnic groups (e.g., younger onset in Native Americans compared with expectations in non-Hispanic whites).[32] On average, more than 80 percent of cases occur in those older than 40 years of age, and a large proportion of affected individuals is asymptomatic.[33] In the United States, the prevalence of undiagnosed diabetes is about equal to that of known cases or approximately 50 percent of all NIDDM in the population.[7,33]

The roles of hormone secretion and action and various pathways of intermediary metabolism in the pathogenesis of diabetes mellitus and its complications have been studied exhaustively for several decades. Two aspects of the pathophysiology of evolving NIDDM, insulin resistance and impaired insulin secretion, have commanded the center of attention as vectors for the myriad factors that may influence glucose homeostasis.[34] Impairment of both β-cell function and insulin action plays an important role in the development of overt symptomatic hyperglycemia through a self-perpetuating cycle, designated *glucose toxicity*.[35,36]

The etiology of type II diabetes is almost certainly multifactorial in most cases and is even less well understood than that of type I diabetes. However, epidemiologic studies are playing an increasingly important role in defining the underlying factors that modulate insulin action and β-cell function. Several epidemiologic studies have identified risk factors (i.e., demographic, genetic, and environmental factors) that are thought to be associated with or play a significant role in the predisposition to NIDDM.[37] For example, age, obesity, family history, racial/ethnic group, exercise level, diet, Western or urban lifestyle, and rural-urban migration are considered to be important risk factors for type II diabetes.[8,37]

There are marked differences in the prevalence of type II diabetes between countries, among different ethnic groups in the same geographic region, and within the same ethnic group undergoing internal or external migration. These points are illustrated graphi-

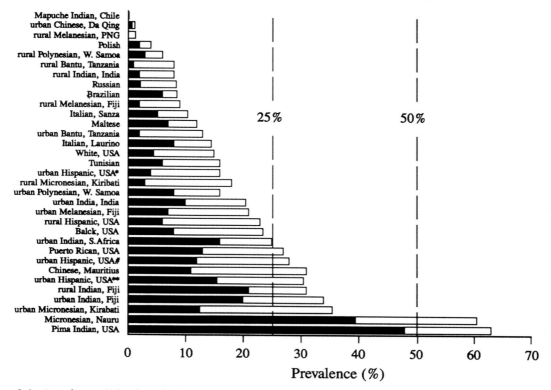

Fig. 2-1. Prevalence (%) of total glucose intolerance (diabetes and impaired glucose tolerance) in selected populations in the age range of 30 to 64 years. Age has been standardized across reporting centers.[37] *, upper income; #, middle income; **low income. ■, Diabetes mellitus; □, impaired glucose tolerance. (Modified from King and Rewers,[38] with permission.)

cally in Figure 2-1. King and Rewers[38] collated data from published reports on the prevalences of NIDDM and impaired glucose tolerance (IGT) in populations around the world in which a 75-g oral glucose tolerance test was used to evaluate glucose tolerance. The data presented in Figure 2-1 and the paper of King and Rewers[38] are adjusted to a standardized distribution of age because of the wide variation in age of the population in various parts of the world. When such adjustments are taken into account, the lowest prevalences have been reported in South American Indians of rural Chile, rural Africa, rural areas of the Indian subcontinent, and several populations in the Far East,[39–41] whereas the highest prevalences of type II diabetes have been identified in the North American Pima Indians and Micronesian population of Nauru.[42,43] Type II diabetes is rare or almost unknown in Polynesia, where

a traditional life-style has been maintained. However, Polynesian populations living in New Zealand have prevalence rates 3 to 10 times those of typical white populations.[44,45] Migrant effects on prevalence is also apparent in other Asian groups with origins in India of Japan.[46,47]

Although considerable progress has been made in identifying epidemiologic risk factors for NIDDM, an interplay between environmental and genetic factors may be of primary importance in most cases. Progress in defining the genetic role in the pathogenesis of NIDDM is reviewed below.

Diabetes Mellitus in Pregnancy

Diabetes mellitus complicating pregnancy is heterogeneous with respect to etiology, duration, severity, and the presence of confounding characteristics such as obesity. Precise classification of the etiology of diabetes mellitus may not be essential for adequate clinical management during pregnancy. However, it is important for optimal genetic counseling of the family concerning risk of diabetes mellitus in their offspring as well as for advising the mother about her expectations after pregnancy.

Differences in definitions and terminology as well as variances in ascertainment of cases have confounded efforts to compare the prevalence and incidence of various types of diabetes mellitus and glucose intolerance during pregnancy in different areas and among various racial/ethnic groups.[5,6] Women who are known to have diabetes mellitus before pregnancy (pregestational diabetes mellitus [PGDM] are often assumed to have type I diabetes, especially if they are receiving treatment with insulin. This may be a valid assumption in populations where the relative prevalence of IDDM is highest (e.g., certain northern European areas such as Sweden[17] or Finland[23]; however, in populations where NIDDM is common, more than half the women with PGDM may have type II rather than type I diabetes mellitus.[48-50] GDM is now commonly defined as "glucose intolerance with onset or first recognition during pregnancy."[2,5,6] Its prevalence generally parallels the incidence of type II diabetes mellitus in a given population. Accordingly, GDM is often viewed as a precursor of NIDDM. Women found to have abnormal glucose tolerance early in pregnancy, especially those with elevated fasting plasma glucose (FPG) concentrations, are likely to manifest diabetes mellitus when they are initially tested postpartum.[51] These subjects may well have NIDDM antedating pregnancy that goes undetected, especially if they are not in a health care system in which screening for glucose intolerance is universally practiced. Furthermore, a certain proportion of women with GDM can be demonstrated to have immunologic or clinical features suggestive of early type I diabetes (see below).

Pregestational Diabetes Mellitus

In the United States, the incidence of PGDM complicating pregnancy has been estimated to be 20 to 50 per 1,000.[52,53] These have been based on review of statewide reports of vital statistics, with amplification and verification by chart review in some instances. However, as indicated above, these estimates include subjects with both type I and type II diabetes mellitus in varying proportions. Furthermore, in such studies, there is substantial evidence for underreporting, especially of those not receiving treatment with insulin. This lack of accurate estimates of the frequency and type of diabetes mellitus complicating pregnancy limits the development of reliable data concerning the frequency of various complications (e.g., fetal morbidities such as major congenital malformations). Similarly, it is difficult to measure their economic impact or to estimate the amount of health care resources that might be required to prevent such complications.

Gestational Diabetes Mellitus

GDM, defined as "carbohydrate intolerance with onset or first recognition during pregnancy," is estimated to occur in approximately 2 to 5 percent of all pregnancies in the United States.[5,6,54] Marked variation has been reported in the prevalence of GDM worldwide. This is summarized in detail in reports to the Second International Workshop Conference on GDM.[55,56] From these detailed reviews, it appears that several factors contribute to this variation, including differences in definition, diagnostic criteria, and methods for screening and ascertainment, as well as the differences in incidence and prevalence of IDDM and NIDDM discussed above. Many additional reports of the prevalence of GDM have been published in the past 5 years. From these, we were able to identify those that used relatively well-defined screening and diagnostic test methods. The prevalences of GDM reported by racial/ethnic group in these studies are summarized in Table 2-1. Although it remains difficult to make direct comparisons among all reports (no attempt has been made to standardize with respect to age as was done in the report of King and Rewers[38]), the marked variation in prevalence of GDM among different racial/ethnic groups is evident in the data from Melbourne,[57,58] Canada,[59] San Francisco,[60] Chicago,[61] Alabama,[62] New York,[63] Yup'ik Eskimo,[64] and Korea.[65] Some indication of a migrant effect on prevalence of GDM is apparent in women of Chinese, Korean, or India subcontinent origin,[58,66] as is the case for NIDDM and IGT in the population at large.[4,38,44-47]

Surveys such as NHANES II[67,68] illustrate that a substantial amount of NIDDM as well as IGT is undiagnosed among persons older than 20 years of age in

Table 2-1. Prevalence of Gestational Diabetes Mellitus by Racial/Ethnic Group

Author/Year	Subjects (Race/Ethnic)	Screening Method (Glucose load/Cutoff)	OGTT/Diagnostic Criteria	GDM Prevalence (%)
Henry et al[57] (1993)	Vietnamese	NA	50 g/1 h ≥9 mmol/L* 2 h ≥7 mmol/L	7.8
Beischer et al[58] (1991)	Vietnam-born	NA	50 g/1 h >9 mmol/L* 2 h >7 mmol/L	7.3
	Chinese			13.9
	Indian subcontinent			15.0
	Australia & New Zealand			4.3
	Africa & Mauritius			9.4
Ranchod et al[59] (1991)	Indian	75 g/1 h/141 mg/dl*	EASD	3.8
			WHO	1.6
Green et al[60] (1990)	White	50 g/>150 mg*	NDDG	1.6
	Black American			1.7
	Hispanic			4.2
	Chinese			7.3
Dooley et al[61] (1991)	White	50 g/≥130 mg*	NDDG	2.7
	Black American			3.3
	Hispanic			4.4
	Other			10.5
Roseman et al[62] (1991)	Black American	100 g/2 h/≥115 mg/dl*	NDDG	2.4
Berkowitz et al[63] (1992)	White	50 g/≥135 mg*	NDDG	2.3
	Black American			3.7
	Hispanic			4.1
Murphy et al[64] (1993)	Yup'ik Eskimo	50 g/1 h/≥140 mg/dl*	NDDG	5.8
Jang et al[65] (1993)	Korean	50 g/≥130 mg*	NDDG	2.1

Abbreviations: WHO, WHO Expert Committee on Diabetes Mellitus, WHO Tech Rep Ser 1985; No. 727, 13, GDM criteria: 2-h value ≥7.8 mmol/L; EASD, Editorial, Glucose tolerance in pregnancy—the WHO and how of testing, Lancet 2:1173, 1988, GDM criteria: fasting ≥5.2 mmol/L, 2h: ≥9.0 mmol/L; NDDG, National Diabetes Data Group: Classification and diagnosis of diabetes mellitus and other categories of glucose intolerance, Diabetes 28:1039, 1979, two or more of the following values had to be present: fasting: ≥105 mg/dl, 1 h: ≥190 mg/dl, 2 h: ≥165 mg/dl, 3 h: ≥145 mg/dl; OGTT, Oral glucose tolerance test; GDM, gestational diabetes mellitus; NA, not applicable.
* Test administered universal for screening.

several racial/ethnic groups in the United States. On the basis of these findings, it has been suggested that the detection of GDM merely represents the discovery of women in the reproductive age range who have pre-existing glucose intolerance.[69] Indeed, there appears to be a correlation between the prevalence of GDM and that of NIDDM in various populations[38] (Table 2-1 and Fig. 2-1). When women have been systematically tested serially for glucose intolerance during pregnancy, a significant proportion of GDM has been confirmed within the first trimester.[69–71] However, repeated testing throughout pregnancy detects additional cases of GDM up to as late as 36 weeks' gestation.[69,71] Furthermore, a large body of evidence indicates that the insulin resistance of late pregnancy is profound[72,73] and plays an important role in the pathogenesis of GDM. Finally, glucose tolerance tests after pregnancy demonstrate normal glucose tolerance

in the great majority of women who had GDM. This preponderance of normal glucose tolerance postpartum would not be expected if testing during pregnancy merely led to the identification of pre-existing glucose intolerance in the female population. However, GDM is followed by relatively rapid progression to NIDDM. Within 5 years, up to 50 percent in several reports[74–76] or even more in at least one study[77] meet the criteria for a diagnosis of diabetes mellitus.

GENETICS

Insulin-Dependent Diabetes Mellitus

The contribution of genetic factors to the etiology of diabetes mellitus has been recognized since ancient times. Initially, such impressions were formed primarily from observing familial aggregation of diabetes. The characteristic clinical features, peak incidence of the disease in youth, and association with various "autoimmune endocrine diseases" helped to identify IDDM as a distinct entity before relatively specific markers of the disease were defined. Up to 90 percent of patients with onset of type I diabetes at younger than 20 years of age have circulating autoantibodies to a variety of protein antigens at the time of diagnosis.[78] The risk of developing IDDM is related strongly to the presence of certain class II human leukocyte (HLA) antigens (i.e., DR3/x, DR4/x, or DR3/DR4) and enhances the individual's risk of type I diabetes that may follow a random environmental event.[79] The presence of DR2 is associated with lower than average risk of IDDM, and it has been considered protective.[80] An even closer association has been found between type I diabetes and class II DQ antigens (Fig. 2-2). Alleles at the DQ locus more precisely localize the association responsible for greater susceptibility to (DQβ1*0204 and DQβ1*0302)

and protection from (DQβ1*0602) type I diabetes. The greatest specificity of risk of IDDM seems to be carried by the amino acid at position 57 on the DQ-β peptide. The presence of aspartic acid at position 57 (Asp-57-positive) is associated with low risk, whereas the risk is very high when another amino acid occupies position 57 (Asp-57-negative).[81]

In the pathogenesis of type I diabetes, the immune response that is postulated to be triggered by an environmental event includes the development of antibodies to several cell surface and cytoplasmic antigens, including insulin,[82] glutamic acid decarboxylase (GAD),[83] and others yet to be identified.[84] The circulating levels of islet cell antibody (ICA), insulin autoantibody (IAA), or GAD antibody can be monitored accurately using standardized immunofluorescent techniques. Levels of ICA greater than 20 Juvenile Diabetes Foundation (JDF) units convey increased risk of the subsequent development of clinical type I diabetes, with the risk in individual persons proportional to the

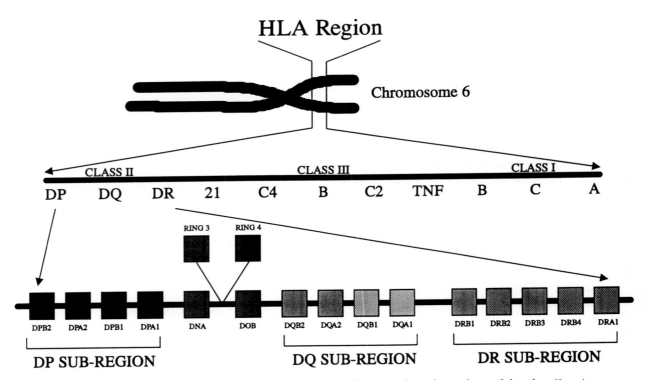

Fig. 2-2. Major histocompatibility complex in humans. This illustrates the relationships of the class II antigens that have been associated with the risk of developing insulin-dependent diabetes mellitus.

antibody titer.[82] With currently available assays of high specificity, only about 0.2 percent of nondiabetic control individuals have a positive ICA (i.e., >20 JDF units). This improved specificity has rendered it plausible to search for "at risk" persons within families or in the general population. The yield of ICA positivity in first-degree relatives of patients with type I diabetes is about 3.0 percent.[85] In children and young adults, ICA is detectable at diagnosis of type I diabetes in about 90 percent of cases.[86] This decreases over time, so that after 5 years of IDDM more than 40 percent of cases have measurable ICA titers.[86] Positive IAA alone does not predict type I diabetes; however, its presence, along with positive ICA, heightens the likelihood of type I diabetes occurring. IAA positivity correlates with age of the individual. In children younger than age 5 years, IAA often develops before the detection of ICA.[87] As immune-mediated destruction of β-cell continues, diminished insulin release can be identified. Clinical diabetes occurs only after function of 75 to 90 percent of β-cells is compromised.

Non-Insulin-Dependent Diabetes Mellitus

There is much evidence that the risk of developing NIDDM is strongly influenced by genetic traits. Maternal factors have been implicated in the inheritance of NIDDM, but the specific mode of transmission of NIDDM remains unclear. Studies in twins have provided some of the strongest evidence for a genetic basis for NIDDM. In monozygotic twins, concordance for type II diabetes has ranged from 55 to 100 percent,[11,88–90] rates that are even higher than those observed for type I diabetes. In family studies among Mexican Americans, the prevalence of diabetes decreased from 28.2 percent in first-degree relatives of the probands to 13.3 percent in second-degree relatives and 11.1 percent in the third-degree relatives when compared with Mexican Americans with no parental history of diabetes.[91] In other studies, persons with both a sibling and a parent with type II diabetes were found to have higher fasting plasma glucose and insulin concentrations than control subjects.[92] Further, it has been reported that the risk of developing type II diabetes is greater if a sibling is the proband rather than a parent.[93–95] Despite higher concordance for diabetes mellitus in twins and the evidence that has been gathered from other family studies for inheritance of NIDDM, the search for specific genetic markers has been largely unsuccessful.[96] There is considerable evidence that genetic factors play an important part in establishing the degree of insulin resistance in individuals. In one particularly illustrative report, Martin and colleagues[97] performed intravenous glucose tests in nondiabetic offspring of two parents with NIDDM. Insulin-independent glucose uptake (S_G) and insulin-sensitivity index (S_I) were estimated with Bergman's MINMOD. Values for S_G and S_I showed no correlation, and there was no clustering of S_G within families. By contrast, values for S_I within families were significantly related and the mean S_I values between families were more widely distributed than the values within a given family. However, the families with the most severe insulin resistance, on average, displayed the greatest degree of intrafamily variation in S_I values, an observation suggesting heterogeneity of a trait with a strong genetic basis. These points are illustrated clearly in Figure 2-3.[97]

Markers and Candidate Genes

As indicated above, there is strong evidence for a major contribution from genetic factors in the etiology of NIDDM. Discovery of the association between certain HLA antigens and IDDM (see above) was an important advance toward the ultimate definition of the etiology of this disorder. By contrast, the search for polymorphic markers for NIDDM has had only limited success to date. Efforts to identify specific genetic defects in NIDDM are hindered by the lack of specific and accurate markers for NIDDM other than the development of arbitrarily defined levels of hyperglycemia, which represents the outcome rather than the cause. This is confounded by the fact that the time at which hyperglycemia first develops, and its severity, may be strongly influenced by factors such as obesity, which may, in part, be environmental in origin. Separation of families or other clusters of subjects into groups on the basis of strict clinical, phenotypic, or physiologic/metabolic characteristics such as insulin sensitivity or insulin secretion is a prerequisite to linking the diabetic syndrome to specific genetic traits.

A few specific genetic defects have been identified in very selective subpopulations of NIDDM patients. In one search for genetic markers of NIDDM, muta-

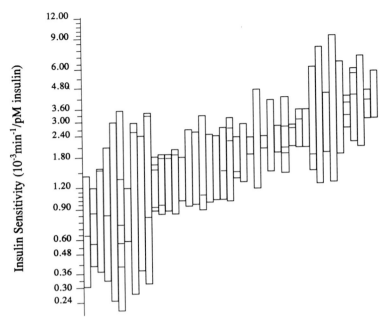

Fig. 2-3. Insulin sensitivity (S_I, $\log_{10}$) in families with two diabetic parents. The 43 families were ranked from lowest to highest according to the midrange of the log of S_I within each family. The midrange is indicated by a small square in the center of the bar. Horizontal lines across the bar, including those at the upper and lower limits, mark the log of S_I for an individual in that family. (Modified from Martin et al,[97] with permission.)

tions in the mitochondrial transfer RNA gene have been recently identified in a large Dutch pedigree in which diabetes mellitus occurs in combination with a sensorineural hearing loss.[98] Inheritance of the syndrome is maternally transmitted and is discussed in more detail below. There is an uncommon variant of NIDDM that is designated maturity onset diabetes of youth (MODY) because it can usually be diagnosed and often requires treatment before 20 to 25 years of age. Distribution of MODY within families conforms to the pattern of an autosomal dominant trait. Two apparently unrelated genetic defects have been described in kindreds with MODY. In the large RW kindred that has been extensively characterized by Fajans[99] over several decades, a marker for MODY has been identified in the adenosine deaminase (ADA) gene on chromosome 20q.[100] No specific metabolic alteration has yet been associated with the ADA defect. Glucokinase is expressed in liver and pancreatic β-cells and plays a key role in the regulation of glucose metabolism in these tissues.[101,102] Several mutations

have been identified within the coding regions of the glucokinase gene in MODY families, mostly of French extraction.[103–105] These alterations of the glucokinase gene are associated with defect in insulin secretion[106] and the presence of MODY. However, screening of several populations of whites and Asian NIDDM subjects indicates a low frequency of mutations in the glucokinase gene or its promoter region. Furthermore, heterogeneity has been noted even in MODY among families with glucokinase mutations. Thus, it is unlikely that mutations of this gene are a major cause of genetic susceptibility to NIDDM.[107,108] Efforts to identify other MODY families or NIDDM subjects with ADA mutations have also been unrewarding.

Association between NIDDM and polymorphism in many other "candidate genes" has been sought, and studies using this approach are continuing at a rapid rate. Impaired nonoxidative disposal of glucose (i.e., storage as glycogen) has been observed commonly in NIDDM subjects. Accordingly, genetic defects in enzymes of glycogen storage and metabolism are being looked for in NIDDM. An association between an allele of glycogen synthase (A$_2$) and NIDDM was reported from Finland among subjects with a severe defect in insulin-stimulated glucose storage.[109] However, the concentration of glycogen synthase protein in muscle biopsies from persons carrying the A$_2$ allele was normal. Thus, the precise mechanism of defective glycogen storage in these subjects remains to be defined. Some association between NIDDM and the glucose transporter genes (GLUT1, GLUT2, and GLUT4) has been postulated, but inconsistent results have been reported in the examination of various populations.[110–112] Markers on chromosome 4q have been associated with insulin resistance in Pima Indians[113] but not in three European white populations (Finnish, United Kingdom, and Welsh).[114] Insulin receptor substrate-1 plays a key role as a mediator of insulin action. A relationship between mutations in this important signaling molecule (Gly-818-Arg, Ser-892-Gly, and Gly-971-Arg) and NIDDM has been sought, and possible subtle associations were found.[115]

The results of studies such as those summarized here demonstrate that progress is being made toward defining the genetic factors that may be responsible for type II diabetes. However, many investigators are convinced that most NIDDM is polygenic in origin[9] and that it will continue to be difficult to define a specific etiology in many cases. Furthermore, although it is certain that specific genetic factors may predispose to NIDDM, it is equally clear that environmental factors such as the level of physical activity or obesity profoundly influences the appearance and course of clinical diabetes. Much work is still needed to gain a better insight into how genetic and environmental factors interact in NIDDM.

Gestational Diabetes Mellitus

Phenotypic Heterogeneity

Epidemiologic studies suggest that a substantial proportion of all adult women with NIDDM may have had GDM.[33,69] Obesity and advanced maternal age increase the risk of GDM,[58,60–62] as is the case for NIDDM. Accordingly, GDM is commonly regarded simply as a forerunner of NIDDM. All cases of GDM do share the fact that they are first recognized during pregnancy, a state of marked "physiologic" insulin resistance. However, this broad definition casts a common title to a very heterogeneous population of subjects.[51,61,116,117] Detailed studies of many GDM subjects have disclosed considerable phenotypic and genotypic heterogeneity. The severity of carbohydrate intolerance at the time of diagnosis represents one form of phenotypic heterogeneity, and it has served as the basis for the use of FPG to subclassify GDM.[5,6,51,116,117] Elevated FPG at diagnosis is associated with a higher risk of diabetes postpartum and at an earlier date.[51,74,77] There is also appreciable heterogeneity in age and weight among women with GDM, although it is well known that women with GDM tend to be older and heavier than unselected populations of pregnant women.[116,117] GDM is also heterogeneous with respect to insulin secretion. Most but not all subjects with GDM have impaired first- and second-phase insulin responses to oral[116–118] or intravenous challenge[72] when compared with age- and obesity-matched normal pregnant women. Although heterogeneity of insulin secretion is substantial, insulin resistance in late gestation is not different in pregnant women with GDM and those with normal carbohydrate metabolism when controlled for age and weight.[72,119]

Genotypic Heterogeneity

Examinations for genetic "markers" suggest that there may also be appreciable genotypic heterogeneity in GDM. In one study, increased DNA polymorphism in regions flanking the insulin receptor gene was significantly associated with GDM risk in black Americans and non-Hispanic whites.[120] A rare form of diabetes mellitus associated with mutations of mitochondrial DNA[98,121] may be initially discovered as GDM. MODY, another uncommon and atypical form of NIDDM, can also present as GDM.

It is also of clinical and prognostic importance to determine if and when GDM represents an early stage of evolving IDDM. We[116,117] and others[122–125] have found an increased occurrence of HLA antigens DR3 and DR4 associated with GDM. The prevalence of ICA in women with GDM has varied with the methods used and the populations tested.[116,117,123–127] On balance, the reports suggest a higher prevalence of ICA among those with more elevated FPG. In recent reports using more specific assays, the prevalence of ICA titers greater than 20 JDF units has not been appreciably higher than in the general obstetric population.[126] Genotypic heterogeneity, possibly related to an admixture of evolving IDDM, is also supported by the finding that HLA-DQβ restriction endonuclease fragments are present with increased frequency in white gravid women with GDM from the Chicago series as in nongravid subjects with IDDM.[128] These findings of immunologic, genetic, and clinical heterogeneity suggest that a small proportion of the gravid women with "onset of first recognition of glucose intolerance during pregnancy" may be exhibiting slowly evolving IDDM. This contention is supported by data from Copenhagen, one of the areas where the incidence and prevalence of IDDM are highest. In that center, a higher than expected number of women with documented IDDM were found to have experienced their initial clinical presentation during pregnancy.[129] Also, those with GDM who progressed to overt clinical diabetes requiring treatment with insulin tended to do so within the first year after the diagnosis of GDM.[130]

MATERNAL INFLUENCES

Data from a variety of sources corroborate that maternal or intrauterine factors may influence the risk of developing both type I and type II diabetes mellitus. There is little, if any, evidence that any form of diabetes mellitus is inherited as an X-linked disorder. However, maternal transmission of diabetes that is linked to mutations in mitochondrial DNA has been described.[98,121] A large pedigree has recently been identified in which diabetes mellitus occurs in combination with a sensorineural hearing loss.[98] Maternal inheritance and a decrease in mitochondrial enzyme activities of the respiratory chain indicate a genetic defect in mitochondrial DNA. An A→G transition has been identified in the mitochondrial gene for tRNA (Leu [UUR] at position 3,243), in persons with the syndrome, but it is absent in controls.[98] Similar findings have also been reported in Japanese subjects with NIDDM.[121]

Insulin-Dependent Diabetes Mellitus

The possibility that IDDM may develop in their offspring is a major concern of couples when one or both has IDDM. Careful review of the patterns of occurrence of IDDM in families has established that offspring of

fathers with IDDM are at significantly higher risk of the development of IDDM than is the case when the mother is the parent with the disease.[131,132] Bleich et al[131] reported that fathers with type I diabetes transmit diabetes to their offsprings two to three times more frequently than mothers with type I diabetes.

The risk of developing type I diabetes in siblings of an IDDM child is increased, but the specific risk is difficult to define. Several epidemiologic studies have reported that a maternal history of diabetes is associated with an increased risk of type II diabetes[133–135] but a lower risk of type I diabetes[131,132] in her children. The mechanism of this "protective" maternal effect is not known. It has been suggested that it may be mediated by alterations in the immunologic system of the fetus that are induced during intrauterine development as a result of the mother's IDDM. No direct evidence has been gathered to support this hypothesis; however, alterations of lymphocyte subsets in children of mothers with IDDM (neonates to children 6 years of age) have been described recently.[136] The changes could not be related to maternal metabolic control or the presence of ICA that were thought to have been transmitted from mother to fetus during intrauterine life. The Pittsburgh group has reported age-specific incidence rates for siblings compared with the general childhood population based on their large Allegheny County registry data for the years 1965 to 1976. Age-specific relative risk varied from a 7- to 18-fold increased risk for siblings.[137] The lifetime cumulative incidence of IDDM in siblings of a child with IDDM in Europid populations is quoted at 5 to 8 percent in contrast to a figure of approximately 0.1 to 0.5 percent in the general population.[138,139] A study from London reported that a sibling of a child with IDDM is approximately 15 to 20 times more likely to develop IDDM before 20 years of age (6 percent) than children from a general population in the same area (0.3 percent).[140]

Non-Insulin-Dependent Diabetes Mellitus and Gestational Diabetes Mellitus

The influence of intrauterine metabolic factors on long-term development of the offspring has been of great interest to many, including our group. Freinkel[141] formulated the hypothesis of "fuel-mediated teratogenesis," which states that maternal fuels may influence development of the fetus by modifying phenotypic gene expression in terminally differentiated, poorly replicating cells. The long-range effects depend on the cells undergoing differentiation, proliferation, or functional maturation at the time of the disturbances in maternal fuel economy. It was postulated that pancreatic β-cells and adipose tissue would be among the tissues vulnerable to functional alterations during later life. The Diabetes in Pregnancy Center was established at Northwestern University to test this hypothesis. Reports from this ongoing study have shown a link between the intrauterine environment and the development of obesity in childhood and IGT in adolescence.[142–144]

In the highly inbred Pima Indian population, maternal diabetes (exclusively type II) is associated with an increased risk of both obesity and the development of NIDDM in young adults.[145,146] We have also observed maternal histories of diabetes more frequently than expected among women with GDM.[147] Cross-sectional epidemiologic studies in Britain[96] and France[148] have shown that individuals with NIDDM more often have had a diabetic mother than a diabetic father. The development of diabetes in the offspring of diabetic rats is influenced by perturbed maternal carbohydrate metabolism, as well as by genetic factors.[149–151]

In Pima Indians, the risk of development of NIDDM is greater if the mother had diabetes during pregnancy rather than developed it after pregnancy.[152] In support of the hypothesis of fuel-mediated teratogenesis, this implies that there is a component of abnormal metabolic milieu in addition to the genetic risk. In our cohort, predisposition to obesity and IGT is linked to prenatal metabolic factors, but not the genetic form of the mother's diabetes (they appear with equal frequency in offspring of mothers with type I, type II, or GDM). The risks of obesity in childhood and IGT in adolescence are independently linked to the presence of fetal hyperinsulinism, which had been documented by a high concentration of amniotic fluid insulin in late pregnancy.[142–144] Further evidence that exposure to excess insulin action in utero can exert long-term effect has been obtained with animal models. Rhesus monkeys made hyperinsulinemic but euglycemic in utero by infusion of insulin into the fetus develop abnormal glucose tolerance as pregnant adults.[153]

Together, these data from humans and primates implicate exposure to excess insulin action in utero in

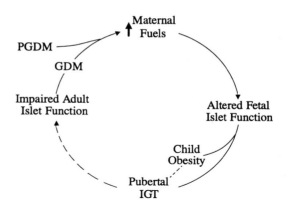

Fig. 2-4. Diabetes begets diabetes: the alterations of maternal fuel metabolism lead to altered fetal islet function (hyperinsulinism). This intrauterine event predisposes to childhood obesity and adolescent impaired glucose tolerance (IGT). Our hypothesis is that it will also lead to impaired adult islet function and IGT and/or gestational diabetes mellitus (GDM).

the predisposition to IGT and putatively to NIDDM. We visualize that the chain of events depicted in Figure 2-4 accounts for our observations. Many of the offspring of diabetic mothers in our study will soon reach childbearing age. If this propensity for glucose intolerance leads to GDM in the second generation, the pattern of perpetuation from generation to generation will be established. This suggests that diabetes mellitus can predispose to more diabetes mellitus, which may contribute to the overall increasing burden of diabetes mellitus in the population. However, this process is potentially preventable by more effectively normalizing metabolism throughout gestation in PGDM and early diagnosis and correction of metabolic disturbances of GDM.

REFERENCES

1. Mazze RS: A systems approach to diabetes care. Diabetes, suppl. 1, 17:5, 1994
2. National Diabetes Data Group: Classification and diagnosis of diabetes mellitus and other categories of glucose intolerance. Diabetes 28:1039, 1979
3. Diabetes Epidemiology Research International Group: Secular trends in incidence of childhood IDDM in 10 countries. Diabetes 39:858, 1990

4. McCart D, Zimmet P: Diabetes 1994 to 2010: Global Estimates and Projections. International Diabetes Institute, Melbourn, Australia, 1994

5. Freinkel N: Summary and recommendations of the Second International Workshop-Conference on Gestational Diabetes Mellitus. Diabetes, suppl. 2, 34:123, 1985

6. Metzger BE, Organizing Committee: Summary and Recommendations of the Third International Workshop-Conference on Gestational Diabetes Mellitus. Diabetes, suppl. 2, 40:197, 1991

7. Harris MI: Diabetes in America: Diabetres Data Compiled 1984. Publication (NIH) 85-1468; VI-1-31. U.S. Department of Health and Human Services, U.S. Government Printing Office, Washington, DC, 1986

8. Bennett PH: Epidemiology of diabetes mellitus. p. 357. In Rifkin H, Porte D (eds): Diabetes Mellitus Theory and Practice. 4th Ed. Elsevier, New York, 1990

9. Rotter JI, Vadheim CM, Rimoin DL: Genetics of diabetes mellitus. p. 378. In Rifkin H, Porte D (eds): Diabetes Mellitus Theory and Practice. 4th Ed. Elsevier, New York, 1990

10. Drash AL: Clinical Care of the Diabetic Child. Year Book Medical Publishers, Chicago, 1987

11. Pyke DA: Diabetes: the genetic connections. Diabetologia 17:333, 1979

12. Keen H, Ekoe JM: The geography of diabetes mellitus. Br Med Bull 40:359, 1984

13. Ko KW, Yang SW, Cho NH: Incidence rate of IDDM in Seoul (1985 to 1988). Diabetes Care 17:1473, 1994

14. Tajima N, LaPorte RE, Hibi I et al: A comparison of the epidemiology of youth-onset insulin-dependent diabetes mellitus between Japan and the United States (Allegheny County, Pennsylvania). Diabetes Care, suppl. 1, 8:17, 1985

15. Cruickshanks KJ, LaPorte RE, Dorman JE et al: The epidemiology of insulin-dependent diabetes mellitus: etiology and diagnosis. p. 332. In Ahmed PI, Ahmed N (eds): Coping with Juvenile Diabetes. Charles C Thomas, Springfield, IL, 1985

16. LaPorte RE, Cruickshanks KJ: Incidence and risk factors for insulin-dependent diabetes. p. 111. In Harris MI, Hamman RF (eds): Diabetes in America. NIH Publ. 85-1468. U.S. Government Printing Office, Washington, DC, 1985

17. Sterky G, Holmgren G, Gustavson KH et al: The incidence of diabetes mellitus in Swedish children 1970–1975. Acta Paediatr Scand 67:139, 1978

18. Joner G, Søvik O: Incidence, age at onset and seasonal variation of diabetes mellitus in Norwegean children 1973–77. Acta Pediatr Scand 70:329, 1981

19. Åkerblom HK, Reunanen A, Käär M-L: The incidence of insulin-dependent diabetes mellitus in 0–4 year-old children in Finland in 1970–80. Nord Council Arct Med Res Rep 26:60, 1980

20. Lestradet H, Besse J: Prevalence et incidence du diabete juvenile insulinodependent en France. Diabetes Metab 3:229, 1977

21. Gleason RE, Kahn CB, Funk IB et al: Seasonal incidence of insulin-dependent diabetes in Massachusetts, 1964–1973. Int J Epidemiol 11:39, 1982

22. LaPorte RE, Fishbein HA, Drash AL et al: The Pittsburgh insulin-dependent diabetes mellitus (IDDM) registry: the incidence of insulin-dependent diabetes in Allegheny County, Pennsylvania (1965–1976). Diabetes 30: 279, 1981

23. Reunanen A, Åkerblom HK, Käär M-L: Prevalence and ten-year (1970–1979) incidence of insulin-dependent diabetes mellitus in children and adolescents. Acta Paediatr Scand 71:892, 1992

24. Rewers M, LaPorte R, Walczak M et al: Apparent epidemic of insulin-dependent diabetes mellitus in midwestern Poland. Diabetes 36:106, 1987

25. Muntoni S, Songini M: Sardinian collaborative group for epidemiology of IDDM. High incidence rate of IDDM in Sardinia. Diabetes Care 15:1317, 1992

26. LaPorte RE, Tajima N, Akerblom HK et al: Geographic differences in the risk of insulin-dependent diabetes mellitus: the importance of registries. Diabetes Care, suppl. 1, 8:101, 1985

27. Patrick SL, Moy CS, LaPorte RE: The world of insulin-dependent diabetes mellitus: what international epidemiologic studies reveal about the etiology and natural history of IDDM. Diabetes Metab Rev 5:571, 1989

28. Yoon J, Austin M, Onodera T et al: Virus induced diabetes mellitus isolation of a virus from the pancreas of a child with diabetic ketoacidosis. N Engl J Med 300:1173, 1979

29. Wagenknecht LE, Roseman JM, Herman WH: Increase incidence of insulin-dependent diabetes mellitus following an epidemic of Coxsackievirus B5. Am J Epidemiol 133:1024, 1991

30. Kostraba JN, Cruickshanks KJ, Lawler-Heavners J et al: Early exposure cow's milk and solid foods in infancy, genetic predisposition and risk of IDDM. Diabetes 42: 288, 1993

31. Dahl-Jorgensen K, Joner G, Hanssen KF: Relationship between cows' milk consumption and incidence of IDDM in childhood. Diabetes Care 14:1081, 1991

32. Bennett PH, Knowler WC, Rushforth NB et al: Diabetes and obesity. p. 507. In Vague J, Vague PH (eds): Excerpta Medica, Amsterdam, 1979

33. Harris MI: Undiagnosed NIDDM: clinical and public health issues. Diabetes Care 16:642, 1993

34. DeFronzo RA, Bonadonna RC, Ferrannini E: Pathogene-

sis of NIDDM. A balanced overview. Diabetes Care 15: 318, 1992

35. Rossetti L, Giaccari A, deFronzo RA et al: Glucose toxicity. Diabetes Care 13:610, 1990

36. Leahy JL, Bonner-Weir S, Weir GC: Beta-cell dysfunction induced by chronic hyperglycemia. Diabetes Care 15: 442, 1992

37. Zimmet PZ: Kelly West Lecture 1991. Challenges in diabetes epidemiology—from West to the rest. Diabetes Care 15:232, 1992

38. King H, Rewers M: Global estimates for prevalence of diabetes mellitus and impaired glucose tolerance in adults. Diabetes Care 16:157, 1993

39. Gupta OP, Dave SH, Joshi MH: Prevalence of diabetes in India. p. 13. In Levine R, Luft R (eds): Advances in Metabolic Disorders. Vol. 9. Academic Press, San Diego, 1978

40. Toyota, Goto Y, Komatsu K et al: Prevalence of diabetes in rural and urban Japan. p. 35. In Baba S, Fukui S, Goto Y (eds): Diabetes Mellitus in Asia. Excerpta Medica, Amsterdam, 1979

41. Shanghai Diabetes Research Cooperative Group: Diabetes mellitus survey in Shanghai. Chin Med J 93:663, 1980

42. Bennett PH, LeCompte PM, Miller M, Rushforth NB: Epidemiological studies of diabetes in the Pima Indians. Recent Prog Horm Res 32:333, 1976

43. Zimmet P, Guinea A, Guthrie W et al: The high prevalence of diabetes mellitus on a Central Pacific island. Diabetologia 13:111, 1977

44. Prior IAM, Davidson F: The epidemiology of diabetes in Polynesians and Europeans in New Zealand and the Pacific. N Z Med J 65:375, 1966

45. Zimmet P: Epidemiology of diabetes and its macrovascular complications in Pacific populations: the medical effects of social progress. Diabetes Care 2:144, 1979

46. Marine N, Edelstein O, Jackson WPU et al: Diabetes hyperglycaemia and glycosuria among Indians, Malays and Africans (Bantu) in Cape Town, South Africa. Diabetes 18:840, 1969

47. Kawate R, Nishimoto Y, Yamakido M: Migrant studies among the Japanese in Hiroshima and Hawaii. p. 526. Waldhäusl WK (ed): Diabetes 1979. Excerpta Medica, Amsterdam, 1980

48. Johnstone FD, Nasrat AA, Prescott RJ: The effect of established gestational diabetes on pregnancy outcome. Br J Obstet Gynaecol 997:1009, 1990

49. Kadiki OA, Reddy MR, Sahli MA et al: Outcome of pregnant diabetic patients in Benghazi (Libya) from 1984 to 1991. Diabetes Res Clin Pract 21:39, 1993

50. Contreras-Soto J, Forsbach G, Vazquez-Rosales J: Noninsulin dependent diabetes mellitus and pregnancy in Mexico. Int J Gynaecol Obstet 34:205, 1991

51. Metzger BE, Bybee DE, Freinkel N et al: Gestational diabetes mellitus. Correlations between the phenotypic and genotypic characteristics of the mother and abnormal glucose tolerance during the first year postpartum. Diabetes, suppl. 2, 34:111, 1985

52. Connell FA, Vadheim, Emanuel I: Diabetes in pregnancy: a population based study of incidence, referral for care and perinatal mortality. Am J Obstet Gynecol 151:598, 1985

53. Wheeler FC, Gollmar CW, Deeb LC: Diabetes and pregnancy in South Carolina: prevalence, perinatal mortality and neonatal morbidity in 1978. Diabetes Care 5:561, 1982

54. Freinkel N, Josimovich J, Conference Planning Committee: American Diabetes Association Workshop-Conference on Gestational Diabetes. Summary and recommendations. Diabetes Care 3:499, 1980

55. Hadden DR: Geographic, ethnic, and racial variations in the incidence of gestational diabetes mellitus. Diabetes, suppl. 2, 34:8, 1985

56. Sepe SJ, Connell FA, Geiss LS et al: Gestational diabetes. Incidence, maternal characteristics, and perinatal outcome. Diabetes, suppl. 2, 34:13, 1985

57. Henry OA, Beischer NA, Sheedy MT, Walstab JE: Gestational diabetes and follow-up among immigrant Vietnam-born women. Aust N Z J Obstet Gynaecol 33:109, 1993

58. Beischer NA, Oats JN, Henry OA et al: Incidence and severity of gestational diabetes mellitus according to country of birth in women living in Australia. Diabetes, suppl. 2, 40:35, 1991

59. Ranchod HA, Vaughan JE, Jarvis P: Incidence of gestational diabetes at Northdale Hospital, Pietermaritzburg. S Afr Med J 80:14, 1991

60. Green JR, Pawson IG, Schumacher LB et al: Glucose tolerance in pregnancy: ethnic variation and influence of body habitus. Am J Obstet Gynecol 163:86, 1990

61. Dooley SL, Metzger BE, Cho N et al: The influence of demographic and phenotypic heterogeneity on the prevalence of gestational diabetes mellitus. Int J Gynaecol Obstet 35:13, 1991

62. Roseman JM, Go RCP, Perkins LL et al: Gestational diabetes mellitus among African-American women. Diabetes Metab Rev 7:99, 1991

63. Berkowitz GS, Lapinski RH, Wein R et al: Race/ethnicity and other risk factors for gestational diabetes. Am J Epidemiol 135:965, 1992

64. Murphy NJ, Bulkow LR, Schraer CD et al: Prevalence of diabetes mellitus in pregnancy among Yup'ik Eskimos, 1987–1988. Diabetes Care 16:315, 1993

65. Jang HC, Cho NH, Min YK et al: Gestational diabetes mellitus (GDM) in Seoul, Korea and Chicago, IL: simi-

larities and differences in racial/ethnic groups. suppl. 1, 42:87A, 1993

66. Cho N, Rim C, Jang S et al: The prevalence of gestational diabetes mellitus: comparison of native Korean, immigrant Korean, and Chicago populations. Am J Epidemiol 12:S6, 1994

67. Harris MI, Hadden WC, Knowler WC et al: Prevalence of diabetes and impaired glucose tolerance and plasma glucose levels in U.S. population aged 20–74 yr. Diabetes 36:523, 1987

68. Harris M: Gestational diabetes may represent discovery of pre-existing glucose intolerance. Diabetes Care 11: 402, 1988

69. Super DM, Edelberg SC, Philipson EH et al: Diagnosis of gestational diabetes in early pregnancy. Diabetes Care 14:288, 1991

70. Lavin JP Jr: Screening of high-risk and general populations for gestational diabetes: clinical application and lost analysis. Diabetes, suppl. 2, 34:24, 1985

71. Jovanovic L, Peterson CM: Screening for gestational diabetes: optimum timing and criteria for retesting. Diabetes, suppl. 2, 34:21, 1985

72. Buchanan TA, Metzger BE, Freinkel N, Bergman RN: Insulin sensitivity and β-cell responsiveness to glucose during late pregnancy in lean and moderately obese women with normal glucose tolerance or mild gestational diabetes. Am J Obstet Gynecol 162:1008, 1990

73. Catalano PM, Tyzbir ED, Roman NM et al: Longitudinal changes in insulin release and insulin resistance in non-obese pregnant women. Am J Obstet Gynecol 165:1667, 1991

74. Metzger BE, Cho NH, Roston SM, Radvany R: Maternal weight and insulin secretion at diagnosis of gestational diabetes mellitus: predictors of glucose tolerance during five year follow-up. Diabetes Care 16:1598, 1993

75. O'Sullivan JB: Long term follow up of gestational diabetes. p. 503. In Camerini-Davalos RA, Cole HS (eds): Early Diabetes in Early Life. Academic Press, San Diego, 1975

76. Mestman JH, Anderson GV, Guadalupe V: Follow-up study of 360 subjects with abnormal carbohydrate metabolism during pregnancy. Obstet Gynecol 39:421, 1972

77. Kjos S, Buchanan T, Peters R et al: Postpartum glucose tolerance testing identifies women with recent gestational diabetes who are at highest risk for developing diabetes within five years. Diabetes, suppl. 1, 43:136A, 1994

78. Marner B, Agner T, Binder C et al: Increased reduction in fasting C-peptide is associated with islet cell antibodies in type I (insulin-dependent) diabetic patients. Diabetologia 28:875, 1985

79. Cahill GF, McDevitt HO: Insulin-dependent diabetes mellitus: the initial lesion. N Engl J Med 304:1454, 1981

80. Erlich HA, Griffith RL, Bugawan TL et al: Implication of specific DQB1 alleles in genetic susceptibility and resistance identification of IDDM siblings with novel HLA-DQB1 allele and unusual DR2 and DR1 haplotypes. Diabetes 40:478, 1991

81. Trucco M: To be or not to be ASP 57, that is the question. Diabetes Care 15:705, 1992

82. Deschamps I, Boitard C, Hors J et al: Life table analysis of the risk of type I (insulin-dependent) diabetes mellitus in siblings according to islet cell antibodies and HLA markers. Diabetologia 35:951, 1992

83. Clare-Salzler MJ, Tobin AJ, Kaufman DL: Glutamate decarboxylatse: an autoantigen in IDDM. Diabetes Care 15:132, 1992

84. Karjalainen J, Martin JM, Knip M et al: A bovine albumin peptide as a possible trigger of insulin dependent diabetes mellitus. N Engl J Med 327:302, 1992

85. Srikanta S, Ganda OP, Rabizadeh A et al: First-degree relatives of patients with type I diabetes mellitus: islet-cell antibodies and abnormal insulin secretion. N Engl J Med 313:462, 1985

86. Ziegler AG, Hillebrand B, Rabi W et al: On the appearance of islet associated autoimmunity in offspring of diabetic mothers: a prospective study from birth. Diabetologia 36:402, 1993

87. Eisenbarth GS: Type I diabetes mellitus. A chronic autoimmune disease. N Engl J Med 314:1360, 1986

88. Barnett AH, Eff C, Leslie RDG et al: Diabetes in identical twins: a study of 200 pairs. Diabetologia 20:87, 1981

89. Gottlieb MS, Root HF: Diabetes mellitus in twins. Diabetes 17:693, 1968

90. Newman B, Selby JV, King MC et al: Concordance for type 2 (non-insulin-dependent) diabetes mellitus in male twins. Diabetologia 30:763, 1987

91. Mitchell BD, Kammerer CM, Reinhart LJ et al: NIDDM in Mexican-American families. Heterogeneity by age of onset. Diabetes Care 17:567, 1994

92. Henriksen JE, Alford E, Handberg A et al: Increased glucose effectiveness in normoglycemic but insulin-resistant relatives of patients with non-insulin-dependent diabetes mellitus. A novel compensatory mechanism. J Clin Invest 94:1196, 1994

93. Leslie RDG, Volkmann HP, Poncher M et al: Metabolic abnormalities in children of non-insulin-dependent diabetics. BMJ 293:840, 1986

94. Beaty TH, Neel JV, Fajans SS: Identifying risk factors for diabetes in first degree relatives of non-insulin dependent patients. Am J Epidemiol 115:380, 1982

95. Iselius L, Lindsten J, Morton NE et al: Genetic regulation of the kinetics of glucose-induced insulin release in man: studies in families with diabetic and non-diabetic probands. Clin Genet 28:8, 1985

96. Alcolado JC, Alcolado R: Importance of maternal history of non-insulin dependent diabetic patients. BMJ 302: 1178, 1991

97. Martin BC, Warram JH, Rosner B et al: Familial clustering of insulin sensitivity. Diabetes 41:850, 1992

98. van den Ouweland JM, Lemkes HH, Ruitenbeek W et al: Mutation in mitochondrial tRNA(Leu)(UUR) gene in a large pedigree with maternally transmitted type II diabetes mellitus and deafness. Nature Gene 1:368, 1992

99. Fajans SS: Scope and heterogeneous nature of maturity-onset diabetes of the young (MODY). Diabetes Care 13: 49, 1990

100. Bell GI, Xiang K, Newman MV et al: Gene for non-insulin-dependent diabetes mellitus (maturity-onset diabetes of the young type) is linked to DNA polymorphism on human chromosome 20q. Proc Natl Acad Sci USA 88:1484, 1991

101. Meglasson MD, Matschinsky FM: Pancreatic islet glucose metabolism and regulation of insulin secretion. Diabetes Metab Rev 2:163, 1986

102. Matschinsky FM: Glucokinase as glucose sensor and metabolic signal generator in pancreatic β-cells and hepatocytes. Diabetes 39:647, 1990

103. Froguel PH, Vaxillaire M, Sun F et al: Close linkage of glucokinase locus on 3 chromosome 7p to early-onset non-insulin dependent diabetes mellitus. Nature 356: 162, 1992

104. Zouali H, Vaxillaire M, Lesage S et al: Linkage analysis and molecular scanning of glucokinase gene in IDDM families. Diabetes 42:1238, 1993

105. Vionnet N, Stoffel M, Takeda J et al: Nonsense mutation in the glucokinase gene cause early-onset non-insulin dependent diabetes mellitus. Nature 356:721, 1992

106. McCarthy MI, Hitchins M, Hitman GA et al: Positive association in the absence of linkage suggests a minor role for the glucokinase gene in the pathogenesis of type 2 (non-insulin-dependent) diabetes mellitus among South Indians. Diabetologia 36:633, 1993

107. Shimokawa K, Sakura H, Otabe S et al: Analysis of the glucokinase gene promoter in Japanese subjects with non-insulin-dependent diabetes mellitus. J Clin Endocrinol Metab 79:883, 1994

108. Cook JTE, Hattersley AT, Christopher P et al: Linkage analysis of glucokinase gene with NIDDM in Caucasian pedigrees. Diabetes 41:1496, 1992

109. Groop LC, Kankuri M, Schalin-Jäntti C et al: Association between polymorphism of the glycogen synthase gene and non-insulin-dependent diabetes mellitus. N Engl J Med 328:10, 1993

110. Schalin-Jantti C, Yki-Jarvinen H, Koranyi L et al: Effect of insulin on GLUT-4 mRNA and protein concentrations in skeletal muscle of patients with NIDDM and their first-degree relatives. Diabetologia 37:401, 1994

111. Mueckler M, Kruse M, Strube M et al: A mutation in the GLUT2 glucose transporter gene of a diabetic patient abolishes transport activity. J Biol Chem 269:17765, 1994

112. Baroni MG, Alcolado JC, Gragnoli C et al: Affected sib-pair analysis of the GLUT1 glucose transporter gene locus in non-insulin-dependent diabetes mellitus (NIDDM): evidence for no linkage. Hum Genet 93:675, 1994

113. Prochazka M, Lillioja S, Tait JF et al: Linkage of chromosomal markers on 4q with a putative gene determining maximal insulin action in Pima Indians. Diabetes 42: 514, 1993

114. Humphreys P, McCarthy M, Tuomilehto J et al: Chromosome 4q locus associated with insulin resistance in Pima Indians. Studies in three European NIDDM population. Diabetes 43:800, 1994

115. Laakso M, Malkki M, Kekalainen P et al: Insulin receptor substrate-1 variants in non-insulin-dependent diabetes. J Clin Invest 94:1141, 1994

116. Freinkel N, Metzger BE, Phelps RI et al: Gestational diabetes mellitus: heterogeneity of maternal age, weight, insulin secretion, HLA antigens, and islet cell antibodies and the impact of maternal metabolism on pancreatic B-cell and somatic development in the offspring. Diabetes, suppl. 2, 34:1, 1985

117. Freinkel N, Metzger BE, Phelps RI et al: "Gestational diabetes mellitus": a syndrome with phenotypic and genotypic heterogeneity. Horm Metab Res 18:427, 1986

118. Hollingsworth DR, Ney D, Stubblefield N et al: Metabolic and therapeutic assessment of gestational diabetes by two-hour and twenty-four-hour isocaloric meal tolerance tests. Diabetes, suppl. 2, 34:81, 1985

119. Catalano PM, Tyzbir ED, Wolfe R et al: Carbohydrate metabolism during pregnancy in control subjects and women with gestational diabetes. Am J Physiol 264:E60, 1993

120. Ober C, Xiang K-S, Thisted R et al: Increased risk for gestational diabetes mellitus associated with insulin receptor and insulin-like growth factor II restriction fragment length polymorphisms. Genet Epidemiol 6:559, 1989

121. Kadowaki T, Kadowaki H, Mori Y et al: A subtype of diabetes mellitus associated with a mutation of mitochondrial DNA. N Engl J Med 330:962, 1994

122. Mawhinney H, Hadden DR, Middleton D et al: HLA antigens in asymptomatic diabetes. A 10-year follow-up study of potential diabetes in pregnancy and gestational diabetes. Ulster Med J 48:166, 1979

123. Rubinstein P, Walker M, Krassner J et al: HLA antigens and islet cell antibodies in gestational diabetes. Hum Immunol 3:271, 1981

124. Budowle B, Huddleston JF, Go RCP et al: Association of HLA-linked factor B with gestational diabetes mellitus in black women. Am J Obstet Gynecol 159:805, 1988

125. Acton RT, Vanichanan CJ, Perkins L et al: Immunogenetic predictors of gestational diabetes in American blacks. p. 207. In Andreani D, Bompiani GD, DiMario U et al (eds): Immunobiology of Normal and Diabetic Pregnancy. John Wiley & Sons, New York, 1990

126. Catalano PM, Tyzbir ED, Sims EAH: Incidence and significance of islet cell antibodies in women with previous gestational diabetes. Diabetes Care 13:478, 1990

127. McEvoy RC, Franklin B, Ginsberg-Fellner F: Gestational diabetes mellitus: evidence for autoimmunity against the pancreatic beta cells. Diabetalogia 34:507, 1991

128. Owerbach D, Carnegie S, Rich C et al: Gestational diabetes mellitus is associated with HLA-DQb-chain DNA endonuclease fragments. Diabetes Res 6:109, 1987

129. Buschard K, Buch I, Molsted-Pedersen L et al: Increased incidence of true type I diabetes acquired during pregnancy. BMJ 294:275, 1987

130. Damm P, Kuhl C, Bertelsen A et al: Predictive factors for the development of diabetes in women with previous gestational diabetes mellitus. Am J Obstet Gynecol 167:607, 1992

131. Bleich D, Polak M, Eisenbarth GS: Decreased risk of type I diabetes in offspring of mothers who acquire diabetes during adrenarchy. Diabetes 42:1433, 1993

132. Pociot F, Norgaard K, Hobolth N et al: A nationwide population-based study of the familial aggregation of type 1 (insulin-dependent) diabetes mellitus in Denmark. Danish Study Group of Diabetes in Childhood. Diabetologia 36:870, 1993

133. Francois R, Picaud JJ, Ruitton-Ugliengo A et al: The newborn of diabetic mothers. Observations on 154 cases, 1958–1972. Biol Neonate 24:1, 1974

134. Amendt P, Michaelis D, Hildmann W: Clinical and metabolic studies in children of diabetic-mothers. Endokrinologie 67:351, 1976

135. Dorner G, Mohnike A: Further evidence for a predominantly maternal transmission of maturity-onset type diabetes. Endokrinologie 68:121, 1976

136. Roll U, Scheeser J, Standl E, Ziegler AG: Alterations of lymphocyte subsets in children of diabetic mothers. Diabetologia 37:1132, 1994

137. Wagener DK, Kuller LH, Orchard TJ et al: Pittsburgh diabetes mellitus study. II. Secondary attack rates in families with insulin-dependent diabetes mellitus. Am J Epidemiol 115:868, 1982

138. Tillil H, Kobberling J: Age-corrected emprical genetic risk estimates for first degree relatives of IDDM patients. Diabetes 36:93, 1987

139. Gamble DR: An epidemiological study of childhood diabetes affecting two or more siblings. Diabetologia 19:341, 1980

140. Bingley PJ, Gale EAM: The incidence of insulin-dependent diabetes in England: a study in the Oxford region 1985-6. BMJ 298:558, 1989

141. Freinkel N: The Banting Lecture 1980: of pregnancy and progeny. Diabetes 29:1023, 1980

142. Metzger BE, Silverman BL, Freinkel N et al: Amniotic fluid insulin as a predictor of obesity. Arch Dis Child 65:1050, 1990

143. Silverman BL, Landsberg L, Metzger BE et al: Fetal hyperinsulinism in offspring of diabetic mothers: association with the subsequent development of childhood obesity. Ann NY Acad Sci 699:36, 1993

144. Silverman BL, Metzger BE, Cho NH: Impaired glucose tolerance in adolescent offspring of diabetic mothers: relationship to fetal hyperinsulinism. Diabetes (in press)

145. Pettitt DJ, Baird HR, Aleck KA et al: Excessive obesity in offspring of Pima Indian women with diabetes during pregnancy. N Engl J Med 308:242, 1983

146. Pettitt DJ, Aleck KA, Baird HA et al: Congenital susceptibility to NIDDM. Role of intrauterine environment. Diabetes 37:622, 1988

147. Martin AO, Simpson JL, Ober C et al: Frequency of diabetes mellitus in mothers of probands with gestational diabetes: possible maternal influence on the predisposition to gestational diabetes. Am J Obstet Gynecol 151:471, 1985

148. Thomas F, Balkau B, Vauzelle-Kervrodan F et al: Maternal effect and familial aggregation in NIDDM. The CODIAB Study. Diabetes 43:63, 1994

149. Gauguier D, Nelson I, Bernard C et al: Higher maternal than paternal inheritance of diabetes in GK rats. Diabetes 43:220, 1994

150. Aerts L, Holemans K, Van Assche FA: Maternal diabetes during pregnancy: consequences for the offspring. Diabetes Metab Rev 6:147, 1990

151. Gauguier D, Nelson I, Bernard C et al: Higher maternal than paternal inheritance of diabetes in GK rats. Diabetes 43:220, 1994

152. Pettitt DJ, Bennett PH, Saad MF et al: Abnormal glucose tolerance during pregnancy in Pima Indian women: long-term effects on the offspring. Diabetes, suppl. 2, 40:126, 1991

153. Susa JB, Sehgal P, Schwartz R: Rhesus monkeys made exogenously hyperinsulinemic in utero as fetuses, display abnormal glucose hemostasis as pregnant adults and have macrosomic fetuses, abstracted. Diabetes, suppl. 1, 42:86A, 1993

3

Prevention and Immunotherapy

JAY S. SKYLER
JENNIFER B. MARKS
MARY JO O'SULLIVAN

The pathogenesis of type I or insulin-dependent diabetes mellitus involves a genetic predisposition to the disease, a putative environmental trigger that in genetically susceptible individuals may activate an immune mechanism, which leads to progressive loss of pancreatic islet β-cells and development of type I diabetes.[1-3] The insidious process of immune-mediated destruction of the pancreatic islet insulin secreting β-cells may precede the overt expression of clinical symptoms by many years, since these become apparent only when most of the β-cells have been destroyed. The possibility of interrupting this pathogenetic sequence by immune intervention offers us the opportunity to alter the natural history of type I diabetes. Such an approach has been eminently successful in animal models of type I diabetes, such as the NOD (nonobese diabetic) mouse and the BB (biobreeding) rat. A variety of immune interventions has been used, some immunosuppressive and some immunomodulatory. Many have been successful in altering the course of type I diabetes in these animal models.

In recent years, immune intervention has been attempted in human type I diabetes as well.[4,5] Human experiments have entailed two basic strategies. The first of these is immune intervention begun shortly after diagnosis of type I diabetes, in an effort to (1) decrease the severity of clinical manifestations, (2) halt destruction of residual β-cells, and (3) perhaps allow some recovery of β-cell function. The second strategy is aimed at prevention or delay of disease onset in susceptible individuals by altering the pathogenetic sequence earlier in its course, before clinical manifestations of type I diabetes. Such intervention is contingent on effective case finding. This involves the screening

of high-risk individuals (e.g., relatives of persons with type I diabetes).

PATHOGENESIS

The main elements in the pathogenetic sequence include (1) a genetic predisposition, conferred principally by genes in the major histocompatability complex (MHC) (i.e., the human leukocyte antigen [HLA] region) on the short arm of chromosome 6, although multiple other gene loci modulate disease risk; (2) nongenetic (environmental) factors that appear to act as triggers in genetically susceptible individuals; and (3) activation of immune mechanisms targeted against pancreatic islet β-cells. The initial immune response appears to engender further secondary and tertiary immune responses, which collectively result in progressive destruction of pancreatic islet β-cells and consequent development of type I diabetes.

The familial predisposition to type I diabetes has long been known. A specific mode of genetic transmission has not been established.[6] There is a higher concordance rate for type I diabetes in monozygotic twins than in dizygotic twins. Type I diabetes is associated with specific HLA region alleles, particularly DR and DQ alleles.[7] There is a strong positive relationship with HLA-DR3 and HLA-DR4 and a strong negative relationship with HLA-DR2. Indeed, more than 90 percent of whites with type I diabetes are HLA-DR3 or HLA-DR4, or both. There is an even stronger relationship of type I diabetes when the DQ loci (DQα and DQβ) are considered together with the DR loci. Thus, the predisposition to type I diabetes in whites is associated with HLA-DR3,DQB1*0201 and with HLA-DR4,DQB1*0302. The strongest association for type I diabetes in whites is with the DQα-DQβ combination DQA1*0501-DQB1*0302. Other DQ alleles appear to confer protection from type I diabetes. For example, DQA1*0201-DQB1*0602 provides protection even in the presence of DQ susceptibility alleles. This suggests that protection is dominant over susceptibility. Because the class II MHC genes regulate the immune response, it has been proposed that the susceptibility and protective alleles could be involved differentially in antigen presentation of peptides that establish and maintain tolerance or influence the immune response.

Environmental factors may initiate the pathogenetic sequence in genetically predisposed animal models. The role of environmental factors in human type I diabetes is uncertain.[8] One potential environmental influence is neonatal and early infancy nutrition.[9] There is a reciprocal relationship between breast feeding and the frequency of type I diabetes. A small prospective Finnish study has suggested that exclusive breast feeding may reduce the likelihood of disease development.[10] It has been proposed that that consumption of cow milk proteins, particularly early in life, may lead to the initiation of the immunologic attack against pancreatic islet β-cells and increase susceptibility to type I diabetes. Alternatively, consumption of breast milk may lead to disease protection.

Several chemical toxins have been shown to have the potential of destroying β-cells. Among these are nitrosourea compounds, including the drug stretozotocin and the rotenticide Vacor (N-3-pyridil-methyl-N-p-nitrophenyl urea).[11] One study suggested that maternal consumption, around the time of conception, of another group of potentially toxic substances—nitrates and nitrites—may influence the eventual development of type I diabetes.[12] The nitrates and nitrites were contained in smoked mutton, consumed disproportionately as part of holiday festivities in Iceland. The notion is that a developing embryo, when exposed to these toxins, suffers an initial β-cell insult, which enhances the risk of diabetes, appearing years later in childhood. Studies in animals support this interpretation.

Exposure to a variety of viruses may influence the development of type I diabetes. Several human viruses can infect and damage islet beta cells in vitro. The potential role of viruses in disease pathogenesis is unclear. Yet, as many as 10 to 12 percent of children with congenital rubella develop type I diabetes.[13] Here, as in the case of maternal periconceptual nitrate/nitrite consumption, the exposure is remote in time from the clinical onset of type I diabetes, being in utero. It is not clear whether this is a direct effect of the virus, whether the virus is initiating an immune mechanism, or whether the involvement is magnified because exposure occurs during embryonic and fetal development.

Environmental factors may be influencing the immune response through molecular mimicry; for example, the homology between a pancreatic β-cell surface protein known as p69 or ICA-69 and a 17-amino-acid sequence (ABBOS) of bovine serum albumin, a major cow milk protein. Likewise, there is homology between several β-cell proteins and viruses, including homology between glutamic acid decarboxylase (GAD) and Coxsackie protein P2-C, homology between insulin and a retrovirus sequence, and homology between a 52-kd islet protein and a rubella protein.

Specific cell-mediated T-lymphocyte immune processes appear to be responsible for the destruction of islet β-cells, although the exact mechanisms involved in the pathogenetic pathway have not yet been clearly defined. Immune activation appears to involve presentation of a diabetogenic peptide (as yet unknown) to the immune system, and activation of a T-helper-1 (Th1) subset of CD4 + T lymphocytes.[14] The cytokines produced by Th1-cell activation are interleukin-2 (IL-2) and interferon-γ (IFN-γ). These cytokines activate cytotoxic T lymphocytes and cytotoxic macrophages to kill islet β-cells by a variety of mechanisms. These killing mechanisms include oxygen free radicals, nitric oxide, destructive cytokines (interleukin-1 [IL-1], tumor necrosis factor-α [TNF-α], tumor necrosis factor-β [TNF-β], and IFN-γ), and CD8 + cytotoxic T lymphocytes that interact with a β-cell autoantigen–MHC class I complex. Once the initial immune destruction commences, secondary and tertiary immune responses also are activated, with virtually the whole immunologic army attacking β-cells.

The hallmark pathologic feature of type I diabetes is mononuclear cell infiltration of the islets (i.e., "insulitis" or "isletitis") in pancreases examined near the time of clinical onset of type I diabetes.[15] This lesion is consistent with a cell-mediated immunoreaction, leading to β-cell destruction, and is similar to the lymphocytic infiltration encountered in other reputed autoimmune conditions including endocrinopathies. Yet, at the time of diagnosis of type I diabetes in both humans and animal models, only a few islets show the classical pathognomonic insulitis lesion. In addition, some intact islets with β-cells can be found, as well as an occasional hyperplastic islet. However, most islets are "pseudoatrophic," small islets both without mononuclear infiltration and devoid of β-cells but with intact glucagon-secreting α-cells and somatostatin-secreting δ-cells. Presumably, these islets have already had their β-cells destroyed, and the immunologic attack on them has abated. Eventually, type I diabetes appears when sufficient β-cells have been destroyed that glucose tolerance can no longer be maintained.

A variety of circulating antibodies to islet cell markers can be detected at diagnosis of type I diabetes in the vast majority of patients.[16,17] These include cytoplasmic islet cell antibodies (ICA), insulin autoantibodies (IAA), antibodies directed against a 64-kd antigen shown to be the enzyme GAD, and a variety of others. Some of these may be antibodies directed against antigen(s) involved in initiating the immune process, but this remains to be established. However, they generally are not thought to mediate β-cell destruction by humoral mechanisms. It is likely that as β-cells are destroyed and multiple antigens are exposed to the immune system, antibodies directed against these components would be generated. Thus, these antibodies serve as markers of immune activity or of β-cell damage and indeed have been found useful in heralding the disease process by their appearance long before that of overt type I diabetes. As β-cell function is lost and "total" diabetes evolves, antibodies tend to decrease in titer or disappear, or both.

Islet immunopathology begins several years before the overt clinical onset of hyperglycemia and type I diabetes.[18,19] This is recognized by the appearance of various antibodies, including ICA, IAA, and anti-GAD antibodies. In individuals destined to develop type I diabetes, a progressive metabolic defect can also be demonstrated, measured as a decline in β-cell function, detected by a decrease in early first-phase insulin release during an intravenous glucose tolerance test. Thus, it is possible to predict the development of type I diabetes by identification of genetic, immunologic, and metabolic markers in asymptomatic individuals.

Currently, screening programs are in place for identifying such individuals among relatives of individuals with type I diabetes, since their empiric risk of type I diabetes (about 3 to 5 percent among first-degree relatives) is about 10-fold that in the general population (prevalence about 0.3 percent). As predictive models are confirmed and screening for genetic markers in the general population becomes feasible, screening may be expanded to society as a whole.

IMMUNOTHERAPEUTIC APPROACHES

Because β-cell destruction is immunologically mediated, attempts have been made to interdict the disease process by immune intervention. This has been done in new-onset type I diabetes in an effort to preserve any residual β-cell function that may be present and is actively being pursued in high-risk individuals in an effort to delay or prevent clinical disease. Studies to date have demonstrated that immune intervention does, indeed, alter the natural history of the disease and have provided convincing support that immune mechanisms are important in type I diabetes pathogenesis. Yet, studies in new-onset diabetes have to date failed to show convincing long-term benefit; perhaps at this stage in the disease process, it may be already too late to preserve sufficient β-cell function to be clinically important.

The interventions that have been used are immunosuppressive or immunomodulating.[4,5] Immunosuppressive agents are cytotoxic by definition, whereas immunomodulating agents act by enhancing or diminishing immune responses, including interrupting or modifying the pathways that mediate β-cell destruction. The earliest studies in human subjects were all conducted in individuals with established diabetes, usually, but not always, of recent onset. Most of these involved insufficient numbers of subjects to draw any firm conclusions, at least with the end points used. Thus, although it is assumed by many that these were apparently ineffective in altering the clinical course of type I diabetes, no firm conclusions can be reached about their potential effectiveness. These early studies used several nonspecific immunosuppressive agents, including glucocorticoids alone and together with antithymocyte globulin, plasmapheresis, methisoprinol, levamisole, ciamexone, γ-globulins, and interferon.

Azathioprine

Azathioprine is an immunosuppressive drug widely used in transplantation and other immune conditions such as rheumatoid arthritis. It is a purine antagonist that prevents the generation of cytotoxic T cells and natural killer (NK) cells. It has been demonstrated to preserve β-cell function in new-onset diabetes in two studies but not in a third.[20–22] In a single subject predicted to be within months of clinical diabetes, azathioprine has been used for more than 5 years without the appearance of diabetes. Although the data available to date in juvenile rheumatoid arthritis subjects show that azathioprine is generally well tolerated and associated with few side effects, it may result in severe leukopenia (but this can be avoided with careful monitoring and dose titration), and there is an unquantitated concern about oncogenic potential. As a consequence of fears about potential toxicity, azathioprine is no longer currently being studied in type I diabetes.

Cyclosporine

Cyclosporine (Cyclosporin A) is a potent immunosuppressive drug that selectively acts on T cells, both helper T cells and cytotoxic T cells. It inhibits the secretion of the cytokine IL-2 by these cells. As a consequence, it suppresses cell-mediated immunity. In double-masked, placebo-controlled clinical trials, it has been shown to preserve β-cell function and reduce insulin requirement when used at the time of clinical onset of type I diabetes.[23–25] Subjects with a shorter duration of symptoms (<6 weeks) before entry had a better chance of response to cyclosporine. Yet, the responses have been transient, ending after withdrawal of cyclosporine or despite continued immunosuppression with cyclosporine.[26–28]

Potential nephrotoxicity is the main concern with cyclosporine usage.[29] Although some is reversible, an irreversible dose-dependent chronic interstitial nephritis may develop. Whether this can be minimized by careful dosage titration, on the basis of both renal function and trough cyclosporine blood or plasma levels, and the potential implications of this remain uncertain. Thus, any long-term potential benefit of immune intervention with cyclosporine must be assessed ver-

sus the risks. The concern is that use of this agent may amount to trading the risk of diabetic nephropathy for the risk of cyclosporine nephropathy. Thus, the toxicity of cyclosporine is such that it cannot safely be considered in usual dosages in either new-onset type I diabetes and especially not in asymptomatic individuals at risk of diabetes.

Nicotinamide

Nicotinamide has been shown to improve β-cell regeneration in models of spontaneous and induced diabetes, to cause an increase in insulin synthesis, and, if administered before onset, to prevent development of clinical diabetes in animal models.[30,31] There are several potential mechanisms by which nicotinamide may be beneficial in preventing β-cell destruction: (1) by restoring β-cell content of nicotinamide adenine dinucleotide (NAD) toward normal by inhibiting poly-adenosine diphosphate-ribose polymerase (a major route of NAD metabolism); (2) by serving as a free radical scavenger, thereby limiting DNA and β-cell damage; or (3) by inhibiting cytokine-induced islet nitric oxide production. As a consequence, nicotinamide has been used in several studies in new-onset diabetes. The results have been mixed, with some studies showing marginal beneficial effects of nicotinamide and others being without effect. Nicotinamide has also been used in prediabetes. No effect was seen in one small pilot study. In two others, subjects given the drug appeared to fare better than did untreated historical control subjects. In a study from Auckland, school children aged 5 to 8 years were randomized by school to receive ICA testing during 1988 to 1991.[32] Of 33,658 children offered testing, 20,195 were tested and 13,463 declined testing. Of those tested, 150 met criteria for treatment with nicotinamide. Meanwhile, another 48,335 school children served as controls and were neither screened nor treated. In 49,000 subject years of follow-up, diabetes developed at a rate of $8.1/10^5$/y in the nicotinamide-treated group. However, in the comparison group, after approximately 322,000 subject years of follow-up, diabetes developed at a rate of $20.1/10^5$/y/ ($P = 0.03$). Among those who refused testing, after 33,000 subject years of follow-up, diabetes developed at a rate of $15.5/10^5$/y. No adverse effects were seen in treated subjects. Given these provocative observations and that nicotinamide is both inexpensive and has a benevolent side effect profile, at least two large multicenter collaborative randomized, prospective, double-masked, controlled clinical trials have been initiated to evaluate the effects of nicotinamide in high-risk relatives of individuals with type I diabetes. These are the European Nicotinamide Diabetes Intervention Trial and the German (Deutsch) Nicotinamide Diabetes Intervention Study.

Insulin

Insulin therapy itself has been shown to delay the development of diabetes and to inhibit the appearance and progression of insulitis in animal models of type I diabetes. Insulin may be acting immunologically—by immunization, tolerization, or immunomodulation. Alternatively, insulin may be acting metabolically—by resting β-cell function, thereby making β-cells less susceptible to immune attack, because actively secreting β-cells are more susceptible to such damage than are resting cells. In contrast with other interventions, which often have generalized effects on the immune system, insulin (1) is β-cell-specific; (2) does not otherwise affect the immune system; (3) is an agent whose effects on people are well understood; and (4) has side effects that are well known and can be controlled.

Several studies have suggested that early and more aggressive insulin treatment may result in preservation of β-cell function, better metabolic control, or a prolonged honeymoon period. However, the results have been inconsistent. In a study from Tampa, intensive insulin therapy in newly diagnosed patients, involving 2 weeks of treatment with intravenous insulin delivered via an artificial pancreas, preserved β-cell function for at least 1 year.[33]

Three pilot studies have investigated the use of insulin in relatives of type I diabetic probands at high risk of diabetes. One such pilot study, from Boston, involved 12 subjects, 5 of whom accepted treatment and 7 who declined and were followed as a comparison group.[34] This study suggested that prophylactic parenteral insulin therapy combining 5 days of insulin by intravenous infusion every 9 months and daily subcutaneous insulin injections could preserve β-cell function and may delay the appearance of diabetes. Subsequently, these investigators joined with colleagues in Denver and continued this approach while enrolling subjects in a randomized fashion with similar results. Another pilot study, from Munich, has randomized 10 similar subjects to a protocol of intravenous insulin for

7 days every 12 months, combined with daily subcutaneous insulin injections for the first 6 months.[35] It, too, suggests that diabetes may be delayed by such intervention. A third pilot study, from Gainesville, has treated a larger group of relatives, some already with onset of glucose intolerance, with daily subcutaneous insulin injections and report the approach safe and the preliminary results encouraging.

These preliminary results suggest that the use of insulin therapy in high-risk relatives has potential benefit in delaying or preventing the evolution to overt clinical diabetes. With this impetus, the United States National Institute of Diabetes and Digestive and Kidney Diseases has initiated the Diabetes Prevention Trial of Type 1 Diabetes (DPT-1), a randomized, controlled, nationwide, multicenter clinical trial, designed to test whether intervention with insulin during the prodromal period of the disease can delay the appearance of overt clinical diabetes. In the "high-risk" group (i.e., ≥50 percent risk over 5 years), the protocol is designed to determine whether parenteral insulin therapy, consisting of periodic courses of continuous intravenous insulin, with accompanying chronic subcutaneous insulin, will delay their expected development of clinical type I diabetes.

Oral Antigen Therapy

Oral ingestion of soluble antigens has been shown to establish immunologic tolerance in experimental animals. As a consequence, the strategy of orally induced antigenic tolerance is being tested in a variety of autoimmune states, including type I diabetes. Oral administration of insulin to young NOD mice results in less insulitis and delays onset of type I diabetes.[36,37] In the DPT-1, the intervention protocol for the "intermediate-risk" group (i.e., 25 to 50 percent risk over 5 years) is being planned as a randomized, placebo-controlled, double-masked, multicenter clinical trial designed to determine whether presentation of an islet cell autoantigen (i.e., orally ingested insulin) to the immune system via the intestinal mucosa could induce disease-relevant immunologic tolerance, thereby delaying the development of type I diabetes.

Adjuvant Therapy

Vaccination with complete Freund's adjuvant or bacillus Calmette-Guerin strain of *Mycobacterium bovis* prevents diabetes in animals,[38] presumably by activating protective components of the immune system, thus decreasing the immune attack on β-cells. A pilot study in new-onset diabetes suggested better preservation of β-cell function, warranting a full-scale clinical trial.[39]

Peptide Therapy

Peptide competitors, which bind to class II MHC molecules and block T-lymphocyte activation, have been used successfully in the treatment of experimental autoimmune diseases in animals, including type I diabetes.[40] Among the peptides that have been used for such vaccination are a peptide of the 60-kd human heat shock protein (hsp60),[41] mycobacterium hsp65,[39] insulin,[37] and insulin B chain.[42] The use of peptide vaccines may prove to be an important means of preventing type I diabetes.

Neonatal and Early Infant Nutrition

As noted earlier, it has been proposed that neonatal and early infancy exposure to cow milk proteins may lead to initiation of the immunologic destruction of β-cells. If this is correct, then the frequency of type I diabetes might be reduced by preventing exposure to cow milk proteins during early life, which would be a "true" primary prevention strategy. This possibility will be tested in a multinational Scandinavian-Canadian randomized prospective trial involving 3,000 to 4,000 infants.[9] In this study, newborns with first-degree relatives with type I diabetes will receive either a formula free of cow milk or a conventional cow milk-based formula. The intervention will be for a 9-month period, with follow-up for 10 years.

Photophoresis

Phototherapy entails extracorporal irradiation with ultraviolet-A light of lymphocytes treated with 8-methoxypsoralen. The treated cells are reinfused into the subject. This approach is being studied in Australia and Sweden, principally in new-onset type I diabetes.[43,44] No clear outcome data have yet emerged.

Monoclonal Antibodies and Related Anti-T-Cell Therapies

Several monoclonal antibodies have been evaluated for potential effectiveness in pilot studies in new-onset type I diabetes.[4] These have included an antiblast anti-body (CBL1), an anti-CD3 antibody (OKT3), an anti-CD4 antibody, an anti-CD5 immunoconjugate coupled to the A chain of ricin toxin (CD5-Plus), a humanized chimeric anti-CD4 antibody, an anti-IL-2 receptor antibody, and an IL-2 receptor (IL-2R) targeted fusion protein, consisting of a diphtheria toxin-related protein linked to IL-2 (DAB$_{486}$-IL-2). Preliminary experience with these agents has generally been suggestive that there is preservation of β-cell function. Unfortunately, full-scale, controlled trials of these or similar therapies have not yet been reported. Other monoclonal antibody strategies are being contemplated.

Other Immunotherapeutic Approaches

Several other immunologic approaches have been tried, generally without much success. Tacrolimus (previously called FK506) is a potent immunosuppressive drug that selectively acts on T lymphocytes to inhibit secretion of IL-2. Although promising in animal models, a small pilot study of tacrolimus in new-onset human type I diabetes was without benefit.[45] Also examined with marginal results have been the thymic hormones thymostimulin and thymopoietin, localized pancreatic irradiation by a linear accelerator, and lymphocyte transfusion.

Ongoing studies are examining linomide, an immunomodulator that upregulates several T-lymphocyte-dependent functions, in new-onset type I diabetes[46]; ketotifen, a potent antihistamine, in high-risk relatives; a combination of antioxidants (which act as free radical scavengers), including nicotinamide, vitamin C, vitamin E, β-carotene, and selenium, in new-onset type I diabetes.[44]

Under consideration for study are sirolimus (previously called rapamycin), an inhibitor of cytokine-mediated signal transduction, which has been effective in preventing diabetes in the NOD mouse[47]; and mycophenolate mofetil, an inhibitor of purine nucleotide synthesis, which has been effective in preventing diabetes in the BB rat.[48]

CONCLUSIONS

Type I diabetes mellitus is an immunologically mediated disease. As a consequence, several immunotherapeutic approaches have been used in an attempt to interdict the disease process. Trials in recent-onset type I diabetes have demonstrated that immune intervention alters the natural history of the disease, with preservation of β-cell function and overall improved metabolic control. Unfortunately, thus far a clear clinical benefit of such intervention has not yet emerged. It may be that by the time of clinical diagnosis there has been such extensive β-cell damage to make it impossible to achieve a clinically meaningful outcome. Therefore, attention has turned to the use of immunotherapeutic strategies for the prevention of type I diabetes in high-risk individuals. Presumably, application of therapy earlier in the course of the disease process, when larger β-cell mass is present, may increase the likelihood of detection of a meaningful therapeutic effect. However, it must be appreciated that such high-risk individuals are asymptomatic and that not all high-risk individuals will show progression to overt clinical disease. As a consequence, it is incumbent that investigations be confined to carefully designed, controlled trials. Moreover, it is desirable to intervene at this point with treatments that are relatively innocuous. If successful, prevention of diabetes could spare these individuals from a lifelong disease associated with morbid complications. Therefore, the conduct of studies is justifiable. If successful in high-risk relatives, a broader approach involving genetic screening in the general population may become warranted. The ultimate goal of prevention of type I diabetes mellitus is an achievable one.

REFERENCES

1. Castano L, Eisenbarth GS: Type-I diabetes: a chronic autoimmune disease of human, mouse, and rat. Annu Rev Immunol 8:647, 1990
2. Atkinson M, Maclaren NK: What causes diabetes? Sci Am 262:61, 1990
3. Rossini AA, Greiner DL, Friedman HP, Mordes JP: Immunopathogenesis of diabetes mellitus. Diabetes Rev 1:43, 1993
4. Skyler JS, Marks JB: Immune intervention in type I diabetes mellitus. Diabetes Rev 1:15, 1993
5. Pozzilli P, Kolb H, Ilkova HM (eds): New trends for prevention and immunotherapy of insulin dependent diabetes mellitus. Diabetes Metab Rev 9:237, 1993
6. Thomson G, Robinson WP, Kuhner MK et al: Genetic heterogeneity, modes of inheritance, and risk estimates for a joint study of caucasians with insulin dependent diabetes mellitus. Am J Hum Genet 43:799, 1988
7. Nepom GT: Immunogenetics and IDDM. Diabetes Rev 1:93, 1993
8. Maclaren N, Atkinson M: Is insulin dependent diabetes mellitus environmentally induced? N Engl J Med 327:348, 1992
9. Akerblom HK, Savilahti E, Saukkonen TT et al: The case for elimination of cow's milk in early infancy in prevention of type I diabetes: the Finnish experience. Diabetes Metab Rev 9:269, 1993
10. Virtanen SM, Rasanen L, Aro A et al: Infant feeding in Finnish children <7 yr of age with newly diagnosed IDDM. Diabetes Care 14:415, 1991
11. Karam JH, Lewitt PA, Young CW et al: Insulinopenic diabetes after rodenticide (Vacor) ingestion. Diabetes 29:971, 1980
12. Helgason T, Jonasson MR: Evidence for a food additive as a cause of ketosis–prone diabetes. Lancet 2:716, 1981
13. Rubinstein P, Walker ME, Fedun B et al: The HLA system in congenital rubella patients with and without diabetes. Diabetes 31:1088, 1982
14. Rabinovitch A: Immunoregulatory and cytokine imbalances in the pathogenesis of IDDM: therapeutic intervention by immunostimulation? Diabetes 43:613, 1994
15. Foulis AK, Liddle CN, Farquharson MA et al: The histopathology of the pancreas in type I (insulin-dependent) diabetes mellitus: a 25 year review of deaths in patients under 20 years of age in the United Kingdom. Diabetologia 29:267, 1986
16. Atkinson M, Maclaren NK: Islet cell autoantigens of IDDM. Diabetes Rev 1:191, 1993
17. Bosi E, Bonifacio E, Bottazzo GF: Autoantigens in IDDM. Diabetes Rev 1:204, 1993
18. Thai AC, Eisenbarth GS: Natural history of IDDM. Autoantigens of IDDM. Diabetes Rev 1:1, 1993
19. Palmer JP: Predicting IDDM: use of humoral markers. Autoantigens of IDDM. Diabetes Rev 1:104, 1993
20. Harrison LC, Colman PG, Dean B et al: Increase in remission rate in newly diagnosed type I diabetic subjects treated with azathioprine. Diabetes 34:1306, 1985
21. Cook JJ, Hudson I, Harrison LC et al: A double-blind controlled trial of azathioprine in children with newly-diagnosed type I diabetes. Diabetes 38:779, 1989
22. Silverstein J, Maclaren N, Riley W et al: Immunosuppression with azathioprine and prednisone in recent onset insulin-dependent diabetes mellitus. N Engl J Med 319:599, 1988
23. Feutren G, Papoz L, Assan R et al: Cyclosporine increases the rate and length of remissions in insulin dependent diabetes of recent onset: results of a multicentre double-blind trial. Lancet 2:119, 1986

24. The Canadian-European Randomized Control Trial Group: Cyclosporine-induced remission of IDDM after early intervention: association of 1 year of cyclosporine treatment with enhanced insulin secretion. Diabetes 37:1574, 1988

25. Skyler JS, Rabinovitch A, Miami Cyclosporine Diabetes Study Group: Cyclosporine in recent onset type I diabetes mellitus: effects on islet beta cell function. J Diabetes Complications 6:77, 1992

26. Bougneres PF, Landais P, Boisson C et al: Limited duration of remission of insulin dependency in children with recent overt type I diabetes treated with low-dose cyclosporine. Diabetes 39:1264, 1990

27. Martin S, Schernthaner G, Nerup J et al: Follow-up of Cyclosporin A treatment in type I (insulin dependent) diabetes mellitus: lack of long-term effects. Diabetologia 34:429, 1991

28. Jenner M, Bradish G, Stiller C et al: Cyclosporin A treatment of young children with newly-diagnosed type I (insulin dependent) diabetes mellitus. Diabetologia 35:884, 1992

29. Myers BD, Ross J, Newton L et al: Cyclosporine associated chronic nephropathy. N Engl J Med 311:699, 1984

30. Pozzilli P, Andreani D: The potential role of nicotinamide in the secondary prevention of IDDM. Diabetes Metab Rev 9:219, 1993

31. Mandrup-Poulsen T, Riemers JI, Andersen HU et al: Nicotinamide treatment in the prevention of insulin-dependent diabetes mellitus. Diabetes Metab Rev 9:295, 1993

32. Elliott RB, Pilcher CC, Stewart A et al: The use of nicotinamide treatment in the prevention of type I diabetes. Ann NY Acad Sci 696:333, 1993

33. Shah SC, Malone JI, Simpson NE: A randomized trial of intensive insulin therapy in newly diagnosed type I insulin-dependent diabetes mellitus. N Engl J Med 320:550, 1989

34. Keller RJ, Eisenbarth GS, Jackson RA: Insulin prophylaxis in individuals at high risk of type I diabetes. Lancet 341:927, 1993

35. Ziegler A, Bachmann W, Rabl W: Prophylactic insulin treatment in relatives at high risk for type I diabetes. Diabetes Metab Rev 9:289, 1993

36. Zhong ZJ, Davidson L, Eisenbarth GS, Weiner HL: Suppression of diabetes in non obese diabetic mice by oral administration of porcine insulin. Proc Nat Acad Sci USA 88:10252, 1991

37. Muir A, Schatz D, Maclaren M: Antigen-specific immunotherapy: oral tolerance and subcutaneous immunization in the treatment of insulin-dependent diabetes. Diabetes Metab Rev 9:279, 1993

38. Vardi P: Adjuvant administration modulates the process of beta cell autoimmunity and prevents IDDM: introduction to human trials. Diabetes Metab Rev 9:317, 1993

39. Shehadeh N, Calcinaro F, Bradley BJ et al: Effects of adjuvant therapy on development of diabetes in mouse and man. Lancet 343:706, 1994

40. Fathman CG: Peptides as therapy of autoimmune disease. Diabetes Metab Rev 9:239, 1993

41. Elias D, Cohen IR: Peptide therapy for diabetes in NOD mice. Lancet 343:704, 1994

42. Muir A, Cornelius J, Ramiya V et al: Insulin B chain immunization activates regulatory T cells and reduces interferon-γ in NOD mouse islets. Diabetes, 43 (suppl. 1): 94A, 1994

43. Harrison LC, Honeyman M, Steele C, Graham M: Photophoresis trial in IDDM: an interim report. Proc Aust Diabetes Soc 91, 1992

44. Ludvigsson J: Intervention at diagnosis of type I diabetes using either antioxidants or photopheresis. Diabetes Metab Rev 9:329, 1993

45. Carroll PB, Khan R, Rilo HL et al: FK506 does not induce long term remission in patients with new onset type I diabetes mellitus. Diabetes, 43 (suppl. 1):94A, 1994

46. Slavin S, Sidi H, Weiss L et al: Linomide, a new treatment for autoimmune diseases: the potential in type I diabetes. Diabetes Metab Rev 9:329, 1993

47. Baeder WL, Sredy J, Sehgal SN et al: Rapamycin prevents the onset of insulin-dependent diabetes mellitus (IDDM) in NOD mice. Clin Exp Immunol 89:174, 1992

48. Hao L, Chan SM, Lafferty K: Mycophenolate mofetil can prevent development of diabetes in BB rats. Ann NY Acad Sci 696:328, 1993

4

Carbohydrate, Lipid, and Amino Acid Metabolism in the Nonpregnant Patient

ROBERT S. SHERWIN
WILLIAM V. TAMBORLANE
WALTER P. BORG

METABOLISM AND DIABETES MELLITUS

Diabetes mellitus may be defined as a syndrome in which a complex interaction of hereditary and environmental factors leads to inadequate action of insulin, due to decreased insulin secretion or resistance of target tissues to its action. Regardless of the pathogenic factors causing the disease, the eventual metabolic consequences of the diabetic syndrome primarily reflect the degree to which there is this absolute or relative deficiency of insulin. Insulin's critical role in the pathophysiology of diabetes derives from its central role in regulating the storage and release of metabolic fuels, namely, glucose, fat, and amino acids.

Insulin Secretion in Diabetes

The deficiency in insulin secretory capacity in diabetes may vary from complete failure to a partial defect that is apparent only in circumstances of increased demands such as physical stress, obesity, pregnancy, or aging. In the typical insulin-dependent (or type I) diabetic patient, insulin secretion is either totally defective or severely impaired; insulin production varies with the duration of the disease. For up to 3 to 5 years, these patients continue to secrete some insulin, despite their requirement for exogenous insulin.[1] The extent to which this residual insulin secretion is maintained appears to be an important factor in determining the stability of long-term metabolic control.[2] Ultimately, endogenous insulin secretion becomes undetectable as residual functioning β-cells are completely destroyed. Abundant evidence now exists that autoimmunity plays a critical role in the pathogenesis of type I (insulin-dependent) diabetes mellitus.[3]

In the patients with type II (non-insulin-dependent) diabetes, the secretory failure is less severe. Basal insulin levels are generally normal or mildly increased, whereas glucose-stimulated insulin secretion is diminished. The magnitude of the insulin secretory defect usually correlates with the severity of fasting hyperglycemia in these patients. In its mildest forms (plasma glucose approximately 140 mg/dl), the β-cell defect involves only the initial secretory phase; the more-delayed insulin response remains intact. In such individuals, the loss of responsiveness to glucose is specific, (i.e., normal responsiveness is maintained to other secretagogues such as β-adrenergic stimulation or amino acids).[4] Consequently, insulin deficiency is much less pronounced during ingestion of mixed meals as compared with glucose.[5] In patients with more severe fasting hyperglycemia (>200 mg/dl), the capacity to respond to increases in circulating glucose is virtually lost. These observations suggest that a specific abnormality in recognition of glucose by the β-cell occurs in the earliest stages of type II diabetes and that this defect advances as the disease progresses.

The initial reports by Yalow and Berson[6] regarding plasma insulin levels in type II diabetes emphasized the presence of hyperinsulinemia. This seeming paradox was subsequently shown to be more apparent than real when total body weight and ambient blood glucose levels are considered. Approximately 80 to 85 percent of type II diabetics are obese. Obesity per se is generally accompanied by hyperinsulinemia and is associated with resistance on the part of target tissues (muscle, liver, adipose tissue) to insulin.[7] When comparison is made between obese type II diabetic patients and appropriate weight-matched nondiabetic control patients, it is apparent that insulin levels in obese diabetic patients are below those observed in obese subjects with normal glucose tolerance.[8] An additional factor contributing to the seeming hyperinsulinemia is the presence of hyperglycemia itself. In other words, when glucose levels are raised in nondiabetic individuals to stimulate the glucose tolerance curve of the diabetic patient, the deficiency of the insulin response in the diabetes becomes more clearly evident.

Insulin Resistance in Diabetes

The biologic action of insulin is not only related to its concentration but is also a function of its ability to activate cellular events. The first step in the cellular action of insulin is the binding of the hormone to a specific receptor on the cell surface. This interaction triggers a cascade of poorly characterized cellular changes, termed *postreceptor events,* leading to a metabolic response. The concentrations of insulin required to activate metabolic processes vary both with respect to the target tissues and the substrates involved. For example, a doubling of systemic insulin levels is sufficient to achieve near-maximal suppression of lipolysis but has a negligible effect on glucose uptake by peripheral tissues (muscle and fat).[9] The insulin concentrations needed to promote protein anabolism or suppress hepatic glucose production fall between these extremes but again are much lower than those that maximally increase peripheral glucose uptake.[10,11] As might be expected from this situation, the consequences of incomplete insulin deficiency differ sub-

stantially among the various insulin-sensitive fuels and target tissues.

In type II diabetic patients, insulin is markedly less effective.[12] The insulin dose-response curve for augmenting glucose uptake in peripheral tissues is shifted to the right (decreased sensitivity) and the maximal response is commonly reduced, particularly in patients with more severe hyperglycemia.[13] Other insulin-stimulated processes, such as inhibition of hepatic glucose production, also show reduced sensitivity to insulin. However, by contrast, hepatic insensitivity is relatively mild and may be readily overcome by larger amounts of insulin.[13] It is generally believed that insulin resistance in type II diabetes results from both a reduction in insulin receptors and postreceptor defect.[14] The causes of insulin resistance in nonobese type II diabetic patients do not appear to be different from their obese counterparts. However, the severity of the resistant state tends to be accentuated by the co-existence of obesity and diabetes. Overall, the available data indicate that insulin resistance contributes importantly to the development of type II diabetes. It remains uncertain, however, whether insulin resistance or the deficiency in insulin secretion is the primary event leading to diabetes in these patients. Regardless, both disturbances undoubtedly interact, thereby magnifying the severity of the metabolic derangement. Interestingly, the ability of insulin to stimulate glucose uptake in peripheral tissues is also impaired in patients with type I diabetes[15] and in animals rendered partially insulin-deficient by subtotal pancreatectomy. This insulin resistance is thought to be mediated by a postreceptor defect and is responsive to intensive insulin therapy.[16] Thus, even in type I diabetes, insulin resistance may contribute to and impair therapeutic measures directed at improving glucose control. The defects in insulin action in diabetes are summarized in Table 4-1.

Table 4-1. Defects in Insulin Secretion and Action in Diabetes

	Type I Diabetes	Type II Diabetes
Insulin secretion	Absent	Impaired (particularly to glucose)
Insulin action	Impaired	Severely impaired (receptor and postreceptor defects)

Table 4-2. Metabolic Actions of Insulin

	Liver	Adipose Tissue	Muscle
Anticatabolic effects	Decreased Glycogenolysis Gluconeogenesis Ketogenesis	Decreased Lipolysis	Decreased Protein breakdown
Anabolic effects	Increased Glycogen synthesis Fat synthesis	Increased Fat synthesis Glycerol synthesis	Increased Glycogen and protein synthesis Glucose uptake

Metabolic Effects of Insulin

Insulin is the primary hormonal factor that controls the storage and metabolism of ingested metabolic fuels. After a meal, augmented secretion of insulin facilitates the uptake and storage of glucose, fat, and amino acids. Conversely, a deficiency of insulin leads to mobilization and endogenous fuels and reduced use of ingested nutrients. The action of insulin involves each of the three metabolic fuels and is manifested in three principal tissues: liver, muscle, and adipose tissue, where insulin exerts both anticatabolic and anabolic effects, which reinforce each other (Table 4-2).

BODY FUEL METABOLISM IN NORMAL SUBJECTS

Postabsorptive State

The period after an overnight fast and preceding the ingestion of the morning meal is referred to as the postabsorptive state. At this time, the concentrations of hormones (insulin and glucagon) and substrates (glucose, amino acids, and fat) that were altered due to meal ingestion during the preceding day have returned to baseline, and the rate of fuel consumption is closely matched by endogenous fuel production. The postabsorptive state thus serves as a useful reference point because it represents the period of transition from the fed to the fasted condition.

After an overnight fast, the decline in circulating insulin leads to a marked reduction of glucose uptake by peripheral insulin-sensitive tissues (e.g., muscle and fat) and a shift toward the mobilization and use of fatty acids as energy-yielding fuels. Glucose consumption, nevertheless, continues in the non-insulin-sensitive tissues (e.g., the brain, renal medulla, formed elements of blood) and in the splanchnic area, so that total glu-

cose use continues at a rate of 200 to 250 g/d.[17] The main site of glucose uptake is the brain, which is critically dependent on an ongoing supply of glucose for oxidative metabolism. Despite the lack of exogenous fuel and the ongoing glucose requirement, blood glucose remains relatively stable as the liver releases glucose at rates sufficient to match those of consuming tissues.

The hepatic processes involved in the release of glucose into the bloodstream consist of glycogenolysis and gluconeogenesis. It has been estimated that approximately 50 to 75 percent of hepatic glucose production in the postabsorptive state is derived from glycogenolysis, with gluconeogenesis contributing the remainder.[18] The resynthesis of glucose from the glycolytic intermediate, lactate, amounts for at least one-half the gluconeogenic component, and the conversion of glycogenic amino acids comprises most of the remainder. Alanine, whose release from muscle and uptake by liver predominates over that of other amino acids, is the main amino acid contributing to glucose synthesis. Conversion of fat-derived glycerol and recycled pyruvate contribute less than 2 percent and 1 percent, respectively, to total glucose production.[18] Fuel homeostasis in the postabsorptive state is summarized in Figure 4-1.

Regarding the hormonal factors regulating glucose metabolism in postabsorptive humans, both glucagon and insulin moderate glucose release by the liver. Perhaps the most compelling evidence that basal glucagon secretion is important in maintaining glucose production in the postabsorptive state derives from studies in which somatostatin is infused to suppress plasma glucagon and circulating insulin is prevented from falling by exogenous insulin infusion. In this circumstance, a sustained 70 to 75 percent reduction in hepatic glucose production occurs, indicating the

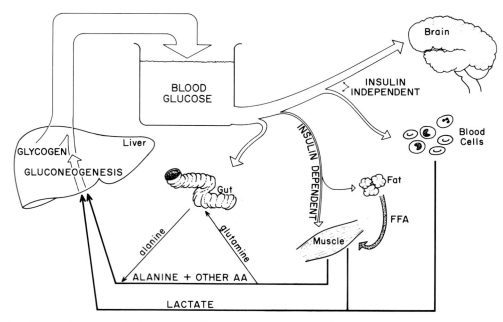

Fig. 4-1. Glucose homeostasis in the postabsorptive state in normal human subjects. FFA, free fatty acid; AA, amino acid(s).

importance of basal concentrations of glucagon in opposing the inhibitory actions on this process.[19] The restraining influence of basal concentrations of insulin on postabsorptive glucose production is also evident when plasma insulin is suppressed by somatostatin and circulating glucagon is maintained at the basal level by exogenous glucagon infusion. Under these conditions, hepatic glucose production promptly increases.[20] Hepatic glucose production appears to be regulated by a "push-pull" system, with the opposing actions of insulin and glucagon balancing each other. In the postabsorptive state, the hormonal regulation of glucose homeostasis is primarily directed at endogenous production of glucose rather than its uptake by tissues.

After overnight fasting, muscle tissue, the main reservoir of body protein, is in negative nitrogen balance as evidenced by a net release of amino acids.[21] This net proteolysis in muscle is facilitated by the decline in circulating insulin to baseline concentrations. Inasmuch as plasma amino acid levels remain relatively constant, amino acid release from muscle must be accompanied by amino acid uptake by nonmuscular tissues (liver and, to a lesser extent, kidney and gut). A

net flux of amino acids thus exists between muscle tissue and nonmuscular tissues where nitrogenous waste products (urea and ammonia) are generated.

Although virtually all amino acids are released by muscle, alanine and glutamine predominate, accounting for more than 50 percent of the total amino acid release.[22] The alanine serves as a substrate for hepatic gluconeogenesis, and glutamine as a precursor for renal ammonia synthesis and as an energy-yielding fuel for the gut. Because alanine and glutamine account for only 10 to 13 percent of the amino acid residues in muscle protein, their release at higher concentrations has been explained on the basis of de novo synthesis in muscle.

The carbon skeleton of alanine is largely derived from pyruvate; it is believed that most of the pyruvate used in alanine synthesis in muscle is formed via glycolysis.[23] The branched chain amino acids (leucine, isoleucine, and valine) appear to be the predominant sources of the nitrogen for alanine formation[24] (Fig. 4-2). In contrast to other amino acids, these amino acids are metabolized to a greater extent in muscle than liver. Furthermore, their oxidation in muscle ap-

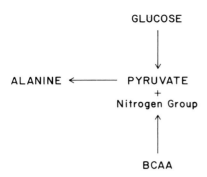

Fig. 4-2. Alanine synthesis in muscle. The carbon skeleton is mainly derived from glucose, whereas branched chain amino acids (BCAA) play an important role in donating the nitrogen group.

pears to be sufficient to provide nearly all the nitrogen required for alanine formation.[25] The apparent coupling between branched chain amino acid catabolism and alanine synthesis suggests that the rate of oxidation of these amino acids may be an important factor, modulating the availability of alanine as a substrate for hepatic gluconeogenesis. Leucine oxidation is inversely correlated with insulin concentration.[26] In contrast to alanine, the carbon skeleton as well as the nitrogen source for glutamine is most likely derived from in situ muscle catabolism of amino acids.[27]

The pattern of amino acid uptake by the splanchnic area (liver and gut) complements that of muscle release (i.e., alanine and glutamine predominate).[28] However, when hepatic and extrahepatic tissues are considered individually, most of the alanine is removed by the liver, whereas glutamine is taken up by the gut.[29] Nevertheless, glutamine contributes to glucose and urea production by the liver, because a portion of the glutamine taken up by the gut is converted to alanine, released directly into the portal vein, and ultimately converted to glucose and urea by the liver (Fig. 4-1). Alanine is thus not only a main vehicle for nitrogen release from muscle but is quantitatively the most important protein-derived precursor for hepatic gluconeogenesis. The rate at which alanine and other amino acids are converted into glucose is in large part determined by the balance between glucagon (stimulatory) and insulin (inhibitory) in the portal vein as well as the availability of glucose precursors generated by muscle. The restraining effects of insulin on

the dissolution of muscle protein and branched chain amino acid oxidation limit the release of glycogenic amino acids by muscle, thereby complementing its restraining effect on hepatic gluconeogenesis.

Finally, the fall in circulating insulin after an overnight fast allows for the release of free fatty acids (FFAs) from adipose tissue depots (Fig. 4-3). Insulin is extremely effective in inhibiting hormone-sensitive lipase within the fat cell, which catalyzes the hydrolysis of stored triglycerides and the liberation of FFAs. This antilipolytic action of insulin occurs at concentrations of insulin well below those necessary to affect glucose transport.[9] The levels of insulin normally present in the postabsorptive state are sufficiently low, however, to permit the flux of FFAs from storage sites to extracerebral tissues, such as muscle, heart, renal cortex, and liver (Fig. 4-3). In these tissues, fatty acids are the principal energy-yielding fuel. The consumption of FFAs by muscle tissue is an important factor in diminishing muscle glucose uptake and oxidation in the postabsorptive state. FFAs act in this way by reducing glycolytic flux as well as entry of glucose-derived pyruvate into the Kreb's cycle (through the pyruvate dehydrogenase step).[30] The rate of lipolysis and the magnitude of the insulin decline in portal blood after an overnight fast is not, however, of sufficient magnitude to stimulate appreciably the rate of hepatic conversion of FFAs to ketones.

Metabolic Adaptation During Short-Term Starvation

Because liver glycogen is limited to about 70 g after an overnight fast,[31] whereas glucose consumption occurs at a rate of approximately 200 to 250 g/d, hepatic glycogen stores are rapidly dissipated very early in the course of fasting. Thus, the initial phase of starvation is characterized by an acceleration of hepatic gluconeogenesis to meet ongoing tissue demands for glucose by the brain. The augmentation of gluconeogenesis and the maintenance of glucose homeostasis are mediated by both hepatic and extrahepatic events. The release of alanine and other glycogenic amino acids from muscle increases,[32] and the rate of hepatic conversion of alanine to glucose accelerates.[21] The enhancement of glucose synthesis from amino acids is not, however, solely a function of increased availability of these precursors, since plasma levels of alanine and

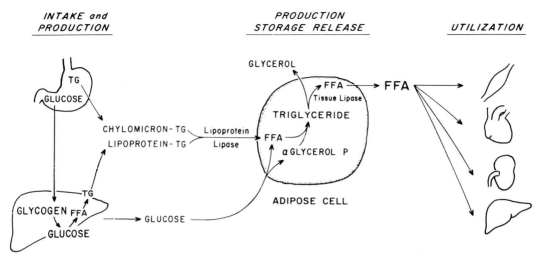

Fig. 4-3. Fat synthesis, storage, and release in normal humans. Normal fat homeostasis is dependent on the action of insulin. Within the liver, insulin stimulates the synthesis of free fatty acids (FFAs) from glucose and their esterification to form triglycerides (TG). Both exogenously derived (dietary) triglycerides (chylomicron-TG) and endogenously synthesized triglycerides (lipoprotein-TG) are sources of fatty acid delivery to adipose tissue. Insulin accelerates the uptake of FFA by adipose tissue by its stimulatory effect on lipoprotein lipase. Fat storage within adipose tissue is also enhanced by insulin's glycerogenic effects. The antilipolytic actions of insulin (inhibition of tissue lipase) enhance fat storage as well, while reducing the availability of circulating fatty acids. FFAs are released from adipose tissue when insulin levels fall and are taken up by muscle, heart, kidney, and liver.

other glycogenic amino acids actually fall despite their increased release from muscle. These observations suggest that intrahepatic gluconeogenic mechanisms are stimulated during short-term fasting. An additional factor contributing to glucose homeostasis at this time is the increased release of FFAs from adipose tissue. Oxidation of fatty acids by muscle spares glucose for use by the brain whereas their oxidation by the liver activates key gluconeogenic enzymes and furnishes the energy and reducing power necessary for glucose synthesis.[33]

These metabolic adaptations (namely, increased gluconeogenesis, amino acid mobilization, and lipolysis) are facilitated by a decline in insulin secretion below postabsorptive levels as well as a modest increase in circulating glucagon levels.[34,35] The former appears to be triggered by a fall in arterial glucose concentration, which inhibits insulin secretion, whereas the rise in glucagon is due to diminution in the rate of glucagon metabolism.[35] Hypoinsulinemia enhances protein breakdown and thus the delivery of glycogenic amino acids from muscle to liver, where increased quantities

of glucose are synthesized under the influence of both the elevation of glucagon and the depression of portal insulin (Fig. 4-4). Hypoinsulinemia further contributes to glucose homeostasis by reducing extracerebral glucose consumption and by increasing the availability of FFAs for oxidative metabolism by muscle and liver.

The progressive rise in blood ketones during starvation is also regulated by insulin and glucagon[36] (Fig. 4-4). The development of hyperketonemia involves three distinct metabolic events: (1) delivery of FFA from adipose tissue, (2) hepatic oxidation of FFAs leading to ketone formation ("ketogenic capacity"), and (3) a reduction in ketone uptake by peripheral tissues. Hypoinsulinemia activates each of these steps, whereas hyperglucagonemia contributes by enhancing ketogenic capacity.[36] Growth hormone may also contribute by promoting lipolysis.[37]

Exercise

As in starvation, during exercise there is a need to generate glucose and FFAs from endogenous sources to meet tissue demands. Because muscle glycogen

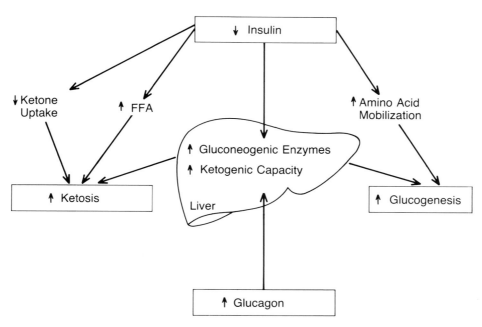

Fig. 4-4. Interaction of insulin suppression and glucagon stimulation in promoting gluconeogenesis and ketosis during starvation. FFA, free fatty acid.

stores are rapidly depleted, energy for working muscle must be supplied from blood-borne fuels (Fig. 4-5). Glucose is supplied by the liver, which may increase its production of glucose three- to fivefold.[38] The rate of hepatic glucose production is precisely regulated to supply enough glucose to keep blood levels from falling despite the increased glucose extraction by working muscle. FFAs are mobilized from adipose tissue at dramatically increased rates to minimize the need for glucose from the liver's limited glycogen stores. As exercise continues for prolonged periods, the consumption of FFAS assumes an increasingly important role in meeting muscle energy requirements[39] (Fig. 4-5). This spares the liver from further demands for glucose production, which, by this time, is occurring to a greater extent from gluconeogenic precursors, including protein-derived amino acids.[39]

Current evidence suggests that the increased consumption of glucose and FFAs by exercising muscle is mediated largely via local nonhormonal mechanisms. A coordinated hormonal and neural response is, however, of critical importance for the production of appropriate quantities of substrates. During exercise,

insulin secretion diminishes in association with the activation of sympathetic nervous system activity. Also, increments in plasma glucagon, epinephrine, growth hormone, and cortisol commonly occur, particularly as the intensity of exercise is increased.[40] These hormonal changes, acting in concert, promote the mobilization of glucose and FFAs from liver and adipose tissue, respectively.

Glucose Ingestion

Glucose ingestion involves a variety of homeostatic mechanisms that act to minimize the rise in plasma glucose and restore normoglycemia. They include (1) suppression of endogenous glucose production by the liver, (2) stimulation of glucose uptake by splanchnic tissues, especially the liver, and (3) stimulation of peripheral glucose uptake, particularly in muscle. These homeostatic processes are activated by a rise in circulating insulin or a rise in blood glucose itself. Specifically, inhibition of hepatic glucose production is exquisitely sensitive to small elevations of portal insulin concentration[10,41] but may also occur in response to

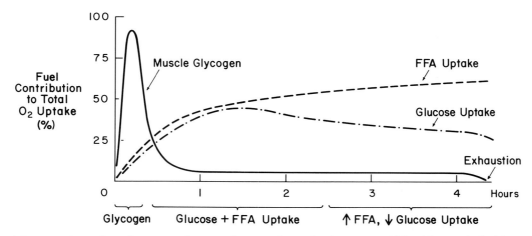

Fig. 4-5. Time-dependent changes in the contribution of muscle glycogen and blood-borne fuels (glucose and free fatty acids [FFAs]) to the energy requirements of leg tissues during bicycle exercise.

hyperglycemia per se, provided that basal insulin levels are maintained.[42] Glucose uptake by splanchnic tissues is stimulated by a rising glucose concentration and to some extent by hyperinsulinemia.[43] The presence of basal amounts of insulin are required for glucose to exert this effect.[44] By contrast, peripheral glucose uptake is promoted by hyperinsulinemia and, to a more limited extent, by the mass effect caused by hyperglycemia itself.[43] Considerably larger amounts of insulin are, however, needed to increase peripheral glucose uptake than are required to suppress hepatic glucose production.[10]

The elevation in plasma glucose caused by ingestion of large glucose loads brings into play each of the above metabolic adjustments. Hepatic glucose production is markedly suppressed for several hours until plasma glucose has returned to baseline. This serves to limit glucose entry into the systemic circulation at a time when the system is overloaded by exogenous glucose. With respect to the uptake of the exogenous glucose load, recent studies indicate that in quantitative terms most of the exogenous glucose load (about two-thirds) is deposited in muscle.[45] The remainder (about one-third) is taken up by splanchnic tissues (e.g., liver and gut). When one considers that the liver also reduces its endogenous production of glucose by more than 50 percent, the net effect is a substantial retention of glucose in the splanchnic area, which approaches in magnitude the amount of glucose deposited in muscle tissue. Thus, the muscle and liver both play a crucial role in the homeostatic response to large glucose meals (Fig. 4-6).

A large (75-g) oral glucose load is, however, not representative of either the magnitude of carbohydrate intake or the amplitude of blood glucose excursions observed in healthy individuals ingesting ordinary meals. In circumstances of mixed meal intake, hexose intake is considerably less and the blood glucose generally varies by no more than 30 mg/dl over 24 hours. This "fine tuning" of blood glucose regulation is determined to a greater extent by the exquisite sensitivity of the liver to small changes in insulin secretion. When small amounts of glucose are consumed, peripheral insulin levels rise modestly (less than twofold). However, because insulin is released directly into the portal vein, portal insulin concentrations rise considerably higher. Consequently, hepatic glucose production is suppressed, whereas peripheral glucose uptake, which requires more insulin to be activated,[10] is only modestly increased.[46] If the quantity of glucose consumed is sufficiently small so that it is compensated for by the reduction in endogenous glucose production, glucose homeostasis is maintained simply by retaining hepatic glycogen stores. Thus, as compared with the liver, muscle and adipose tissue are involved to a more limited extent in the metabolic adjustment to very small glucose loads. This phenomenon is a direct consequence

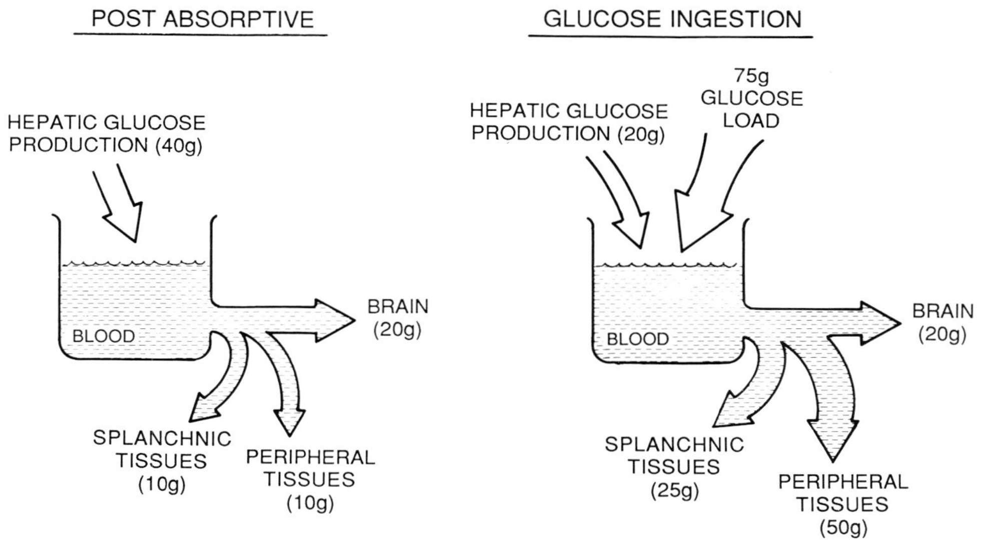

POST ABSORPTIVE

GLUCOSE INGESTION

HEPATIC GLUCOSE
PRODUCTION (40g)

BLOOD

BRAIN
(20g)

SPLANCHNIC
TISSUES
(10g)

PERIPHERAL
TISSUES
(10g)

HEPATIC GLUCOSE
PRODUCTION (20g)

75g
GLUCOSE
LOAD

BLOOD

BRAIN
(20g)

SPLANCHNIC
TISSUES
(25g)

PERIPHERAL
TISSUES
(50g)

Fig. 4-6. Cumulative rates of hepatic glucose production and glucose disposal by non-insulin-dependent tissues (brain), the splanchnic bed, and peripheral insulin-sensitive tissues during a 4-hour period either in the postabsorptive state (fast) or after ingestion of a 75-g glucose load in normal subjects. After glucose ingestion, hepatic glucose production is reduced (by 50 percent) and glucose uptake by splanchnic (2.5-fold) and peripheral (5-fold) tissues is increased.

of the disparity of the dose-response curves of hepatic and peripheral tissues to insulin.[10]

Protein Ingestion

Because muscle is in negative nitrogen balance in the fasting state, repletion of muscle nitrogen depends on a net uptake of amino acids in response to protein feeding. The transfer of amino acids from the gut to muscle after protein ingestion is facilitated by the action of insulin.

In normal healthy subjects, ingestion of a pure protein meal is followed by a large output of amino acids from the splanchnic bed, involving predominantly the branched chain amino acids.[47] Valine, isoleucine, and leucine together account for more than 60 percent of the total amino acids entering the systemic circulation, even though they contribute only 20 percent of the total amino acids in the protein meal (Fig. 4-7). The glycogenic amino acids, however, are for the most part deposited within the splanchnic area.[47] Simultaneous with the release of amino acids from the splanchnic bed, peripheral muscle exchange of most amino acids

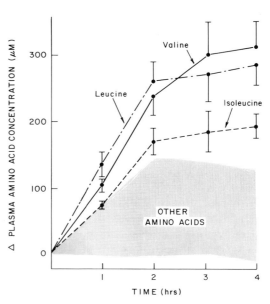

Fig. 4-7. Changes in plasma amino acids after ingestion of a pure protein meal. Increments in the branched chain amino acids (leucine, isoleucine, and valine) exceed those of other amino acids. (Based on unpublished data.)

reverts from the net output observed in the basal state to a net uptake. As in the case of splanchnic exchange, the net uptake of amino acids across peripheral muscle tissue is most marked for the branched chain amino acids. The latter account for more than half the total peripheral amino acid uptake in the first hour and for nearly 90 percent at 2 to 3 hours.[47] Leucine, isoleucine, and valine thus constitute the main substrate for the immediate repletion of muscle nitrogen after protein intake. Furthermore, because the branched chain amino acids comprise only 20 percent of the amino acid residues in muscle protein,[25] it is likely that these amino acids are not solely used for protein synthesis but are catabolized within muscle. Thus, as in the fasting state they provide a source of energy for muscle. Interestingly, the high intracellular levels of branched chain amino acids in muscle induced by protein feeding may have importance beyond delivery of nitrogen. There is evidence that the branched chain amino acids have a regulatory role in stimulating protein synthesis.[48]

Fat Metabolism

The rise in plasma insulin that normally accompanies the consumption of mixed meals accelerates the removal of ingested triglyceride by adipose tissue and serves to promote triglyceride synthesis in liver and adipose tissue (Fig. 4-3). In the liver, a significant proportion of the dietary carbohydrate taken up is used for triglyceride formation. In humans, the liver is quantitatively a far more important site of conversion of dietary carbohydrate into fat than is adipose tissue. However, both exogenously derived (or dietary) triglycerides (chylomicron-TG) and endogenously synthesized triglycerides (lipoprotein-TG) provide a source of FFA for triglyceride synthesis in adipose tissue. Insulin accelerates the uptake of FFA by adipose tissue by virtue of its stimulatory effect on lipoprotein lipase, an enzyme that breaks down circulating triglycerides.[49] Triglyceride storage within adipose tissue is also enhanced by insulin's glycerogenic effects. A large proportion of insulin-mediated glucose uptake in the fat cell is used for the formation of α-glycerophosphate, which is necessary for the esterification of fatty acids to form triglycerides. The antilipolytic actions of insulin (inhibition of hormone-sensitive lipase) also enhance fat storage while reducing FFA concentra-

tions. The net effect of the antilipolytic, fat synthetic, and glycerogenic actions of meal-stimulated insulin elevations is to increase total fat storage and reduce circulating FFAs and ketone bodies.

Role of Gender in Glucose Homeostasis

Assessment of metabolism has generally been performed without regard to the sex steroid hormonal milieu. Recently, however, several lines of evidence indicate the existence of gender-related differences in fuel metabolism. In response to exogenous insulin infusions, the rates of total whole-body glucose uptake or glucose uptake per unit of insulin have been shown to be greater in males than females.[50–52] Furthermore, the response to extended fasting is notably influenced by the sex of the individual. Whereas the fall in circulating glucose in normal men is gradual and glucose levels rarely fall below 50 mg/dl, in nonobese women the process is accelerated and plasma glucose often decreases to the 40 to 50-mg/dl range after 48 to 72 hours.[53] Although the explanation for these differences has not been established, it has been suggested that the smaller muscle mass of women than men leads to the reduction in insulin-stimulated glucose uptake, as well as the changes seen during fasting in females. With respect to the latter, it has been demonstrated that the generation of amino acids from muscle is diminished in fasted females. In keeping with this, the fasting-induced decline in circulating alanine is more pronounced in women than in men.[53] The greater decline in glucose concentrations leads to greater suppression of insulin secretion and, in turn, to a more pronounced rise in blood ketones in fasted women. Despite the evidence that women achieve a lower glucose level during fasting than men, the literature contains conflicting data regarding the effect of the gender on counterregulatory response to hypoglycemia. Several reports have demonstrated that epinephrine, norepinephrine, and growth hormone responses to hypoglycemia and other stimuli were significantly higher in males.[54,55] By contrast, other investigators have failed to demonstrate such differences.[56]

Another situation in which there is variation in the sex hormones milieu is the follicular and luteal phases of the menstrual cycle in women. Assessment of carbohydrate metabolism under hyperglycemic conditions have demonstrated greater glucose uptake in the preovulatory period.[57–59] However, no detectable differences in the basal rate of glucose turnover, insulin-stimulated glucose uptake, or the insulin-induced suppression of hepatic glucose production has been observed between two phases of the menstrual cycle.[60–62] Also, the counterregulatory hormone responses to hypoglycemia are similar in the follicular and luteal phase of the cycle.[63]

BODY FUEL METABOLISM IN DIABETES
Metabolic Dysfunction

The metabolic alterations observed in diabetes primarily reflect the degree to which there is an absolute or relative deficiency of insulin. Viewed in the context of the role of insulin as the main storage hormone, a minimal deficiency results in a diminished ability to increase effectively the storage reservoir of body fuels, because of inadequate disposal of ingested foodstuffs (e.g., postprandial hyperglycemia, hyperaminoacidemia, and elevated triglycerides). In its most severe form (diabetic ketoacidosis), there is overproduction of glucose and marked acceleration of catabolic processes (lipolysis and proteolysis).

Postabsorptive State

After an overnight fast, substrate homeostasis in the patient with diabetes resembles that observed during starvation in nondiabetic individuals. Thus, diabetes might be thought of as a state of "accelerated starvation," a situation not unlike that seen in normal pregnancy. This should not be surprising considering that the hormonal milieu of diabetes and starvation share many common features, namely, insulin deficiency in association with relative or absolute glucagon and growth hormone excess. The principal difference from the metabolic standpoint is that blood glucose in the diabetic patient is elevated rather than reduced as it is in the case during starvation. Such discrepancies may be due to the persistence of liver glycogen stores in the diabetic that allow glycogenolysis to be maintained in conjunction with increased rates of gluconeogenesis.

In the patient with glucose intolerance, relative insulin deficiency is apparent (by definition) only after meal ingestion, when augmented glucose uptake by peripheral insulin-sensitive tissue is required to compensate for increased glucose entry into the circulation. The postabsorptive glucose level is normal because basal insulin secretion is adequate to prevent glucose overproduction by the liver, a process that is very sensitive to minor increments of insulin.

When absolute or relative insulin deficiency occurs in the basal state, an elevation in fasting blood glucose ensues. In patients with type II diabetes, normal or even increased basal levels of insulin may be maintained but only at the expense of fasting hyperglycemia. In such patients, hepatic glucose production (as determined by radioactive tracers) may be normal but is generally increased in proportion to the magnitude of the blood glucose elevation.[64] Because only mild hyperglycemia in normal individuals is sufficient to inhibit hepatic glucose production,[46] the type II diabetic patient with fasting hyperglycemia is always in a state of relative or absolute glucose overproduction. In patients with type I diabetes, portal insulin deficiency is invariably present, and thus hepatic glucose production is more consistently elevated. In this situation, the insulin deficiency leads to hypersecretion of glucagon and growth hormone, which further accentuate glucose overproduction.[65,66] Because glucose uptake (in contrast to glucose production) in the postabsorptive state largely occurs in non-insulin-sensitive tissues, it is not unexpected that total body glucose uptake tends to be increased under fasting conditions as a result of the mass action of hyperglycemia. This underscores the crucial role that the liver plays in determining the fasting glucose level in diabetes (Fig. 4-8).

The increased hepatic glucose production accompanying diabetes is characterized by an alteration in the relative contribution of glycogenolysis and gluconeogenesis to total hepatic glucose production. In type I diabetes, the presence of glucagon and the absence of a restraining effect of insulin increase the hepatic uptake of glycogenic substrates and facilitate their conversion to glucose in the liver. As a result, gluconeogenesis accounts for a substantially larger proportion of hepatic glucose production in such patients as compared with that in normal subjects; the relative contribution of gluconeogenesis is increased twofold.[67] By contrast, the magnitude and pattern of amino acid release from muscle in hyperglycemic type I diabetic

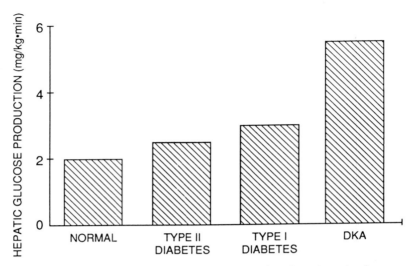

Fig. 4-8. Influence of diabetes and diabetic ketoacidosis (DKA) on hepatic glucose production.

subjects is similar to healthy controls,[67] implying that changes in intrahepatic process rather in muscle are primarily responsible for augmented gluconeogenesis in diabetes. Nevertheless, it is possible that increased recycling of glycolytic intermediates (e.g., lactate) may occur as well. Because FFAs are oxidized at an accelerated rate in the muscle of diabetic patients (as a result of their high circulating levels), glucose-derived pyruvate cannot readily enter the Kreb's cycle. Similar changes have also been reported in type II diabetes.[68] The presence of increased gluconeogenesis in type II diabetes is consistent with the finding that greater amounts of insulin are necessary to inhibit gluconeogenesis as compared with glycogenolysis in liver.[69]

In the extreme situation of total insulin lack, an ever-increasing fasting blood glucose level fails to elicit a secretory response. The absence of insulin together with the excessive release of a variety of counterregulatory hormones (glucagon, catecholamines, growth hormone, and cortisol) that ensues causes hepatic glucose production to increase threefold or more above normal, largely as a consequence of accelerated gluconeogenesis. Because of the hypoinsulinemia and the insulin resistance produced by the elevated levels of insulin-antagonistic hormones, compensatory increases in glucose disposal (other than renal) are virtually paralyzed. The clinical correlate of this sequence of events is profound hyperglycemia, as is observed

in diabetic ketoacidosis or nonketotic hyperosmolar coma.

In the postabsorptive state, patients with insulin-dependent diabetes exhibit hyperaminoacidemia. Examination of individual amino acid levels reveals that the increment in circulating amino acids in these patients is due almost entirely to a rise in the branched chain amino acids (leucine, isoleucine, and valine)[67] (Fig. 4-9). By contrast, plasma alanine levels may be reduced, particularly when insulin deficiency is severe and hepatic removal of alanine is accelerated.[70] The specific tissue site accounting for this rise in plasma branched chain amino acids has not been fully clarified. For example, there is no demonstrable increase in the net release of branched chain amino acids from either leg[67] or splanchnic tissues in these subjects.[70] Nevertheless, recent studies using radioactive tracers demonstrate that the delivery of branched chain amino acids into the circulation is augmented in poorly controlled type I diabetic individuals.[71] Considering that the branched chains are essential amino acids, these studies imply that total body protein breakdown is increased in such patients even though they show only moderate insulin deficiency. Such changes are not usually discerned in the clinical setting, perhaps because compensatory increases in protein synthesis may minimize the loss of body protein. This is not the case if insulin deficiency becomes more severe, as evidenced

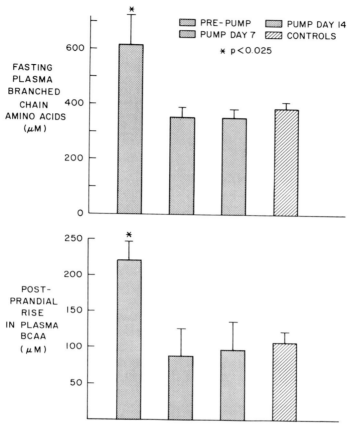

Fig. 4-9. Fasting and postprandial increments (after mixed meal ingestion) of total branched chain amino acids (BCAA) in type I diabetic patients and healthy controls. The diabetic patients were studied before (during poor control) and after 7 and 14 days of intensive insulin therapy using a portable pump. (Based on the data of Tamborlane et al.[102])

by the stunted growth of young diabetic patients in the preinsulin era and the marked protein wasting of the diabetic individual in ketoacidosis.

The elevated circulating levels of branched chain amino acids also lead to an acceleration of leucine, isoleucine, and valine oxidation in the diabetic state.[71] In diabetic animals, oxidation of branched chain amino acids is increased by 50 percent.[26] The increased in situ catabolism of these amino acids provides muscle tissue with the nitrogen groups necessary for alanine synthesis,[24] thereby increasing substrate availability for gluconeogenesis. In this way, the accelerated breakdown of amino acids in muscle contributes indirectly to hyperglycemia in diabetes.

The abnormalities of branched chain amino acid metabolism described for insulin-dependent patients may not be evident in patients with type II diabetes. This may be because the metabolism of branched chain amino acids is more sensitive to the action of insulin than is peripheral glucose metabolism.[11]

In addition to hyperglycemia and hyperaminoacidemia, the levels of FFAs are frequently elevated in postabsorptive diabetic patients.[72] This phenomenon appears to be a consequence of accelerated mobilization of body fat stores and can primarily be attributed to deficiency of insulin. In type II diabetic subjects, FFA elevations occur in the presence of normal or increased levels of insulin,[72] suggesting resistance to insulin's inhibitory effect on lipolysis. The increased availability of FFAs leads to their oxidation by muscle tissues and in turn causes a concomitant diminution in the rate of glucose oxidation.[30] Although FFAs cannot be directly converted to glucose, they promote hyperglycemia in diabetes by providing the liver with energy-yielding fuel and the necessary cofactors to support gluconeogenesis and by interfering with glucose consumption by muscle.[73]

In type II diabetes, the presence of endogenous insulin secretion allows for sufficient levels of insulin in the portal vein to suppress ketogenic processes in the liver. In the patient with type I diabetes, however, mobilized FFAs are very readily converted to ketone bodies. Lack of insulin in the portal circulation and the presence of glucagon suppresses fat synthesis in the liver and thus intrahepatic levels of malonyl co-enzyme A. The latter together with increased availability of carnitine stimulates the activity of hepatic acylcarnitine transferase. This enzyme facilitates the transfer of long chain fatty acids into mitochondria, where they are broken down via β-oxidation and converted to ketone bodies.[36] By virtue of its inhibitory effect on ketone turnover, hypoinsulinemia in the type I diabetic individual enhances the magnitude of the ketosis for any given level of increased ketone production.[74] As a result, blood ketones are generally elevated in type I diabetic patients (Fig. 4-10), although usually not to the extent that acid-base balance is affected.

Finally, patients with diabetes commonly exhibit elevated fasting concentrations of lipoproteins. Most striking is the elevation in very low-density lipoprotein (VLDL) triglyceride, which may be seen in milder forms of type II diabetes as well as in insulin-deficient patients. It would appear that the mechanism responsible for hypertriglyceridemia varies in these groups. In the former situation, elevated portal insulin levels may promote VLDL triglyceride synthesis, and in the latter circumstance, lipoprotein lipase, an insulin-sensitive enzyme, is deficient, leading to decreased triglyceride removal from the circulation.[75–77]

Glucose Ingestion

The ingestion of glucose triggers a variety of homeostatic responses in nondiabetic subjects (see above) that are directed toward minimizing the rise in blood glucose concentrations. They include suppression of endogenous glucose production, as well as the uptake of the exogenous glucose load, by splanchnic and peripheral tissues (mainly muscle). Because these responses are largely dependent on insulin, diabetes, even in its mildest forms, is invariably accompanied by postprandial hyperglycemia.

Patients with impaired glucose tolerance appear to have relatively intact insulin secretory responses to glucose but demonstrate reduced sensitivity to insulin.[13] Postprandial hyperglycemia in these patients mainly derives from a reduction in glucose uptake by peripheral tissues. A similar pattern is observed in type II diabetic subjects with fasting hyperglycemia, although the magnitude of the pancreatic defect is more pronounced.[78] This is because (1) insulin secretory response is markedly reduced in these patients and

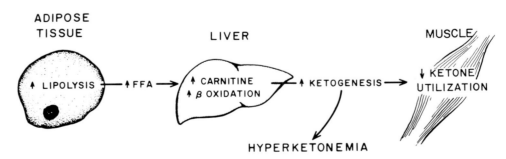

Fig. 4-10. The development of hyperketonemia in diabetes is a consequence of three distinct metabolic events: (1) accelerated delivery of free fatty acids (FFAs) from adipose tissue, (2) augmented β-oxidation of FFAs to ketones as a result of elevated cartinine levels and reduced concentrations of malonyl co-enzyme A, and (3) a reduction in ketone use in muscle. Each of these processes is reversed by the action of insulin.

(2) the magnitude of the defect in insulin action on peripheral tissues is greater (these patients can no longer overcome the defect with larger amounts of insulin and thus presumably have an impairment in postreceptor processing of the insulin signal).[13] However, patients with type II diabetes have sufficient levels of insulin in their portal circulation to allow the rising glucose level itself to suppress glucose production and promote glucose uptake by the liver. This tends to reduce the postprandial glucose excursion somewhat, at least as compared with insulin-deficient type I diabetic patients. The type I diabetic individual characteristically shows the most marked and prolonged elevations in blood glucose concentration after ingestion of carbohydrate. These individuals, because they fail to secrete insulin even in the postabsorptive state, have considerably lower portal insulin levels than patients with type II diabetes. This loss of the portal-peripheral insulin gradient is not readily reversed by conventional subcutaneous insulin therapy. Consequently, the insulin-deprived liver fails to reduce its glucose production or take up glucose in response to a rising circulating glucose level.[67] In addition, glucose uptake by peripheral tissues is grossly impaired because of the lack of an insulin secretory response and the development of insulin resistance at the postreceptor level after chronic insulin deprivation.[15] The net result of this multifaceted disturbance is a gross defect in metabolic glucose disposal that is only partially compensated for by increased renal glycosuria (Table 4-3).

In normal subjects, the rise in plasma insulin caused by glucose ingestion also inhibits lipolysis, which in turn decreases the availability of FFAs for oxidation in muscle. This facilitates glucose uptake and oxidation because the oxidation of FFAs interferes with glycolysis and the movement of glucose-derived pyruvate into the Kreb's cycle.[73] In type II diabetic subjects, despite the availability of some insulin, there is much less suppression of lipolysis during glucose ingestion because of insulin resistance.[72] Similar changes are observed in type I diabetic patients, largely because of hypoinsulinemia (although resistance to insulin may also contribute). The failure of diabetic patients to suppress fat oxidation during consumption of glucose contributes to the peripheral insulin resistance of diabetes and acts to block the oxidation of glucose that enters muscle tissue.

Protein Ingestion

In addition to the increased use of amino acids for gluconeogenesis and release of branched chain amino acids in the postabsorptive state, repletion of muscle nitrogen is impaired in the type I diabetic patient. After ingestion of a protein meal, the net splanchnic release of individual amino acids in insulin-dependent diabetic subjects is similar to that observed in healthy controls.[47] Although the systemic delivery is not altered, postprandial elevations in arterial amino acids are exaggerated.[47] This protein-induced hyperaminoacidemia is solely accounted for by the branched chain amino acids (Fig. 4-9). In contrast to the ongoing net uptake of branched chain amino acids by muscle tissues seen in normal subjects, in diabetic individuals a net uptake is only transiently observed.[47] As a consequence, the total uptake of these amino acids by muscle is decreased, resulting in their accumulation in plasma. Type I diabetes thus may be viewed as a disorder of protein tolerance as well as glucose tolerance. This view is in keeping with the known capacity of insulin to inhibit the net release of branched chain amino acids from muscle tissue.[79] Because the capacity to release insulin in response to systemic hyperaminoacidemia is commonly intact in patients with type II diabetes,[5] it is unlikely that comparable defects in protein disposal would occur in such patients. This, however, has not been fully investigated.

Protein feeding also produces abnormalities in glucose regulation in the insulin-deficient diabetic subjects. In normal subjects, protein ingestion induces a modest rise in insulin secretion, which offsets the stimulatory effects of glucagon (and the amino acid load itself) on hepatic glucose production.[47] As a result,

Table 4-3. Homeostatic Response to Glucose Ingestion in Diabetes

	Impaired Glucose Tolerance	Type II Diabetes	Type I Diabetes
Suppression of glucose production	NL	NL ↓	↓ ↓
Stimulation of splanchnic glucose uptake	NL	NL	↓ ↓
Stimulation of peripheral glucose uptake	↓	↓ ↓	↓ ↓

Abbreviations: NL, normal; NL ↓, normal or below normal.

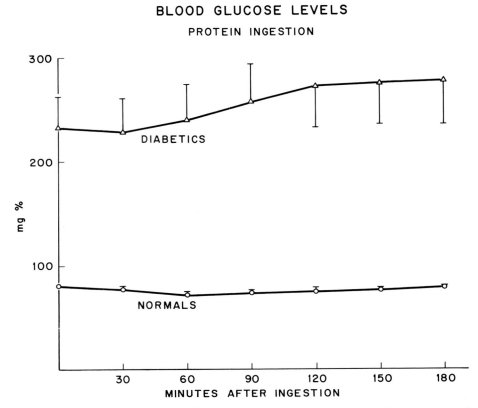

BLOOD GLUCOSE LEVELS
PROTEIN INGESTION

Fig. 4-11. Hyperglycemic effect of protein feeding in patients with type I diabetes. (Based on unpublished data.)

blood glucose levels remain at basal values. By contrast, in diabetic subjects protein ingestion produces a large (albeit transient) increase in hepatic glucose production due to the rise in glucagon in a setting in which insulin is deficient.[47] Consequently, there is a substantial increase in blood glucose (Fig. 4-11). This exaggerated glucose response in this setting also partly reflects the failure to metabolize the glucose released by the liver due to the failure of insulin secretion.

Fat Ingestion

Consumption of fat-containing foods leads to the formation of chylomicrons, which provide a means of transferring triglycerides from the gut to adipose tissue. The ultimate disposal of exogenous triglycerides (like endogenous triglycerides) is regulated by the activity of insulin-sensitive lipoprotein lipase. Conse-

quently, postprandial elevations of plasma triglycerides may be increased or prolonged in insulin-deficient diabetic patients because of deficient triglyceride removal. This situation is most evident during ingestion of carbohydrate-containing mixed meals, when the discrepancies between insulin levels in nondiabetic and diabetic individuals are most pronounced.

Exercise

The rapid fall in blood glucose levels commonly observed in diabetic patients after vigorous exercise has traditionally been the basis for recommending exercise to diabetic patients. This acute glucose-lowering action is much more pronounced in insulin-treated diabetic subjects and occurs only if insulin therapy is sufficient to prevent marked hyperglycemia (i.e., >300 mg/dl) or ketosis.[80] The importance of insulin availability in mediating the exercise-induced fall in glucose levels is underscored by two observations in insulin-treated patients. First, it is well recognized that the magnitude of the decline in blood glucose is increased if exercise coincides with the time of the peak action of the insulin preparation used. Second, exercise may accelerate insulin absorption from its injection site, and when this occurs, the falling blood glucose is more pronounced.[81]

Recently, studies using regional catheters and radiolabeled glucose have helped elucidate the mechanism of the glucose-lowering effect of acute exercise in diabetes. Normally, physical exercise causes a marked increase in glucose uptake by muscle.[38] Blood glucose levels nevertheless remain stable, because hepatic glucose production increases to match exactly the rate of glucose consumption. This process is mediated by a decline in circulating insulin and by an activation of the sympathetic nervous system as well as counterregulatory hormone release.[40] In the diabetic individual receiving insulin exogenously, the circulating level of the insulin may, at times, be inappropriately high and fail to decline during exercise. Consequently, this "finely tuned" homeostatic mechanism is disturbed. Exogenous hyperinsulinemia has been shown to potentiate the stimulatory effect of exercise on glucose uptake.[82] Even more important, the compensatory increase in glucose release from the liver is blocked under these conditions, resulting in a fall in glucose concentration (Fig. 4-12).

The usefulness of the acute glucose-lowering effect of intermittent exercise in type I diabetes is limited, because the effect is relatively short-lived (generally several hours) after exercise is terminated. Unless exercise is regular and of appropriate intensity and duration, there is little long-term "carry-over" effect that can be expected to aid in diabetic care. Furthermore, the magnitude of the fall is not easily titrated, so hypoglycemia is a frequent complication of vigorous exercise. The rapid rise in counterregulatory hormones that ensues, coupled with the increased responsiveness of the diabetic individual to these hormones[66] and a tendency to overeat when hypoglycemic symptoms occur, often leads to a rebound increase in blood glucose to hyperglycemic levels. Thus, if the diabetic subject is unable to adjust her diet and insulin dose, acute intermittent exercise may cause large fluctuations in blood glucose levels rather than improve glycemic control.

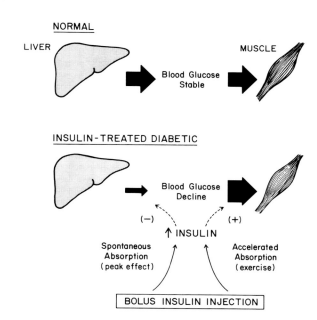

Fig. 4-12. Mechanism of exercise-induced hypoglycemia in insulin-treated diabetic patients. The failure of insulin levels to fall during exercise and the potential for insulin to rise because of accelerated absorption prevents the normal compensatory increase in hepatic glucose production and may potentiate glucose uptake by exercising muscle. The net effect is a reduction in blood glucose levels.

In poorly regulated ketotic diabetic individuals, exercise accentuates hyperglycemia and may increase ketonemia as well, particularly if exercise is prolonged.[83] This may be explained by the low levels of insulin in these patients and because that poor control causes an exaggerated release of counterregulatory hormones in response to exercise.[84] These hormonal changes (coupled with the diabetic's hyperresponsiveness to counterregulatory hormones[66]) potentiate the exercise-induced increase in hepatic glucose production as well as lipolysis and ketone production by the liver (Fig. 4-13). Because the stimulation of glucose uptake in muscle occurs independent of insulin (namely, local factors, as described above), glucose consumption by exercising muscle is relatively unaffected during poor control and thus does not contribute to a rise in blood glucose levels.[85]

The differences in the rate of gluconeogenesis between nondiabetic and type I diabetic subjects are fur-

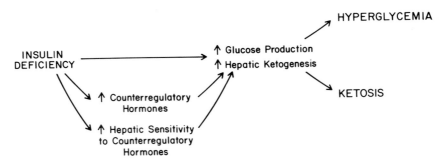

Fig. 4-13. Mechanism of exercise-induced hyperglycemia and ketosis in poorly controlled type I diabetic patients.

ther increased during exercise. During short-term exercise, the compensatory elevation in hepatic glucose production in nondiabetics is mediated by an acceleration of glycogenolysis; gluconeogenesis remains unchanged.[38] By contrast, the diabetic individual demonstrates a rapid increase in gluconeogenesis that is only seen in normal subjects when exercise is extended for prolonged periods (2 to 4 hours).[80] Thus, the effect of exercise in insulin-deficient diabetic patients is to exaggerate the excessive rate of gluconeogenesis that characterizes diabetes.

Glucose Counterregulation

The main risk of insulin therapy in diabetes is hypoglycemia. It is now appreciated that patients with diabetes are more vulnerable to hypoglycemia, not only because they are unable to normally synchronize insulin delivery with meal ingestion and activity but also because the hormonal responses that normally protect against hypoglycemia are defective. In normal subjects, insulin administration produces a rapid decline in plasma glucose concentration. The glucose fall is due to a suppression of hepatic glucose production and a rise in peripheral glucose uptake.[86] The former process is more sensitive to insulin (see above), and this is mainly responsible for hypoglycemia when insulin elevations are relatively small.[87] Glucose recovery requires the reversal of these responses—most important, a stimulation of hepatic glucose production. Once circulating glucose levels fall below 60 to 70 mg/dl, secretion of glucagon and epinephrine is triggered and endogenous insulin secretion is suppressed. These

hormonal changes combine to promote glucose production and return the plasma glucose level toward normal.[88]

In type I diabetes, insulin levels are incapable of responding to physiologic signals and the glucagon response to hypoglycemia is lost.[89] Although some patients retain the ability to release glucagon during hypoglycemia early in the course of their disease,[90] the ultimate failure of glucagon secretion to this particular stimulus is a consistent finding in patients who have had type I diabetes for several years.[89,91] As a result, such patients are largely dependent on epinephrine for acute glucose counterregulation (Table 4-4). Consequently, they may show impaired glucose recovery when β-adrenergic blocking agents are administered[92] or when there is coexisting autonomic neuropathy.[93] Some long-standing diabetic patients show defective catecholamine secretion in response to hypoglycemia without overt clinical evidence of diabetic neuropathy,[94] and more important, intensive insulin therapy aimed at normalizing blood glucose levels may itself diminish epinephrine responses to hypoglycemia.[95] The latter may be especially important during pregnancy, when such treatment regimens have become standard clinical practice.

Table 4-4. Hormonal Defense Mechanisms Against Acute Hypoglycemia

Hormone Secretion	Normal	Type I Diabetes
Insulin	↓	—
Epinephrine	↑	↑
Glucagon	↑	—

Effect of Intensive Insulin Therapy on Body Fuel Metabolism

As described above, poorly controlled diabetes is characterized by a variety of metabolic and hormonal abnormalities that may contribute to the long-term complications of the disease. The introduction of improved methods for quantifying blood glucose control and delivering insulin in a more physiologic manner with multiple injections or portable infusion pumps has recently allowed investigators to examine the extent to which these abnormalities may be reversed by systemic insulin delivery.

Many studies have shown that intensive insulin treatment restores blood glucose levels to near-normal values.[96–98] Because these regimens provide a relatively constant basal level of insulin throughout the night in amounts sufficient to restrain hepatic glucose production, they normalize postabsorptive glucose concentrations. Postprandial glucose elevations are also dramatically reduced but not consistently normalized. In nondiabetic patients, fluctuations in blood glucose are minimized by the concomitant suppression of endogenous glucose production from the liver.[46] This fails to occur in conventionally treated type I diabetic subjects because, in this situation, the liver is less sensitive to small increments in circulating insulin[99] and unable to respond to the inhibitory effects of hyperglycemia per se on glucose production.[67] After intensive insulin therapy, these abnormalities are corrected,[42,99] and therefore the endogenous contribution to circulating glucose levels can be effectively suppressed. In addition, the premeal bolus doses of insulin allow for adequate portal insulin levels to promote glucose uptake by splanchnic tissues. As noted above, this process requires some insulin but is mainly driven by the magnitude of hyperglycemia.[44] The anticipated result is the restoration of the liver's capacity to handle administered glucose. However, the rise in circulating insulin after subcutaneous hormone injection is delayed, and peak levels are lower as compared with normal subjects.[100] Furthermore, peripheral resistance to the action of insulin is only partially reversed by intensive insulin therapy.[101] It is, therefore, unlikely that peripheral glucose uptake in response to glucose ingestion is restored to normal. Because this is the main site of exogenous glucose disposal,[45] it is not unexpected that postprandial glucose levels commonly exceed normal values.

With respect to other insulin-sensitive fuels, the elevated basal concentrations of branched chain amino acids are reduced to normal in conjunction with improved glucose regulation (Fig. 4-9). Tracer studies have demonstrated that the accelerated leucine delivery into plasma observed during conventional treatment is decreased,[71] accounting for the observed changes in circulating amino acids. Furthermore, intensive treatment of type I diabetes reverses the excessive postprandial levels of branched chain amino acids after ingestion of mixed meals (Fig. 4-9) and the decreased clearance of intravenously administered leucine seen in conventionally treated patients.[100,102] Similarly, increased levels of FFAs and triglycerides are reduced toward normal.[100,102]

Elevations in growth hormone and glucagon concentrations observed during 24-hour monitoring in patients with poorly controlled diabetes are diminished after institution of strict glycemic control.[65,103] In addition, excessive increments in catecholamines and growth hormone during mild exercise are reversed[90] (Fig. 4-14). It follows, therefore, that some of the metabolic benefits of intensive insulin regimens may be derived from their counterregulatory hormone-lowering effects. This may be particularly true with regard to growth hormone. When growth hormone was infused as hourly intravenous pulses to a group of diabetic subjects who were intensively treated using a portable insulin pump, serum growth hormone was raised to levels similar to those observed in poorly controlled diabetes. Under these conditions, glycemic control markedly deteriorated while circulatory fatty acids, ketones, and branched amino acids also increased.[65] Thus, growth hormone elevations can themselves reproduce the entire spectrum of poor diabetic control despite previously optimized insulin treatment. This serves to emphasize the multifactorial nature of the metabolic disturbances of diabetes as well as the primary role of insulin deficiency in initiating them.

Role of Insulin-like Growth Factor 1 Deficiency

The classical studies of Froesch and colleagues demonstrated that somatomedin C, the putative mediator of growth hormone's somatotrophic actions, exerted metabolic effects in vitro that closely resembled those of insulin. Hence, its redesignation as insulin-like

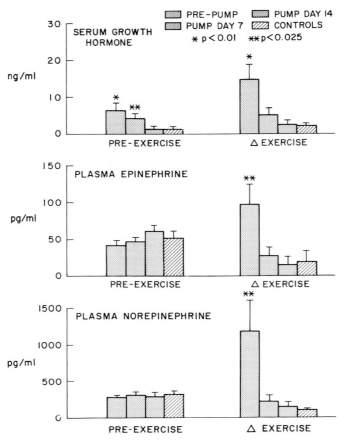

Fig. 4-14. Resting levels and exercise-induced increments of growth hormone, epinephrine, and norepinephrine in diabetic and healthy control subjects. The diabetic patients were studied before (during poor control) and after 7 and 14 days of intensive insulin treatment using a portable pump. (Based on the data of Tamborlane et al.[84])

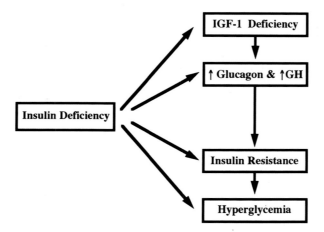

Fig. 4-15. Hypothetical role of insulin-like growth factor-1 (IGF-1) deficiency in the pathology of insulin-dependent diabetes mellitus. GH, growth hormone.

growth factor 1 (IGF-1). Later studies of Zapf and Guler clearly established IGF-1's unique position as the only naturally occurring hypoglycemic hormone besides insulin. The bulk of data indicates that conventionally treated insulin-dependent diabetes mellitus (IDDM) patients have subnormal levels of IGF-1,[104,105] especially during puberty. It has been suggested that raised growth hormone levels in IDDM are, in part, a compensatory attempt to overcome a block in IGF-1 synthesis caused by insulin deficiency and poor metabolic control.[65] Although it is uncertain whether IGF-1 deficiency has direct adverse metabolic effects in IDDM, to the extent that it contributes to growth hormone hypersecretion, it undoubtedly contributes to diabetic hyperglycemia (see above). Furthermore, it is conceivable that IGF-1 deficiency plays a role in the hyperglucagonemia of poorly controlled IDDM. Thus, it is intriguing to speculate that insulin resistance associated with poorly controlled IDDM may, in part, be due to IGF-1 deficiency, which in turn promotes growth hormone and glucagon hypersecretion (Fig. 4-15).

REFERENCES

1. Block MB, Mako ME, Steiner DF, Rubenstein AH: Circulating C-peptide immunoreactivity: studies in normals and diabetic patients. Diabetes 21:1013, 1972
2. Shima K, Tanaka R, Morishita S et al: Studies on the etiology of "brittle" diabetes: relationship between diabetic instability and insulinogenic reserve. Diabetes 26:717, 1977
3. Rashba EJ, Reich EP, Janeway CA, Sherwin RS: Type 1 diabetes mellitus: an imbalance between effector and regulatory T cells? Acta Diabetol 30:61, 1993
4. Robertson RP, Porte D Jr: The glucose receptor: a defector mechanism in diabetes mellitus distinct from the beta adrenergic receptor. J Clin Invest 52:870, 1973
5. Coulston GLA, Chen Y-DI, Reaven GM: Does day-long absolute hypoinsulinemia characterize the patient with non-insulin-dependent diabetes mellitus. Metabolism 32:754, 1983
6. Yalow RS, Berson SA: Immunoassay of endogenous plasma insulin in man. J Clin Invest 39:1157, 1960
7. Lockwood DH, Amatruda TM: Cellular alterations responsible for insulin resistance in obesity and type II diabetes mellitus. Am J Med 75:23, 1983
8. Kipnis DM: Insulin secretion in normal and diabetic individuals. Ann Intern Med 16:103, 1970
9. Zierler L, Rabinowitz D: Effects of very small concentrations of insulin on forearm metabolism: persistence of its action on potassium and free fatty acids without its effect on glucose. J Clin Invest 43:950, 1964
10. Rizza R, Mandarino L, Gerich J: Dose-response characteristics for effects of insulin on production and utilization of glucose in man. Am J Physiol 240:E630, 1981
11. Fukagawa NK, Minaker KL, Rowe JE et al: Insulin-mediated reduction of whole body protein breakdown: dose-response effects on leucine metabolism in postabsorptive man. J Clin Invest 76:2306, 1985
12. DeFronzo RA, Ferrannini E, Koivisto V: New concepts in the pathogenesis and treatment of non-insulin-dependent diabetes mellitus. Am J Med 74:52, 1983
13. Olefsky TM, Ciaraldi TP, Kolterman OG: Mechanism of insulin resistance in non-insulin-dependent (type II) diabetes. Am J Med 79:12, 1985
14. Kolterman OG, Gray RS, Griffin J et al: Receptor and postreceptor defects contribute to the insulin resistance in non-insulin-dependent diabetes mellitus. J Clin Invest 68:957, 1981
15. DeFronzo RA, Hendler R, Simonson D: Insulin resistance is a prominent feature of insulin-dependent diabetes. Diabetes 31:795, 1982
16. Scarlett JA, Gray RS, Griffin J et al: Insulin treatment reverses the insulin resistance of type II diabetes mellitus. Diabetes Care 5:353, 1982
17. Saccà L, Vigorito C, Cacala M et al: Mechanisms of epinephrine-induced glucose intolerance in normal humans: role of the splanchnic bed. J Clin Invest 69:284, 1982
18. Felig P: The glucose-alanine cycle. Metabolism 22:179, 1973
19. Cherrington AD, Liljenquist JE, Shulman GI et al: Importance of hypoglycemia-induced glucose production during isolated glucagon deficiency. Am J Physiol 236:E263, 1979
20. Sherwin RS, Tamborlane W, Hendler R et al: Influence of glucagon replacement on the hyperglycemic and hyperketonemic response to prolonged somatostatin infusion in normal man. J Clin Endocrinol Metab 45:1104, 1977
21. Felig P: Amino acid metabolism in man. Annu Rev Biochem 44:933, 1975
22. Felig P, Pozefsky T, Marliss E, Cahill GF Jr: Alanine: key role in gluconeogenesis. Science 167:1003, 1970
23. Chang TW, Goldberg AL: The origin of alanine produced in skeletal muscle. J Biol Chem 253:3677, 1967
24. Haymond MW, Miles TM: Branched chain amino acids as a major source of alanine nitrogen in man. Diabetes 31:86, 1982
25. Odessey R, Khairallah EA, Goldberg AL: Origin and possible significance of alanine production by skeletal muscle. J Biol Chem 249:7623, 1974

26. Buse MG, Herlong HF, Weigand DA: The effects of diabetes, insulin, and the redox potential on leucine metabolism by isolated rat hemidiaphragm. Endocrinology 98:1166, 1976

27. Chang TW, Goldberg AL: The metabolic fates of amino acids and the formation of glutamine in skeletal muscle. J Biol Chem 253:3685, 1978

28. Felig P, Owen OE, Wahren J, Cahill GH Jr: Amino acid metabolism during prolonged starvation. J Clin Invest 48:584, 1969

29. Elwyn D, Parikh HC, Shoemaker WC: Amino acid movements between gut, liver and periphery in unanesthetized dogs. Am J Physiol 215:1260, 1968

30. Randle P, Garland JPB, Hales CN, Newsholme EA: The glucose-fatty acid cycle: its role in insulin sensitivity and the metabolic disturbances of diabetes mellitus. Lancet 1:785, 1963

31. Hultman E, Nilsson LH: Liver glycogen in man: effect of different diets and muscular exercise. Adv Exp Med Biol 11:143, 1971

32. Pozefsky T, Tancredi RG, Moxley RT et al: Effects of brief starvation on muscle amino acid metabolism in nonobese man. J Clin Invest 57:444, 1976

33. Cahil GF Jr: Starvation in man. N Engl J Med 282:668, 1970

34. Cahill GH Jr, Herrera MG, Morgan AP et al: Hormone-fuel interrelationships during fasting. J Clin Invest 45:1751, 1966

35. Fisher M, Sherwin RS, Hendler R, Felig P: Kinetics of glucagon in man: effects of starvation. Proc Natl Acad Sci USA 73:1734, 1976

36. McGarry JD, Wright P, Foster D: Hormonal control of ketogenesis: rapid activation of hepatic ketogenic capacity in fed rats by anti-insulin serum and glucagon. J Clin Invest 55:1202, 1975

37. Sherwin RS, Shulman GI, Hendler R et al: Effect of growth hormone on oral glucose tolerance and circulating metabolic fuels in man. Diabetologia 24:155, 1983

38. Wahren J, Felig P, Ahlborg G, Jorfeldt L: Glucose metabolism during leg exercise in man. J Clin Invest 50:2715, 1978

39. Ahlborg G, Felig P, Hagenfeldt L et al: Substrate turnover during prolonged exercise in man. J Clin Invest 53:1080, 1974

40. Galbo G, Richter J, Hilsted J et al: Hormonal regulation during prolonged exercise. Ann NY Acad Sci 301:72, 1977

41. Steele R: Influence of glucose loading and/or injected insulin on hepatic glucose output. Ann NY Acad Sci 82:420, 1959

42. Saccà L, Hendler R, Sherwin RS: Hyperglycemia inhibits glucose production in man independent of changes in glucoregulatory hormones. J Clin Endocrinol Metab 47:1160, 1978

43. DeFronzo RA, Ferrannini E, Hendler R et al: Influence of hyperinsulinemia, hyperglycemia, and the route of glucose administration on splanchnic glucose exchange. Proc Natl Acad Sci USA 75:5173, 1977

44. Saccà L, Cicala M, Trimarco B et al: Differential effects of insulin on splanchnic and peripheral glucose disposal after an intravenous glucose load in man. J Clin Invest 70:117, 1982

45. Katz LK, Glickman MG, Rapoport S et al: Splanchnic and peripheral disposal of oral glucose in man. Diabetes 32:675, 1983

46. Felig P, Wahren J: Influence of endogenous insulin secretion on splanchnic glucose and amino acid metabolism in man. J Clin Invest 50:1702, 1971

47. Wahren J, Felig P, Hagenfeldt J: Effect of protein ingestion on splanchnic and leg metabolism in normal man and in patients with diabetes mellitus. J Clin Invest 57:987, 1976

48. Buse MG, Reid SS: Leucine: a possible regulator of protein turnover in muscle. J Clin Invest 56:1250, 1975

49. Sadur CN, Eckel RH: Insulin stimulation of adipose tissue lipoprotein lipase: use of the euglycemic clamp technique. J Clin Invest 69:1119, 1982

50. Yki-Jarvinen H: Sex and insulin sensitivity. Metabolism 33:1011, 1984

51. Hale PJ, Wright JV, Nattrass M: Differences in insulin sensitivity between normal men and women. Metabolism 34:1133, 1985

52. Arslanian SA, Heil BV, Becker DJ, Drash AL: Sexual dimorphism in insulin sensitivity in adolescents with insulin-dependent diabetes mellitus. J Clin Endocrinol Metab 72:920, 1991

53. Haymond MW, Kan IE, Clarke WL et al: Differences in circulating gluconeogenic substrates during short-term fasting in men, women, and children. Metabolism 31:33, 1982

54. Diamond MP, Jones T, Caprio S et al: Gender influences counterregulatory hormone responses to hypoglycemia. Metabolism 42:1568, 1993

55. Frankenhaeuser M, Dunne E, Lundberg U: Sex differences in sympathetic-adrenal medullary reactions induced by different stressors. Psychopharmacology 47:1, 1976

56. Amiel SA, Maran A, MacDonald IA: Sex differences in counterregulatory hormone responses but not glucose kinetics during insulin induced hypoglycemia. Diabetes, suppl. 1, 40:2221, 1991

57. Diamond MP, Simonson DC, DeFronzo RA: Menstrual cyclicity has a profound effect on glucose homeostasis. Fertil Steril 52:204, 1989

58. Valdes CT, Elkind-Hirsch KE: Intravenous glucose tolerance test insulin sensitivity changes derived during the menstrual cycle. J Clin Endocrinol Metab 72:642, 1991

59. Singh BM, Nattrass M: Alterations in insulin action during the menstrual cycle in normal women. Diabetes Nutr Metab 2:39, 1989

60. Diamond MP, Jacob RJ, Connolly-Diamond M, DeFronzo RA: Glucose metabolism during the menstrual cycle: assessment by the euglycemic, hyperinsulinemic clamp technique. J Reprod Med 38:417, 1993

61. Yki-Jarvinen H: Insulin sensitivity during the menstrual cycle. J Clin Endocrinol Metab 59:350, 1984

62. Toth EL, Suthijumroom A, Crockford PM, Ryan EA: Insulin action does not change during the menstrual cycle in normal women. J Clin Endocrinol Metab 64:74, 1987

63. Diamond MP, Grainger DA, Rossi G et al: Counter-regulatory response to hypoglycemia in the follicular and luteal phases of the menstrual cycle. Fertil Steril 60:988, 1993

64. DeFronzo RA, Simonson D, Ferrannini E: Hepatic and peripheral insulin resistance: a common feature in non-insulin-dependent and insulin-dependent diabetes. Diabetologia 23:313, 1982

65. Press M, Tamborlane WV, Sherwin RS: Importance of raised growth hormone levels in mediating the metabolic derangements of diabetes. N Engl J Med 310:810, 1984

66. Shamoon H, Hendler R, Sherwin RS: Altered responsiveness to cortisol, epinephrine, and glucagon in insulin-infused juvenile-onset diabetics: a mechanism for diabetic instability. Diabetes 29:284, 1980

67. Wahren J, Felig P, Cerase E, Luft R: Splanchnic and peripheral glucose and amino acid metabolism in diabetes mellitus. J Clin Invest 51:1870, 1972

68. Shulman GI, Rothman DL, Jue T et al: Direct quantitation of muscle glycogen synthesis in normal men and non insulin-dependent diabetics by ^{13}C nuclear magnetic resonance spectroscopy. N Engl J Med 322:223, 1990

69. Chiasson JL, Liljenquist JE, Finger FE, Lacy WW: Differential sensitivity of glycogenolysis and glucogenogenesis to insulin infusion in dogs. Diabetes 25:283, 1976

70. Nikou D, Philippidis H, Palaiologos G: Serum alanine concentration in diabetic children under insulin treatment. Horm Metab Res 7:207, 1975

71. Gertner J, Press M, Mathews D, Tamborlane WV: Improvements in leucine kinetics with continuous subcutaneous insulin infusion. Diabetes, suppl 1, 33:2A, 1984

72. Greenfield M, Kolterman O, Olefsky J, Reaven GM: Mechanism of hypertriglyceridemia in diabetic patients with fasting hyperglycemia. Diabetologia 18:441, 1980

73. Ferrannini E, Barrett EJ, Bevilacqua S, DeFronzo RA: Effect of fatty acids on glucose production and utilization in man. J Clin Invest 72:1737, 1983

74. Sherwin RS, Hendler R, Felig P: Effect of diabetes mellitus and insulin on the turnover and metabolic response to ketones in man. Diabetes 26:776, 1976

75. Bagdad JD, Porte D Jr, Bierman EL: Acute insulin withdrawal and the regulation of plasma triglyceride removal in diabetic subjects. Diabetes 17:127, 1968

76. Nikkila EA, Huttunen JK, Ehnholm C: Postheparin plasma lipoproteinlipase and hepatic lipase in diabetes mellitus: relationship to plasma triglyceride metabolism. Diabetes 26:11, 1977

77. Tobey TA, Greenfield M, Kraemer F, Reaven GM: Relationship between insulin resistance, insulin secretion, very low density lipoprotein kinetics, and plasma triglyceride levels in normotriglyceridemic man. Metabolism 30:165, 1981

78. DeFronzo RA, Gunnarsson R, Björkman O et al: Effects of insulin on peripheral and splanchnic glucose metabolism in non-insulin-dependent (type II) diabetes mellitus. J Clin Invest 76:149, 1985

79. Pozefsky T, Felig P, Tobin J et al: Amino acid balance across the tissues of the forearm in postabsorptive man: effects of insulin at two dose levels. J Clin Invest 48:2273, 1969

80. Wahren J, Hagenfeldt L, Felig P: Splanchnic and leg exchange of glucose, amino acids, and free fatty acids during exercise in diabetes mellitus. J Clin Invest 55:1303, 1975

81. Koivisto VA, Felig P: Effects of leg exercise on insulin absorption in diabetic parents. N Engl J Med 298:79, 1978

82. DeFronzo R, Felig P, Ferrannini E et al: Synergistic interaction between exercise and insulin on peripheral glucose uptake. J Clin Invest 69:1468, 1981

83. Berger M, Berchtold P, Cüppers HJ et al: Metabolic and hormonal effects of muscular exercise in juvenile type diabetes. Diabetologia 13:355, 1977

84. Tamborlane WV, Sherwin RS, Koivisto V et al: Normalization of the growth hormone and catecholamine response to exercise in juvenile-onset diabetics treated with a portable insulin infusion pump. Diabetes 28:785, 1979

85. Wahren J, Felig P, Hagenfeldt L: Physical exercise and fuel homeostasis in diabetes mellitus. Diabetologia 14:213, 1978

86. Garber AJ, Cryer PE, Santiago JV et al: The role of adrenergic mechanisms in the substrate and hormonal response to insulin-induced hypoglycemia in man. J Clin Invest 58:7, 1976

87. Saccà L, Sherwin R, Hendler R, Felig P: Influence of continuous physiologic hyperinsulinemia on glucose

kinetics and counterregulatory hormones in normal and diabetic humans. J Clin Invest 63:849, 1979

88. Rizza RA, Cryer PE, Gerich JE: Role of glucagon, catecholamines and growth hormone in human glucose counterregulation. J Clin Invest 64:62, 1979

89. Gerich JE, Langlois M, Noacco C et al: Lack of glucagon response to hypoglycemia in diabetes: evidence for an intrinsic pancreatic alpha cell defect. Science 182:171, 1973

90. Colli G, De Feo P, Compagnucci P et al: Abnormal glucose counterregulation in insulindependent diabetes mellitus: interaction of anti-insulin antibodies and impaired glucagon and epinephrine secretion. Diabetes 32:134, 1983

91. Bolli G, De Feo P, Compagnucci P et al: Important role of adrenergic mechanisms in acute glucose counterregulation following insulin-induced hypoglycemia in type I diabetes: evidence for an effect mediated by beta-adrenoreceptors. Diabetes 31:641, 1982

92. Popp DA, Shah SD, Cryer PE: Role of epinephrine-mediated β-adrenergic mechanisms in hypoglycemic glucose counterregulation and post-hypoglycemic hyperglycemia in insulin-dependent diabetes mellitus. J Clin Invest 69:315, 1982

93. Hoeldtke RD, Boden G, Shuman CR, Owen OE: Reduced epinephrine secretion and hypoglycemia unawareness in diabetic autonomic neuropathy. Ann Intern Med 96:459, 1982

94. Kleinbaum J, Shamoon H: Impaired counterregulation of hypoglycemia in insulin-dependent diabetes mellitus. Diabetes 32:493, 1983

95. Simonson DC, Tamborlane WV, DeFronzo RA, Sherwin RS: Intensive insulin therapy reduces counterregulatory hormone responses to hypoglycemia in patients with type I diabetes. Ann Intern Med 103:184, 1985

96. Pickup JC, Keen H, Parsons JA et al: Continuous subcutaneous insulin infusion: improved blood glucose and intermediatry metabolite control in diabetics. Lancet 1: 1255, 1979

97. Tamborlane WV, Sherwin RS, Genel M, Felig P: Reduction to normal of plasma glucose in juvenile diabetes by subcutaneous administration of insulin with a portable infusion pump. N Engl J Med 300:573, 1979

98. Champion MC, Shephard GAA, Rodger NW, Dupre J: Continuous subcutaneous infusion of insulin in the management of diabetes mellitus. Diabetes 29:206, 1980

99. Amiel SA, Tamborlane WV, Simonson DC, Sherwin RS: Defective glucose counterregulation after strict glycemic control of insulin-dependent diabetes mellitus. N Engl J Med 316:1376, 1987

100. Verdonk C, Tamborlane W, Hendler R et al: Does insulin treatment of diabetes cause hyperinsulinemia and hypoaminoacidemia? Clin Res 29:425A, 1981

101. Simonson DC, Tamborlane WV, Sherwin RS et al: Improved insulin sensitivity in patients with type I diabetes mellitus after CSII. Diabetes, suppl. 3, 34:80, 1985

102. Tamborlane WV, Sherwin RS, Genel M, Felig P: Restoration of normal lipid and amino-acid metabolism in diabetic patients treated with a portable insulin-infusion pump. Lancet 1:1258, 1979

103. Raskin P, Pietri A, Unger R: Changes in glucagon levels after four to five weeks of glucoregulation by portable insulin infusion pumps. Diabetes 29:1033, 1979

104. Amiel SA, Sherwin RS, Hintz RL et al: Effect of diabetes and its control on insulin-like growth factors in the young subjects with type I diabetes. Diabetics 33:1175, 1987

105. Tan K, Baxter RE: Serum insulin-like growth factor I levels in adult diabetic patients: the effect of age. J Clin Endocrinol Metab 63:651, 1986

5

Metabolic Changes During Normal and Diabetic Pregnancies

THOMAS A. BUCHANAN

Millennia of evolution have provided mammals, including humans, with a carefully orchestrated set of metabolic changes during pregnancy that serve to enhance maternal metabolic efficiency and the delivery of nutrients to the fetus during feeding, while at the same time accentuating the mother's ability to use her own stored fat as an energy source during fasting. The changes appear to be initiated in large part by the fetoplacental unit through the metabolic effects of several placental hormones. However, the overall impact of those hormones on maternal metabolism is modified by the pancreatic B cells and their secretion of insulin. In women with limited B-cell secretory capacity (e.g., women with diabetes mellitus), maternal metabolic responses to pregnancy are abnormal in ways that can be detrimental to both the mother and her developing infant. This chapter reviews normal maternal metabolism during pregnancy and the metabolic abnormalities that occur in women with diabetes mellitus. The impact of those metabolic abnormalities on fetal development are discussed in Chapters 6 to 9.

NORMAL PREGNANCY
Metabolic Changes During Feeding
Glucose Metabolism: Insulin Resistance and Hyperinsulinemia

From the standpoint of relevance to diabetes mellitus, the metabolic changes of pregnancy that occur during the first 5 to 6 hours after a meal (i.e., in the "fed state")

are dominated by a single characteristic: resistance to the glucose-lowering effects of insulin. The resistance was first demonstrated more than 30 years ago by Burt,[1] who reported a blunted hypoglycemic effect when exogenous insulin was given to pregnant as compared with nonpregnant women. Insulin resistance has subsequently been quantified by measuring the amount of glucose required to maintain normal blood glucose levels during 2- to 3-hour insulin infusions ("euglycemic clamps"[2])[3,4] and by using computer analysis to measure the effect of insulin on glucose disappearance after an intravenous glucose injection ("minimal model" analysis[5]).[6] In both settings, insulin action during the third trimester of pregnancy has been reported to be reduced by 50 to 70 percent below nonpregnant levels, indicating that late normal pregnancy is characterized by marked insulin resistance compared with many other conditions[5] (Fig. 5-1).

The physiologic changes responsible for the insulin resistance of pregnancy are not known with certainty, but the changes appear to be related to the metabolic effects of several hormones that are elevated in the maternal circulation during pregnancy. Those hormones include human placental lactogen (HPL), progesterone, prolactin, and cortisol. Evidence to support an impact of those hormones on insulin action in pregnancy comes from three sources. First, the pattern of insulin resistance during pregnancy tends to parallel the growth of the fetoplacental unit and the levels of hormones secreted by the placenta.[4,7,8] Second, administration of hormones such as HPL,[8,9] progester-

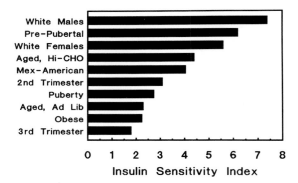

Fig. 5-1. Range of insulin sensitivity in people with normal glucose tolerance. Whole-body insulin sensitivity index (min^{-1} per μU/ml) was measured with the Bergman minimal model technique[5] in 10 groups of people with normal glucose tolerance. Note the wide range of insulin sensitivity despite the relatively narrow range of circulating glucose concentrations among the groups. Hi-CHO, data collected after ingestion of a high-carbohydrate diet; Ad Lib, data collected on an unrestricted diet. (Adapted from Bergman,[5] with permission.)

Table 5-1. Effect of Hormones Elevated During Pregnancy on Insulin Binding and Glucose Uptake in Rat Adipocytes Studied In Vitro[a]

Source of Adipocytes	In Vitro Exposure	Insulin Binding	Glucose Transport
No hormonal exposure in vitro			
Control	None	Normal	Normal
Pregnant	None	Normal	Decreased
Hormonal exposure in vitro: normal glucose uptake			
Control	HCG	Normal	Normal
Control	Estradiol	Increased	Normal
Hormonal exposure in vitro: impaired glucose uptake			
Control	HPL	Normal	Decreased
Control	Progesterone	Decreased	Decreased
Control	Prolactin	Normal	Decreased
Control	Cortisol	Decreased	Decreased
Control	All hormones	Normal	Decreased

[a] Abbreviations: HCG, human chorionic gonadotropin; HPL, human placental ketogen; All hormones, studies performed after exposure to all six hormones in combination.

[a] Adipocytes were isolated from parametrial fat of virgin control rats or term pregnant rats. Insulin binding studies and glucose transport studies were performed in vitro in the absence of added hormones (adipocytes from control and pregnant rats) or in the presence of the hormones listed in physiologic concentrations, singly or in combination (adipocytes from control rats only). Effects of pregnancy and hormones on insulin binding and glucose transport are expressed relative to control adipocytes that were not exposed to pregnancy hormones in vitro.

(Data from Ryan and Enns.[12])

one,[10,11] or glucocorticoids[9] to nonpregnant individuals induces metabolic changes (e.g., hyperinsulinemia without hypoglycemia) that are consistent with a blunting of insulin action. Third, in vitro exposure of insulin target cells such as adipocytes to hormones that are elevated during pregnancy has been reported to impair insulin-mediated glucose uptake by those cells[12] (Table 5-1). Thus, it seems likely that the progressive insulin resistance of pregnancy results in large part from the metabolic actions of hormones secreted by the fetoplacental unit. As a result, one of the main forces exerted by the conceptus on maternal metabolism results in a blunting of insulin's action on glucose uptake in insulin target tissues (i.e., skeletal muscle and adipose tissue). Maternal factors such as increased food intake, adiposity, and inactivity may contribute to the insulin resistance of pregnancy as well.

The cellular determinants of insulin resistance during pregnancy are not known. The major steps involved in insulin-mediated glucose uptake are summarized in Figure 5-2. In theory, one or more of those steps could be impaired in pregnant individuals. In fact, insulin binding to surface receptors of circulating blood cells has generally been reported to be normal in pregnant women,[13–16] whereas several groups[17–19] have reported a decrease in the binding of insulin to adipocytes from pregnant as compared with nonpregnant women. Binding of insulin to skeletal muscle, the target tissue that is quantitatively most important for total-body insulin-mediated glucose uptake, has been reported to be similar in nonpregnant and pregnant women,[20] suggesting that much of the whole-body insulin resistance of pregnancy occurs at postbinding steps of insulin action. The earliest postbinding step, autophosphorylation of the cytoplasmic portion of the insulin receptor, has been reported to be normal in skeletal muscle tissue from pregnant women.[20] Likewise, the total content of insulin-sensitive glucose transport molecules (GLUT 4; molecules that are stimulated by insulin to move from vesicles in the cytoplasm to the cell surface where they mediate glucose transport into insulin target cells [Fig. 5-2]) has been reported to be normal in skeletal muscle from pregnant women.[21] Thus, it seems likely that the reduction in insulin-mediated glucose transport that occurs in skel-

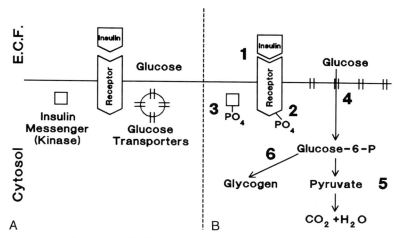

Fig. 5-2. Major steps in insulin-mediated glucose disposition in insulin target cells. **(A)** In the unstimulated condition, insulin receptors and cytoplasmic messengers are not phosphorylated and GLUT 4 transporters (glucose transport molecules) reside in cytoplasmic vesicles. **(B)** Stimulation by binding of insulin to transmembrane receptor (step 1, receptor binding) causes the intracellular portion of the receptor to be phosphorylated (step 2, autophosphorylation). Phosphorylated receptors catalyze the phosphorylation of other intracellular proteins (step 3, kinase activation), which themselves may act as kinases. Activation of the receptor is associated with movement of GLUT 4 transporters to the cell surface, where they transport glucose into the cell (step 4, glucose transport). The steps linking receptor activation and transporter translocation have not been delineated. Once inside the cell, glucose is rapidly phosphorylated, then either metabolized for energy (step 5, glycolysis stimulation) or stored as glycogen (step 6, glycogen synthase activation).

etal muscle during pregnancy results from inefficient coupling between activation of insulin cell surface receptors and the translocation of GLUT 4 molecules to the cell surface (steps 3 and 4 in Fig. 5-2). Our current understanding of that coupling is far from complete, so that it is not possible to determine the precise cellular mechanisms underlying the insulin resistance of pregnancy. However, data from animal[22] and human[23] studies indicate that elevations of circulating free fatty acid (FFA) levels may reduce insulin-mediated glucose uptake and enhance hepatic glucose production. Thus, the elevated FFA levels that occur during normal pregnancy[24] may be involved in the pathogenesis of insulin resistance, as originally proposed by Randle.[25]

In normal individuals, pancreatic B cells respond to insulin resistance by increasing their insulin output under basal conditions and after stimulation by secretagogues such as glucose. This plasticity of B-cell function allows for the maintenance of normal circulating glucose levels in the face of the wide variations in insu-

lin action depicted in Figure 5-1. As originally described by Bergman et al,[26] the magnitude of enhanced B-cell responsiveness to glucose is a hyperbolic function of insulin action in nonpregnant individuals.[26,27] In other words, a halving of insulin action is associated with a doubling of insulin secretion in people with normal glucose tolerance. Buchanan et al[6,28] reported a similar relationship between B-cell function and insulin action in pregnant and nonpregnant women (Fig. 5-3). The latter finding is consistent with the concept that the hyperinsulinemia of pregnancy is largely the result of pancreatic B-cell compensation for physiologic insulin resistance, although there is in vitro evidence that placental hormones such as progesterone may exert a small direct effect to enhance B-cell insulin release as well.[29] Because of the normal capacity for B cells to increase their insulin secretion in response to insulin resistance, glucose tolerance normally deteriorates only slightly by late pregnancy[30] despite the marked insulin resistance present at that stage of gestation.

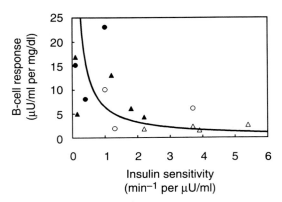

Fig. 5-3. Relationship between insulin action and pancreatic B-cell function in pregnant and nonpregnant women with normal glucose tolerance. Measurements were made with the minimal model technique.[5] Symbols denote individual women; line is a hyperbolic fit of the data, as originally proposed by Bergman et al.[26] Open triangles, lean nonpregnant; open circles, obese nonpregnant; closed triangles, lean pregnant; closed circles, obese pregnant. (Data from Buchanan et al.[28])

Adaptive Significance of Insulin Resistance

As a result of the fed-state changes in glucose metabolism described above, normal pregnancy can be viewed as a progressive condition of insulin resistance, hyperinsulinemia, and mild postprandial hyperglycemia. The adaptive advantages of such a condition may be twofold. First, as suggested by Freinkel et al,[31] the mild postprandial hyperglycemia serves to increase the amount of time that maternal glucose levels are elevated above basal after a meal, thereby increasing the flux of ingested nutrients from mother to fetus and enhancing *fetal* anabolism. Second, to the extent that insulin resistance in skeletal muscle is more pronounced than resistance in adipose tissue,[32] the former resistance may favor the shunting of ingested nutrients toward adipose tissue, thereby promoting *maternal* anabolism and energy storage during feeding as well.

Lipids and Amino Acids

As documented by Phelps et al,[24] pregnancy is associated not only with alterations in glucose metabolism but also with altered concentrations of lipids and amino acids in the circulation. In the fed state, FFA release from adipose tissue is suppressed by the antilipolytic actions of insulin so that FFA levels are only slightly higher in pregnant as compared with nonpregnant individuals during the first 2 to 3 hours after feeding (Fig. 5-4). However, as discussed below, the stimulation of lipolysis that occurs during pregnancy leads to an increase in circulating FFA levels when insulin levels fall after completion of food absorption from the gut. Thus, fasting and postabsorptive FFA levels tend to be increased in pregnant as compared with nonpregnant women[24] (Fig. 5-4). Triglyceride concentrations in pregnant women are increased 1.5- to 2-fold above nonpregnant levels by the third trimester.[24] The hypertriglyceridemia of late pregnancy appears to result from a combination of three factors[33]: (1) increased circulating FFAs and hyperinsulinemia, which combine to promote triglyceride production by the liver[34]; (2) increased food intake, resulting in increased appearance of chylomicrons from the gut; and (3) reduced activity of lipoprotein lipase in adipose tissue, resulting in reduced clearance of triglycerides from the circulation. The first factor can account for much of the increase in fasting triglycerides that occurs by late pregnancy, whereas all three factors are likely to contribute to hypertriglyceridemia in the fed state. As a result of these three factors, triglyceride concentrations are higher around the clock in third-trimester pregnant women as compared with nonpregnant women[24] (Fig. 5-4).

Unlike glucose and lipids, circulating concentrations of most amino acids are reduced in pregnant as compared with nonpregnant individuals.[24] The pattern of circulating amino acids in the third trimester (Fig. 5-4) reveals a lowering of postprandial as well as fasting concentrations. The mechanisms underlying the hypoaminoacidemia of pregnancy are not well worked out.[35] The lowering of fasting amino acid concentrations is discussed below in relation to the fasting hypoglycemia of pregnancy. Mechanisms that might contribute to the postprandial hypoaminoacidemia of pregnancy include accelerated maternal uptake of amino acids in response to postprandial hyperinsulinemia, alterations in the distribution volume for amino acids as a result of fluid accumulation during pregnancy, and increased amino acid use by the fetus during late pregnancy. However, existing data indicating that amino acid turnover is not increased in the third trimester as compared with early pregnancy[36] do not

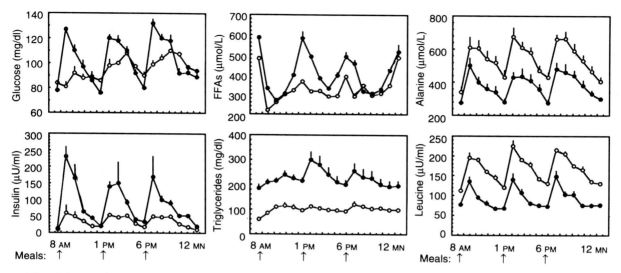

Fig. 5-4. Profiles of plasma glucose, insulin, free fatty acids (FFAs), triglycerides, and two representative amino acids in eight nonpregnant women (open circles) and eight pregnant women with normal glucose tolerance studied during the third trimester (closed circles). Women were given liquid formula meals at arrows, and blood was collected hourly from indwelling venous catheters. (Adapted from Phelps et al,[24] with permission.)

favor a role for fetal "siphoning" of amino acids as a cause for hypoaminoacidemia in human pregnancies.

Metabolic Changes During Fasting

The metabolic changes that occur during fasting in pregnant women are similar in character to the changes that occur during fasting in nonpregnant individuals (see Ch. 4). However, the changes occur more rapidly and to a greater degree during pregnancy. Thus, Freinkel[37] has referred to the metabolic profile of fasted pregnant women as "accelerated starvation." The two major components of accelerated starvation are (1) a reduction in circulating glucose concentrations and (2) accelerated lipolysis and ketogenesis.

Lowered Fasting Glucose

The main alteration in glucose metabolism that occurs during pregnancy under postabsorptive and fasted conditions (i.e., >5 hours after eating) is an exaggerated lowering of circulating glucose concentrations. This lowering was first demonstrated by Felig and Lynch[38] in their studies of prolonged fasting during

the second trimester, when the fetal mass is relatively small compared with the mass of the mother. Subsequent studies by those investigators[39] indicate that reduced availability of alanine, an important substrate for gluconeogenesis, is involved in the lowered plasma glucose levels during prolonged fasting in the second trimester.

Studies of normal women during the third trimester indicate that the propensity of fasting hypoglycemia is more pronounced than at earlier stages of gestation. Metzger et al[40] reported that plasma glucose concentrations after an overnight fast were approximately 10 mg/dl lower in pregnant than in nonpregnant women and that glucose fell by an additional 8 to 10 mg/dl in the pregnant but not the nonpregnant women when both groups postponed breakfast for 6 hours. We have observed a similar decline in plasma glucose in women with gestational diabetes mellitus (GDM) during the third trimester,[41] and we recently demonstrated that the decline is due to an abrupt fall in endogenous glucose production after about 15 hours of fasting.[42] Kalhan et al[43] studied alanine turnover in normal women after an overnight fast in the third trimester. Those investigators reported that whole-body rates of alanine production and use were similar to rates in nonpregnant women but that the pregnant group exhibited a reduction in the efficiency of alanine incorporation into glucose, possibly related to the higher fasting insulin levels in the pregnant women.

Taken together, the available data suggest a complex physiology underlying the fasting hypoglycemia of pregnancy. During mid-pregnancy, the hypoglycemia occurs after prolonged fasting and appears to be related to a reduced supply of gluconeogenic substrates, especially alanine. The mechanisms underlying the substrate deficiency are not fully known but may involve an effect of placental hormones to limit amino acid release from skeletal muscle.[44,45] Later in pregnancy, relative hypoglycemia is present after an overnight fast and progresses rapidly during a brief (i.e., 4- to 6-hour) extension of such a fast. At that stage, increased glucose use by the fetus in combination with relative hyperinsulinemia, which curbs gluconeogenesis, may combine to lower plasma glucose levels rapidly when exogenous calories are not ingested.

Accelerated Lipolysis and Ketogenesis

In their studies of fasting in mid-pregnancy, Felig and Lynch[38] demonstrated that women who fasted for up to 84 hours during the second trimester exhibited an exaggerated increase in circulating ketone concentrations compared with nonpregnant women who fasted for a similar period. Subsequently, Metzer et al[40] reported that a much shorter (i.e., 18-hour) fast during the third trimester was associated with a brisk rise in circulating ketone and FFA concentrations in pregnant but not in nonpregnant women. The mechanisms underlying the accelerated fat catabolism of pregnancy have not been well studied in humans. However, in vitro data[46] indicate that placental hormones such as HPL provide a direct stimulation of lipolysis and FFA release from adipose tissue. This lipolytic effect can be expected to increase in parallel with HPL levels during gestation, providing an increasing drive toward lipolysis as pregnancy progresses. The drive normally is counterbalanced by the antilipolytic effects of insulin, and the progressive enhancement of insulin secretion during pregnancy can be expected to compensate for the progressive stimulation of lipolysis, at least during feeding. As insulin levels fall during fasting, the lipolytic effect of HPL and related hormones is unmasked,

allowing circulating FFA levels to rise. Those FFAs serve as a primary energy source for skeletal and cardiac muscle, and they provide the substrate for ketone production in the liver when insulin levels are low. The ketones can be used directly by the central nervous system as an energy source, reducing the amount of glucose that must be produced via muscle breakdown and gluconeogenesis.

Adaptive Significance

The simultaneous changes in glucose and fat metabolism associated with fasting in pregnancy may serve to minimize the impact of the increased energy demands of gestation on maternal protein stores. Although maternal protein catabolism clearly occurs during fasting,[47] the magnitude of the protein loss will be curbed to the extent that amino acid release from muscle is restrained by the hormonal effects of pregnancy.[44,45] The restraint can be expected to minimize the catabolism of muscle to form glucose, especially during prolonged fasting. At the same time, accelerated fat catabolism provides an alternate energy source to glucose in the form of ketones and FFAs derived from adipose tissue. Because the mass of adipose tissue increases significantly during the first half of gestation,[48] the accelerated lipolysis of late pregnancy allows the mother to take advantage of an expanded, noncarbohydrate energy source at a time when her ability to convert her protein stores to glucose is limited. Together, the coordinated changes of "accelerated starvation" afford the mother some protection against uncontrolled protein catabolism while allowing her to provide energy for herself and her fetus. Like the insulin resistance of pregnancy, the important adaptive effects of accelerated fat catabolism appear to be mediated in large part by the conceptus, through the elaboration of placental hormones.

Impact on Maternal Nutrient Concentrations

The integrated effect of the maternal metabolic adaptations described above is reflected in the patterns of circulating glucose, insulin, triglycerides, FFAs, and amino acids during pregnancy. Those concentrations, modified to the maximum degree by the metabolic changes of the third trimester, are depicted in Figure

5-4. It can be seen that the patterns of glucose, insulin, and FFAs represent an exaggeration of the normal swings between fed-state anabolism and fasting catabolism that occur in nonpregnant individuals. During feeding, glucose and insulin levels rise rapidly as a result of the marked insulin resistance and compensatory hyperinsulinemia of late pregnancy. The hyperinsulinemia is sufficient to minimize but not to eliminate postprandial hyperglycemia. The hyperinsulinemia also counterbalances the lipolytic effects of placental hormones, thereby suppressing circulating FFA and ketone concentrations during feeding. Between meals, glucose levels fall more rapidly and to lower levels in pregnant as compared with nonpregnant women. The fall in glucose is associated with a fall in circulating insulin concentrations, leaving the lipolytic effects of placental hormones unopposed. As a result, there is a brisk rise in circulating FFA concentrations between meals; ketone concentrations rise as well, especially when the period of fasting is extended to more than 14 hours. Unlike the exaggerated cyclicity of glucose, insulin, and FFAs, circulating triglycerides and amino acids exhibit more constant changes during late pregnancy. Triglycerides concentrations are higher and concentrations of nearly all amino acids are lower in pregnant as compared with nonpregnant women.

The metabolic changes of pregnancy appear to be mediated in large part by the effects of placental hormones and, thus, represent the adaptive impact of the conceptus on maternal metabolism. That impact increases in magnitude during pregnancy and abates rapidly on delivery of the fetus and placenta. Maternal insulin plays a critical role in modulating the maternal response to the metabolic impact of the fetus and placenta. Lack of an adequate maternal insulin response during feeding will lead to an exaggeration of postprandial glucose and amino acid excursions. More-severe insulin deficiency will leave the lipolytic and ketogenic effects of placental hormones unopposed. Thus, as discussed below, the relative or absolute insulin deficiency that occurs in patients with diabetes mellitus can be expected to cause important alterations in concentrations of many nutrients in the maternal circulation. The impact of maternal diabetes on fetal development is thought to result in large measure from the impact of those maternal nutrients on the intrauterine environment and on fetal development, as discussed in Chapters 6 to 8, 23, and 24.

DIABETES MELLITUS IN NONPREGNANT INDIVIDUALS
Pathogenesis and Classification

Stated most simply, the pathogenesis of diabetes mellitus involves an imbalance between the amount of insulin that can be produced by the pancreas and the amount that is required to suppress hepatic glucose production and stimulate peripheral glucose use. Current diagnostic criteria for diabetes in nonpregnant individuals[49,50] require either marked fasting hyperglycemia (venous serum or plasma glucose $\geq$140 mg/dl) or marked glucose intolerance (venous glucose $\geq$200 mg/dl 2 hours after a 75-g glucose challenge). Thus, people with overt diabetes generally have a rather marked imbalance between insulin secretion and insulin action. However, the types and relative contributions of defects in insulin secretion and insulin action that lead to diabetes in individual patients may vary considerably, so that diabetes mellitus must be considered a physiologically and genetically heterogeneous group of disorders that have in common a single clinical manifestation: hyperglycemia.

At least two general types of diabetes have been identified[49]: type I diabetes (also known as insulin-dependent diabetes mellitus [IDDM]) and type II diabetes (non-insulin-dependent diabetes mellitus [NIDDM]). IDDM results from immune destruction of the pancreatic B cells,[51] which leads to a complete or nearly complete absence of endogenous insulin secretion and a strong propensity to develop diabetic ketoacidosis. IDDM generally occurs in young, lean individuals, and most patients have evidence of an active autoimmune process (i.e., circulating autoantibodies to pancreatic islet cell antigens[52] or to insulin itself[53]) at the time their hyperglycemia becomes symptomatic. The autoimmune process has been shown to antedate the development of hyperglycemia by several years,[51] and pancreatic B-cell reserve may be limited during that "prediabetic" period of chronic autoimmunity. Thus, patients who are in the predictable phase of IDDM may develop mild-to-moderate hyperglycemia when they encounter the normal insulin resistance of pregnancy; those patients account for some cases of gestational diabetes (see below).

The term *type II diabetes* (NIDDM) was initially developed to describe patients who do not have a marked propensity to develop ketoacidosis in the absence of insulin treatment.[49] As our understanding of the pathogenesis of diabetes has improved, NIDDM has come to denote patients who develop hyperglycemia in the absence of pancreatic B-cell autoimmunity. Patients with NIDDM often are obese and older than 40 years of age at diagnosis, although the disease can occur at almost any age and in lean patients. Hyperglycemia in patients with NIDDM results from an imbalance between the amount of insulin required to maintain normal blood glucose levels and the amount of insulin that can be produced by the pancreas.[54] One or the other defect may dominate the pathogenesis of hyperglycemia in some patients. For example, an autosomal dominant form of NIDDM with a young age of onset (referred to by Fajans[55] as "maturity-onset diabetes of the young" [MODY]) has been linked to an abnormal gene for the B-cell enzyme glucokinase in some families.[56] The genetic abnormality leads to a prominent defect in insulin secretion and, thus, to hyperglycemia in the face of normal insulin action. In other patients with NIDDM, discrete mutations of genes coding for cell surface insulin receptor molecules have been reported.[57] Those patients manifest severe insulin resistance, which dominates the pathogenesis of their hyperglycemia. Although severe isolated abnormalities of insulin secretion or insulin resistance account for a few cases of NIDDM, most patients appear to have less-severe combined defects in insulin secretion and action underlying their hyperglycemia.[54] A large body of evidence indicates that a component of the insulin resistance may be inherited[58,59] and present long before the development of hyperglycemia.[60-63] The insulin resistance may be worsened by environmental factors such as overeating, inactivity, and high-fat diets. The B-cell defect may not be apparent before the onset of hyperglycemia. In fact, many people who eventually develop NIDDM manifest a combination of insulin resistance, *hyper*insulinemia, and mild glucose intolerance before the onset of overt hyperglycemia.[60-63] That combination suggests that the B-cell defect is a relatively late development in the pathogenesis of NIDDM, following years of B-cell compensation for insulin resistance (Fig. 5-5). However, Lillioja et al[64] recently reported that a combination of insulin resistance and inappropriately low insulin secretion is a better predictor of NIDDM in nondiabetic individuals than is either abnormality alone in a population with a very high prevalence of NIDDM. That observation supports the concept that two abnormalities are present early on in many patients who develop NIDDM: insulin resis-

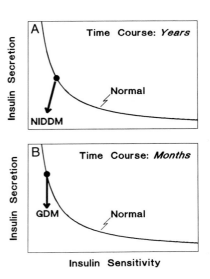

Fig. 5-5. Schematic representations of pathogenesis of **(A)** non-insulin-dependent diabetes mellitus (NIDDM) and **(B)** gestational diabetes mellitus (GDM). In each figure, the curve represents the normal hyperbolic relationship between insulin sensitivity and pancreatic B-cell responsiveness. Hyperglycemia results when pancreatic B cells cannot compensate for chronic (NIDDM) or acute (GDM) insulin resistance, so that B-cell function falls off the line (arrows).

tance and limited B-cell reserve to compensate for the insulin resistance.

At least two findings suggest that the B-cell defect in patients with NIDDM is functional rather than anatomic. First, patients generally have normal or slightly reduced numbers of B cells in their pancreatic islets. Second, the B-cell defect may be worsened by hyperglycemia and ameliorated by treatments that lower blood glucose levels.[65] The latter observation suggests that intermittent hyperglycemia may be involved in the progressive decline of B-cell function as patients develop overt hyperglycemia, a process referred to as *glucose toxicity.*[66] The amount of insulin secreted from the abnormal B cells is not sufficient to maintain normal circulating glucose concentrations but is sufficient to suppress ketosis under most circumstances. Thus, the patients are "non-insulin-dependent" regarding the risk of ketoacidosis, and many patients can be treated with a diet or an oral hypoglycemic agent when they are not pregnant. However, some nonpregnant patients and virtually all pregnant patients with NIDDM require insulin treatment to achieve acceptable glycemic control. *Insulin-treated* is the preferred term for those patients. The genetic and cellular abnormalities that underline the insulin resistance and B-cell abnormalities in most patients with NIDDM are not known and are likely to vary considerably among patients, especially patients from different ethnic groups.

Effect of Diabetes on Circulating Nutrients

Although the hallmark of diabetes mellitus is hyperglycemia, diabetes is associated with abnormalities of lipid and amino acid metabolism as well. When blood glucose levels are high, reflecting relative or absolute insulin deficiency, levels of circulating lipids and many amino acids are often elevated as well. Elevated triglyceride concentrations may result from two abnormalities related to diabetes.[67] Patients with mild NIDDM may have sufficient insulin resistance and hyperglycemia in the face of a moderate B-cell defect to cause portal vein hyperinsulinemia. The increased hepatic exposure to insulin increases hepatic triglyceride production,[34] leading to elevated triglyceride concentrations in the peripheral circulation. Patients with more severe NIDDM or with IDDM may have a prominent degree of insulin deficiency. In those patients, reduced activity of lipoprotein lipase results from the insulin deficiency[67] and leads to reduced clearance of triglycerides from the circulation. Elevated FFA and ketone concentrations may result from severe insulin deficiency, which leads to unrestrained lipolysis in adipose tissue and unrestrained ketogenesis in the liver. Insulin normally promotes protein anabolism by stimulating amino acid uptake into tissues such as muscle and by suppressing proteolysis and amino acid release into the circulation. These functions of insulin may be impaired in poorly controlled diabetes, leading to elevated amino acid concentrations in the circulation. Thus, diabetes must be viewed as a disorder of multiple circulating nutrients in addition to glucose, and the abnormalities of nonglucose nutrients may contribute to the impact of maternal diabetes on the fetus.[68]

DIABETIC PREGNANCY
Classification

The classification of diabetes in pregnancy proposed by White[69] relates fetal risks to the duration of maternal diabetes, the age of onset of that disease, and the presence or absence of maternal vascular complications. Although the White classification has been used widely in the past, our current understanding of the pathogenesis of diabetes, the impact of pregnancy on maternal diabetes, and the effects of diabetes on the fetus allow a somewhat simplified classification of diabetes during pregnancy. From the standpoint of the metabolic impact of pregnancy on maternal diabetes, the most important distinctions to be made are (1) between pregestational diabetes (i.e., diabetes diagnosed before pregnancy) and gestational diabetes (diabetes first detected during pregnancy); and (2) between pregestational IDDM and pregestational NIDDM. The remainder of this chapter is devoted to the maternal metabolic abnormalities that occur during pregnancy in those conditions.

Metabolic Changes in Pregestational Diabetes

The metabolic impact of pregnancy has predictable effects on patients with pre-existing diabetes mellitus. Relative or absolute insulin deficiency leaves the metabolic effects of the fetoplacental unit on maternal carbohydrate, fat, and amino acid metabolism unchecked. As a result, concentrations of glucose, fatty acids, ketones, triglycerides, and many amino acids may be elevated in the maternal circulation. As discussed in Chapter 9, those metabolites can alter embryonic and fetal development, leading to many of the perinatal complications of maternal diabetes. Restoration of a normal relationship between circulating insulin levels and maternal insulin needs can greatly reduce the impact of maternal diabetes on intrauterine development from conception onward. Thus, provision of insulin in a physiologic pattern (Fig. 5-4) and in sufficient amounts to normalize maternal intermediary metabolism is a general goal of therapy for diabetes in pregnant women. Glucose is the most readily measured of the metabolites affected by maternal diabetes, and glucose provides a "benchmark" for assessment of metabolic regulation in diabetic pregnancies. However, other metabolites may have an effect on embryonic[70] and fetal[71-73] development, which may explain why careful glycemic control does not invariably eliminate fetal complications in diabetic pregnancies.

Pregestational IDDM

Patients with IDDM have a virtual absence of endogenous insulin secretion. Therefore, they require exogenous insulin treatment not only to regulate their blood glucose levels but also to suppress fat catabolism and prevent ketoacidosis. Because patients with IDDM generally have normal insulin sensitivity before pregnancy, the insulin resistance of pregnancy leads to a substantial increase in the amount of insulin required to maintain normoglycemia. Rudolf et al[74] and Jovanovic and Peterson[76] reported that insulin requirements in pregnant women with IDDM increase two- to threefold during pregnancy; most of the increase occurred during the last half of gestation.[74] The rapidly changing insulin requirements dictate that pregnant patients be seen or contacted frequently for review of blood glucose levels and adjustment of insulin doses. In my clinic, telephone contact at 3- to 7-day intervals and clinic visits every 1 to 2 weeks are used to facilitate insulin management. Several reports[76-68] indicate that normalization of maternal glucose levels with intensive insulin treatment of patients with IDDM normalizes circulating levels of ketones, FFAs, triglycerides, and several amino acids as well.

The progressive stimulation of fat catabolism in pregnancy places women with IDDM at increased risk for ketoacidosis, which results when lipolysis and ketogenesis progress unchecked by the counterbalancing effects of insulin. Although ketoacidosis may develop over the course of several days in nonpregnant patients with IDDM, ketoacidosis may develop within 12 to 24 hours in pregnant patients who fail to take their insulin or who develop an intercurrent illness. The risk for ketoacidosis may be especially prominent during the latter half of pregnancy, when the stimulation of fat catabolism is most prominent. Thus, care providers must maintain a high index of suspicion for ketoacidosis when patients with IDDM fail to take their insulin or develop an intercurrent illness and have persistent fasting or premeal hyperglycemia of 200 mg/dl or greater. Measurement of urinary ketone concentrations should be performed in those settings as a screening test for ketoacidosis. Moderate or large ketonuria warrants measurement of serum electrolytes. Ketoacidosis is diagnosed on the basis of hyperglycemia, a low bicarbonate level (usually but not invariably with an increase in the unmeasured anion gap[80]), and elevated serum ketone concentrations. Treatment, including intravenous fluids, intravenous insulin, and correction of electrolyte abnormalities, must be instituted rapidly and should be undertaken as described for nonpregnant patients.[80] Careful monitoring of fetal well-being is indicated in patients with ketoacidosis, because the condition has been associated with high fetal mortality rates.[82]

The careful regulation of blood glucose concentrations that is required during pregnancy (see Ch. 11) places diabetic patients at increased risk of hypoglycemia.[82] The risk can be particularly great in patients with IDDM for several reasons (Table 5-2). First, most patients with IDDM lose the ability to secrete glucagon in response to hypoglycemia within 2 to 5 years after the onset of diabetes.[83] Those patients are dependent on epinephrine release to mediate a spontaneous recovery from a hypoglycemic episode.[84] Second, many patients with long-standing IDDM have subnormal epinephrine responses to hypoglycemia.[83] Those patients are left with little or no ability to stimulate hepatic glucose production and recover from a hypoglycemic episode spontaneously.[84] Third, strict glucose control lowers the threshold for epinephrine release in response to hypoglycemia.[85] Thus, patients who achieve very good glycemic control may have few, if any, of the typical sympathetic symptoms (tremor, palpitations, sweating) before the onset of neuroglycopenic symptoms (confusion, lethargy) when hypoglycemia occurs. Finally, some patients have poorly developed self-management skills. Those patients increase their risk of severe hypoglycemia through improper insulin doses, poor timing of meals and exercise, and failure to perform self-glucose monitoring. As a result of their risk of severe hypoglycemia, patients with IDDM need special education when beginning a program of aggressive blood glucose regulation. Three areas that should be stressed in the education are (1) patients and their family members must learn to recognize and treat the earliest symptoms of hypoglycemia; (2) at

Table 5-2. Factors Predisposing to Severe Hypoglycemia in Patients With IDDM

Impaired glucagon response to hypoglycemia
Reduced epinephrine response to hypoglycemia
Lowered threshold for glucose counterregulation
Poor diabetes self-management skills

least one household member should learn how to inject glucagon to treat hypoglycemia causing unresponsiveness; and (3) self-glucose monitoring should be used liberally to detect incipient hypoglycemia before it becomes severe.

Pregestational NIDDM

The metabolic impact of pregnancy on patients with NIDDM relates predominantly to the effect of insulin resistance on blood glucose regulation. Patients with NIDDM often enter pregnancy with some degree of insulin resistance, so that their total daily insulin requirements may be 50 to 100 percent greater than the requirements of women with IDDM.[86] However, both groups exhibit an increase in insulin requirements, especially during the latter half of gestation,[86] so that total daily requirements in women with NIDDM may reach 1.5 to 2.0 U/kg body weight by the third trimester.[86] Blood glucose regulation is critical to normal fetal development in all diabetic pregnancies, so that patients with NIDDM will need frequent contact for assessment of blood glucose levels and adjustment of exogenous insulin doses. Weekly or every-other-week assessments are used in my clinic for patients with NIDDM. Although sulfonylurea agents can ameliorate the B-cell defect and the hyperglycemia in patients with NIDDM, the effects of those agents on fetal development in humans have not been well studied and the agents are not currently recommended for use during pregnancy.

Patients with NIDDM are not at high risk of ketoacidosis. However, the accelerated lipolysis and ketogenesis of pregnancy have an important implication for the dietary treatment of patients with NIDDM during pregnancy. Caloric restriction and weight loss have been shown to improve insulin sensitivity and ameliorate the hyperglycemia of nonpregnant patients with NIDDM.[87,88] However, for reasons reviewed earlier in this chapter, caloric restriction during pregnancy frequently leads to ketonuria and mild ketonemia in the absence of hyperglycemia ("starvation ketosis"). Although starvation ketosis does not pose any significant risk to mothers, at least three studies have linked ketonuria or mild ketonemia during pregnancy to impaired motor and intellectual development of young children.[89–91] Thus, it appears prudent to avoid starvation ketosis by avoiding marked caloric restriction when treating pregnant women with NIDDM. Studies in

women with gestational diabetes (below) indicate that mild caloric restriction (to about 25 kcal/kg actual body weight/d, as compared with a 30- to 32-kcal/kg weight-maintaining diet) may lower glucose levels without inducing ketonuria.[92] Such mild caloric restriction may be used to treat pregnant women with NIDDM, provided that urinary ketone monitoring is used to allow the detection and treatment of ketosis that may develop in occasional patients.

Metabolic Changes in Gestational Diabetes

The diagnosis of GDM is given to all women who are discovered to have glucose intolerance for the first time during pregnancy.[49,75,93] Ideally, the process by which the diagnosis is made involves two steps[49,75,93]: (1) screening of all pregnant women with a relatively simple 1-hour glucose tolerance test that identifies a group of patients (generally 15 to 25 percent of pregnant women[94]) who have some risk of GDM; and (2) performance of a more-complicated 3-hour glucose tolerance test in those women to identify the subset (generally 2 to 5 percent of all pregnant women[95–97]) who meet the current diagnostic criteria for GDM.[49] Thus, the process by which GDM is diagnosed represents one of the few instances in clinical medicine in which relatively young people are evaluated routinely for abnormal glucose tolerance. Women who fail that evaluation are the women in the population who are least able to maintain normal glucose tolerance in the face of the metabolic challenges of pregnancy. Those women impart to their infants an increased risk of perinatal complications related to fetal hyperinsulinemia and excessive growth, as discussed in Chapter 6. Available data indicate that elevations of maternal glucose, amino acids, fatty acids, and triglycerides may be involved in the genesis of excessive fetal growth associated with maternal GDM.[71–73] In addition to the fetal risks, women with GDM incur an increased risk of developing diabetes when they are not pregnant,[98] as discussed in the remainder of this chapter.

The rates at which women with a history of GDM develop diabetes after pregnancy vary widely among published studies.[98] Much of the variation may result from the use of different criteria to diagnose GDM or nonpregnant diabetes in published reports. A review of studies in which National Diabetes Data Group crite-

Table 5-3. Rates of Diabetes after Pregnancies Complicated by Gestational Diabetes[a]

Investigators	Ethnicity of Patients[b]	Length of Follow-up (y)	Diabetes Rate (%)
Metzger et al[108]	W, B, H	5	50
Kjos et al[99]	H	5	54
O'Sullivan[100]	W, B	28	50

[a] Gestational diabetes mellitus and postpregnancy diabetes were diagnosed by National Diabetes Data Group criteria.[49]

[b] Ethnicity refers to the major ethnic groups included in the study populations: W, white; B, black; H, Hispanic.

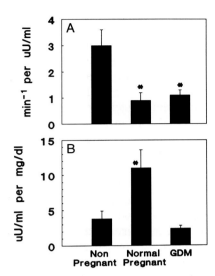

Fig. 5-6. **(A)** Insulin sensitivity and **(B)** first-phase insulin release in nonpregnant, normal pregnant, and gestational diabetic (GDM) women. Measurements were made with Bergman's minimal model technique.[5] All three patient groups consisted of lean and obese whites, blacks, and Hispanics. Pregnant women were studied during the third trimester. Asterisks denote significant differences from the nonpregnant group. (Data from Buchanan et al.[28])

ria[49] have been used to diagnose GDM and postpregnancy diabetes (Table 5-3) suggests that 50 percent or more of women with a history of GDM will develop diabetes during their lifetime. Whether the risk of subsequent diabetes differs among women with GDM from different ethnic groups is not clear, although the data of Kjos et al[99] suggest that Hispanic women with prior GDM are at greater risk of subsequent diabetes (i.e., >50 percent 5 years after pregnancy and increasing by about 10 percent annually) than are white and black women with prior GDM (about 50 percent 28 years after the index pregnancy[100]). A difference among ethnic groups in postpregnancy diabetes rates would not be surprising in view of the well-known ethic differences in prevalence rates of NIDDM[101] and GDM.[96]

Available data on insulin action and pancreatic B-cell function indicate that limited insulin secretory capacity is a common mechanism underlying the hyperglycemia of GDM. Buchanan et al,[6] Catalano et al,[4] and Cousins et al[102] have reported that insulin sensitivity is reduced below nonpregnant levels to a similar degree in normal pregnant women and women with mild-to-moderate GDM (i.e., fasting plasma glucose levels ≤130 mg/dl) when both groups were studied during the third trimester (Fig. 5-6). However, data from Cousins et al,[102] Catalano et al,[4] and Ward et al[103,104] indicate that women who develop GDM are more insulin-resistant than normal women when studied early in pregnancy or after pregnancy, when the normal women are not affected by the severe physiologic insulin resistance of late gestation. Those findings suggest that women who develop GDM may encounter two types of insulin resistance: (1) the reversible insulin resistance that occurs in all pregnancies and that is severe by the third trimester; and (2) the less severe, chronic insulin resistance that is found in many people who are at risk of NIDDM. The former type of insulin resistance cay be expected to place significant demands on the pancreatic B cells of all women during late pregnancy and may contribute to the pathogenesis of GDM in women with limited B-cell reserve. The latter type of insulin resistance may contribute to the pathogenesis of GDM in women who present during early or mid-pregnancy. The cellular and genetic abnormalities that underlie the chronic form of insulin resistance in women with GDM or with a history of that disease are not known, although Garvey et al[105] recently reported an abnormality in the intracellular localization of GLUT 4 transporter molecules in adipocytes from some women with GDM. That abnormality could contribute to an underlying impairment of insulin-mediated glucose disposal in those women and, thus, to their chronic insulin resistance.

Unlike insulin action, B-cell function has been shown to differ markedly between women with GDM and normal pregnant women during late pregnancy.[4,6,106,107] At that stage, normal pregnant women manifest insulin responses to nutrients that are two to three times the responses of nonpregnant women[6] (Fig. 5-6). By contrast, women with GDM have been shown to have much lower insulin responses, despite a similar degree of insulin resistance[4,6] (Fig. 5-6). Thus, existing data suggest that failure of B-cell compensation for the insulin resistance of pregnancy is a common mechanism underlying the hyperglycemia of women with GDM. In that regard, the pathogenesis of GDM may be viewed as a temporally compressed version of the pathogenesis of many cases of NIDDM (Fig. 5-5). Thus, pregnancy appears to provide a "pancreatic stress test" that, in combination with routine glucose screening during pregnancy, allows the detection of young women with limited B-cell reserve who are at increased risk of developing diabetes when they are not pregnant. Indeed, impaired B-cell responsiveness to glucose during pregnancy has been linked to an in-

creased risk of the development of diabetes after pregnancies complicated by GDM.[108–110]

The preceding discussion suggests that GDM is a disorder of homogeneous pathogenesis. However, that is not the case. The diagnosis of GDM encompasses all women whose glucose levels exceed statistically defined thresholds of normality for pregnancy. Because circulating glucose concentrations are distributed in a unimodal rather than a bimodal fashion in most populations (Fig. 5-7), the distinction between normal and abnormal glucose tolerance in pregnancy is made by drawing a line across a continuum of circulating glucose concentrations (Fig. 5-7). As a result, the diagnosis of GDM is likely to identify a significant number of women with a true genetic risk of subsequent diabetes, as well as some women whose glucose tolerance is simply at the upper end of the normal distribution for the population. That concept is supported by two

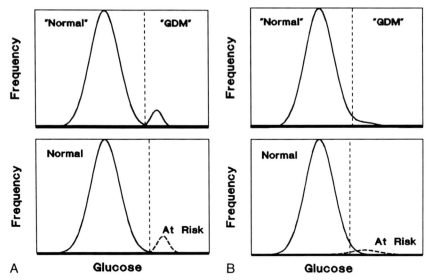

Fig. 5-7. Theoretical representation of the diagnosis of gestational diabetes mellitus (GDM) in populations exhibiting **(A)** bimodal and **(B)** unimodal distributions for plasma glucose. In the top two panels, the solid lines represent the population distribution of glucose and the vertical dashed lines represent "cutoff" points for the diagnosis of GDM. The cutoff point is based on bimodality in Fig. A and on 95 percent confidence intervals in Fig. B. In the bottom two panels, the dashed portions of the population distribution for glucose represent subsets of people at true genetic risk of subsequent diabetes. The distinction between normal and at-risk groups is made precisely by plasma glucose measurements in the population with a bimodal distribution. However, in the population with a unimodal distribution, the distinction is less clear, so that some normal individuals are given the diagnosis of GDM. The phenomenon depicted in this figure may explain why a subset of women with GDM do not go on to develop diabetes when they are not pregnant.

findings. First, we have reported that approximately 25 percent of a group of white, black, and Hispanic women with GDM had insulin secretory responses to glucose that were normal for their degree of insulin resistance in late pregnancy.[28] Those women had mild GDM and might be expected to be at low risk of diabetes when they are not pregnant.[97,99,108,111] Second, as indicated by the long-term follow-up studies of O'Sullivan,[100] a significant number of women with GDM may never develop diabetes after pregnancy. Thus, not all women with GDM can be regarded as truly abnormal in their regulation of circulating glucose concentrations.

A second level of complexity in the pathogenesis of GDM is likely to exist among patients who are truly abnormal in the sense that they will develop diabetes at some time after pregnancy. The hyperglycemia of those women during and after pregnancy could result from any of the abnormalities that lead to hyperglycemia in nonpregnant individuals (see discussion of pregestational diabetes, above). Thus, some women with GDM may have evolving autoimmune diabetes (IDDM) with partial destruction of pancreatic B cells that is first detected as glucose intolerance during pregnancy. In most studies in the United States, the prevalence of circulating immune markers such as anti-islet cell antibodies is low in women with GDM (i.e., in the range of 3 to 8 percent[112,113]), suggesting that autoimmune B-cell dysfunction is an uncommon contributor to GDM and postpregnancy diabetes among those women. Most patients with GDM have nonimmune B-cell dysfunction and are probably at risk of NIDDM. Limited B-cell reserve and some degree of chronic insulin resistance most likely contribute to the development of NIDDM in those women (Fig. 5-5), although direct studies of the mechanisms involved in the development of NIDDM in women with prior GDM are lacking.

The pathogenesis of GDM detailed above has significant implications for the treatment of women with that disease during and after pregnancy. The basic approach to the treatment should be to maintain a balance between total-body insulin requirements and the supply of insulin available to the tissues. During pregnancy, maintenance of that balance is challenged by the physiologic insulin resistance of pregnancy. That insulin resistance may be critical to the normal course of pregnancy, and it may be both difficult and unwise

to reverse the resistance. Thus, increasing the insulin supply with exogenous insulin appears to be the most logical approach to treatment of GDM during pregnancy, because sulfonylurea drugs (direct simulators of insulin secretion) are not recommended during pregnancy. Insulin treatment is administered during pregnancy to mitigate fetal complications of GDM and, except for the report of O'Sullivan,[114] there is little evidence that such treatment averts subsequent maternal diabetes. Aerobic exercise[115,116] and mild caloric restriction[92] have been reported to lower circulating glucose concentrations during pregnancy in women with GDM, but the mechanisms for those beneficial effects have not been determined.

Maintenance of a normal balance between insulin sensitivity and B-cell function after pregnancy in women who have had GDM should reduce the risk of subsequent diabetes in those women. Although specific techniques to prevent or delay diabetes have not been defined, sufficient information exists to allow some recommendations for the routine care of women with recent GDM. To the extent that the pathogenesis of GDM and NIDDM are similar regarding failure of B-cell compensation for insulin resistance (Fig. 5-5), it seems prudent to recommend measures that minimize insulin resistance be initiated in women who have had GDM. At the present time, measures that have been shown to improve insulin action in nonpregnant individuals include weight loss in obese people,[117,118] chronic aerobic exercise,[119,120] and avoidance of a high fat content in the diet.[121] Thus, those measures should be part of the standard management of women with a history of GDM. Additional approaches, such as the administration of pharmacologic agents to enhance insulin secretion[122,123] or to improve insulin action[124–126] in patients at risk of NIDDM, as well as interventions to suppress the immune system in the subset of patients with evolving autoimmune diabetes, remain experimental.

SUMMARY

The metabolic demands of the developing fetus dictate that maternal metabolism must change markedly during pregnancy to allow efficient nutrient storage during feeding and rapid use of the stored nutrients with minimal catabolism of maternal protein during fasting.

The changes that have evolved to serve those functions appear to be mediated to a large extent by hormones secreted from the fetoplacental unit. The three most prominent changes are progressive insulin resistance, accelerated fat catabolism, and fasting hypoglycemia.

Insulin secretion from pancreatic B cells normally modulates the impact of the fetoplacental unit on maternal metabolism. Because insulin demands increase during pregnancy, women with overt or incipient diabetes mellitus (i.e., women with limited B-cell secretory reserve) are not able to make sufficient insulin to modulate normally the metabolic impact of the fetus and placenta. As a result, those women develop significant and predictable metabolic abnormalities of intermediary metabolism that can threaten fetal and maternal well-being. Women with overt diabetes antedating pregnancy will develop progressive metabolic decompensation unless they receive aggressive insulin therapy to mitigate the metabolic impact of pregnancy. Apparently normal women with a covert limitation of B-cell function may also develop metabolic abnormalities (i.e., GDM) during pregnancy. Those women may warrant antidiabetic treatment to maintain fetal well-being, and they are at increased risk of developing diabetes when they are not pregnant.

REFERENCES

1. Burt RL: Peripheral utilization of glucose in pregnancy. III. Insulin tolerance. Obstet Gynecol 2:658, 1956
2. DeFronzo RA, Tobin JD, Andres R: Glucose clamp technique: a method for quantifying insulin secretion and resistance. Am J Physiol 237:E214, 1979
3. Ryan EA, O'Sullivan MJ, Skyler JS: Insulin action during pregnancy. Studies with the euglycemic glucose clamp technique. Diabetes 34:380, 1985
4. Catalano PM, Tyzbir ED, Wolfe RR et al: Carbohydrate metabolism during pregnancy in control subjects and women with gestational diabetes. Am J Physiol 264:E60, 1993
5. Bergman RN: The Lilly Lecture 1989. Toward a physiological understanding of glucose tolerance: minimal model approach. Diabetes 38:1512, 1989
6. Buchanan TA, Metzger BE, Freinkel N, Bergman RN: Insulin sensitivty and B-cell responsiveness to glucose during late pregnancy in lean and moderately obese women with normal glucose tolerance or mild gestational diabetes. Am J Obstet Gynecol 162:1008, 1990
7. Freinkel N: The Banting Lecture 1980. Of pregnancy and progeny. Diabetes 29:1023, 1980
8. Samaan N, Yen SCC, Gonzalez D: Metabolic effects of placental lactogen in man. J Clin Endocrinol Metab 28:485, 1968
9. Kalkhoff RK, Richardson BL, Beck P: Relative effects of pregnancy human placental lactogen and prednisolone on carbohydrate tolerance in normal and subclinical diabetic subjects. Diabetes 18:153, 1969
10. Beck P: Progestin enhancement of the plasma insulin response to glucose in rhesus monkeys. Diabetes 18:146, 1969
11. Kalkhoff RK, Jacobson M, Lemper D: Progesterone, pregnancy and the augmented plasma insulin response. J Clin Endocrinol 31:24, 1970
12. Ryan EA, Enns L: Role of gestational hormones in the induction of insulin resistance. J Clin Endocrinol Metab 67:341, 1988
13. Gratcos JA, Nufeld N, Kumar D et al: Monocyte insulin binding studies in normal and diabetic pregnancies. Am J Obstet Gynecol 141:611, 1980
14. Moore O, Kolterman O, Weyant J et al: Insulin binding in human pregnancy: comparison to the postpartum, luteal and follicular states. J Clin Endocrinol Metab 52:937, 1981
15. Tsibris J, Raynor L, Buhi W: Insulin receptors in circulating erythrocytes and monocytes from women on oral contraceptives and pregnant women near term. J Clin Endocrinol Metab 51:711, 1980
16. Pauvilai G, Drobney EC, Domont L, Baumann G: Insulin receptors and insulin resistance in human pregnancy: evidence for a postreceptor defect in insulin action. J Clin Endocrinol Metab 54:247, 1982
17. Pagano G, Cassader M, Massobrio M et al: Insulin binding to human adipocytes during late pregnancy in healthy, obese and diabetic state. Horm Metab Res 12:177, 1980
18. Hjolland E, Pedersen O, Espersen T, Klebe JG: Impaired insulin receptor binding and postbinding defects of adipocytes from normal and diabetic pregnant women. Diabetes 35:598, 1986
19. Ciraldi TP, Kettel M, El-Roeiy A et al: Mechanisms of cellular insulin resistance in human pregnancy. Am J Obstet Gynecol 170:635, 1994
20. Damm P, Handberg A, Kuhl C et al: Insulin receptor binding and tyrosine kinase activity in skeletal muscle from normal pregnant women and women with gestational diabetes. Obstet Gynecol 82:251, 1993
21. Garvey WT, Maianu L, Hancock JA et al: Gene expression of GLUT4 in skeletal muscle form insulin-resistant patients with obesity, IGT, GDM, and NIDDM. Diabetes 41:465, 1992

22. Seyffert WA, Madison LL: Physiologic effects of metabolic fuels on carbohydrate metabolism. I. Acute effect of elevation of plasma free fatty acids on hepatic glucose output, peripheral glucose utilization, serum insulin and glucagon levels. Diabetes 16:765, 1967

23. Bonadonna RC, Groop LC, Simonson DC, DeFronzo RA: Free fatty acid and glucose metabolism in human aging: evidence for operation of the Randle cycle. Am J Physiol 266:501, 1994

24. Phelps RL, Metzger BE, Freinkel N: Diurnal profiles of glucose, insulin, free fatty acids, triglycerides, cholesterol, and individual amino acids in late normal pregnancy. Am J Obstet Gynecol 140:730, 1981

25. Randle PJ, Hales CN, Garland PB, Newsholme EA: The glucose-fatty acid cycle: its role in insulin sensitivity and the metabolic abnormalities of diabetes mellitus. Lancet 1:785, 1963

26. Bergman RN, Phillips LS, Cobelli C: Physiologic evaluation of factors controlling glucose tolerance in man. Measurement of insulin sensitivity and beta-cell sensitivity from the response to intravenous glucose. J Clin Invest 68:1456, 1981

27. Kahn SE, Prigeon RL, McCulloch DK et al: Quantification of the relationship between insulin sensitivity and B-cell function in human subjects: evidence for a hyperbolic function. Diabetes 42:1663, 1993

28. Buchanan TA: Carbohydrate metabolism in pregnancy: normal physiology and implications for diabetes mellitus. Isr J Med Sci 27:432, 1991

29. Howell SL, Tyhurst M, Green IC: Direct effects of progesterone on rat islets of Langerhans in vivo and in tissue culture. Diabetologia 13:579, 1977

30. Lind T, Billewicz WZ, Brown G: A serial study of the changes occurring in the oral glucose tolerance test during pregnancy. J Obstet Gynaecol Br Commonw 80:1033, 1973

31. Freinkel N, Metzger BE, Nitzan M: Facilitated anabolism in late pregnancy: some novel maternal compensations for accelerated starvation. p. 474. In Malaisse WJ, Pirart J (eds): Proceedings of the VIII Congress of the International Diabetes Federation, International Congress Series, Exerpta Medica, Amsterdam, 1974

32. LeTurque A, Ferre P, Burnol A-F et al: Glucose utilization rates and insulin sensitivity in vivo in tissues of virgin and pregnant rats. Diabetes 35:172, 1986

33. Herrera E, Gomez-Coronado D, Lasuncion MA: Lipid metabolism in pregnancy. Biol Neonate 51:70, 1987

34. Topping DL, Mayes PA: The immediate effect of insulin and fructose on the metabolism of the perfused liver. Biochem J 126:295, 1972

35. Kalhan SC, Assel BG: Protein metabolism in pregnancy. p. 163. In Cowett RM (ed): Principles of Perinatal-Neonatal Metabolism. Springer Verlag, New York, 1991

36. DeBenoist B, Jackson AA, Hall J: Whole-body protein turnover in Jamaican women during pregnancy. Hum Nutr Clin Nutr 39C:167, 1985

37. Freinkel N: Effects of the conceptus on maternal metabolism during pregnancy. p. 679. In Leibel BS, Wrenshall GA (eds): On the Nature and Treatment of Diabetes. Exerpta Medica, Amsterdam, 1965

38. Felig P, Lynch V: Starvation in human pregnancy: hypoglycemia, hypoinsulinemia and hyperketonemia. Science 170:990, 1970

39. Felig P, Kim YJ, Lynch V, Hendler R: Amino acid metabolism during starvation in human pregnancy. J Clin Invest 51:1195, 1972

40. Metzger BE, Ravnikar V, Vilesis R, Freinkel N: Accelerated starvation and the skipped breakfast in late normal pregnancy. Lancet 1:588, 1982

41. Buchanan TA, Metzger BE, Freinkel N: Accelerated starvation in late pregnancy: a comparison between obese women with and without gestational diabetes mellitus. Am J Obstet Gynecol 162:1015, 1990

42. Bruschetta H, Buchanan TA, Steil GM et al: Reduced glucose production accounts for the fall in plasma glucose during brief extension of an overnight fast in women with gestational diabetes. Clin Res 42:27A, 1994

43. Kalhan SC, Gilfillian CA, Tserng KY, Savin SM: Glucose-alanine relationship in normal human pregnancy. Metabolism 37:152, 1988

44. Morrow PG, Marshall WP, Kim H-J, Kalkhoff RK: Metabolic response to starvation. I. Relative effects of pregnancy and sex steroid administration in the rat. Metabolism 30:268, 1981

45. Morrow PG, Marshall WP, Kim H-J, Kalkhoff RK: Metabolic response to starvation. II. Effects of sex steroid administration to pre- and post-menopausal women. Metabolism 30:274, 1981

46. Turtle JR, Kipnis DM: The lipolytic action of human placental lactogen in isolated fat cells. Biochim Biophys Acta 144:583, 1967

47. Metzger BE, Freinkel N: Regulation of maternal protein metabolism and gluconeogenesis in the fasted state. p. 303. In Camerini-Davalos R, Cole H (eds): Early Diabetes in Early Life. Academic Press, San Diego, 1975

48. Hytten FE, Leitch I: The Physiology of Human Pregnancy. 2nd Ed. Blackwell Scientific Publications, Oxford, 1971

49. National Diabetes Data Group: Classification and diagnosis of diabetes mellitus and other categories of glucose intolerance. Diabetes 29:1039, 1979

50. WHO Expert Committee on Diabetes Mellitus: Second Report. Technical Report Series 646. World Health Organization, Geneva, 1980

51. Eisenbarth GS: Type I diabetes mellitus: a chronic autoimmune disease. N Engl J Med 314:1360, 1986

52. Bosi E, Bonifacio E, Botazzo GF: Autoantigens in IDDM. Diabetes Rev 1:204, 1993

53. Srikanta S, Ricker AT, McCulloch DK et al: Autoimmunity to insulin, beta cell dysfunction and development of insulin dependent diabetes mellitus. Diabetes 35:139, 1986

54. DeFronzo RA, Bonadonna RC, Ferrannini E: The pathogenesis of NIDDM: a balanced overview. Diabetes Care 15:318, 1992

55. Fajans SS, Floyd J, Tattersall R et al: The various faces of diabetes in the young. Arch Intern Med 136:194, 1976

56. Froguel PH, Zouali H, Vionnet N et al: Familial hyperglycemia due to mutations in glucokinase: definition of a subtype of diabetes mellitus. N Engl J Med 328:697, 1993

57. Flier JS: Lilly Lecture 1991. Syndromes of insulin resistance: from patient to gene and back again. Diabetes 41:1207, 1991

58. Bogardus C, Lillioja S, Nyomba L et al: Distribution of in vivo insulin action in Pima Indians as a mixture of three normal distributions. Diabetes 38:1423, 1989

59. Eriksson J, Franssila-Kallunki A, Ekstrand A et al: Early metabolic defects in persons at increased risk for non-insulin-dependent diabetes mellitus. N Engl J Med 231:337, 1989

60. Warram JH, Martin BC, Krolewski AS et al: Slow glucose removal rate and hyperinsulinemia preceded the development of type II diabetes in the offspring of diabetic parents. Ann Intern Med 113:909, 1990

61. Martin BC, Warram JH, Krolewski AS et al: Role of glucose and insulin resistance in development of type 2 diabetes mellitus: results of a 25-year follow-up study. Lancet 340:925, 1992

62. Haffner SM, Stern MP, Mitchell BD et al: Incidence of type II diabetes in Mexican Americans predicted by fasting insulin and glucose levels, obesity, and body fat distribution. Diabetes 39:283, 1990

63. Saad MF, Knowler WC, Petrtitt DJ et al: The natural history of impaired glucose tolerance in Pima Indians. N Engl J Med 319:1500, 1988

64. Lillioja S, Mott DM, Spraul M et al: Insulin resistance and insulin secretory dysfunction as precursors of non-insulin-dependent diabetes mellitus. N Engl J Med 329:1988, 1993

65. Hideki H, Nagulesparan M, Klimes I et al: Improvement of insulin secretion but not insulin resistance after short term control of plasma glucose in obese type II diabetics. J Clin Endocrinol Metab 54:217, 1982

66. Leahy JL, Bonner-Weir S, Weir GC: B-cell dysfunction induced by chronic hyperglycemia: current ideas on mechanism of impaired glucose-induced insulin secretion. Diabetes Care 15:442, 1992

67. Howard BV: Lipoprotein metabolism in diabetes mellitus. J Lipid Res 28:613, 1987

68. Freinkel N, Metzger BE: Pregnancy as a tissue culture experience: the critical implications of maternal metabolism for fetal development. p. 3. In Pregnancy Metabolism, Diabetes and the Fetus. Ciba Foundation Symposium no. 63. Exerpta Medica, Amsterdam, 1979

69. White P: Pregnancy complicating diabetes. Am J Med 7:609, 1949

70. Sadler TW, Hunter ES III, Wynn RE, Phillips LS: Evidence for multifactorial origin of diabetes-induced embryopathies. Diabetes 38:70, 1989

71. Kalkhoff RK: Impact of maternal fuels and nutritional state on fetal growth. Diabetes, suppl. 2, 40:61, 1991

72. Metzger BE. Biphasic effects of maternal metabolism on fetal growth. Quintessential expression of fuel-mediated metabolism. Diabtes, suppl. 2, 40:99, 1991

73. Knopp RH, Bergelin RO, Wahl PW, Walden CE: Relationship of infant birth size to maternal lipoproteins, apoproteins, fuels, hormones, clinical chemistries, and body weight at 36 weeks gestation. Diabetes, suppl. 2, 34:71, 1985

74. Rudolf MC, Coustan DR, Sherwin RS et al: Efficacy of the insulin pump in the home treatment of pregnant diabetics. Diabetes 30:891, 1981

75. Jovanovic L, Peterson CM: Optimal insulin delivery for the pregnant diabetic patient. Diabetes Care, suppl. 1, 5:24, 1982

76. Potter JM, Reckless JPD, Cullen DR: The effect of continuous subcutaneous insulin infusion and conventional insulin regimes on 24-hour variation of blood glucose and intermediary metabolites in the third trimester of diabetic pregnancy. Diabetologia 21:534, 1981

77. Hertz RH, King KC, Kalhan SC: Management of third-trimester diabetic pregnancies with the use of continuous subcutaneous insulin infusion therapy: a pilot study. Am J Obstet Gynecol 149:256, 1984

78. Reece EA, Coustan DR, Sherwin RS et al: Does intensive glycemic control in diabetic pregnancies result in normalization of other metabolic fuels? Am J Obstet Gynecol 165:126, 1991

79. Adrogue HJ, Wilson H, Boyd AE et al: Plasma acid-base patterns in diabetic ketoacidosis. N Engl J Med 307:1603, 1982

80. Foster DW, McGarry JD: The metabolic derangements and treatment of diabetic ketoacidosis. N Engl J Med 309:159, 1983

81. Montoro MN, Meyers VP, Mestman JH et al: Outcome of pregnancy in diabetic ketoacidosis. Am J Perinatol 10:17, 1993

82. Diabetes Control and Complications Trial Research Group: Epidemiology of severe hypoglycemia in diabetes control and complications trial. Am J Med 90:450, 1991

83. Bolli GB, Dimitriadis GD, Pehling GB et al: Abnormal glucose counterregulation after subcutaneous insulin in insulin-dependent diabetes mellitus. N Engl J Med 310:1706, 1984

84. Cryer PE: Glucose counterregulation in man. Diabetes 30:261, 1981

85. Amiel SA, Sherwin RS, Simonson DC, Tamborlane WV: Effect of intensive insulin therapy on glycemic thresholds for counterregulatory release. Diabetes 37:901, 1988

86. Langer O, Anyaegbunam A, Brustman L et al: Pregestational diabetes: insulin requirements throughout pregnancy. Am J Obstet Gynecol 159:616, 1988

87. Henry RR, Schaeffer L, Olefsky JM: Glycemic effects of intensive calorie restriction and refeeding in noninsulin dependent diabetes mellitus. J Clin Endocrinol Metab 61:917, 1985

88. Wing RR: Behavioral treatment of obesity. Its application to type II diabetes. Diabetes Care 16:193, 1993

89. Churchill JA, Berendez HW, Nemore J: Neuropsychological deficits in children of diabetic mothers. Am J Obstet Gynecol 105:257, 1966

90. Stehbens JA, Baker GL, Kitchell M: Outcome at ages 1, 3, and 5 years of children born to diabetic women. Am J Obstet Gynecol 127:408, 1977

91. Rizzo T, Metzger BE, Burns WJ, Burns K: Correlation between antepartum maternal metabolism and intelligence of offspring. N Engl J Med 325:911, 1991

92. Knopp RH, Magee MS, Raisys V, Benedetti T: Metabolic effects of hypocaloric diets in management of gestational diabetes. Diabetes, suppl. 2, 40:165, 1991

93. Metzger BE, Conference Organizing Committee: Summary and recommendations of the third international workshop-conference on gestational diabetes. Diabetes, suppl. 2, 40:197, 1991

94. Sacks DA, Abu-Fadil S, Karten GJ et al: Screening for gestational diabetes with the one-hour 50-g glucose test. Obstet Gynecol 70:89, 1987

95. O'Sullivan JB, Mahan CM: Criteria for the oral glucose tolerance test in pregnancy. Diabetes 13:278, 1964

96. Dooley SL, Metzger BE, Cho N: Gestational diabetes: influence of race on disease prevalence and perinatal outcome in a U.S. population. Diabetes, suppl. 2, 40:25, 1991

97. Kjos SL, Buchanan TA, Montoro M et al: Serum lipids within 36 months of delivery in women with recent gestational diabetes mellitus. Diabetes, suppl. 2, 40:142, 1991

98. O'Sullivan JB: Diabetes after GDM. Diabetes, suppl. 2, 40:131, 1991

99. Kjos SL, Buchanan TA, Peters R et al: Postpartum glucose tolerance testing identifies women with recent gestational diabetes who are at highest risk for developing diabetes within five years. Diabetes, suppl. 1, 43:136A, 1994

100. O'Sullivan JB: The Boston gestational diabetes studies: review and perspectives. p. 287. In Sutherland HW, Stowers JM, Pearson DWM (eds): Carbohydrate Metabolism in Pregnancy and the Newborn. Springer-Verlag, London, 1989

101. Stern MP: Diabetes in Hispanic Americans. p. 1X1. In Harris MI, Hamman RF (eds): Diabetes in America. NIH Publication 85-1468, USPHS, Bethesda, MD, 1985

102. Cousins L, Rea C, Crawford M: Longitudinal characterization of insulin sensitivity and body fat in normal and gestational diabetic pregnancies. Diabetes, suppl. 1, 37: 251A, 1988

103. Ward WK, Johnston CLW, Beard JC et al: Abnormalities of islet B-cell function, insulin action and fat distribution in women with a history of gestational diabetes: relation to obesity. J Clin Endocrinol Metab 61:1039, 1985

104. Ward WK, Johnston CLW, Beard JC et al: Insulin resistance and impaired insulin secretion in subjects with a history of gestational diabetes mellitus. Diabetes 34:861, 1985

105. Garvey WT, Maianu L, Zhu J-H et al: Multiple defects in the adipocyte glucose transport system cause cellular insulin resistance in gestational diabetes. Diabetes 42: 1773, 1993

106. Yen SCC, Tsai CC, Vela P: Gestational diabetogenesis: quantitative analysis of glucose-insulin interrelationship between normal pregnancy and pregnancy with gestational diabetes. Am J Obstet Gynecol 111:792, 1971

107. Fisher PM, Sutherland HW, Bewsher PD: The insulin response to glucose infusion in gestational diabetes. Diabetologia 19:10, 1980

108. Metzger BE, Bybee DE, Freinkel N et al: Gestational diabetes mellitus. Correlations between the phenotypic and genotypic characteristics of the mother and abnormal glucose tolerance during the first year postpartum. Diabetes, suppl. 2, 43:111, 1985

109. Damm P, Kuhl C, Bertelsen A, Molsted-Pedersen L: Predictive factors for the development of diabetes in women with previous gestational diabetes mellitus. Am J Obstet Gynecol 167:607, 1992

110. Metzger BE, Cho NH, Roston SM, Radvany R: Prepregnancy weight and antepartum insulin secretion predict glucose tolerance five years after gestational diabetes mellitus. Diabetes Care 16:1598, 1994

111. Catalano PM, Vargo KM, Bernstein IM, Amini SB: Incidence and risk factors associated with abnormal postpartum glucose tolerance in women with gestational diabetes. Am J Obstet Gynecol 165:914, 1991

112. Freinkel N, Metzger BE, Phelps RL et al: Gestational diabetes mellitus: heterogeneity of maternal age, weight, insulin secretion, HLA antigens, and islet cell antibodies and the impact of maternal metabolism on pancreatic B-cell function and somatic growth in the offspring. Diabetes, suppl. 2, 34:1, 1985

113. Catalano PM, Tyzbir ED, Simms EAH: Incidence and significance of islet cell antibodies in women with previous gestational diabetes. Diabetes Care 13:478, 1990

114. O'Sullivan JB: Insulin treatment and high risk groups. Diabetes Care 3:482, 1980

115. Bung P, Artal R, Khodiguiab N, Kjos S: Exercise in gestational diabetes. An optional therapeutic approach? Diabetes, suppl. 2, 40:182, 1991

116. Jovanovic-Peterson L, Peterson CM: Is exercise safe or useful for gestational diabetic women? Diabetes, suppl. 2, 40:179, 1991

117. Friedman JE, Dohm GL, Leggett-Frazier N et al: Restoration of insulin responsiveness in skeletal muscle of morbidly obese patients after weight loss. J Clin Invest 39:701, 1992

118. Franssila-Kallunki A, Rissanen A, Ekstrand A et al: Effects of weight loss on substrate oxidation, energy expenditure, and insulin sensitivity in obese individuals. Am J Clin Nutr 55:356, 1992

119. Krotkiewski M, Lonnroth P, Bjorntorp P: The effects of physical training on insulin secretion and effectiveness and on glucose metabolism in obesity and type 2 diabetes mellitus. Diabetologia 28:881, 1985

120. Koivisto VA, DeFronzo RA: Physical training and insulin sensitivity. Diabetes Metab Rev 1:445, 1986

121. Swinburn BA, Boyce VL, Bergman RN et al: Deterioration in carbohydrate metabolism and lipoprotein changes induced by modern, high-fat diet in Pima Indians and caucasians. J Clin Endocrinol Metab 73:156, 1991

122. Sartor G, Schersten B, Carlstrom S et al: Ten-year follow-up of subjects with impaired glucose tolerance: prevention of diabetes by tolbutamide and diet regulation. Diabetes 29:41, 1980

123. Stowers J: Treatment of chemical diabetes with chlorpropamide and associated mortality. Adv Metab Disord, suppl. 2, 2:549, 1973

124. Landin K, Tengborn L, Smith U: Treating insulin resistance in hypertension with metformin reduces both blood pressure and metabolic risk factors. J Intern Med 229:181, 1991

125. Widen EIM, Eriksson JG, Groop LC: Metformin normalizes nonoxidative glucose metabolism in insulin-resistant, normoglycemic first-degree relatives of patients with NIDDM. Diabetes 41:354, 1992

126. Nolan JJ, Ludvik B, Beerdsen P, Joyce M: Metabolic effects of troglitazone in subjects with impaired glucose tolerance and insulin resistance. Diabetes, suppl. 1, 43:49A, 1994

6

Diabetes and Fetal Growth

JOHN B. SUSA
ODED LANGER

CONTROL OF HUMAN FETAL GROWTH

Although embryonic cell proliferation is occurring at a very rapid rate and embryonic weight is increasing rapidly during the period of organ embryogenesis, 95 percent of the eventual weight of the human and non-human primate fetus is gained during the second half of gestation.[1] Human placental and fetal weights are similar until the rapid growth phase begins in the fetus at approximately 20 weeks' gestation. The disparity between fetal and placental weight gain during this period can be viewed as suggestive evidence that factors other than the placental transport functions are involved in controlling fetal growth.

The development of the fertilized ovum into a term human infant involves 44 cellular divisions.[2] The control of such a process is understandably complex and is influenced by many factors. During the early phases of organ embryogenesis, control is exercised primarily by the genome. Beyond this point, however, the ultimate growth of the fetus is controlled by a multitude of factors. Fetal growth requires the uninterrupted transfer of nutrients and oxygen from mother to fetus. The uptake of nutrients and oxygen by the placenta and their subsequent use by this organ as well as their transfer to the fetus for its use are controlled by maternal, placental, and fetal determinants.[1] The activity of those growth-promoting factors is influenced by the availability of nutrients in the maternal and fetal circulation. The availability of nutrients is influenced by maternal nutritional factors or aberrant metabolic states, the most common of which is diabetes mellitus.

Specific growth-promoting factors that directly influence fetal growth have been difficult to identify.

Growth hormone of maternal origin appears to have little influence on fetal growth, as demonstrated by the fact that normal birthweight is obtained after maternal hypophysectomy in a variety of animals[3] and in humans.[4] A correlation exists between infant birthweight and maternal undernutrition when maternal growth factors are dramatically suppressed; however, newborn birthweight is reduced by only up to 20 percent.[5] It is thus unlikely that specific maternal growth factors play a significant role in the transplacental regulation of fetal growth.

Uteroplacental Factors

A maternal factor that may play a role in the control of fetal growth is uteroplacental blood flow. If nutrients and oxygen cannot be delivered in adequate amounts to the fetus, fetal growth may be retarded.[1] The precise mechanism by which uteroplacental blood flow affects fetal growth is not clear because the reduction of uteroplacental perfusion is not necessarily accompanied by a reduction in placental-fetal blood flow.[6] Although it is generally accepted that maternal diabetes can alter uteroplacental circulation as a secondary effect of maternal vasculopathy, the effect of maternal diabetes on the fetal-placental circulation is less clearly understood. Altered placental architecture consisting of hyper- and hyporamification of the terminal villi is a well-established phenomenon in diabetic gestations.[7] It follows logically that these changes may affect placental vascular volume and resistance and, thus, modulate fetal-placental flow.

Studies using Doppler[8,9] have demonstrated a relationship between maternal diabetes, glycemic profile, and alterations in fetal blood flow to the placenta as measured by umbilical vein flow rates. When controlled for gestational age and estimated fetal weight, fetal-placental blood flow was 20 to 25 percent greater in diabetic pregnancies when compared with normal controls. Likewise, the overall maternal glycemic profile in diabetic women correlated with fetal-placental blood flow. In circumstances of either long-term maternal hypo- or hyperglycemia, fetal-placental blood flow was reduced and placental resistance increased when compared with euglycemic control. These changes in flow correlated only with overall maternal glycemic profile and did not appear to be affected by acute changes in maternal glucose levels, consistent with a mechanism of chronic structural changes rather than acute vasoreactive changes in the placenta.

The above studies suggest that long-term maternal glycemic control plays an important role in the establishment of normal placental architecture and adequate fetal-placental blood flow. Similarly, decreased fetal-placental blood flow as a result of suboptimal maternal glycemic control may be a mechanism by which uteroplacental insufficiency evolves and fetal death occurs in the poorly controlled diabetic woman. The critical exposure period and glucose levels required to prevent these placental changes, however, remain to be determined by further study.

A "volume hypothesis" has been proposed that states that the uteroplacental blood flow per unit of time exerts a greater influence on fetal outcome than the concentration of nutrients and oxygen in the intervillous blood. Despite some animal models in which uteroplacental blood flow is severely limited by uterine artery ligation and intrauterine growth retardation produced,[10] alteration of uteroplacental blood flow in humans has not yet been clearly associated with human fetal growth retardation; nevertheless, the decreased birthweight of the infant of the hypertensive mother is often attributed to reduced placental flow.

Placental factors, including size and increased villous area, are related to rapid fetal growth.[11,12] The mechanism by which this process is controlled is, however, not clear. Placental pathology clearly limits nutrient and oxygen transfer and thus retards fetal growth.[13] Nevertheless, fetal growth retardation is not always associated with small placentas and with obvious lesions. Other factors indicating placental dysfunction at a biochemical level may also be involved. Human placental lactogen possesses growth hormone-like activity and is a possible growth factor of placental origin. Its concentration in the maternal circulation increases with gestation. It mobilizes maternal lipid stores, thus sparing maternal glucose so that sufficient glucose is available for fetal metabolism.[14] However, human placental lactogen and another growth hormone homologue of placental origin, human chorionic gonadotropin, are found at very low levels in the fetal circulation.[15] It is, therefore, doubtful that either hormone directly supports fetal growth. Because growth hormone exerts its growth-stimulating action by stimulating somatomedin synthesis and release, growth hormones such as placental hormones prolactin, placental lactogen, or chorionic gonadotropin may exert their influence via a similar mechanism. Placental lactogen is equipotent as growth hormone in elevating insulin-like growth factor I (IGF-I) in hypophysectomized rats.[16]

Metabolic Substrate Factors

Maternal diabetes is characterized by increased plasma concentrations of glucose, free fatty acids, triglycerides, and some amino acids.[17] Maternal plasma concentrations of glucose, triglycerides, and the amino acids alanine, serine, and isoleucine are correlated with the birthweight of the infants of diabetic mothers (IDM). Pedersen[18] first proposed an explanation of the pathophysiology of the infant of the diabetic mother, which has become known as the hyperglycemia-hyperinsulinemia hypothesis.[19] In its simplest form, the hypothesis proposes that maternal hyperglycemia results in fetal hyperglycemia, with fetal insulin hypersecretion and fetal hyperinsulinemia, and subsequently in hypertrophy of fetal tissue. The hyperinsulinemia in the presence of hyperglycemia, abruptly terminated at birth, is responsible for many of the characteristic features of the fetus and the IDM. With the recognition that the concentrations of other nutrients are also elevated in the pregnant diabetic woman and her fetus and that these nutrients can also stimulate pancreatic hypersecretion of insulin, the Pedersen hypothesis has been modified and widely accepted.[20]

Further expansion of the Pedersen hypothesis was suggested regarding growth-delayed fetuses.[21] Similarly, excess of substrate (glucose) will result in fetal hyperinsulinemia; and inadequate substrate delivery to the fetus will be reflected in fetal hypoinsulinemia, resulting in growth delay and smaller fetuses. Indeed, several clinical studies have demonstrated the association between relative maternal oral glucose tolerance test (OGTT) hypoglycemia and intrauterine growth retardation (IUGR) infants.[22–25] In addition, it was shown that IUGR infants are characterized by hypoinsulinemia, hypoglycemia, and low insulin glucose index.[26] Finally, tight glycemic control is not free of complications. There was a 20 percent incidence of small-for-gestational-age (SGA) infants in patients with mean blood glucose of 87 mg/dl or less and an approximate 8 percent incidence when the level of glycemia was 87 to 95 mg/dl.[27] This finding may represent fetal nutritional deprivation resulting in growth delay-related abnormalities. Thus, although tight glycemic control is desirable, the care provider must be alert to preventing overtreatment, which could predispose to IUGR.

EFFECT OF HYPERINSULINEMIA: AN ANIMAL MODEL

Maternal diabetes has been produced by streptozotocin injection in the pregnant rhesus *(Macaca mulatta)* monkey.[28] The infants born to these monkeys are macrosomic and exhibit the selective organomegaly characteristic of human IDMs.[29] These infants appear to be metabolically similar to human IDMs, with demonstrable hyperglycemia and hyperinsulinemia. Although the pregnant, glucose-intolerant rhesus monkey model provides experimental verification of the Pedersen hypothesis, it does not provide direct experimental evidence that fetal hyperinsulinemia results in fetal overgrowth. The hyperinsulinemic fetus in this model is also hyperglycemic, and hence, the effect of excess substrate on fetal growth cannot be excluded.

The fetus of the diabetic rhesus monkey mother shares many features in common with its human counterpart. In addition, the fetus is of sufficient size, 450 g at birth, to permit adequate blood sampling. The growth-stimulating effect of insulin in the nonhuman primate fetus can only be confirmed when experimental fetal hyperinsulinemia is produced while maternal metabolic substrate concentrations are undisturbed and fetal substrate concentrations are at approximately normal levels. Because the primate placenta is impermeable to insulin,[30] fetal hyperinsulinemia can be produced by the delivery of insulin to the fetal component of the maternal-fetal unit. Even with the marked fetal hyperinsulinemia and attendant increase in fetal substrate use, fetal glucose concentration may be maintained by increased glucose delivery by the mother to the fetus. Isolated hyperinsulinemia in the fetal rhesus monkey has been produced by surgically implanting an insulin-delivering minipump in the fetus during the last third of pregnancy.[31,32]

Our earliest rhesus studies were performed by the delivery of 19 U/d of sodium pork insulin for 21 days.[31] These studies produced macrosomia, with fetal plasma insulin levels in the supraphysiologic range as high as 5,300 μU/ml. Because fetal plasma insulin levels that high may be clinically irrelevant to IDMs, fetal hyperinsulinemia with insulin concentrations comparable with those that may be reached in infants of human mothers with poorly controlled diabetes[33,34] was subsequently produced in the rhesus by the delivery of 4.75 U/d of insulin.

Table 6-1 summarizes the effect of chronic experimentally produced hyperinsulinemia on the rhesus fetus. In the low-dose-treated group, the insulin concentration of 340 ± 208 μU/ml is comparable with insulin levels reported in human IDMs.[35,36] The high-dose-treated group have insulin concentrations higher than that observed in the IDMs. Insulin-treated fetuses are approximately 100 g heavier than their age-matched controls. The excess weight for these two groups over controls was 23 percent for the low dose and 27 percent for the high dose, which compares with a 22 percent increase in one group of IDMs.[33] During this stage of gestation, the fetal rhesus monkey gains weight at the approximate rate of 5 g/d.[37] At implant, fetal weight is estimated from normal gestational age/weight data to be approximately 260 g. After 21 days, the controls had gained 112 g compared with 200 g for the low-dose- and 224 g for the high-dose-treated groups. This represents an approximate doubling of weight gain to 10 g/d.

The placental weight was also increased by insulin treatment but only significantly so in the high-dose-treated group. Although birthweight was increased by insulin treatment, skeletal growth was not altered as evidenced by the lack of effect on crown–heel length or head circumference. Figure 6-1 shows the birthweight ratio (actual birthweight/expected birthweight). A highly significant correlation exists between birthweight ratio and natural logarithm of

Table 6-1. Effects of Chronic Hyperinsulinemia on Fetal Rhesus Monkey Size

Insulin Dose (U/d)	Day	Gestational Age (day)	Fetal Plasma Insulin (μU/ml)	Fetal Weight (g)	Placental Weight (g)	Crown–heel Length (cm)	Head Circumference (cm)
Control 0 (N = 9)	21.0 ± 0	142 ± 5	28 ± 12	372 ± 54	92.4 ± 12.0	29 ± 2	19 ± 1
Low dose 4.75 (N = 10)	19 ± 1	145 ± 3	340 ± 208[a]	459 ± 53[a]	124.6 ± 39.5	28 ± 2	18 ± 1
High dose 19.0 (N = 10)	20 ± 1	141 ± 4	3625 ± 1700[b,c]	474 ± 48[b]	141.6 ± 50.8[d]	28 ± 2	18 ± 1

[a] Low dose versus control, $P < .005$.
[b] High dose versus control, $P < .001$.
[c] High dose versus low dose, $P < .005$.
[d] High dose versus control, $P < .01$.
(From Susa et al,[35] with permission.)

plasma insulin concentration. The logarithmic nature of this correlation is consistent with the fact that it is possible to saturate the growth-promoting system in the fetus. The mechanism by which this occurs is not clear but may be related to the availability and numbers of insulin receptors or the limitation placed on growth because of the placental inability to transfer nutrients at a sufficiently rapid rate to make up for the fetal compartment's accelerated use rate.

Figure 6-2 summarizes the effects of hyperinsulinemia on fetal organ weight. The panel on the left is for the fetal rhesus, the panel on the right is for the

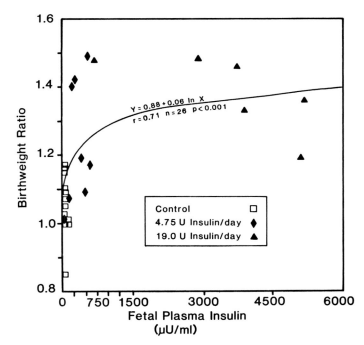

Fig. 6-1. Correlation between fetal birthweight ratio and fetal umbilical artery plasma insulin. Controls are represented by open squares (□), fetuses receiving 4.75 U/d of insulin by closed diamonds (◆), and fetuses receiving 19.0 U/d of insulin by closed triangles (▲). (From Susa et al,[35] with permission.)

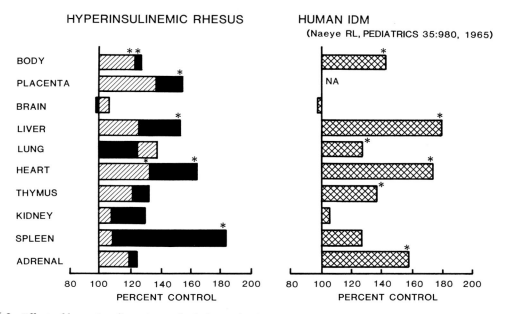

Fig. 6-2. Effect of hyperinsulinemia on fetal rhesus body and organ weights in low-dose- and high-dose-treated animals compared with body and organ weights of human infants of diabetic mothers (IDMs). Shaded area, 4.75 U/d insulin; block area, 19.09 U/d insulin. (Human IDM data from Naeye.[38])

human IDM. The similarity between these two groups is obvious. The human infants were presumably carried by mothers whose diabetes was in poor control during their entire pregnancy. These infants represent the extreme in consequences of maternal diabetes, with birthweights 141 percent of normal.[38] Although insulin levels are unavailable, they are likely to be as high or even higher than those reported by other investigators. After only 3 weeks of hyperinsulinemia produced by 19 U/d of insulin, organomegaly very similar to the human IDM was produced in the fetal rhesus, with significantly increased body, heart, liver, and spleen weight. The lower-dose insulin treatment produced only significant weight gain and cardiomegaly.

In a recent postmortem study of human IDMs from a Scandinavian population, total body weight and heart weight were increased.[39] This is identical to the effect of 4.5 U/d of insulin treatment on the fetal rhesus monkey. These studies have demonstrated that this level of hyperinsulinemia is capable of stimulating growth to a rate very similar to that observed during the third trimester in the human fetus of the diabetic mother.

The above experiments have not permitted the mea-surement of substrate transfer from mother to fetus. The reduced umbilical artery plasma glucose concentration suggests that increased fetal glucose use is a consequence of in utero hyperinsulinemia. The measurement of substrate concentrations alone cannot identify the potentially increased fetal glucose use rates and placental transfer rates. Studies in the chronically catheterized fetal sheep have, however, documented increased fetal glucose uptake after short-term[40,41] and long-term[42] insulin infusion.

In several different animal systems using either in vivo or in vitro experiments, short-term insulin administration has resulted in increased uptake of glucose and synthesis of glycogen and fat.[43,44] Total hepatic lipid content, although slightly higher in our high-dose insulin-treated fetal rhesus group, was not significant. A similar but nonsignificant elevation of lipid concentration was also found in the fetuses of streptozotocin-induced diabetic rhesus monkeys.[45] Protein, RNA, and DNA concentrations in the livers were not different. The increased liver mass in these fetuses cannot be accounted for solely by the glycogen increase, which only represents a 1.5 percent increase in total weight.

That protein/DNA ratios are similar suggests that insulin stimulates hyperplasia of hepatic parenchymal and hematopoietic cells. Microscopic examination of fetal livers indicates that parenchymal and hematopoietic cells are the same size. Thus, the increased liver weight is the result of cell proliferation rather than an increase in size.

In vitro experiments have proved that insulin stimulates incorporation of labeled amino acids into protein of human fetal tissue maintained in organ culture.[43] In vivo experiments have also documented increased fetal uptake of amino acids and protein synthesis as well as decreased protein catabolism in response to insulin.[44] The concentration of several amino acids is reduced in the plasma of hyperinsulinemic IDMs at birth and at 2 hours of age.[46] In hyperinsulinemic rhesus fetus studies, a negative logarithmic correlation between amino acid and insulin concentration is consistent with these effects. The lack of effect of hyperinsulinemia on muscle (heart and psoas) DNA, RNA, and protein concentration is the same as in liver. The increased muscle mass must, therefore, be due to hyperplasia. Consistent with this conclusion are the results of microscopic examination of skeletal muscle fibers, including computer-assisted cross-sectional area determination, which confirms that the mean fiber area in the hyperinsulinemic fetuses is the same

as in controls.[47] We interpret these data as evidence that hyperinsulinemia in the absence of elevated growth substrate concentrations stimulates cellular proliferation; when fetal growth substrates are also elevated, both hyperplasia and hypertrophy have been reported.[38]

Although the rhesus fetus normally contains little visible fat, increased deposits of adipose tissue in the thoracic cavity, perinephric region, and pericardium are found in hyperinsulinemic fetuses. The hyperinsulinemic fetus on the right in Figure 6-3 illustrates the difference in the amount of adipose tissue compared with a control fetus of the same gestational age, 143 days. Livers of fetuses of pregnant rhesus monkeys with streptozotocin-induced diabetes have an increased rate of lipogenesis and of triglyceride synthesis.[45] In our hyperinsulinemic fetal rhesus studies, we have found increased activity of hepatic fatty acid synthase in both high- and low-dose-treated fetuses.[32] The stimulation of lipid synthesis during hyperinsulinemia explains the 50 to 60 percent more fat found in the IDM.

Chronic, euglycemic, exogenously produced hyperinsulinemia in the rhesus monkey fetus results in fetal macrosomia and attenuated insulin secretion to a variety of secretagogues at birth and during infancy.[48–50] Because pregnancy imposes significant stress to normal glucose homeostasis, we tested the hypothesis that

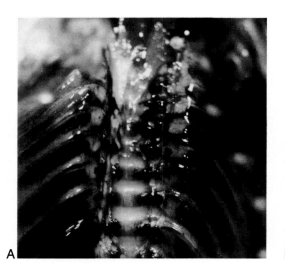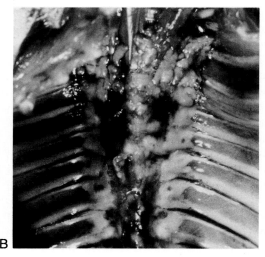

Fig. 6-3. Thoracic cavity adipose tissue in (**A**) a control and (**B**) a hyperinsulinemic rhesus fetus at 143 days' gestation. (From Susa and Schwartz,[86] with permission.)

glucose tolerance would be reduced in animals that had been made hyperinsulinemic in utero, and their offspring, the second generation, would consequently be macrosomic. Rapid intravenous glucose tolerance tests (GTTs) were performed 2 weeks before term in eight control and five pregnant rhesus monkeys that had been hyperinsulinemic in utero.

The five experimental animals delivered 11 live fetuses. The weight of these fetuses was significantly higher (518 ± 78 g) than the control fetuses (454 ± 43 g). Maternal fasting plasma glucose in the experimental group is significantly elevated at 68 ± 12 compared with 57 ± 8 mg/dl. Although glucose disappearance rates in both groups are not significantly different, they are significant negative linear correlations between fetal weight and glucose disappearance rate, as well as integrated insulin secretion. These studies demonstrate that fetal hyperinsulinemia can adversely affect glucose metabolism in adult females during pregnancy and place the second-generation progeny at risk of fetal macrosomia. These nongenetic and transgenerational effects are consistent with the in utero fuel/hormone-mediated teratogenesis hypothesis.[51]

EFFECT OF INSULIN-LIKE GROWTH FACTORS

Like insulin, IGF-I and IGF-II exert their biologic effects via receptor-mediated processes. Because of the structural homology between insulin and IGF-I and IGF-II, low-affinity binding exists between IGFs and insulin receptors.[52] Homology also exists between the type I IGF receptor, which has a higher affinity for IGF-I than for IGF-II, and the insulin receptor, with the consequence that cross binding is possible with insulin binding to the IGF-I receptor with lower affinity, however, than for IGF-I or IGF-II. A second IGF receptor that is not structurally homologous to the insulin or IGF-I receptor binds IGF-II with an affinity much higher than for IGF-I and binds insulin very poorly.[53] The relative ratio of these various receptors is tissue-specific and, as a result, the relative potencies of IGF-I and IGF-II differ from those of insulin, depending on the tissue being studied.[54]

Given the relative insulin-like potency and the 2,000 to 3,000-fold higher plasma concentration of the IGFs, most of the plasma IGF activity must exist in an inactive form, otherwise permanent hypoglycemia would result. The carrier protein may play a vital role in controlling the biologic action of plasma IGFs because it abolishes the acute insulin-like action of the free polypeptides, restricts their permeability through membranes, and interferes with receptor binding.[52,55–57] It is possible that these factors act locally, before they are bound by carrier proteins, by autocrine or paracrine processes rather than the classical endocrine mechanism. Therefore, the plasma levels of these IGFs do not necessarily reflect their physiologic expression or activity.

Although it has not yet been proved, evidence is accumulating consistent with the hypothesis that IGFs do indeed influence fetal growth. Four lines of evidence point to this possibility. First are the studies that demonstrate that IGFs are capable of stimulating the proliferation of fetal cells from various species, including humans. Second, both type I and II IGF receptors have been identified and partially purified from fetal tissues. The third line of evidence comes from studies that show that fetal plasma IGFs are of fetal origin, since they are not transported from mother to fetus by the placenta, and several studies have demonstrated the direct synthesis of IGFs by fetal fibroblasts, limb bud mesenchyma, intestine, heart, brain, kidney, liver, and lung. Finally, although IGF concentrations in fetal plasma are low compared with adults, positive correlations between plasma IGFs and newborn weight, length, and placental weights have been observed.[58]

Several studies have investigated the relationship between birthweight and plasma concentration of growth factors believed to be involved in the control of fetal growth in humans. In a study in which IGF-I and IGF-II and their binding proteins were measured in utero by cord puncture between 20 and 37 weeks' gestation or taken at delivery between 38 and 42 weeks, IGF-I levels were significantly increased in fetuses whose weights were higher than the mean weight. Conversely, those SGA fetuses had significantly reduced IGF-I levels, whereas IGF-II levels did not correlate with weight.[59] Both fetal umbilical IGF-I and insulin concentrations are elevated in IDMs and low in IUGR neonates.[60] In a study of more than 500 pregnancies, both IGF-I and IGF-II were found to correlate with fetal growth and weight, with IGF-I levels correlating best with weight. However, by 36 weeks' gestation, IGF-I levels have reached their peak and begin to decline while fetal weight gain continues. Consistent with the hypothesis that hyperinsulinemia is responsible for fetal overgrowth are the elevated plasma C-peptide and presumably insulin levels found in large-for-gestational-age (LGA) fetuses.[61]

Although there is abundant evidence that IGF-I and IGF-II receptors are present in the fetus, their role in the control of fetal growth has not been experimentally established. The introduction of an inactivated IGF-II gene yields heterozygous progeny that are growth-retarded, weighing only 60 percent of normal birthweight. The difference in weight persists into adulthood. This study provides the first direct evidence that IGF-II plays a physiologic role in fetal growth.[62] A line of transgenic mice has been produced that overexpress IGF-I in most tissue and have plasma levels of IGF-I that are approximately 50 percent higher than normal.[63] Newborn pups from this line are of normal weight and size compared with controls and continue to be similar to controls until 1.5 months of age. From that point on, the transgenic animals become heavier than the control animals so that at 6 months they weigh 25 percent more than the controls. These studies confirm that IGF-I is a potent stimulator of postnatal growth but not of fetal growth.

Mouse embryos from two lines of mice bred for having low and high adult IGF-I levels have been transplanted into a neutral line of mice at day 4 of gestation. At day 19 of gestation, the fetuses were delivered and weighed. As expected, mean fetal weight and litter size were negatively correlated. Embryos from the high IGF-I line weighed more than those of the low IGF-I line, irrespective of litter size. Because IGF-I, insulin, or metabolic substrate levels were not measured in the fetuses, it is premature to suggest that these studies provide direct evidence that IGF-I plays a key role in controlling fetal growth.[64]

The hyperinsulinemic fetal rhesus model has been used to study changes in IGF levels associated with hyperinsulinemia.[65] No significant increase in total fetal IGFs measured by a radioreceptor assay was found when grouped data were compared. However, regression analysis revealed a significant correlation between fetal insulin and total fetal IGF, with IGF levels being increased only when very high insulin levels were present. The macrosomia in these monkey fetuses correlates with both insulin and IGFs. The linear relationship between fetal birthweight ratio and IGFs

up to 0.5 U/ml in control and hyperinsulinemic fetuses is consistent with the possibility that IGFs influence normal fetal growth. Excess fetal weight in humans and monkeys is present even when IGF levels are in the normal range when hyperinsulinemia is present. This is consistent with the hypothesis that excess insulin is responsible for the excess weight gain of the fetus carried by the mother with diabetes during pregnancy.

FETUS OF THE PREGNANT WOMAN WITH DIABETES

Although genetic factors are the major controlling factors of fetal growth during the first half of gestation,[66,67] other factors become more important in controlling growth during the last trimester. During the last trimester, nutritional, hormonal, metabolic, and environmental factors become of prime importance. In fact, adequacy of nutrient supply to the fetus ultimately controls the increase of fetal weight from approximately 1.6 kg to 3.2 kg during the 3-month period. It is during this interval that the growth rate of the fetus carried by a diabetic mother is most susceptible to alteration and during this interval that the root cause of the macrosomia of these fetuses may be found.

Many studies have confirmed that when gestational age is taken into account, the IDM has excessive body weight compared with control infants. Pedersen[18] reports that the weight increase is approximately 500 g for a series of 122 live births. In a much larger series of 1,809 deliveries in Karlsburg, the weight of IDMs exceeded the age-matched control weight by 500 to 600 g from 34 to 39 weeks' gestation.[19] Even though autopsy data are skewed to those diabetic pregnancies with greater morbidity, increased body weight was found in a small series of 30 IDMs of at least 36 weeks' gestational age.[38] In an autopsy study that tried to account for maternal complications in a population of pregnant diabetic women in Sweden, the birthweight was increased overall. Diabetic mothers with more severe complications such as angionephropathy or hypertensive disorders (or both) delivered infants whose birthweights were lower than normal.[39]

There is disagreement on the effect of maternal diabetes on fetal length. Naeye[38] reported that body length of IDMs at autopsy was 112 percent of control. Farquhar[68] also reported increased length in the IDMs delivered in Boston and Edinburgh. Autopsy data obtained in Sweden[39] indicated no increase in birth length in the IDMs. Although no increase in length in relation to gestational age was found, those infants who were heavier also tended to be longer and vice versa. These data suggest that birth length is a function of birthweight but not necessarily influenced by maternal diabetes. Pedersen compared the birth length of IDMs with weight-matched controls over a weight range of 2,250 to 5,100 g and found no significant difference between the two groups. A correlation of weight to length was identical to infants of nondiabetic mothers over the entire weights and gestational ages studied.[69] These findings are consistent with the hypothesis that the increased growth of the IDMs manifests itself as increased fetal weight due to overnutrition rather than to length-increasing stimuli.

Evidence has been obtained that insulin-sensitive tissue growth rate is accelerated in the fetus of the diabetic mother when assessed by ultrasound measurement of abdominal diameter as compared with biparietal diameter, an example of insulin-insensitive tissue.[70] There are other clinical fetal macrosomia syndromes in which fetal hyperinsulinemia has been reported.[43] These include the Beckwith-Wiedeman syndrome, infant giants, B-cell hyperplasia or adenomatosis, and nesidioblastosis. By contrast, IUGR and insulinopenia are associated with transient neonatal diabetes mellitus and pancreatic agenesis.

More than 100,000 LGA infants are born each year in the United States.[71] These pregnancies are characterized by increased maternal and neonatal morbidity and mortality.[72] The definition of fetal macrosomia is not clear and varies between 4,000 to 4,536 g.[73–75] The most common definition in use is a birthweight equal to or greater than 4,000 g. However, a more appropriate approach would be to define large infants as LGA when the 90th percentile or greater for a given gestational age is used as the threshold for abnormality.

Two types of macrosomic infants can be identified: (1) constitutional macrosomia, which represents the genetic drive to growth—this infant is LGA (≥90th percentile) already in the second trimester and will continue to grow on its own growth curve during pregnancy; and (2) metabolic macrosomia, which represents diabetic fetopathy as a result of abnormal glucose metabolism—this infant is characterized by increased liver and spleen size (greater abdominal circumference) and normal head size (head circumference). In addition, this infant suffers from an enlarged heart and increased subcutaneous fat.[76,77]

Clinical studies have demonstrated that large infants may be associated with even a mild degree of hyperglycemia. It was shown that with a positive glucose screening (>140) and normal OGTT results, there was a significantly higher rate of macrosomia.[78] Furthermore, for women who were nondiabetic (normal GTT by the National Diabetes Data Group), a direct association was found between the 2-hour glucose values and macrosomia.[79] In our studies, women with one abnormal value on the GTT were metabolically (level of glycemia) similar to subjects with gestational diabetes mellitus (GDM) before treatment but had a 30 percent rate of large infants.[80] In another study, patients with one abnormal value on the OGTT were randomized into treated and untreated groups. Macrosomia resulted in 6 percent versus 12 percent in the treated and untreated groups of infants, respectively.[81]

Langer et al[27] found that the rate of macrosomia increased significantly as blood glucose levels increased. There was a 12-fold higher relative risk in the rate of macrosomia for patients with mean blood glucose of more than 114 mg/dl when compared with patients with mean blood glucose levels of less than 81 mg/dl. Also, there was a fourfold increase when patients with mean blood glucose levels of more than 114 mg/dl were compared with those subjects with mean blood glucose levels of 95 mg/dl.[27]

CONCLUSION

The mechanism by which insulin stimulates fetal growth is not yet clear. It may cause its effect by altering metabolic substrate entry into cells and subsequently diverting their metabolic fate into anabolic processes such as lipogenesis, glycogenesis, and protein synthesis. It may also exert its growth-promoting effect by influencing other endocrine, paracrine, and autocrine systems, which produce other growth factors that then stimulate growth. The unraveling of the mechanism of insulin's stimulation of fetal overgrowth is not yet possible.

Figure 6-4 illustrates the relationship between fetal birthweight and fetal plasma insulin concentration. The birthweight ratio of human infants of diabetic and

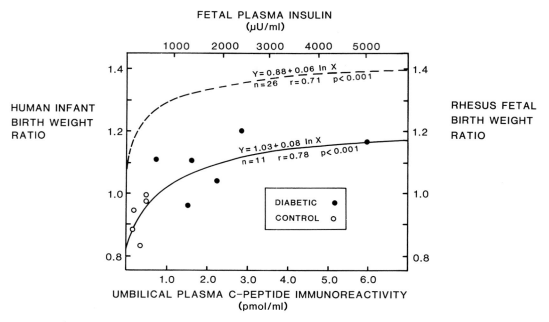

Fig. 6-4. Correlation of human infant birthweight ratio on the left ordinate with human umbilical plasma C-peptide immunoreactivity on the lower abscissa, represented by the solid line, described by $y = 1.03 + 0.08 \ln x$, compared with the correlation of rhesus fetal birthweight ratio on the right ordinate with rhesus umbilical artery plasma insulin concentration on the upper abscissa, represented by the dashed line, described by $y = 0.88 + 0.06 \ln x$. (From Susa and Schwartz,[86] with permission.)

nondiabetic mothers is plotted as the solid line against the fetal C-peptide immunoreactivity, which reflects fetal insulin levels. Even in this small population, a highly significant logarithmic correlation exists. The similarity between human and nonhuman primate birthweight ratio after fetal hyperinsulinemia is apparent when the logarithmic correlation, plotted as a dashed line, between rhesus birthweight ratio and plasma insulin concentration is compared with the human data.

The animal model that produces a fetopathy most similar to that of the human IDM is the streptozotocin-diabetic pregnant rhesus monkey. The rhesus and human fetus develop glucose-responsive insulin secretion and tissue insulin sensitivity during the last third of gestation. Fetal macrosomia is the result of fetal hyperinsulinemia during the latter part of the diabetic pregnancy. Other human clinical conditions such as Beckwith-Wiedeman syndrome, infant giants, nesidioblastosis, and islet adenomatosis are also associated with excess fetal weights. In utero hyperinsulinemia is

common to all these macrosomia syndromes. Much of the fetopathy found in these syndromes can be produced by experimentally inducing hyperinsulinemia by the direct infusion of insulin into the fetal rhesus monkey.

Differences between the human diabetes, animal models of diabetes, or animal studies designed to investigate specific elements of the disease state much be recognized, since they are not identical pathologic states. Table 6-2 summarizes the similarities in pathophysiology found in two human fetal macrosomia syndromes and their two nonhuman primate models. The concordance between the human and nonhuman primates illustrates the value of the animal models. The similarities justify the extrapolation of data and conclusions derived from nonhuman primate experiments to help clinical scientists better understand human pathology such as diabetes during pregnancy.

The association between the level of glycemia and neonatal morbidity, mainly fetal macrosomia and its consequences, provides the foundation for under-

Table 6-2. Similarities in Pathophysiology of Fetal Macrosomia Syndromes

	Human		Nonhuman Primate	
	IDM	Islet Adenomatosis	STZ Diabetes	Primary Hyperinsulinemia
Fetal hyperglycemia	+	−	+	−
Fetal hyperinsulinemia	+	+	+	+
Fetal macrosomia	+	+	+	+
Fetal organomegaly	+	+	?	+
Placental hyperplasia	+	?	+	+
Intrauterine death	+	+	+	+
β-Cell hyperplasia	+	+	+	−
Congenital anomalies	+	?	−	−

Abbreviations: IDM, infant of a diabetic mother; STZ, streptozotocin.
(From Susa and Schwartz,[86] with permission.)

standing the rationale for treatment of the pregnant diabetic patient. Also, it supports the Pedersen hypothesis that maternal hyperglycemia results in fetal hyperinsulinemia and macrosomia. Finally, the importance of tight glycemic control on perinatal outcome has been demonstrated.[82–85] Although a direct relationship exists between the tight glycemic control and macrosomia, it is not yet clear what threshold should be targeted to prevent macrosomia.

ACKNOWLEDGMENTS

We are indebted to our colleagues, particularly Dr. Robert Schwartz, for their valuable support and advice. Research support has been provided by the National Institutes of Health (HD-11343 and RR-00168), the Hood Foundation, and the Rhode Island Hospital Research Fund.

REFERENCES

1. Vorherr H: Factors influencing fetal growth. Am J Obstet Gynecol 142:577, 1982
2. Milner RDG, Hill DJ: Fetal growth control: the role of insulin and related peptides. Clin Endocrinol 21:415, 1874
3. Jost A: Endocrine factors in fetal development. Triangle 5:189, 1962
4. Little B, Smith OW, Jessiman AG et al: Hypophysectomy during pregnancy in a patient with cancer of the breast. J Clin Endocrinol 18:425, 1958
5. Stein Z, Suser M, Rush D: Prenatal nutrition and birth weights: experiments and quasi-experiments in the past decade. J Reprod Med 21:287, 1978
6. Rosenfeld CR: Considerations of the uteroplacental circulation in intrauterine growth. Semin Perinatol 8:42, 1984
7. Honda M, Toyoda C, Nakabayashi M, Omori Y: Quantitative investigations of placental terminal villi in maternal diabetes mellitus by scanning and transmission electron microscopy. Tohoku J Exp Med 167:247, 1992
8. Elliott BD, Langer O, Valdez M: Fetal placental blood flow is affected by maternal profile in diabetic pregnancies. Am J Obstet Gynecol 170:313A, 1994
9. Elliott BD, Langer O: Fetal placental blood flow in a population at risk for growth abnormalities and placental insufficiency. Am J Obstet Gynecol 170:314A, 1994
10. Dawes GS: Foetal and Neonatal Physiology: The Placental and Foetal Growth. Year Book Medical Publishers, Chicago, 1968
11. Behrman RE: Placental function and malnutrition. Am J Dis Child 129:425, 1975
12. Molteni RA, Stys SJ, Battaglia FC: Relationship of fetal and placental weight in human beings: fetal/placental weight ratios at various gestational ages and birth weight distributions. J Reprod Med 21:327, 1978
13. Resnik R: Maternal diseases associated with abnormal fetal growth. J Reprod Med 21:315, 1978
14. Porter DG: Fetal-maternal relationships: the actions and control of certain placental hormones. Placenta 1:259, 1980
15. Kastrup KW, Andersen JH, Lebech P: Somatomedin in newborns and the relationship to human chorionic so-

matotropin and fetal growth. Acta Paediatr Scand 67:757, 1978

16. Hurley TW, D'Ercole AJ, Handwerger S et al: Ovine placental lactogen induces somatomedin: a possible role in fetal growth. Endocrinology 101:1635, 1977

17. Freinkel N: Of pregnancy and progeny. Diabetes 19:1023, 1980

18. Pedersen J: Weight and length at birth of infants of diabetic mothers. Acta Endocrinol 16:330, 1954

19. Gödel E, Amendt P, Amendt U, Albrecht G: Diabetes und schwangershafteine klinische und statistiche analyse von 1800 schwangershaften und entbindungen aus den jahren 1952 vix 1971. 3. Mitteelung: Geburtsgewichtsperzentilwerte von neugenborenen diabertischer Mütter und weitere untersuchungen zun gebertsgewicht. Abl Gynäh 97:1435, 1975

20. Freinkel N, Metzger BE: Pregnancy as a tissue culture experience: the critical implications of maternal metabolism for fetal development. p. 3. In Ciba Foundation Symposium no. 63: Pregnancy, Metabolism, Diabetes and the Fetus. Excerpta Medica, Amsterdam, 1979

21. Langer O: Prevention of macrosomia. p. 333. In Oats JN (ed): Diabetes in Pregnancy. WB Saunders, Philadelphia, 1991

22. Abell DA: The significance of abnormal glucose tolerance (hyperglycaemia and hypoglycaemia) in pregnancy. Br J Obstet Gynaecol 86:214, 1979

23. Langer O, Damus K, Maiman M et al: A link between relative hypoglycemia-hypoinsulinemia during oral glucose tolerance tests and intrauterine growth retardation. Am J Obstet Gynecol 155:711, 1986

24. Sokol RJ, Kazzi GM, Kalhan SC, Pillay SK: Identifying the pregnancy at risk for intrauterine growth retardation: possible usefulness of the intravenous glucose tolerance test. Am J Obstet Gynecol 143:220, 1982

25. Khouzami VA, Ginsburg DS, Daikoku NH, Jonson JWC: The glucose tolerance test as a means of identifying intrauterine growth retardation. Am J Obstet Gynecol 139:423, 1981

26. Economides DL, Nicolaides KH: Blood glucose and oxygen tension levels in small-for-gestational-age fetuses. Am J Obstet Gynecol 160:385, 1989

27. Langer O, Levy J, Brustman L et al: Glycemic control in gestational diabetes mellitus—how tight is tight enough: small for gestational age versus large for gestational age? Am J Obstet Gynecol 161:646, 1989

28. Mintz DH, Chez RA, Hutchinson DL: Subhuman primate pregnancy complicated by streptozotocin-induced diabetes mellitus. J Clin Invest 51:837, 1972

29. Cheek DB, Hill DE: Changes in somatic growth after ablation of maternal or fetal pancreatic beta cells. p. 299. In Cheek DB (ed): Fetal and Postnatal Cellular Growth. Wiley, New York, 1975

30. Adam PAJ, Teramo K, Räiha N et al: Human fetal insulin metabolism early in gestation. Diabetes 18:409, 1969

31. Susa JB, McCormick KL, Widness JA et al: Chronic hyperinsulinemia in the fetal rhesus monkey. Effects on fetal growth and composition. Diabetes 28:1058, 1979

32. McCormick KL, Susa JB, Widness JA et al: Chronic hyperinsulinemia in the fetal rhesus monkey. Effects on hepatic enzymes active in lipogenesis and carbohydrate metabolism. Diabetes 28:1064, 1979

33. Widness JA, Susa JB, Garcia JF et al: Increased erythropoiesis and elevated erythropoietin in infants born to diabetic mothers and in hyperinsulinemic rhesus fetuses. J Clin Invest 67:637, 1981

34. Kühl C, Andersen GE, Hertel J, Molsted-Pedersen L: Metabolic events in infants of diabetic mothers during the first 24 hours after birth. I. Changes in plasma glucose, insulin and glucagon. Acta Paediatr Scand 71:19, 1982

35. Susa JB, Neave C, Sehgal PK et al: Chronic hyperinsulinemia in the rhesus monkey fetus. Effects of physiologic hyperinsulinemia on fetal growth and composition. Diabetes 33:656, 1984

36. Susa JB, Gruppuso PA, Widness JA et al: Chronic hyperinsulinemia in the rhesus monkey. Effects of physiologic hyperinsulinemia on fetal substrates, hormones, and hepatic enzymes. Am J Obstet Gynecol 150:415, 1984

37. Mellits ED, Hill DE, Kallman CH: Growth of visceral organs in the fetus. p. 20a. In Cheek DB (ed): Fetal and Postnatal Cellular Growth. Wiley, New York, 1975

38. Naeye RL: Infants of diabetic mothers: a quantitative morphologic study. Pediatrics 35:980, 1965

39. Hultquist GT, Olding LB: Endocrine pathology of infants of diabetic mothers. Acta Endocrinol Scand, suppl. 241:97, 1981

40. Simmons MA, Jones MD, Battaglia FC, Meschia G: Insulin effect on fetal glucose utilization. Pediatr Res 12:90, 1978

41. Hay WW, Meznarich HK, Sparks MA et al: The effect of insulin on fetal glucose utilization and oxidation. Pediatr Res 18:294a, 1984

42. Carson BS, Phillips AF, Simmons MA et al: Effects of a sustained insulin infusion upon glucose uptake and oxygenation of the ovine fetus. Pediatr Res 14:147, 1980

43. Hill DE: Fetal effects of insulin. Obstet Gynecol Ann 11:133, 1982

44. Persson B: Insulin as a growth factor in the fetus. p. 213. In Ritzen M (ed): The Biology of Normal Human Growth. Raven Press, New York, 1981

45. Reynolds WA, Chez RA: Observations on the tissue lipids of infants born to diabetic monkeys. Lipid composition of tissue. p. 323. In Cheek DB (ed): Fetal and Postnatal Cellular Growth. Wiley, New York, 1975

46. Hertel J, Andersen GE, Brandt NJ et al: Metabolic events in infants of diabetic mothers during the first 24 hours

after birth. III. Changes in plasma amino acids. Acta Paediatr Scand 71:33, 1981

47. Martins EA, Neave C, Susa JB, Singer DB: The effect of insulin on the size of skeletal muscle fibers of fetal rhesus monkey. Pediatr Pathol 6:377, 1985

48. Susa JB, Boylan JM, Sehgal PK, Schwartz R: Impaired insulin secretion in the neonatal rhesus monkey after chronic hyperinsulinemia in utero. Proc Soc Exp Biol Med 194: 209, 1990

49. Susa JB, Boylan JM, Sehgal P, Schwartz R: Impaired insulin secretion following i.v. glucose in neonatal rhesus monkeys that had been chronically hyperinsulinemic in utero. Proc Soc Exp Biol Med 199:327, 1992

50. Susa JB, Boylan JM, Sehgal P, Schwartz R: Persistence of impaired insulin secretion in infant rhesus monkeys that had been hyperinsulinemic in utero. J Clin Endocrinol Metab 75:265, 1992

51. Susa JB, Sehgal P, Schwartz R: Rhesus monkeys made exogenously hyperinsulinemic in utero as fetuses, display abnormal glucose homeostasis as pregnant adults and have macrosomic fetuses. Diabetes, suppl. 2, 42:86A, 1993

52. Zapf J, Schmid C, Froesch ER: Biological and immunological properties of insulin-like growth factors (IGF) I and II. Clin Endocrinol Metab 13:3, 1984

53. Hill DJ, Milner RDG: Insulin as a growth factor. Pediatr Res 19:879, 1985

54. Nissley SP, Rechler MM: Somatomedin/insulin-like growth factor tissue receptors. Clin Endocrinol Metab 13:43, 1984

55. Hintz RL: Plasma forms of somatomedin and the binding protein phenomenon. Clin Endocrinol Metab 13:31, 1984

56. Hill DJ, Clemmons DR: Similar distribution of insulin-like growth factor binding proteins -1, -2, -3 in human fetal tissues. Growth Factors 6:315, 1992

57. McCusker RH, Busky WH, Dehoff MH et al: Insulin-like growth factor (IGF) binding to cell monolayers is directly modulated by the addition of IGF-binding proteins. Endocrinology 129:939, 1991

58. Underwood LE, D'Ercole AJ: Insulin and insulin-like growth factors/somatomedins in fetal and neonatal development. Clin Endocrinol Metab 13:60, 1984

59. Lassarre C, Hardouin S, Daffos F et al: Serum insulin-like growth factors and insulin-like growth factor binding proteins in the human fetus. Relationships with growth in normal subjects and in subjects with intrauterine growth retardation. Pediatr Res 29:219, 1991

60. Delmis J, Drazancic A, Ivanisevic M et al: Glucose, insulin, HGH and IGF-1 levels in maternal serum, amniotic fluid and umbilical venous serum: a comparison between late normal pregnancy and pregnancies complicated by diabetes and fetal growth retardation. J Perinat Med 20:47, 1992

61. Verhaeghe J, Van Bree R, Van Herek E et al: C-peptide, insulin-like growth factors I and II, and insulin-like growth factor binding protein-1 in umbilical cord serum: correlations with birth weight. Am J Obstet Gynecol 169: 89, 1993

62. DeChiara TM, Eftratiadis A, Robertson EJ et al: A growth-deficient phenotype in heterozygous mice carrying an insulin-like growth factor-II gene disrupted by targeting. Nature 345:78, 1990

63. Mathews LS, Hammer RE, Behringer RR et al: Growth enhancement of transgenic mice expressing human insulin-like growth factor-I. Endocrinology 123:2827, 1988

64. Gluckman PD, Morel PCH, Ambler GR et al: Elevating maternal insulin-like growth factor-I in mice and rats alters the pattern of fetal growth by removing maternal constraint. J Endocrinol 134:R1, 1992

65. Susa JB, Widness JA, Hintz R et al: Somatomedins and insulin in diabetic pregnancies: effects on fetal macrosomia in the human and rhesus monkey. J Clin Endocrinol Metab 58:1099, 1984

66. Persson PH, Grennert L, Gennser G: Impact of fetal and maternal factors on the normal growth of the biparietal diameter. Acta Obstet Gynecol Scand, suppl. 78:21, 1978

67. Weingold AB: Intrauterine growth retardation: obstetrical aspects. J Reprod Med 14:244, 1975

68. Farquhar JW: Maternal hyperglycaemia and foetal hyperinsulinemia in diabetic pregnancy. Postgrad Med J 38: 612, 1962

69. Pedersen J: The Pregnant Diabetic and Her Newborn. 2nd Ed. Williams & Wilkins, Baltimore, 1977

70. Ogata ES, Sabbagha R, Metzger BE et al: Serial ultrasonography to assess evolving fetal macrosomia. Studies in 23 pregnant diabetic women. JAMA 243:2405, 1980

71. United States Bureau of Vital Statistics: Vital statistics for the United States. Vol 1. Natality. USBVS, Washington, DC, 1970

72. Langer O: Diabetes in pregnancy. p. 979. In Merkatz IR, Cherry SH (eds): Medical, Surgical and Gynecologic Complications of Pregnancy. 4th Ed. Williams & Wilkins, Baltimore, 1991

73. Sack RA: The large infant. Am J Obstet Gynecol 104:195, 1969

74. Golditch IM: The large fetus: management and outcome. Obstet Gynecol 52:26, 1978

75. Modanlou HD, Dorchester WL, Thorosian A et al: Macrosomia—maternal, fetal and neonatal implications. Obstet Gynecol 55:420, 1980

76. Langer O, Kozlowski S, Brustman L: A longitudinal study: different abnormal growth patterns in diabetes in pregnancy. Isr J Med Sci 27:516, 1991

77. Langer O, Kagan-Hallet K: Diabetic vs. non-diabetic infants: a quantitative morphological study. Proceedings of the 38th Annual Meeting of the Society for Gynecologic Investigation, San Antonio, Texas, 1992

78. Leikin EL, Jenkins JH, Pomerantz GA, Klein L: Abnormal glucose screening tests in pregnancy: a risk factor for fetal macrosomia. Obstet Gynecol 69:570, 1987

79. Tallarigo L, Giampietro O, Penno G et al: Relation of glucose tolerance to complications of pregnancy in non-diabetic women. N Engl J Med 315:989, 1986

80. Langer O, Brustman L, Anyaegbunam A: The significance of one abnormal glucose tolerance test value on adverse outcome in pregnancy. Am J Obstet Gynecol 157:758, 1987

81. Langer O, Anyaegbunam A, Brustman L, Divon M: A prospective randomized study: management of women with one abnormal value (OGTT) reduces adverse outcome in pregnancy. Am J Obstet Gynecol 161:593, 1989

82. Roversi GD, Gargiulo M, Nicolina U et al: A new approach to the treatment of diabetic pregnancy women. Am J Obstet Gynecol 135:567, 1979

83. Coustan DR, Imarah J: Prophylactic insulin treatment of gestational diabetes reduces the incidence of macrosomia, operative delivery, and birth trauma. Am J Obstet Gynecol 150:834, 1984

84. Langer O: Management of gestational diabetes. Clin Perinatol 30:603, 1993

85. Langer O, Mazze RS: The relationship between large-for-gestational-age infants and glycemic control in women with GDM. Am J Obstet Gynecol 159:1478, 1988

86. Susa JB, Schwartz R: Effects of hyperinsulinemia in the primate fetus. Diabetes, suppl. 2, 34:36, 1985

7
Fetal Lung Development

SUSAN H. GUTTENTAG
ROBERTA A. BALLARD

Development and maturation of the fetal lung into a functioning organ at birth is influenced by the metabolic and hormonal milieu in which it develops. In diabetic pregnancy, abnormalities of this environment result in delayed fetal lung maturation. This was first suggested by Gellis and Hsia[1] in 1959 when they observed increased respiratory disease in infants of diabetic mothers (IDMs). Reports of increased risk of respiratory distress syndrome (RDS) in IDMs soon followed at a time when RDS became associated with pulmonary surfactant deficiency.[2,3] With the advent of methods to analyze surfactant components, it is now possible to predict the risk of RDS for an IDM. This, along with a better understanding of the effects of diabetic pregnancy on fetal lung maturity, has had a significant impact on reducing the risk of RDS to IDMs.

MATURATION OF THE FETAL LUNG

Fetal lung development includes structural development (formation of the tracheobronchial tree and alveoli) and functional development (cellular differentiation of the respiratory epithelium and the manufacture and secretion of surfactant). Complete reviews of this subject can be found elsewhere.[4,5] The laryngotracheal diverticulum evaginates from the primitive foregut at 4 weeks' gestation, ultimately giving rise to the larynx, trachea, bronchi, and pulmonary epithelium. By the end of the 24th week of gestation, branching of the tracheobronchial tree has extended to the respiratory bronchioles and alveolar ducts. The columnar respiratory epithelium thins to a more cubodial appearance by 24 weeks. At this point, vascularization of the primitive acinus is developed enough

to allow gas exchange in some infants. Progressive thinning of the alveolar interstitium and further acinar development followed by formation of alveoli continue through 36 weeks.

Differentiation of the respiratory epithelium begins as early as 20 to 24 weeks' gestation. Type I epithelial cells take on a more flattened appearance, comprising as much as 96 percent of the alveolar surface area at maturity. Type II epithelial cells are characterized by their cubodial appearance and the presence of lamellar bodies in the apical cytoplasm. Glycogen is found in large amounts within type II cell cytoplasm and decreases as lamellar bodies become more numerous. The lamellar body is the intracellular storage site of the tightly wound surfactant phospholipids. Although detectable by mid-gestation in human fetal lungs, surfactant is not usually excreted into the lung liquid and hence into amniotic fluid until after 30 weeks' gestation.

Changes in endogenous hormone concentration during development modulate the process of fetal lung maturation. In particular, endogenous glucocorticoids play an important role in normal fetal lung maturation, and this is the basis for exogenous glucocorticoid therapy in preterm labor to accelerate fetal lung maturity.[6] Thyroid hormone also seems to play a role in normal fetal lung maturation, whereas β-agonists appear to stimulate surfactant synthesis and cause release of surfactant.

Pulmonary surfactant is a complex mixture of lipids, phospholipids, and protein that possesses surface active properties.[6,7] The major component of surfactant is phospholipid (75 percent by weight), with the most abundant phospholipid being phosphatidylcholine (PC), predominantly disaturated PC (DSPC) (Fig. 7-1). Phosphatidyglycerol (PG), present as 8 percent of the

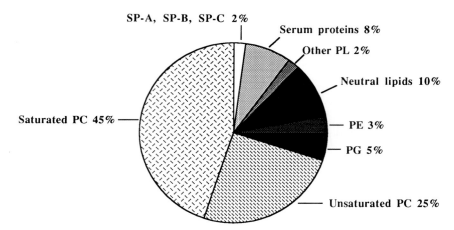

Fig. 7-1. Components of human pulmonary surfactant (given as a percentage by weight). PL, phospholipids; PE, phosphatidylethanolamine.

phospholipid fraction, appears late in gestation and may play an important role in ordering and disordering the phospholipid monolayer.[8] The presence of PG in amniotic fluid correlates well with fetal lung maturity.

The surfactant phospholipids exist in several intracellular and extracellular forms and are densely packed into lamellar bodies that, when extruded from the type II alveolar cell, unravel their lamellar structure. Tubular myelin exists in the liquid hypophase as a lattice structure from which the phospholipid monolayer arises (Fig. 7-2). Each intermediate form is essential to the proper functioning of surfactant in the alveolus. Absence of any of these components has been linked to RDS, suggesting that phospholipid alone is insufficient for monolayer film formation and reduced surface tension.[9]

By weight, 5 to 10 percent of pulmonary surfactant is protein. Although most are serum proteins (i.e., albumin), at least four proteins are unique to surfactant: surfactant proteins A, B, C, and D (SP-A, SP-B, SP-C, and SP-D).[7] The surfactant proteins contribute to the proper functioning of surfactant in several ways, including facilitating the adsorption of phospholipids to the air–liquid interface of the alveolus, enhancing the surface tension-reducing ability of the phospholipids, and participating in the recycling of surfactant. Each of the surfactant proteins has unique functions, suggesting that their presence is essential to the proper functioning of pulmonary surfactant.

SP-A, a glycoprotein synthesized by the alveolar type II cell and bronchiolar Clara cell, is detected in human amniotic fluid by the 30th week of gestation.[10] Amniotic fluid SP-A concentration correlates well with surfactant phospholipid concentration during the third trimester. Absence of SP-A from amniotic fluid is associated with an increased incidence of RDS in preterm infants. However, it is of interest that commercially produced replacement surfactants do not generally contain SP-A, yet function very well in surfactant replacement therapy.

SP-B is a lipophilic protein synthesized by the alveolar type II cell and bronchiolar Clara cell. It is packaged with lipids in lamellar bodies and appears in amniotic fluid in the third trimester. SP-C is a true proteolipid containing two palmitic acid residues and is only synthesized by alveolar type II cells. SP-B and SP-C are present in differing concentrations in all naturally derived surfactant replacement preparations and appear to be essential for normal surfactant function. More complete reviews of the surfactant proteins can be found elsewhere.[11,12]

RESPIRATORY DISTRESS SYNDROME

Whereas structural lung immaturity can contribute to respiratory distress in the very-low-birthweight infant, deficiency of surfactant and, in some instances, abnor-

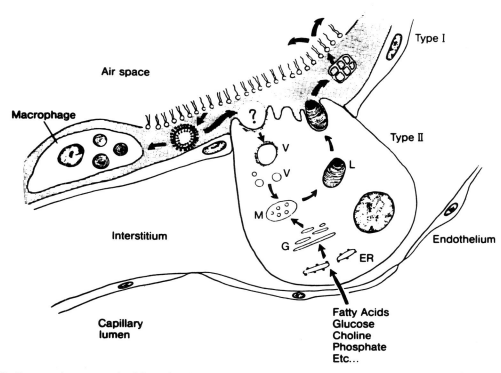

Fig. 7-2. Proposed events in the life cycle of surfactant. Secreted surfactant forms tubular myelin, which generates a monolayer of saturated phosphatidycholine at the aqueous interface. Phospholipid leaving the monolayer may be ingested by macrophages or recycled into the type II cell as vesicles. ER, endoplasmic reticulum; G, golgi apparatus; M, multivesicular body; L, lamellar bodies; V, vesicles. (From Ballard,[4] with permission.)

mal surfactant, is primarily responsible for the clinical entity RDS.[13,14] The absence of functional surfactant in the alveolus leads to progressive, generalized atelectasis and results in restrictive pulmonary disease. The clinical syndrome is one of increasing work of breathing manifested as tachypnea and grunting as the affected infant attempts to maintain alveolar inflation. In severe cases, this leads to respiratory failure requiring ventilatory assistance as the disease progresses. The radiographic appearance, described as "ground glass," is homogeneous in distribution with progressive loss of lung volume. Before surfactant therapy was available, the disease typically worsened over the first 24 to 48 hours after birth, with improvement beginning after 72 hours. With the advent of surfactant therapies, the disease can be at least modified if not eradicated within the first 24 hours of life.

In early studies of diabetic pregnancy, the diagnosis of RDS was often complicated by transient tachypnea of the newborn (TTNB), which may have a similar initial clinical presentation. TTNB, or delayed clearance of fetal lung fluid, is generally distinguished from RDS by its shorter and less dramatic clinical course, with resolution of symptoms typically within 24 hours. These infants often require oxygen therapy but seldom require ventilatory assistance. Radiographically, excessive fluid is noted by the presence of engorged lymphatics of the lungs manifested as thickening of the fissures and pleural effusions, as well as pulmonary vascular haziness. Delayed clearance of lung water is more common in the preterm infant, particularly if delivered by cesarean section without labor. Therefore, there is often a component of TTNB contributing to neonatal respiratory disease.

Variables that through differing mechanisms affect the timing of surfactant maturation can markedly influence the incidence of RDS in a study population. Gender plays an important role in the incidence of RDS.[15,16] It has been suggested that fetal androgens delay the appearance of surfactant proteins and the increase in surfactant production in fetal type II alveolar cells.[17] This may explain the higher incidence of RDS in preterm male infants compared with females of similar gestational age. Race appears to play a role as well, resulting in lower RDS rates among black preterm infants, although the mechanism has yet to be defined.

Antenatal events can similarly influence RDS rates in a population. Elective preterm delivery alone will place an infant at increased risk of developing RDS. However, the risk may be modified by antenatal stressors that can promote early fetal lung maturation, such as maternal hypertension, placental vascular compromise, infection, and prolonged or preterm rupture of membranes.[18]

Route of delivery can influence the risk of respiratory disease, depending on the presence or absence of labor. The hormonal changes that occur during labor have an effect on the risks of both TTNB and RDS. Hormonal fluctuations at term, especially increases in catecholamines with labor, decrease fetal lung fluid volumes by reducing production and subsequently by increasing absorption. TTNB is increased in abdominal delivery without labor largely because the catecholamine stimulation of adrenergic receptors in the lung does not occur. RDS may also be increased in the absence of these catecholamine effects that normally promote surfactant release from pulmonary type II cells. Conversely, premature labor can stimulate both lung liquid mobilization and surfactant secretion through adrenergic receptors. In the presence of these potentially competing effects, it is difficult to assess the role of delivery route on the incidence of respiratory disease.

AMNIOTIC FLUID INDICES OF LUNG MATURITY

Antenatal assessment of surfactant maturity and the ability to predict the likelihood of RDS prenatally became possible in the 1970s.[19–22] In the preterm fetus, lung fluid is secreted in excess of its rate of reabsorption. This coupled with normal fetal breathing movements results in a net efflux of lung fluid into the amniotic fluid, which can be sampled and analyzed. In 1978, Kulovich, Hallman, and Gluck[22] showed that preterm infants who developed RDS had decreased amounts of surfactant phospholipid in amniotic fluid before delivery. Amniotic fluid levels of sphingomyelin and DSPC (lecithin) remain nearly equal until the third trimester when the amount of DSPC (lecithin) increases dramatically, typically after 35 weeks' gestational age. An amniotic fluid lecithin/sphingomyelin (L/S) ratio will begin to rise at this time. L/S ratios exceeding 2:1 are associated with fetal lung maturity and a reduced risk of RDS in uncomplicated pregnancies, and this typically occurs after 35 weeks' gestation. Other markers of surfactant sufficiency include amniotic fluid PG, detectable after 35 weeks' gestation,[21] and SP-A, first noted at 30 weeks then rising toward term.[10]

DIABETIC PREGNANCY AND FETAL LUNG MATURITY

In evaluating the impact of maternal diabetes on fetal lung maturation, it is important that investigators control for the factors mentioned above. Earlier studies describing rates as high as 37 percent (Table 7-1) seldom reported such critical variables as gender, race, or presence of labor in their control or study populations and tended to confuse the literature on RDS in

Table 7-1. Incidence of RDS in Infants of diabetic Mothers

Authors	Years	No. of Infants	Cesarean Section (%)	RDS (%)
Gellis and Hsia[1]	1940–56	711	72	33[a]
Usher et al[3]	1940–65	146	49	16[a]
Hubbell and Drorbaugh[2]	1956–64	473	70	27[a]
Robert et al[23]	1958–68	805	73	23[a]
Gabbe et al[24]	1971–75	260	55	6
Kitzmiller et al[25]	1975–76	147	70	7.6
Coustan et al[26]	1975–79	73	49	2.7
Drury et al[27]	1979–82	125	20	2.4
Dudley and Black[28]	1978–83	104	46	0

Abbreviation: RDS, respiratory distress syndrome.
[a] Percentages given represent infants with respiratory disease. Most of these infants were diagnosed as RDS or possible RDS.

diabetic pregnancy. In the following discussion, we highlight those studies that attempted to control for such variables and attempt to answer some important questions affecting management in the diabetic pregnancy.

Is RDS Risk Increased in Diabetic Pregnancy

In 1976, Robert et al[23] reported the outcome of 805 diabetic pregnancies over a 10-year period, comparing them with a cohort of 10,152 nondiabetic women. The uncorrected relative risk for developing RDS was 23.7. This is similar to other uncontrolled studies of the time. Their systematic analysis of potential confounding variables appears in Table 7-2. They found that the estimated gestational age (EGA) at delivery had an effect on the incidence of RDS in diabetic pregnancies as in nondiabetic pregnancies. After 38.5 weeks' EGA, RDS rates were not increased in diabetic pregnancies over control rates. Before 38.5 weeks' EGA, there remained an increased incidence of RDS over rates in nondiabetic pregnancy (Fig. 7-3). It should be remember, however, that management of diabetic pregnancies in this and other studies from the 1970s included elective delivery at ≤37 weeks for White's class B, C, D, and F diabetic pregnancies, which comprised 97.4 percent of the cohort. As expected, vaginal delivery was associated with a lowered risk of RDS in diabetic pregnancy, but abdominal delivery did not fully account for the risk differences between diabetic and nondiabetic cohorts. After controlling for all confounding variables, the relative risk of RDS for diabetic pregnancy with preterm delivery was still 5.6-fold higher than for nondiabetic pregnancies.

Table 7-2. Confounding Variables for Respiratory Distress Syndrome in Diabetic Pregnancy

Factors	Risk of RDS	Diabetic Cohort (%)	Nondiabetic Cohort (%)
Gestational age[1]			
30.5–32.4	↑	3	1
32.5–34.4	↑	8	1
34.5–36.4	↑	50	4
36.5–38.4	↓	35	13
38.5+	↓	2	80
Route of delivery			
Vaginal	↓	27	95
Cesarean section	↑	73	5
Absence of labor	↑	59	3
Type of labor			
Spontaneous	↓	18	83
Induced	0	23	14
None	↑	59	3
Birthweight (g)			
<3,000	↑	47	29
>3,000	↓	53	71
Infant sex			
Male	↑	49	52
Female	↓	51	48
Apgar score (5 min)			
<8	↑	44	18
9 or 10	↓	56	82
Antepartum hemorrhage	↑	1	7
Presence of hydramnios	↑	81	3
Maternal anemia	↑	8	4
Maternal age[b] (y)			
<20	↓	4	14
20–34	↑	85	77
>35	↓	11	9

[a] Median gestational age for diabetic cohort, 36 weeks; for nondiabetic cohort, 40 weeks.
[b] Median maternal age for diabetic cohort, 27 years; for nondiabetic cohort, 24 years.
(From Robert et al,[23] with permission.)

What Are the Mechanisms Leading to RDS in IDMs

An increased incidence of RDS implies that lung development in IDMs is altered from normal. What is it about diabetic pregnancy that predisposes to delayed fetal lung maturity? To attempt to answer this question, we must consider the metabolic and hormonal milieu in maternal diabetes that may influence the developing fetus. In 1961, Pederson and Osler[29] proposed that fetal macrosomia resulted from transplacental transport of glucose from a hyperglycemic mother to her fetus with its intact, functional pancreas. Fetal hyperglycemia thus resulted in fetal hyperinsulinemia and subsequently increased glycogen and fat deposition. Neonatal β-cell hyperplasia appeared to be the result of chronic hyperglycemia in diabetic pregnancy.[30] This became the basis for examining the roles of glucose and insulin in IDM-associated RDS. However, in addition to the primary effects of insulin and glucose, other metabolites and hormones may be altered in diabetic pregnancy secondarily influencing fetal lung maturity.

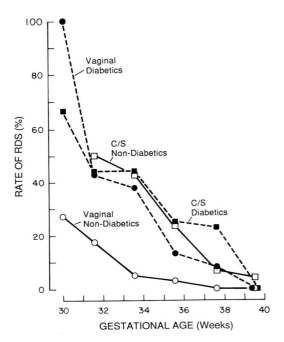

Fig. 7-3. Incidence of respiratory distress syndrome (RDS) according to gestational age and mode of delivery in diabetic and nondiabetic patients. (From Robert et al,[23] with permission.)

There are several methods of investigating these mechanisms, both in vitro and in vivo, and advantages and disadvantages to each. Although lung epithelium in culture seems the most direct way to investigate the effects of hormones on fetal lung, results of in vitro experiments can be difficult to interpret or to translate into whole animal effects. The concentrations of hormone used are often greater than may exist in situ. Changes in intracellular pool sizes and turnover rates of the surfactant components can be very difficult to assess. Options for in vivo experiments include chemical (streptozotocin, alloxan) and genetic (db mouse, BW rat) induction of diabetes in breeding or pregnant animals. This can produce highly variable degrees of maternal glycemia. Infusion pumps in chronically instrumented pregnant animals permit precise titration of maternal glucose and insulin levels, which is not possible in chemical and genetic models. The usefulness of an animal model depends on its success in duplicating the key features of human diabetic pregnancy, namely, fetal macrosomia, fetal hyperinsuli-

nemia with neonatal hypoglycemic episodes, and maternal glucose intolerance.

How Do the Hormonal Changes in Diabetic Pregnancy Delay Fetal Lung Maturity

Abnormalities in fetal lung maturation must be explained in the context of the role that endogenous hormones play in normal fetal lung maturation. Fetal lung maturity might be delayed either due to the presence of an abnormal inhibitor or due to the absence of a normal stimulator of fetal lung development. Alterations in the hormonal milieu of diabetic pregnancy present possibilities in both of the cases. Known inhibitors of cell differentiation and maturation in fetal lungs present in diabetic pregnancy include insulin, glucose, myoinositol, and β-hydroxybutyrate. Evidence also suggests that endogenous glucocorticoid[31] and thyroid hormone levels[32] may be suppressed by diabetes.

How Does Insulin Affect Fetal Lung Maturation

Insulin receptors are present on type II cells, and receptor numbers increase late in gestation in fetal rats and rabbits.[33] Unlike adult tissues, evidence suggests that increased insulin levels may increase receptor numbers in IDMs. Thus, the fetal lung is very susceptible to the effects of insulin. Lung cell culture studies have demonstrated little effect of lower insulin concentrations on choline incorporation into PC,[34] whereas higher concentrations appeared to decrease PC, DSPC, and PG production as well as impair glucose use. Low insulin concentrations have had similar effects on phospholipid production in explants[35,36] but also decreased type II cell number and the number of lamellar bodies per type II cell, suggesting that cell differentiation had been impaired.

The effect of insulin in the presence of glucocorticoid is more remarkable. Insulin may block the effects of glucocorticoid on cell cultures[34] and explants.[35] Insulin may abolish the glucocorticoid-induced rise in choline incorporation into PC and DSPC[37,38] and the expected rise in SP-A.[36] This evidence suggests that insulin may delay fetal lung maturation in two ways: through direct action on type II cells via insulin receptors (type II cell culture studies) and indirectly via lung fibroblasts (explant studies) probably by interfering with fibroblast pneumatocyte factor (FPF) stimulation of type II cells.[39]

An insulin-induced delay in fetal lung maturation is further supported by in vivo experiments. The hyperinsulinemic and euglycemic offspring of matings between db heterozygote females (db/+) and normal males are macrosomic and show delayed lung maturation. The lungs of these offspring show increased incorporation of label into DSPC but reduced incorporation of label into PG.[40] Morphologically, their lungs appear less mature than controls despite their increased size due to macrosomia. Low-dose streptozotocin (STZ) in rats produces euglycemic, hyperinsulinemic, macrosomic offspring.[41] In these animals, total lung DSPC is decreased but bronchoalveolar wash DSPC is unaffected. More significant decreases in phospholipids were noted by Merritt et al[42] and Neufeld and Melmed[43] in alloxan-treated rabbits whose offspring were hyperinsulinemic. Finally, chronic insulin infusion into fetal lambs produced tracheal fluid that contained 26 times less surface active material than controls.[44] Regardless of the method used, it is clear that insulin can delay fetal lung maturity.

How Does Hyperglycemia Affect Fetal Lung Maturation

Hyperglycemia can delay fetal lung maturation independently of insulin concentration. Possible mechanisms may relate to excessive or decreased bioavailability of important precursors for phospholipid production and surfactant protein modifications. Excessive amounts of glycogen noted in type II cells of hyperglycemic animals with normal insulin levels supports this notion.[41,45–47] In type II cell culture experiments, high glucose concentrations decrease incorporation of label into PC,[38] PG, and DSPC.[37] Insulin added to high glucose medium results in an additive effect on type II cells, significantly reducing both PG and DSPC production. High-dose STZ given to pregnant animals produces fetuses that are hyperglycemic with low-to-normal insulin levels. The fetal lungs exhibit abnormal lung morphology late in gestation, including reduction in basement membrane foot processes,[48] increased glycogen content,[41,47] and decreased numbers of type II alveolar cells and numbers of type II cell lamellar bodies.[47] Biochemically, there are more sig-

nificant aberrations late in gestation, with reduced production of DSPC, PC, and PG.[46,49–52] In rabbit fetuses of alloxan-treated mothers with no significant difference in lung phospholipid content, lung deflation stability (a reflection of surface activity) is reduced. Steroid administration in late gestation corrects the deficit,[53] suggesting that a steroid-inducible factor other than phospholipid may be responsible for the observed impaired alveolar stability. Surfactant protein production is inhibited in STZ pregnancy, with significant reductions of SP-A, SP-B, and SP-C,[54,55] which may explain altered alveolar stability in other models in which phospholipids are not affected.

How Do Other Hormones Altered in Diabetic Pregnancy Affect Lung Maturation

In addition to hyperinsulinemia and hyperglycemia, other metabolic and hormonal abnormalities exist during diabetic pregnancy that may result in altered fetal lung maturation. The transfer of substrates such as butyrate from mother to fetus depends on the concentration of substrate in the maternal circulation. β-Hydroxybutyrate has been shown to inhibit SP-A expression in fetal lung explants.[56] Maternal β-hydroxybutyrate levels are elevated in STZ-treated maternal rats,[41] and their fetuses show delayed SP-A accumulation.[54] More important, evidence exists that, at delivery, human infants of mothers with gestational diabetes have higher than normal β-hydroxybutyrate levels,[57] with levels paralleling maternal glycemia. This suggests an important role of β-hydroxybutyrate in delaying fetal lung maturation in poorly controlled diabetic pregnancy. Another metabolite that may play a role in diabetic pregnancy is myoinositol.[5] Myoinositol enhances surfactant phosphatidylinositol (PI) synthesis preferentially over PG synthesis. In rat and rabbit fetuses, plasma myoinositol levels are higher than in adults, and fetal levels fall toward term. This occurs at the same time that surfactant PG synthesis is increasing and PI synthesis is decreasing. In STZ and glucose infusion models of diabetic pregnancy, fetal hyperglycemia and hyperinsulinemia have been associated with persistently elevated fetal plasma myoinositol. The delayed appearance of PG in amniotic fluid (and the persistence of elevated PI levels) seen in human diabetic pregnancy may well be due to increased fetal myoinositol as a result of inadequately controlled maternal hyperglycemia.

As mentioned previously, it is equally possible that delayed fetal lung maturation results from a lack of stimulation by factors known to increase surfactant production late in gestation, as suggested by the results of insulin/cortisol experiments discussed above. Fetal levels of corticosterone, the primary endogenous glucocorticoid in the rat, are lower in STZ pregnancy.[31] This suggests that lower glucocorticoid levels may fail to stimulate surfactant component expression, contributing to delays in fetal lung maturity in STZ-induced diabetic pregnancy as well as in other models. However, studies clarifying the role of glucocorticoids in fetal rat lung development are inconsistent. Thyroid hormone deficiency may also contribute to delayed fetal lung maturation. IDMs have low cord triiodothyronine (T_3) levels.[32] Neufeld and Melmed[43] showed improvements in fetal lung maturity parameters when alloxan-induced diabetic rabbits were treated with a T_3 analog that crosses the placenta. Treatment did not have adverse effects on the pregnant alloxan rabbits. This suggests that therapy to correct deficiencies in endogenous hormones associated with diabetic pregnancy may help to normalize fetal lung maturation.

In summary, insulin and glucose inhibit aspects of fetal lung maturity, and the effects of both are additive. Other substances such as β-hydroxybutyrate and myoinositol may contribute to inhibition of surfactant component production. Impaired type II cell differentiation, morphologically and biochemically, results in decreased availability of surfactant components necessary for alveolar stabilization during air breathing. It is difficult to determine which components and which mechanisms are most critical in delaying fetal lung maturation in diabetic pregnancy. They do, however, suggest new avenues of investigation into prevention and treatment to reduce the risk of RDS in this population.

How Does White's Classification of Diabetes Mellitus in the Mother Affect RDS Risk in the Infant

Because the severity of diabetes varies with White's classification, both in terms of maternal complications and glycemic control, the effects on fetal lung development can be highly variable. The mix of patients in a study population can therefore affect the interpretation of results. Class B and C diabetic individuals represent a group of patients without end organ damage but with varying duration of diabetes. Consequently, fetal lung development and the risk of RDS in this group are difficult to assess or predict. Class B and C diabetic subjects dominate most study populations. The incidence of RDS in these groups has been reported by some to be higher than normal,[58,59] whereas others noted no differences.[60] In some cases among class B and C diabetics, additional stressors such as hypertension can accelerate fetal lung maturation.[61,62] Maternal glycemic control can be highly variable in this population as well. These factors may explain the controversy over the incidence of RDS in these groups.

Class D, F, and R diabetic individuals have some evidence of microvascular compromise resulting in end organ damage. Such vascular damage can present an independent stressor on the IDM. Placental compromise results in a higher incidence of intrauterine growth retardation and accelerated fetal lung maturation in this population, especially when associated with hypertension. These stressors tend to promote acceleration of fetal lung maturation. In their initial report of 27 diabetic pregnancies, Cunningham and colleagues[63] showed that class D diabetic pregnancies had the highest mean amniotic fluid PG levels, suggesting accelerated fetal lung maturation. Unlike class B and C diabetic pregnancies, class D through R diabetic pregnancies tend to be underrepresented in the literature, often as little as 15 percent of the diabetic study population, but they can potentially influence the interpretation of results in studies that analyze whole-population RDS risk.

Finally, RDS risk is elevated in infants of women with gestational diabetes[64,65] for several possible reasons. Individuals with gestational diabetes are more difficult to identify reliably as a population compared with class B through R diabetic patients, since they do not exhibit glucose intolerance before pregnancy. The interpretation of glucose tolerance testing is central to identifying these patients, and authors differ in the criteria used.[66] Testing is often performed only once and late in pregnancy, leaving little room for therapeutic intervention. Furthermore, there is disagreement on appropriate therapeutic goals for gestational diabetes, and patient compliance can be difficult.[67] This may lead to inadequate glycemic control, which has been shown to have an adverse effect on RDS risk.

How Does Maternal Glycemic Control Affect RDS Risk

Goals for glycemic control have changed in response to evidence showing that poor control leads to increased fetal morbidity and mortality. Table 7-3 shows that efforts to improve glycemic control improve fetal outcome. Karlsson and Kjellmer[65] in 1972 showed that within their strict control cohort, those pregnancies with mean blood glucose values of less than 100 mg/dl had lower mortality rates and a lower incidence of RDS. These results were echoed in subsequent studies attempting to lower fasting blood glucose goals even farther.[28,68–70] Improvements in glycemic control can improve amniotic fluid testing results as well as RDS incidence. McMahon et al.[71] showed no significant differences in amniotic fluid SP-A levels or in RDS incidence in a population of insulin-dependent diabetic gravidas who were strictly controlled and hospitalized when necessary to maintain tight glycemic control. In latter studies such as by Crombach et al,[72] strict control was associated with an increased number of episodes of maternal hypoglycemia but did not adversely affect fetal well-being. In most studies cited throughout this chapter, most of the diabetic study populations are made up of class B through R diabetic subjects who most often have been identified early in pregnancy.

Table 7-3. Maternal Glycemia and Neonatal Morbidity and Mortality in Diabetic Pregnancy

Authors	Population Characteristics[a]	Glycemic Goals[b]	Morbidity and Mortality
Dudley and Black[28]	$n = 104$ A = 0, B = 65, C = 18, D = 16, F = 2, R = 3	FBG <90 1-h postprandial BG < 145 in 93 of 104 patients Hb A_{1c} <0.8	No RDS
Karlsson and Kjellmer[65]	$n = 179$ Group I A = 7, B = 20, C = 29, D = 23, F + R = 5 Group II A = 13, B = 29, C = 31, D = 19, F + R = 4	Group I BG <150 Elective delivery at 35–37 wk Group II Keep BG as low as possible Aim for term delivery	RDS Mean BG <100 = 9/52 Mean BG >100 = 33/115, $P < .05$ Mortality rates Group I = 21.4% Group II = 9.4%, $P < .01$ Mean BG <100 = 2/52 Mean BG >100 = 21/115, $P < .05$
Tabsch et al[79]	$n = 95$ 93% B + C 7% D–R	FBG <100 Mean BG <120	RDS 3.9% of diabetic patients 1.5% of controls
Farrell et al[68]	$n = 40$ 14.8% A 52.6% B 31.6% C	Mean daily BG = 167 Hb A_{1c} 10.9% for controls 11.1% for diabetic patients	No RDS
Crombach et al[72]	$n = 112$	Euglycemia achieved in 9% from 1971–1980 79% from 1982–1988	Mortality 20.9% from 1971–1980 2.9% from 1982–1988 Morbidity 30–90% decrease in all morbidity except malformation rate
Kjos et al[74]	$n = 584$ 90% A 6% B 4% C–R	FBG <105	No RDS No TTNB
Piper and Langer[70]	$n = 289$ 100% A	2-h postprandial BG <105	RDS Total cases <37 wk 6/97 <34 wk, poor control = 4/14 <24 wk, good control = 25/207

[a] Letters refer to White's classification.
[b] All glucose measurements given as milligrams per deciliter.
Abbreviations: FBG, fasting blood glucose; BG, blood glucose; RDS, respiratory distress syndrome; Hb A_{1c}, hemoglobin A_{1c}; TTNB, transient tachypnea of the newborn.

Early, strict glycemic control in this population offers the greatest potential benefit in decreasing fetal morbidity and mortality.

In summary, diabetic patient populations exhibit significant variability in disease detection rates, severity, duration, and glycemic control, all of which have an effect on fetal lung maturity and RDS risk. Analysis of whole-population risk can be misleading in the face of such variability and should be considered when weighing the significance of study results. Future investigations should strive to control as many variables as possible, as well as to subanalyze results by White's classification to assure meaningful interpretations.

How Does Diabetic Pregnancy Alter Amniotic Fluid Fetal Lung Maturity Profiles

The L/S ratio, despite modifications in procedure since first described, has remained a specific as well as a sensitive marker of fetal lung maturity.[58,73–75] Its widespread use has contributed to an overall decrease in the number of preterm deliveries of IDMs. However, its usefulness in predicting RDS risk in the context of diabetic pregnancy has remained the topic of much debate. Several well-controlled studies show that the maturation of the L/S ratio does not differ in diabetic versus control pregnancies. In a study of 132 diabetic pregnancies of White's class B through R, Tchobroutsky et al[76] found no delay in the L/S ratio rise either between classes B and C diabetic patients and classes D, F, and R diabetic patients, or when each group was compared with accepted normal profiles. Kulovich and Gluck[64] included class A diabetic subjects in a similar study and found similar results. The controversy arises when the L/S ratio is used to predict the likelihood of RDS in an individual case. Several investigators have reported IDMs with RDS despite an L/S ratio of 2 to 3:1.[75,77–79]

If amniotic fluid PG is added to the fetal lung maturity profile, the significance of a single L/S ratio can be better interpreted.[63,74,80] As mentioned previously, PG is a late but sensitive and specific marker of fetal lung maturity. In diabetic pregnancies, the appearance of PG in amniotic fluid is delayed compared with nondiabetic pregnancy.[63,64,73,77] Hallman and Teramo,[80] in a study of 88 diabetic pregnancies, showed that with L/S of 2 or greater, amniotic fluid PG levels were lower than in gestational age-matched nondiabetic controls. Only 4 of the 88 infants developed RDS, and all had an L/S ratio of 2 to 3:1 but were PG-negative. Interestingly, the same amniotic fluid L/S ratio results were reported for 5 other infants who developed TTNB. Kulovich and Gluck[64] reported significantly delayed PG for class A IDMs when compared with controls and with other classes of IDM before 37 weeks' EGA. In two separate studies, Cunningham and colleagues also showed delayed PG appearance in diabetic pregnancy, with only 17 percent of amniotic fluid samples being positive for PG when L/S was 2 to 2.9:1.

Although not commonly performed, assays of amniotic fluid surfactant proteins, specifically SP-A, can be used in the assessment of fetal lung maturity. Amniotic fluid SP-A is detectable in amniotic fluid after 30 weeks' gestation, and levels may rise as early as 33 weeks. In a study of 10 diabetic pregnancies at 33 to 36 weeks' EGA, Katyal et al[81] reported that amniotic fluid SP-A measuring less than 2.1 μg/ml accurately predicted all cases (diabetic or nondiabetic) of RDS, regardless of L/S ratio. Three of the four IDMs developing RDS had L/S ratios greater than 2:1. In a later study by Snyder et al,[10] all reported amniotic fluid SP-A levels (diabetic and control) were greater than 2 μg/ml at delivery and no infants developed RDS. Most of the diabetic subjects studied were class A, eligible for short-term glycemic control due to diagnosis in the third trimester.

Although no single test of fetal lung maturity appears to be perfect in identifying IDMs at risk of RDS, a combination of tests appears to afford the greatest measure of confidence in establishing fetal lung maturity before delivery. Most often, the L/S ratio and amniotic fluid PG will suffice, although measurements of amniotic fluid SP-A may lend additional diagnostic certainty.

What Is the Bottom Line for Clinical Management

Diabetic pregnancy before the 1980s resulted in a significantly increased incidence of RDS. As management strategies such as those listed in Table 7-4 have evolved, that risk has decreased significantly. Preventive measures that have contributed to lowering the risk of RDS include aggressive maternal glycemic control regardless of White's classification, appropriate timing of the delivery using the vaginal route whenever possible, and liberal use of a profile amniotic fluid

Table 7-4. Prevention of RDS in IDMs

Detection
    Improved identification of gestational diabetes
Management
    Optimal glycemic and metabolic control
    Treatment of complications (e.g., preterm labor, infections, toxemia)
    Determination of fetal lung maturity by amniotic fluid phospholipid profile
    Early detection and management of fetal compromise
    Vaginal delivery when appropriate
Acceleration of fetal lung maturity
    Antenatal steroids
    Antenatal TRH

Abbreviations: RDS, respiratory distress syndrome; IDMs, infants of diabetic mothers; TRH, thyrotropin-releasing hormone.

analysis for markers of fetal lung maturity (both the L/S ratio and amniotic fluid PG level and occasionally SP-A presence). Like the clinical evidence, experimental observations support aggressive metabolic control of diabetic mothers to eliminate hyperglycemia and the resultant fetal hyperinsulinemia. Therapeutic interventions that reduce ketosis and normalize myoinositol levels, both consequences of poor glycemic control, would similarly reduce their effects on fetal lung maturity.

There are instances in which improvements in management are still needed. Unless gestational diabetic patients are aggressively sought out and managed, this group has the potential of predominating in the future as continuing at high risk for RDS.

Should Hormonal Therapy Be Used in Diabetic Pregnancies

There will still be occasions when delivery is indicated in the face of known fetal lung immaturity. In such cases, maternal therapies to accelerate fetal lung maturation should be considered. Recommendations of the National Institutes of Health Consensus Conference on Antenatal Steroids (1994) include administration of glucocorticoids when the fetus is younger than 34 weeks or has evidence of immature lungs and there is no specific maternal contraindication. Although maternal diabetes does not preclude glucocorticoid use, glucocorticoids may exacerbate glycemic control, leading to severe hyperglycemia and even ketoacidosis. This does not mean that glucocorticoids should not be used but rather that they should be used with caution. The role of combined hormone therapy with thyrotropin-releasing hormone (releases both thyroid hormones and prolactin) is currently being investigated and may provide additional benefit in these high-risk pregnancies.

CONCLUSION

Diabetic pregnancy is associated with a higher incidence of respiratory disease, especially RDS, in the premature newborn. Clinical and basic science research have led to a better understanding of the epidemiology and pathophysiology of both RDS and diabetic pregnancy and have provided some solutions to this problem. Obstetric management of diabetic pregnancy before the 1980s contributed significantly to RDS risk by promoting early, abdominal delivery of the gravid diabetic patient. Derangements in the metabolic and hormonal milieu of the developing fetus in poorly controlled diabetic pregnancy clearly delay fetal lung maturity, further increasing the risk of RDS. Improvements in obstetric management aimed at controlling maternal glycemia and eliminating metabolic and hormonal abnormalities, as well as efforts to promote vaginal delivery with mature amniotic fluid fetal lung profiles, have resulted in a dramatic decrease in the incidence of RDS among IDMs. Continued advances, including hormone therapy to accelerate fetal lung maturation when delivery is indicated despite known fetal lung immaturity, are likely to further reduce this risk.

REFERENCES

1. Gellis SS, Hsia DY-Y: The infant of diabetic mother. Am J Dis Child 97:1, 1959
2. Hubbell JP Jr, Drorbaugh JE: Infants of diabetic mothers: neonatal problems and their management. Diabetes 14:157, 1965
3. Usher R, Allen A, McLean F: Risk of respiratory distress syndrome related to gestational age, route of delivery, and maternal diabetes. Am J Obstet Gynecol 11:826, 1971
4. Ballard PL: Monographs on Endocrinology: Hormones and Lung Maturation. Springer-Verlag, New York, 1986

5. Boubon JR, Farrell PM: Fetal lung development in the diabetic pregnancy. Pediat Res 19:253, 1985

6. Ballard PL: Hormonal regulation of pulmonary surfactant. Endocr Rev 10:165, 1989

7. Possmayer F: A proposed nomenclature for pulmonary surfactant-associated proteins. Am Rev Respir Dis 138:990, 1988

8. Yu S, Possmayer F: Role of bovine pulmonary surfactant-associated proteins in the surface-active property of phospholipid. Biochim Biophys Acta 1046:233, 1990

9. deMello D, Chi E, Doo E, Lagunoff D: Absence of tubular myelin in lungs of infants dying with hyaline membrane disease. Am J Physiol 127:131, 1987

10. Snyder JM, Kwun JE, O'Brien JA et al: The concentration of the 35-kDa surfactant apoprotein in amniotic fluid from normal and diabetic pregnancies. Pediatr Res 24:728, 1988

11. Weaver TE, Whitsett JA: Function and regulation of expression of pulmonary surfactant-associated proteins. Biochem J 273:249, 1991

12. Hawgood S, Shiffer K: Structures and properties of the surfactant-associated proteins. Annu Rev Physiol 53:375, 1991

13. Jobe A, Ikegami M: Surfactant for the treatment of respiratory distress syndrome. Am Rev Respir Dis 136:1256, 1987

14. Nogee L, deMello D, Dehner L, Colten H: Brief report: deficiency of pulmonary surfactant protein B in congenital alveolar proteinosis. N Engl J Med 328:406, 1993

15. Naeye R, Freeman R, Blanc W: Nutrition, sex and fetal lung maturation. Pediatr Res 8:200, 1974

16. Torday JS, Nielsen HC: The sex difference in fetal lung surfactant production. Exp Lung Res 12:1, 1987

17. Ballard PL: Glucocorticord Effects In Vivo. p. 57. In Monographs on Endocrinology: Hormones and Lung Maturation. Springer-Verlag, New York, 1986

18. Liggins G: Adrenocortical-related maturational events in the fetus. Am J Obstet Gynecol 126:931, 1976

19. Gluck L, Kulovich MV, Borer RC et al: Diagnosis of the respiratory distress syndrome by amniocentesis. Am J Obstet Gynecol 109:440, 1971

20. Gluck L, Kulovich MV, Borer RC, Keidel WN: The interpretation and significance of the lecithin/sphingomyelin ratio in amniotic fluid. Am J Obstet Gynecol 120:142, 1974

21. Hallman M, Kulovich MV, Kirkpatrick E et al: Phosphatidylinositol and phosphatidylglycerol in amniotic fluid: indices of lung maturity. Am J Obstet Gynecol 125:613, 1976

22. Kulovich MV, Hallman M, Gluck L: The lung profile. I. Normal pregnancy. Am J Obstet Gynecol 135:57, 1979

23. Robert MF, Neff RK, Hubbell JP et al: Association between maternal diabetes and the respiratory-distress syndrome in the newborn. N Engl J Med 294:357, 1976

24. Gabbe S, Mestman J, Freeman R et al: Management and outcome of pregnancy in diabetes mellitus, classes B to R. Am J Obstet Gynecol 129:723, 1977

25. Kitzmiller J, Cloherty J, Younger M et al: Diabetic pregnancy and perinatal morbidity. Am J Obstet Gynecol 131:560, 1978

26. Coustan D, Berkowitz R, Hobbins J: Tight metabolic control of overt diabetes in pregnancy. Am J Med 68:845, 1980

27. Drury M, Stronge J, Foley M et al: Pregnancy in the diabetic patient: timing and mode of delivery. Obstet Gynecol 62:279, 1983

28. Dudley D, Black D: Reliability of lecithin/sphingomyelin ratios in diabetic pregnancy. Obstet Gynecol 66:521, 1985

29. Pedersen J, Osler M: Hyperglycemia as the cause of characteristic features of the foetus and newborn of diabetic and control mothers. Dan Med Bull 8:78, 1961

30. Steinke J, Driscoll S: The extractable insulin content of pancreas from fetuses and infants of diabetic and control mothers. Diabetes 14:573, 1965

31. Gewolb I, Warshaw J: Fetal and maternal corticosterone and corticosteroid binding globulin in the diabetic rat gestation. Pediatr Res 20:155, 1986

32. Wilker R, Fleischman A, Saenger P et al: Thyroid hormone levels in diabetic mothers and their neonates. Am J Perinatol 3:259, 1984

33. Ballard PL: Other Hormones. p. 299. In Monographs on Endocrinology: Hormones and Lung Maturation. Springer-Verlag, New York, 1986

34. Smith BT, Giroud CJP, Robert M, Avery ME: Insulin antagonism of cortisol action on lecithin synthesis by cultured fetal lung cells. J Pediatr 87:953, 1975

35. Gross I, Walker Smith GJ, Wilson CM et al: The influence of hormones on the biochemical development of fetal rat lung in organ culture. II. Insulin Pediatr Res 14:834, 1980

36. Snyder JM, Mendelson CR: Insulin inhibits the accumulation of the major lung surfactant apoprotein in human fetal lung explants maintained in vitro. Endocrinology 120:1250, 1987

37. Bourbon J, Rieutort M, Engle M, Farrell P: Utilization of glycogen for phospholipid synthesis in fetal rat lung. Biochim Biophys Acta 712:382, 1982

38. Engle M, Langan S, Sanders R et al: The effects of insulin and hyperglycemia on surfactant phospholipid biosynthesis in organotypic cultures of type II pneumocytes. Biochim Biophys Acta 753:6, 1983

39. Carlson KS, Smith BT, Post M: Insulin acts on the fibroblast to inhibit glucocorticoid stimulation of lung maturation. J Appl Physiol 57:1577, 1984

40. Lawrence S, Warshaw J, Nielsen HC: Delayed lung maturation in the macrosomic offspring of genetically determined diabetic (db/+) mice. Pediatr Res 25:173, 1989

41. Bourbon JR, Pignol B, Marin L et al: Maturation of fetal rat lung in diabetic pregnancies of graduated severity. Diabetes 34:734, 1985

42. Merritt T, Curbelo V, Gluck L, Clements R: Alterations in fetal lung phosphatidylinositol metabolism associated with maternal glucose intolerance. Biol Neonate 39:217, 1981

43. Neufeld N, Melmed S: 3,5-dimethyl-3'-isopropyl-L-thyronine therapy in diabetic pregnancy. J Clin Invest 68:1605, 1981

44. Warburton D, Lew C, Platzker A: Primary hyperinsulinemia reduces surface active material flux in tracheal fluid of fetal lambs. Pediatr Res 15:1422, 1981

45. Sosenko IRS, Frantz ID, Roberts RJ, Meyrick B: Morphologic disturbance of lung maturation in fetuses of alloxan diabetic rabbits. Am Rev Respir Dis 122:687, 1980

46. Rieutort M, Farrell P, Engle M et al: Changes in surfactant phospholipids in fetal rat lungs from normal and diabetic pregnancies. Pediatr Res 20:650, 1986

47. Gewolb I, Rooney S, Barrett C et al: Delayed pulmonary maturation in the fetus of the streptozotocin-diabetic rat. Exp Lung Res 8:141, 1985

48. Grant M, Cutts N, Brody J: Lung basement membrane alterations and type II cell development in fetuses of diabetic rats. Fed Proc 41:859, 1983

49. Boutwell W, Goldman A: Depressed biochemical lung maturation and steroid uptake in an animal model of infant of diabetic mother. Pediatr Res 13:355, 1979

50. Tyden O, Berne C, Eriksson U: Lung maturation in fetuses of diabetic rats. Pediatr Res 14:1192, 1980

51. Eriksson U, Tyden O, Berne C: Glycogen content and lipid biosynthesis in the lungs of fetuses of diabetic rats. Biol Res Prog 4:103, 1983

52. Tsai M, Josephson M, Brown D: Fetal rat lung phosphatidylcholine synthesis in diabetic and normal pregnancies: a comparison of prenatal dexamethasone treatments. Exp Lung Res 4:315, 1983

53. Sosenko IRS, Hartig-Beeckmen I, Frantz ID: Cortisol reversal of functional delay of lung maturation in fetuses of diabetic rabbits. J Appl Physiol 49:971, 1980

54. Guttentag SH, Phelps DS, Stenzel W et al: Surfactant protein-A expression is delayed in fetuses of streptozotocin-treated rats. Am J Physiol 262:L489, 1992

55. Guttentag SH, Phelps DS, Warshaw JB, Floros J: Delayed hydrophobic surfactant proteins (SP-B, SP-C) expression in fetuses of streptozotocin-treated rats. Am J Respir Cell Mol Biol 7:190, 1992

56. Nichols K, Floros J, Dynia D et al: Regulation of surfactant protein A mRNA by hormones and by butyrate in cultured fetal rat lung. Am J Physiol 259:L488, 1990

57. Persson B: Newborn fuel homeostasis and metabolic abnormalities in infants of diabetic mothers. Mead Johnson Symp Perinat Dev Med 13:45, 1978

58. Mueller-Heubach E, Caritis S, Edelstone D, Turner J: Lecithin/sphingomyelin ratio in amniotic fluid and its value for the prediction of neonatal respiratory distress syndrome in pregnant diabetic women. Am J Obstet Gynecol 130:28, 1978

59. Cruz A, Buhi W, Birk S, Spellacy W: Respiratory distress syndrome with mature lecithin/sphingomyelin ratio: diabetes mellitus and low Apgar scores. Am J Obstet Gynecol 126:78, 1976

60. Gabbe S, Lowensohn R, Mestman J et al: Lecithin/sphingomyelin ratio in pregnancies complicated by diabetes mellitus. Am J Obstet Gynecol 128:757, 1977

61. Aubry R, Rourke J, Almanza R et al: The lecithin/sphingomyelin ratio in a high-risk obstetric population. Obstet Gynecol 47:21, 1976

62. Yambao T, Clark D, Smith C, Aubry R: Amniotic fluid phosphatidylglycerol in stressed pregnancies. Am J Obstet Gynecol 141:191, 1981

63. Cunningham M, Desai N, Thompson S, Greene J: Amniotic fluid phosphatidylglycerol in diabetic pregnancies. Am J Obstet Gynecol 131:719, 1978

64. Kulovich MV, Gluck L: The lung profile. II. Complicated pregnancy. Am J Obstet Gynecol 135:64, 1979

65. Karlsson K, Kjellmer I: The outcome of diabetic pregnancies in relation to the mother's blood sugar level. Am J Obstet Gynecol 112:213, 1972

66. Coustan D: Methods of screening for and diagnosing of gestational diabetes. Clin Perinatol 20:593, 1993

67. Langer O: Management of gestational diabetes. Clin Perinatol 20:603, 1993

68. Farrell P, Engle M, Curet L et al: Saturated phospholipids in amniotic fluid of normal and diabetic pregnancies. Obstet Gynecol 64:77, 1984

69. Mimouni F, Miodovnik M, Whitsett J et al: Respiratory distress syndrome in infants of diabetic mothers in the 1980s: no direct adverse effect of maternal diabetes with modern management. Obstet Gynecol 69:191, 1987

70. Piper J, Langer O: Does maternal diabetes delay fetal pulmonary maturity? Am J Obstet Gynecol 168:783, 1993

71. McMahon MJ, Mimouni F, Miodovnik M et al: Surfactant associated protein (SAP-35) in amniotic fluid from diabetic and nondiabetic pregnancies. Obstet Gynecol 70:94, 1987

72. Crombach G, Wolff F, Klein W et al: [Pregnancy outcome with intensified insulin therapy in manifest diabetes.] Geburtshilfe Frauenheilkd 50:263, 1990

73. Cunningham M, McKean H, Gillispie D, Greene J: Improved prediction of fetal lung maturity in diabetic pregnancies: a comparison of chromatographic methods. Am J Obstet Gynecol 142:197, 1982

74. Kjos S, Walther F, Montoro M et al: Prevlance and etiology of respiratory distress in infants of diabetic mothers: predictive value of fetal lung maturation tests. Am J Obstet Gynecol 163:898, 1990

75. Lowensohn R, Gabbe S: The value of lecithin/sphingomyelin ratios in diabetes: a critical review. Am J Obstet Gynecol 134:702, 1979

76. Tchobroutsky C, Amiel-Tison C, Cedard L et al: The lecithin/sphingomyelin ratio in 132 insulin-dependent diabetic pregnancies. Am J Obstet Gynecol 130:754, 1978

77. Curet L, Olson R, Schneider J, Zachman R: Effect of diabetes mellitus on amniotic fluid lecithin/sphingomyelin ratio and respiratory distress syndrome. Am J Obstet Gynecol 135:10, 1979

78. O'Neil G, Davies IJ, Siu J: Palmitic/stearic ratio of amniotic fluid in diabetic and nondiabetic pregnancies and its relationship to development of respiratory distress syndrome. Am J Obstet Gynecol 132:519, 1978

79. Tabsch K, Brinkman C, Bashore R: Lecithin:sphingomyelin ratio in pregnancies complicated by insulin-dependent diabetes mellitus. Obstet Gynecol 59:353, 1982

80. Hallman M, Teramo K: Amniotic fluid phospholipid profile as a predictor of fetal maturity in diabetic pregnancies. Obstet Gynecol 54:703, 1979

81. Katyal SL, Amenta JS, Singh G, Silverman JA: Deficient lung surfactant apoproteins in amniotic fluid with mature phospholipid profile from diabetic pregnancies. Am J Obstet Gynecol 148:48, 1984

8

Pathology of Fetuses and Infants Born to Diabetic Mothers

DON B. SINGER

After insulin therapy was introduced in 1922 and in the subsequent four decades, conception in diabetic women was often normal, but as many as one-third of these pregnancies ended in fetal death, neonatal death, or significant neonatal morbidity.[1,2] In the past three decades, perinatal mortality and morbidity have been substantially reduced, mainly through efforts to control glucose metabolism throughout gestation or even before conception. Placental abnormalities are reduced to the point that it is difficult to identify changes that can be attributed strictly to maternal diabetes. The reader should be aware that good control of glucose homeostasis in the gravida can reduce or eliminate many of the conditions and pathologic lesions described in this chapter (Table 8-1).

MACROSOMIA

Macrosomia is a classic feature of fetuses and infants born to diabetic mothers (IDMs)[3,4] (Fig. 8-1). Macrosomia may even occur when diabetic mothers have pregnancy-induced hypertension, a condition usually associated with small babies.[5]

An exception to the general rule that maternal diabetes leads to fetal macrosomia is when babies are born to mothers with severe diabetes complicated by vascular disease[6] or when there is significantly elevated glycosylated hemoglobin early in pregnancy.[7] In these latter conditions, fetal growth is often retarded.

In large IDMs, both the weight and the length are

increased as much as 10 to 15 percent.[6] Skin-fold thickness is also increased, and when compared with normal infants, the amount of truncal adipose tissue is increased.[8] Most of the extra adipose tissue develops in the last 10 weeks of gestation.

Visceral organs are heavier than normal, especially the heart, liver, and kidneys. To a lesser extent, the lungs, spleen, thymus, and adrenal glands are enlarged. However, the brain is usually appropriate in weight for the gestational age or may be smaller than expected.[9] In the enlarged tissues and organs, both hyperplasia and hypertrophy account for the increased size.[6,10] Total body water is less than normal.[11] Placentomegaly is also a feature of maternal diabetes mellitus. The increased weight occurs in all classes of maternal diabetes mellitus except those with vascular disease.[12,13]

The Pedersen hypothesis, proposed in 1961, is still considered the most plausible explanation for macrosomia. This hypothesis states that maternal hyperglycemia leads to fetal hyperglycemia, which in turn stimulates the fetal pancreas to produce excessive amounts of insulin.[14] Insulin is known to be one of the main growth factors for fetal tissues. Susa and colleagues[15,16] demonstrated this experimentally by implanting insulin capsules subcutaneously in fetal rhesus monkeys. Markedly increased fetal growth occurred even though the maternal glucose levels remained within the normal range.

In clinical situations, macrosomia is virtually eliminated when the maternal blood glucose levels are

Table 8-1. Major Pathologic Conditions and Lesions Associated with Fetuses and Infants Born to Mothers With Diabetes Mellitus

Macrosomia

Hypoxia

Polycythemia and thrombosis

Respiratory distress syndrome

Pancreatic islet hyperplasia, hypertrophy, and insulitis

Placental immaturity and infarcts

Umbilical cord edema and single umbilical artery

Spontaneous abortion

Congenital malformations

  Caudal anomalies, microcephaly, ear anomalies, cardiac ventricular septal defect and asymmetric septal hypertrophy, vertebral and rib defects, small left colon syndrome

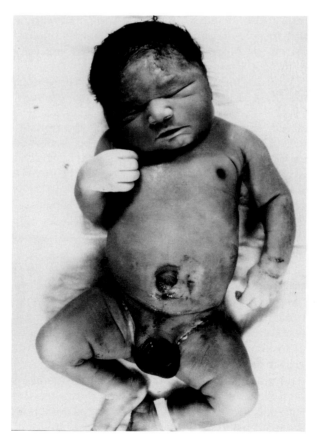

Fig. 8-1. Infant of diabetic mother with macrosomia. The cherubic face and stocky appearance are characteristic of such infants.

maintained in the normal range.[17,18] Early and strict control of maternal glucose levels also tends to reduce the placental weights to essentially normal values.[19] Although some investigators have shown that fetal macrosomia may not be ameliorated by good maternal glucose control,[20] most reports indicate that maintaining serum glucose levels in the normal range usually results in babies and placentas of normal size.

HYPOXIA

The demands for oxygen are increased in macrosomic fetuses. This is particularly evident in the last weeks of gestation, when acquisition of fetal mass accelerates. When the demand for oxygen exceeds the supply, asphyxia is the result. This may account for the increased death rate observed in macrosomic fetuses in the 37th to 42nd weeks of gestation. These deaths are often unexplained except for subtle findings of asphyxia such as pleural and thymic petechiae or aspirated meconium.

Excessive erythropoiesis in the liver of macrosomic IDMs is another clue that hypoxia is present.[21] Shannon and colleagues[22] have proved that excessive erythropoiesis is not a primary condition in IDMs but requires the presence of hypoxia.

Asphyxia may result in characteristic lesions in the brain. Those areas of the fetal and neonatal brain that are particularly susceptible to hypoxia are the hippocampus, the basal ganglia, and the reticular substance of the brain stem. Edema of the neuropil, pyknosis of neurons, peripheral dispersion of Nissl substance in the neuronal cytoplasm, increased oligodendrogliocytes, and enlarged astrocytes are all features of hypoxia. Untreated hypoglycemia may produce identical lesions, and it is impossible to distinguish this etiology from that of hypoxia. Despite the foregoing, follow-up studies of children born to mothers with either pregestational diabetes or gestational diabetes show normal neuropsychological development at 5 years of age.[23]

In severe asphyxia, lesions occur in the kidney, adrenal, and liver. Any of these organs may show foci of necrosis. The kidney may have acute tubular necrosis, cortical necrosis, or medullary hemorrhage. The last mentioned is a lesion that is peculiar to neonates with hypoxia or shock, whether or not the mother has diabetes. The liver may show isolated cell necrosis or larger patches of necrosis with an irregular distribution in the hepatic lobules. The adrenal glands may have either focal or diffuse necrosis or medullary hemorrhage.

POLYCYTHEMIA AND THROMBOSIS

Chronic fetal hypoxia may also account for the polycythemia that occurs in IDMs. Hematocrits in excess of 65 volumes percent can result in another one of the fetal and neonatal hazards in these babies, namely, intravascular thrombosis. Thrombosis has been described in the arterial system, including the aorta, but is particularly prone to occur in the veins. In the kidney, thrombi can propagate from venules to large renal veins and the inferior vena cava, with the possibility that pulmonary embolus can develop.[24] (Fig. 8-2).

Nappi and colleagues[25] have suggested that endothelial cells in IDMs are subject to increased trauma due to accentuated clot retraction. The resulting endothelial lesions may lead to thrombosis at the sites of injury.[25] A further hazard of fetal polycythemia is an increased number of destroyed red blood cells and hyperbilirubinemia after birth. Excessive jaundice is common in neonates born to diabetic mothers.

RESPIRATORY DISTRESS SYNDROME AND HYALINE MEMBRANE DISEASE

Respiratory distress syndrome with morphologically characteristic hyaline membranes occurs with increased frequency in IDMs[26] (Fig. 8-3). This is true whether or not the infant is delivered by cesarean section. The maturation of surfactant-producing cells is altered in these fetuses. Although the lecithin/sphingomyelin ratio may be normal, the production of phos-

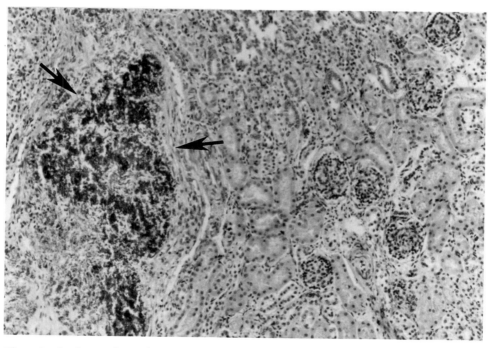

Fig. 8-2. Thrombosis of a renal vein (arrows). This thrombus is partially calcified. Such thrombi propagate from renal venules to renal veins to the inferior vena cava and have the potential to embolize to the pulmonary arteries. (Hematoxylin and eosin stain, original magnification × 125.)

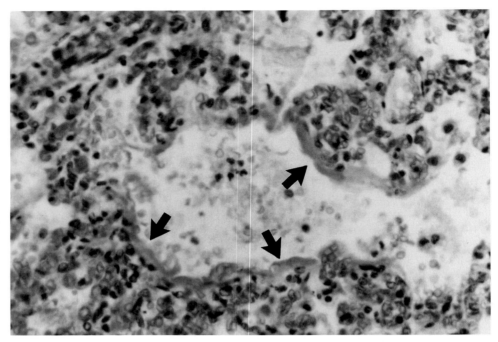

Fig. 8-3. Hyaline membranes (arrows) line the alveolar duct in the lung of this infant of a diabetic mother. The disease is clinically and pathologically similar to that seen in infants of nondiabetic mothers, except that infants of diabetic mothers tend to be larger and with slightly more advanced gestational ages. (Hematoxylin and eosin stain, original magnification × 250.)

phatidyl glycerol (PG) is frequently delayed beyond 36 weeks' gestational age.[27,28] As in other infants, administration of steroids may stimulate maturation of the granular pneumocyte in the fetus of a diabetic mother or IDM so that adequate quantities and quality of surfactant material are produced and respiratory distress is avoided. Good control of maternal glucose levels also eliminates the increased frequency of respiratory distress in these infants.[29]

PANCREATIC ISLET HYPERPLASIA AND HYPERTROPHY

Normal fetuses and neonates have smaller pancreatic islets than do older children and adults, but they also have more islet tissue per total pancreatic volume than do older individuals.[30] The small clusters of islet cells are scattered inconspicuously throughout the pancreas. This normal feature should not be confused with nesidioblastosis, a pathologic condition with a similar appearance that occurs in children and adults.[31]

Enlarged islets in the neonate and fetus are usually defined as having average diameters greater than 250 μm or individual islets with diameters greater than 400 μm. Many conditions are associated with islet hyperplasia and hypertrophy, including Beckwith-Wiedemann syndrome, hereditary tyrosinemia, leprechaunism, Zellweger syndrome, some cases of fetal growth retardation, infant giantism, and erythroblastosis fetalis.[30]

Enlarged islets of Langerhans and an increase in their numbers were noted in the pancreas of an IDM by Gray and Feemster in 1926.[32] This has proved to be a hallmark for maternal diabetes in fetal or neonatal autopsies, so much so that when the other conditions are ruled out, the diagnosis of maternal diabetes can

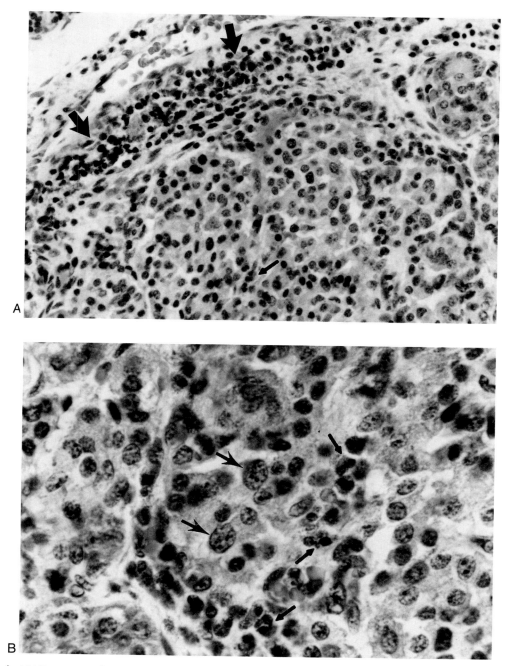

Fig. 8-4. **(A)** Pancreatic islet of Langerhans from an infant of a diabetic mother. Eosinophils and other inflammatory cells (arrows) surround and invade the islet. (Hematoxylin and eosin stain, original magnification × 250.) **(B)** Portion of pancreatic islet of Langerhans with eosinophilic infiltrate (small arrows) and enlarged nuclei of insulin-producing cells (large arrows). (Hematoxylin and eosin stain, original magnification × 500.)

be suggested on this basis alone. When such islets also have enlarged nuclei in the insulin-producing β-cells, the suggestion that maternal diabetes is present is strengthened. If eosinophils surround and invade the islets, the diagnosis of maternal diabetes is virtually certain[33] (Fig. 8-4). Charcot-Leyden crystals, the breakdown products of eosinophils, have been identified in some cases.[34] Other inflammatory cells, such as lymphocytes, macrophages, and neutrophils, may also surround and invade islets in IDMs and fetuses of diabetic mothers. As Salafia[35] pointed out, insulitis in these cases may be a response to anti-insulin antibodies circulating from the mother's blood to the fetus. The enlarged and numerous islets with or without insulitis may persist for 3 or 4 months.

Experimental data in rats are contradictory to the observations in humans. In the pancreases of fetuses born to spontaneously diabetic BB rats or to dams with streptozotocin-induced diabetes, β-cells have reduced insulin granules compared with controls. Furthermore, insulin levels are decreased in the plasma of these fetuses when compared with normal fetuses. Islet β-cells show ultrastructural signs of increased cellular metabolic activity, with prominent Golgi apparatus and profiles of endoplasmic reticulum.[36]

PLACENTAL PATHOLOGY

Many different placental lesions, with a variety of pathogeneses, are described in cases of maternal diabetes mellitus. The descriptions include small placentas, large placentas, focal infarcts, extensive infarcts, accelerated maturation with premature senescence, persistent immaturity, angiopathies including mild capillary dilation, chorangiomatosis and sclerosis of fetal arteries, hydropic villi, fibrotic villi, paddle-shaped villi, excessive sprouting of syncytiotrophoblast, increased erythropoiesis, and villous basement membranes that are thickened, thinned, split, or entirely normal.[9,13,19,37–45]

Using scanning electron microscopy, Honda and colleagues[46] have recently shown that the diameter of terminal villi is significantly reduced in placentas from fetuses of diabetic mothers. These same investigators showed that the ramification pattern of villi was reduced in placentas when mothers had severe diabetes with retinopathy and when their babies weighed less than control babies. Syncytial knots were more frequent and the trophoblast basement membranes were thicker in placentas from diabetic mothers. Capillary basement membranes, however, were thinner in Jirkovska's study.[47]

Villous immaturity is one of the more constantly reported findings in placentas from diabetic mothers (Fig. 8-5). Immaturity is characterized by large and plump villi in which a loose stroma is prominent. Syncytial trophoblast is less prominent and cytotrophoblast is more prominent than in normal placentas of the same gestational age. Villous capillaries are small, centrally placed in the stroma, and reduced in number. Syncytial-capillary membranes are infrequently found. Arizawa and colleagues[48] correlated such immaturity with mildly elevated maternal levels of glycosylated hemoglobin, whereas Greco and colleagues[49] found that functional immaturity was expressed by increased β-human chorionic gonadotropin and decreased placental alkaline phosphatase, pregnancy specific β-1-glycoprotein, and human placental lactogen. They demonstrated these functional proteins in the immature regions by immunohistochemical techniques.[49] Emmrich[50] recently proposed that villous immaturity, if pronounced, may be used as a suggestive diagnosis of maternal diabetes, provided other causes of immaturity, such as fetal hydrops or erythroblastosis fetalis, are clinically ruled out.

Morphometric studies of the placenta have provided some insight into the pathophysiology of maternal diabetes mellitus. Teasdale[51] found placentas from class A diabetic mothers were heavier, had more parenchymal and villous tissue, more cells and more surface exchange area than did placentas from normal mothers. In my own studies,[19] placentas were somewhat larger in 20 diabetic cases than in 20 normal cases (553 g versus 497 g), but this was not statistically significant. The body weights of IDMs were greater than weights of control infants by an average of 160 g (3,520 g versus 3,360 g), again without statistical significance although the ratio of body weight to ideal weight, defined as the 50th percentile of normal distribution for gestational age, was significantly greater in the diabetic group than in the control group (1.18 versus 1.02, $P < .01$). In our studies, the average surface area of villi was slightly increased in placentas from diabetic pregnancies when compared with controls (7.08 versus 6.63 m²) as was the average surface area of villous capillaries (8.28 ver-

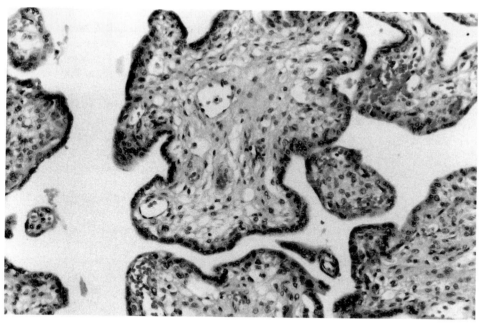

Fig. 8-5. Immature villi in placenta from infant of a diabetic mother. The characteristic features are large villi with few syncytial knots. Villous capillaries are centrally placed in the abundant stroma. (Hematoxylin and eosin stain, original magnification × 125.)

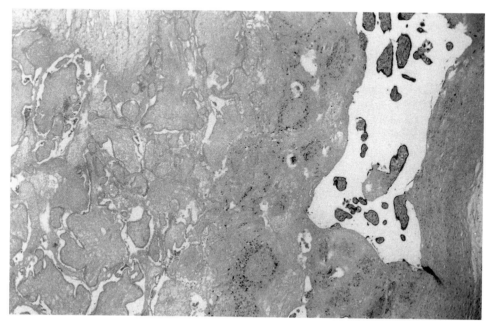

Fig. 8-6. Microscopic appearance of placental infarct. The villi are represented by ghost outlines. Such infarcts are fairly common in placentas from diabetic mothers. (Hematoxylin and eosin stain, original magnification × 125.)

sus 7.56 m^2), but these differences were not significant. We found no statistical differences in the amount of syncytial trophoblast, cytotrophoblast, or villous stroma when comparing placentas from diabetic mothers with those from normal mothers. At the ultrastructural level, no differences were found in trophoblast endoplasmic reticulum, mitochondria, pinocytotic vesicles, or secretory granules.[19]

Perhaps placental infarcts comprise the lesions predicted by Lister[52] when he made the following comment nearly 30 years ago: "in diabetes mellitus even though the disease is well controlled, there would be a morphologic feature expressed in the placenta." In our studies, placental infarcts were five times more numerous in diabetic cases than in the controls.[19] The sizes of the infarcts were small, in aggregate comprising less than 1 percent of the placental volume, but all were detectable with unaided visual examination.

Infarcts suggest ischemia (Fig. 8-6). Ischemia may be on the basis of maternal vascular spasm or due to the slightly larger mass of placental tissue that requires perfusion. Fibrinoid deposits between the villi, however, were not increased in our cases, nor were they in cases reported by Haust.[9]

Atherosis of maternal arteries in the decidua basalis associated with placentas from diabetic mothers was described by Benirschke and Driscoll[37] many years ago. The earliest histologically convincing lesion is fibrinoid necrosis of the arterial wall with a perivascular infiltrate of mononuclear inflammatory cells. Lipophages in the intima tend to occlude the lumen of these vessels in the late stages of the process. Khong[53] revisited this subject and found that atherosis is not observed in maternal diabetes mellitus unless the pregnancies are complicated by pre-eclampsia.

UMBILICAL CORD EDEMA AND SINGLE UMBILICAL ARTERY

The umbilical cord is occasionally edematous in fetuses of diabetic women. The edematous cords can weigh as much as 50 g or more and can measure 4 cm or more in diameter. Watery Wharton's jelly freely exudes from the cut surface. Few other conditions are associated with such pronounced edema of the umbilical cord.

Single umbilical artery is said to be three to six times

as common in these cases as in those without maternal diabetes, but the relationship to other congenital malformations in the same infants is not yet established.[13,37]

SPONTANEOUS ABORTION

Early spontaneous abortion, although known to be a special hazard in diabetic women,[54] has rarely been evaluated carefully by pathologic techniques. In a recent report, Bendon and colleagues[55] found that spontaneous abortuses in diabetic women with relatively mild disease had decidual changes that were indistinguishable from controls. However, more severely affected diabetic individuals (i.e., those with retinopathy) had significant decidual congestion, and fibrin clots were noted in the decidual veins.[55] Elevated serum glycosylated hemoglobin values are also associated with increased spontaneous abortion in diabetic mothers.[56]

CONGENITAL MALFORMATIONS

The association of maternal diabetes and congenital malformations has intrigued investigators for many years.[34,57] Mølsted-Pedersen and colleagues[58] suggested that IDMs were at greater risk of lethal and major malformations, especially when maternal vascular disease complicated the diabetes. Elevated maternal glycosylated hemoglobin values are associated with increased frequency of congenital malformation in the offspring.[59] Conversely, strict control of maternal serum glucose levels results in malformation rates comparable with those in the general population.[60,61]

Neave[62] performed the most extensive survey of malformations in offspring of diabetic patients. Among 2,592 diabetic mothers, he found an increased frequency of malformations (13.1 percent) in IDMs compared with the offspring of either 1,262 diabetic men (1.8 percent) or 1,212 nondiabetic women (5.3 percent). Those mothers with mild diabetes (class A) had fetuses and infants with no increase in malformations. Similar findings were reported from the National Collaborative Perinatal Project, in which 567 "overt" diabetic mothers and 372 "gestational" diabetic mothers were studied.[63]

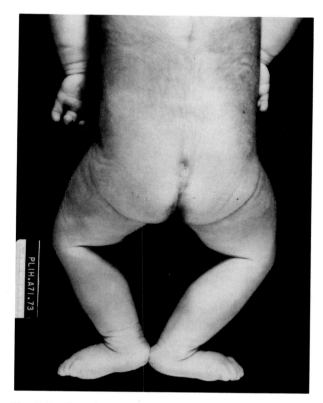

Fig. 8-7. Short femurs, representing a mild form of caudal regression, in an infant born to a diabetic mother. Caudal regression is rare but is overrepresented among infants of diabetic mothers compared with the general population.

The rare caudal regression lesions, also described under names such as sacral dysgenesis, sacral agenesis, or caudal dysgenesis, are strongly associated with maternal diabetes.[64] Maldevelopment or absence of the sacrum or coccyx occurs with or without hypoplastic femurs, dislocated hips, defects of tibias or fibulas, or other lower limb malformations. (Fig. 8-7). Affected babies often have anomalies in other organ systems. Experimental data bearing on these anomalies are provided by Styrud and Eriksson,[65] who placed rat embryos in culture media containing diabetic rat serum. Lower somite numbers were found in these embryos, and this developmental defect may correspond to the caudal lesions noted in human fetuses of diabetic mothers and IDMs.

Although not as vividly associated with maternal diabetes as the caudal-limb anomalies, other malforma-

tions tend to cluster within certain organ systems. These include the central nervous system, alimentary tract, cardiovascular system, genitourinary system, skeletal system, and the umbilical cord. Five anomalies that are most likely to have occurred in fetuses of diabetic mothers are microcephaly, ear deformities, cardiac ventricular septal defects, single umbilical artery, and rib and vertebral anomalies. In Neave's series, 22 percent of the malformed fetuses of diabetic mothers and IDMs had one or more of these malformations. Single umbilical artery was found seven times more frequently in IDMs than in control infants.[62]

The neonatal small left colon syndrome is another anomaly found predominantly in IDMs.[66] The small bowel becomes distended, as does the colon proximal to the splenic flexure. The lumenal diameter of the descending colon is abruptly or gradually reduced to 0.5 cm or less. This can be confused with Hirschsprung's disease, but ganglion cells are morphologically present. Although the etiology of small left colon syndrome is unknown, dysfunctional ganglion cells have been suggested as a cause.[9]

Transient hypertrophic cardiomyopathy is accepted as a fetal and neonatal complication of maternal diabetes, especially when the diabetes is poorly controlled.[67,68] This lesion is characterized as septal hyper-

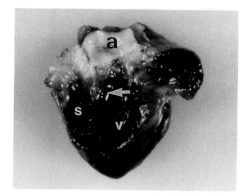

Fig. 8-8. Septal hypertrophy in the heart from a rhesus monkey fetus. The opened aorta (a) and left ventricle (v) and the hypertrophic septum (s) are marked. The septum bulges (white arrow) into the left ventricle just below the aortic valve. An insulin pump was implanted subcutaneously a few weeks before delivery to simulate the hyperinsulinemia in human fetuses of diabetic mothers.

trophy, producing a shelf of muscle bulging into the left ventricle just below the aorta (Fig. 8-8). Some cases have focal myocardial necroses or disarray of myocardial fibers, but other cases do not show such lesions. The glycogen content of the myocardium is normal. The septal hypertrophy is usually not sufficiently severe to result in death and resolves to a normal cardiac anatomy in 2 to 6 months. However, deaths have, on occasion, been attributed to septal hypertrophy in IDMs. The pathophysiologic basis for death is presumably similar to that found in familial hypertrophic cardiomyopathy or idiopathic hypertrophic subaortic stenosis.[67,69]

SUMMARY

Fetuses born to diabetic mothers and IDMs have a wide range of structural and biochemical abnormalities that can be reduced or eliminated by improved control of maternal glucose metabolism. Fetal and placental macrosomia, hypoxia, perinatal polycythemia and thrombosis, and respiratory distress syndrome respond favorably to maternal treatment. Direct histologic studies of pancreatic islets have not been reported from fetuses or neonates born to "well-controlled" diabetic mothers, but fetal insulin production is reduced and hypoglycemia is avoided in such babies.

Placental infarcts and fetal malformations are persistent complications of maternal diabetes, even when maternal glucose metabolism is reasonably well controlled. Fetal malformations can be reduced to levels found in the normal population only when early (i.e., preconceptional) and strict glucose control is established.

REFERENCES

1. Henley WE: Diabetes and pregnancy. NZ Med J 46:386, 1947
2. White P: Diabetes mellitus in pregnancy. Clin Perinatol 1:331, 1974
3. Warren S: The Pathology of Diabetes Mellitus. 2 Ed. Lea & Febiger, Philadelphia, 1938
4. Oates JN, Abell DA, Beischer NA, Broomhall GR: Maternal glucose tolerance during pregnancy with excessive size infants. Obstet Gynecol 55:184, 1980
5. Goldkrand JW, Lin JY: Large for gestational age: dilemma of the infant of the diabetic mother. J Perinatol 7:282, 1987
6. Naeye RL: Infants of diabetic mothers: a quantitative morphologic study. Pediatrics 35:980, 1965
7. Pedersen JF, Mølsted-Pedersen L, Mortensen HB: Fetal growth delay and maternal hemoglobin A1c in early diabetic pregnancy. Obstet Gynecol 64:351, 1984
8. Fee BA, Weil WB Jr: Body compositon of infants of diabetic mothers by direct analysis. Ann NY Acad Sci 110:869, 1963
9. Haust D: Maternal diabetes mellitus effects on the fetus and placenta. p. 201. In Naeye RL, Kissane JM, Kaufman N (eds): Perinatal Diseases. Williams & Wilkins, Baltimore, 1981
10. Martins EA, Neave C, Susa JB, Singer DB: Effect of insulin on the size of skeletal muscle fibers of fetal rhesus monkeys. Pediat Pathol 6:377, 1986
11. Osler M, Pedersen J: The body composition of newborn infants of diabetic mothers. Pediatrics 26:985, 1960
12. Salafia CM, Silberman L: Placental pathology and abnormal fetal heart rate patterns in gestational diabetes. Pediat Pathol 9:513, 1989
13. Driscoll SG: Pathology of pregnancy complicated by diabetes mellitus. Med Clin North Am 49:1053, 1965
14. Pedersen J, Osler M: Hyperglycemia as the cause of characteristic features of the foetus and newborn of diabetic mothers. Dan Med Bull 8:78, 1961
15. Susa JB, McCormick KL, Widness JA et al: Chronic hyperinsulinemia in the fetal rhesus monkey. Effects on fetal growth and composition. Diabetes 28:1058, 1979
16. Susa JB, Neave C, Sehgal P et al: Chronic hyperinsulinemia in the fetal rhesus monkey. Effects of physiologic hyperinsulinemia on fetal growth and composition. Diabetes 33:656, 1984
17. Clarson C, Tevaarwerk GJ, Harding PG et al: Placental weight in diabetic pregnancies. Placenta 10:275, 1989
18. Nelson RL: Diabetes and pregnancy: control can make a difference. Mayo Clin Proc 61:825, 1986
19. Singer DB: The placenta in pregnancies complicated by diabetes mellitus. Perspect Pediat Pathol 8:199, 1984
20. Small M, Cameron A, Lunan CB, MacCuish AC: Macrosomia in pregnancy complicated by insulin-dependent diabetes mellitus. Diabetes Care 10:594, 1987
21. Singer DB: Hepatic erythropoiesis in infants of diabetic mothers. A morphometric study. Pediat Pathol 5:471, 1986
22. Shannon K, Davis JC, Kitzmiller JL et al: Erythropoiesis in infants of diabetic mothers. Pediatr Res 20:161, 1986
23. Persson B, Gentz J: Follow-up of children of insulin-de-

pendent and gestational diabetic mothers. Neuropsychological outcome. Acta Paediatr Scand 73:349, 1984

24. Oppenheimer EH, Esterly J: Thrombosis in the newborn: comparison between infants of diabetic and nondiabetic mothers. J Pediatr 67:549, 1965

25. Nappi C, Cerbone AM, Papa R et al: Increased retraction of fibrin clots by endothelial cells of infants of diabetic mothers. Biol Res Preg Perinatol 6:141, 1985

26. Robert MF, Neff RK, Hubbell JP et al: Association between maternal diabetes and the respiratory distress syndrome in the newborn. N Engl J Med 294:357, 1976

27. Cunningham MD, Desai NS, Thompson SA, Greene JM: Amniotic fluid phosphatidylglycerol in diabetic pregnancies. Am J Obstet Gynecol 131:719, 1978

28. Hallman M, Gluck L: Development of the fetal lung. J Perinat Med 5:3, 1977

29. McMahan MJ, Mimouni F, Miodovnik M et al: Surfactant associated protein (SAP-35) in amniotic fluid from diabetic and nondiabetic pregnancies. Obstet Gynecol 70:94, 1987

30. Jaffe R, Hashida Y, Yunis EJ: The endocrine pancreas of the neonate and infant. Perspect Pediat Pathol 7:137, 1982

31. Hahn von Dorsche H, Reiher H, Hahn HJ: Quantitative-histologic studies of human fetal pancreas from metabolically healthy and insulin-dependent diabetic women. Acta Anat 118:139, 1984

32. Gray SH, Feemster L: Compensatory hypertrophy and hyperplasia of islands of Langerhans in the pancreas of a child born of a diabetic mother. Arch Pathol 1:348, 1926

33. Naeye RL, Sims EAH, Welsh GW, Gray MJ: Newborn organ abnormalities: a guide to abnormal maternal glucose metabolism. Arch Pathol 81:552, 1966

34. Driscoll SG, Benirschke K, Curtis GW: Neonatal deaths among infants of diabetic mothers. Am J Dis Child 100:818, 1960

35. Salafia C: The fetal, placental, and neonatal pathology associated with maternal diabetes mellitus. p. 143. In Reece EA, Coustan DR (eds): Diabetes Mellitus in Pregnancy: Principles and Practice. Churchill Livingstone, New York, 1988

36. Verhaeghe J, Peeters TL, Vandeputte M et al: Maternal and fetal endocrine pancreas in the spontaneously diabetic BB rat. Biol Neonat 55:298, 1989

37. Benirschke K, Driscoll SG: The Pathology of the Human Placenta. Springer-Verlag, New York, 1967

38. Fox H: Pathology of the placenta in maternal diabetes mellitus. Obstet Gynecol 34:792, 1969

39. Jones CJP, Fox H: Placental changes in gestational diabetes: an ultrastructural study. Obstet Gynecol 48:274, 1976

40. Naeye R: The outcome of diabetic pregnancies. A prospective study. Ciba Found Symp 63:227, 1978

41. Ornoy A, Crone K, Altshuler G: Pathologic features of the placenta in fetal death. Arch Pathol Lab Med 100:367, 1976

42. Becker V: Abnormal Maturation of Villi. University Park Press, Baltimore, 1975

43. Okudaira Y, Hirota K, Cohen S, Strauss L: Ultrastructure of the human placenta in maternal diabetes mellitus. Lab Invest 15:910, 1966

44. Emmrich P, Fuchs V, Heinke P et al: The epithelial and capillary basal laminae of the placenta in maternal diabetes mellitus. Lab Invest 35:87, 1976

45. Zacks S, Blazer A: Chorionic villi in normal pregnancy, pre-eclamptic toxemia, erythroblastosis and diabetes mellitus. Obstet Gynecol 22:149, 1963

46. Honda M, Toyoda C, Nakabayashi M, Omori Y: Quantitative investigations of placental terminal villi in maternal diabetes mellitus by scanning and transmission electron microscopy. Tohoku J Exp Med 167:247, 1992

47. Jirkovska M: Comparison of the thickness of the capillary basement membrane of the human placenta under normal conditions and in type 1 diabetes. Func Dev Morphol 1:9, 1991

48. Arizawa M, Nakayama M, Kidoguchi K: Correlation of placental villous immaturity and dysmaturity with clinical control of maternal diabetes. Acta Obstet Gynaecol Japonica 43:595, 1991

49. Greco MA, Kamat BR, Demopoulos RI: Placental protein distribution in maternal diabetes mellitus; and immunocytochemical study. Pediat Pathol 9:679, 1989

50. Emmrich P: Pathologie der plazenta. IV Reifungsstorungen der Plazenta unter besonderen klinischen Bedingungen. Zentr, Pathol 137:2, 1991

51. Teasdale F: Histomorphometry on the placenta of the diabetic woman: class A diabetes mellitus. Placenta 2:241, 1981

52. Lister VM: The ultrastructure of the placenta in abnormal pregnancy: I. Preliminary observations on the fine structure of the human placenta in cases of maternal diabetes. J Obstet Gynaecol Br Commonw 72:203, 1965

53. Khong TY: Acute atherosis in pregnancies complicated by hypertension, small-for-gestational age infants, and diabetes mellitus. Arch Pathol Lab Med 115:722, 1991

54. Sutherland HW, Pritchard CW: Increased incidence of spontaneous abortion in pregnancies complicated by diabetes mellitus. Am J Obstet Gynecol 155:135, 1986

55. Bendon RW, Mimouni F, Khoury J, Miodovnik M: Histopathology of spontaneous abortion in diabetic pregnancies. Am J Perinatol 7:207, 1990

56. Miodovnik M, Skillman C, Holroyde JC et al: Elevated maternal glycohemoglobin in early pregnancy and spontaneous abortion among insulin-dependent diabetic women. Am J Obstet Gynecol 153:439, 1985

57. Gellis SA, Hsia DY: The infant of the diabetic mother. Am J Dis Child 97:1, 1959

58. Mølsted-Pedersen L, Tygstrup I, Pedersen J: Congenital malformations in newborn infants of diabetic women. Correlation with maternal diabetic vascular complications. Lancet 1:1124, 1964

59. Reece EA, Hobbins JC: Diabetic embryopathy: pathogenesis, prenatal diagnosis and prevention. Obstet Gynecol Surv 41:325, 1986

60. Fuhrmann K, Reiher H, Semmler K et al: Prevention of congenital malformations in infants of insulin-dependent diabetic mothers. Diabetes Care 6:219, 1983

61. Hod M, Merlob P, Friedman S et al: Prevalence of congenital anomalies and neonatal complications in the offspring of diabetic mothers in Israel. Isr J Med Sci 27:498, 1991

62. Neave C: Congenital malformation in offspring of diabetics. Prespect Pediatr Pathol 8:213, 1984

63. Chung CS, Myrianthopoulos NC: Factors affecting risks of congenital malformations. II. Effects of maternal diabetes. Birth Defects 11:23, 1975

64. Rusnak SL, Driscoll SG: Congenital spinal anomalies in infants of diabetic mothers. Pediatrics 35:989, 1965

65. Styrud J, Eriksson UJ: Development of rat embryos in culture media containing different concentrations of normal and diabetic rat serum. Teratology 46:473, 1992

66. Davis WS, Allen RP, Favara BE, Slovis TL: Neonatal small left colon syndrome. AJR 120:322, 1974

67. Gutgesell HP, Speer ME, Rosenberg HS: Characterization of the cardiomyopathy in infants of diabetic mothers. Circulation 61:441, 1980

68. Morriss FH Jr: Infants of diabetic mothers: fetal and neonatal pathophysiology. Perspect Pediat Pathol 8:223, 1984

69. McMahon JN, Berry PJ, Joffe HS: Fatal hypertrophic cardiomyopathy in an infant of a diabetic mother. Pediat Cardiol 11:211, 1990

9

Congenital Malformations: Epidemiology, Pathogenesis, and Experimental Methods of Induction and Prevention

E. ALBERT REECE
ULF J. ERIKSSON

Most neonatal problems have gradually declined during this century. The clinical significance of birth defects, therefore, has now assumed greater importance because mortality rates attributed to congenital malformations have decreased far less than other causes of death.[1] Thus, the relative impact of major congenital malformations has continued to grow.[2,3] Congenital anomalies occur in about 3 percent of all infants born in the United States, accounting for about 21 percent of infant mortality.[2,3] The causes are heterogeneous, and some categorization has been proposed. Kalter and Warkany[3] divided malformations into those (1) caused by single major mutant genes, (2) due to interaction between hereditary tendencies and genetic factors, (3) associated with chromosomal aberrations, (4) attributed to discrete environmental factors, and (5) with no identified causes.

Diabetes mellitus is one of the most common maternal illnesses resulting in anomalous offspring.[4–21] The frequency of major congenital anomalies among infants of diabetic mothers (IDMs) has been estimated at 6 to 10 percent, representing a two- to threefold increase over the frequency in the general population and accounting for 40 percent of all perinatal deaths among these infants.[22–32]

These congenital malformations have become a serious problem with both social and financial implications. Despite extensive human and animal studies, the precise pathogenesis remains unknown, as several reviews have shown.[24,28,33–37]

Unfortunately, the origin of the dysmorphogenesis dates back to a very early developmental period when the pregnancy is hardly recognizable.[38] However, current clinical and experimental evidence suggest that the maternal metabolic milieu has a direct influence on the embryo during a critical and vulnerable developmental period in early pregnancy.[39,50] Clinical and experimental studies have also implicated alterations in maternal metabolic fuels (i.e., manifested as hyperglycemia, hyperketonemia, or altered branched chain amino acid [BCAA] levels) to be involved in the induction of congenital malformations during the critical phase of organogenesis.[40,41,48,49,51–54]

In particular, in experimental studies, increased ambient concentration of glucose,[55–64] β-hydroxybutyrate,[59,61,64–75] or BCAA[64,74] has been shown to cause embryonic dysmorphogenesis in vitro. Furthermore, experimental hyperglycemia and hyperketonemia result in a deficiency state of arachidonic acid[76–79] and certain prostaglandins.[80,81] Increased ambient glucose concentration may also cause hyperaccumulation of sorbitol,[82–86] decreased concentration of myoinositol (MI)[80,84,86–92] as well as increased generation of free oxygen radicals[63,64,74,92] in embryonic tissue in con-

Table 9-1. Etiologic Factors Associated with Diabetic Embryopathy

Altered metabolic fuels
Maternal hyperglycemia
Maternal hyperketonemia
Maternal hypoglycemia
Free oxygen radicals
Somatomedin inhibitors
Genetic susceptibility
Other maternal factors

(From Reece et al,[35] with permission.)

junction with the induction of embryonic dysmorphogenesis (Table 9-1).

This chapter reviews much of the available information on diabetic embryopathy, provides a brief summary of neural tube development and yolk sac function during organogenesis, discusses experimental studies of induction and prevention of hyperglycemia-related malformations, and examines possible pathogenic mechanisms of embryopathy, with special regard to the function of the yolk sac and the transport of nutrients and antioxidants from mother to embryo.

DIABETES-RELATED BIRTH DEFECTS IN HUMAN EPIDEMIOLOGY

Statistical analysis reveals a shift in the percentages of assigned causes of infant deaths and demonstrates that the contribution made by congenital malformations is formidable and has now become a recognized public health problem.[1–3] Maternal diabetes mellitus is one of the known causes of congenital malformations, which, at the present time, accounts for about one-half of the perinatal mortality among offspring of diabetic women.[8,20,21,28,38] Before the discovery of insulin, the outcome of diabetic pregnancies was extremely poor. In fact, Duncan in 1882[93] reported a dismal picture of rapid death for both mother and fetus, with a perinatal mortality rate of 70 percent and maternal mortality in the range of 30 to 40 percent.[94] After the introduction of insulin, maternal mortality rates declined precipitously, but the perinatal mortality rate declined very slow, eventually reaching the present rate of 4 to 13 percent.[6,13,14,21,24,26,29,31,95,96] This decline in mortality

and morbidity is thought to result from a combination of improved protocols for insulin administration, centralization of care, and aggressive perinatal/neonatal management.[19–21,43,47] Unfortunately, the incidence of congenital malformations among IDMs has not changed and, at the present time, accounts for a relatively greater proportion of morbidity and mortality of IDMs than previously.[2,11,16,26–28,31,94,96]

The first association between congenital malformations and diabetes in pregnancy is credited to Lecorche in 1885.[97] Since that time, there has been controversy regarding the incidence and potential causes of anomalous development. In the preinsulin and early insulin periods, White[98] reported that the diabetes-related malformation rate was 3.4 percent, a figure that she later recognized was understated.[99–101] In a personal discussion that one of us had with Dr. White a few years before her death, she recalled noting an increased malformation rate in offspring of diabetics, even in the early to mid-1920s. Although the association between maternal diabetes and birth defects was recognized, the magnitude and potential causality were not appreciated until Pedersen[6] demonstrated that the incidence of malformation was three times higher than in the nondiabetic population.

The results of the perinatal collaborative project derived from hospitals throughout the United States were reported by Chung and Myrianthopoulos in 1975,[25] in which they analyzed 47,000 nondiabetic pregnancies, 372 pregnancies of women with gestational diabetes mellitus (GDM) and 577 overtly diabetic pregnancies, and demonstrated that 17 percent of the infants of overt diabetes and 8.4 percent of those of nondiabetic women had malformations. However, the malformation rate in the offspring of the nondiabetic mother was higher than is usually seen in other series. It is possible that minor malformations were included. In any event, the difference was statistically significant. In 1976, Soler and co-workers[26] reported having studied 701 diabetic pregnancies between 1950 and 1974, whereas Drury and co-workers[7] reported 300 diabetic pregnancies studied between 1969 and 1976. They found malformation rates of 8 and 6.4 percent, respectively, in IDMs compared with 1 to 2 percent in the general population.[7,26] In Scandinavia, slightly lower malformation rates have been reported in diabetic pregnancy,[17,19,20] whereas in the United States, the incidence of malformations varies considerably, from almost 20 percent in the Atlanta Birth Defect Case Control study[32] to almost normal levels in a recent study of prepregnancy control in California.[21] In most studies, however, the frequency of malformations observed during the neonatal period among IDMs ranges from 4 to 13 percent.[6,13,14,21,23,24,26,29,31,33,40,95,96,102,103]

The issue of GDM being associated with congenital anomalies is controversial.[15,23,104,105] Prospective studies have suggested the possibility of increased rates of malformations in offspring of women with GDM.[7,23] Adashi and co-workers[104] in an 18-month study surveyed 113 diabetic pregnancies: 81 diet-controlled women with GDM, 6 women with insulin-requiring GDM, and 26 women with pregestational insulin-dependent diabetes mellitus (IDDM). The rate of congenital malformation was 5.3 percent in the diet-controlled GDM group, compared with no malformations in offspring of women with either GDM or pregestational diabetes receiving insulin.[104] Several other studies, however, do not support this increased rate of structural anomalies.[16,23,25] Hadden[16] reported comparable rates of anomalies between women with GDM and the general population. Other studies also report the lack of increased risk of fetal abnormalities in infants of mothers with GDM.[23,25] It is possible that the results of the former study is somewhat skewed because of the few women with IDDM.

TYPES OF BIRTH DEFECTS

Structural Abnormalities

Great diversity in the types of malformations are observed among IDMs, and analysis of collected data from many centers reveal no diabetes-specific anomalies.[23,24,28,35,38,106–110] Data suggest that these defects are indistinguishable from malformations related to other genetic or environmental causes.[111] Despite these data, some authors have erroneously suggested that caudal regression syndrome was pathognomonic of a diabetes-induced malformation.[23,28,38]

Diabetes-related malformations are major anomalies, which often involve multiple organs, causing disability or death.[23,25,35,65] The most frequent types of malformations found in IDMs involve the central nervous

Table 9-2. Congenital Anomalies in IDMs

Skeletal and Central Nervous System
    Caudal regression syndrome
    Neural tube defects excluding anencephaly
    Anencephaly with or without herniation of neural elements
    Microcephaly
Cardiac
    Transportation of the great vessels with or without ventricular septal defect
    Ventricular septal defects
    Coarctation of the aorta with or without ventricular septal or patent ductus arteriosus
    Atrial septal defects
    Cardiomegaly
Renal Anomalies
    Hydronephrosis
    Renal agenesis
    Ureteral duplication
Gastrointestinal
    Duodenal atresis
    Anorectal atresia
    Small left colon syndrome
Other
    Single umbilical artery

(From Reece and Hobbins,[110] with permission.)

system and cardiovascular, gastrointestinal, genitourinary, and skeletal systems[23–25,35] (Table 9-2).

Malformations of the Central Nervous System

Neural axis malformations constitute a significance proportion of abnormalities of IDMs.[1,22–25,40,112–116] The most common types in this group are (1) anencephaly, (2) acrania, (3) meningocele, (4) meningomyelocele, (5) arrhinencephaly, (6) microcephaly, and (7) holoprosencephaly. Malformations of the central nervous system can involve any aspect of the neural axis.[23–25,28,40,113–119] Some authors report a much higher incidence of anencephaly than meningocele: Kucera[24] reported a 6:1 ratio, whereas Chung and Myrianthopoulos[25] had an 8:1 ratio. Barr et al[117] and Miller et al[40] found holoprosencephaly, a relatively rare defect, to be increased in IDMs. The overall incidence of neural tube defects among offspring of IDDM women is considerably higher than in nondiabetic individuals.[115] Mills[28] reported a threefold difference, whereas Milunsky[115] found a 20-fold increase among IDMs. Zacharias et al[116] found, in a predominantly black indigent inner-city population, that the incidence of neural tube defects among diabetic offspring was significantly higher than in nondiabetic individuals. These various studies demonstrate that neural tube defects are increased in diabetic pregnancies irrespective of the socioeconomic status or ethnic background of the populations studied.

Cardiac Anomalies

There is a general agreement that an increased incidence of cardiac anomalies occurs among offspring of women with IDDM.[24,28,35,120,121] The types of malformations vary with different studies. The most frequent types of cardiac anomalies are (1) ventricular septal defect, (2) transposition of the great vessels, (3) coarctation of the aorta, (4) single ventricle, (5) hypoplastic left ventricle, and (6) pulmonic valve atresia.[4,22,24,28,35,108,120,121] Mølsted Pedersen et al[22] demonstrated a direct relationship between the overall rate of congenital heart disease in IDMs and an increasing degree of maternal vascular complications. Neave,[108] in a prospective study, demonstrated a positive correlation between the severity of malformations and the duration of maternal diabetes mellitus. Rowland et al,[121] in a series of 470 IDMs, reported an incidence of congenital heart disease of approximately 4 percent in these patients. This represents a fivefold higher incidence than that seen in the general populations (8 per 1,000). Mølsted Pedersen et al,[22] in a series of 853 IDMs, found an incidence of only 1.7 percent. Similar diversity in the various types of cardiac malformations has also been reported.[22] For example, Rowland et al[121] found 50 percent of the cardiac anomalies to be transposition of the great vessels, ventricular septal defect, and coarctation of the aorta, whereas Herre and Horky[120] found 73 percent of congenital heart disease being accounted for by aortic abnormalities.[120,121] Kucera[24] and Mills[28] reported an increased frequency of situs inversus, whereas Driscoll[4] and Mølsted Pedersen[22] showed ventricular septal defect to be the most common single cardiac anomaly.

Despite these diversities in the types and incidences of cardiac anomalies, the overall rate of occurrence is significantly higher than in the general population.

Renal Anomalies

An increased rate of genitourinary anomalies among IDMs was first noted by Kucera.[24] The most frequent types of renal anomalies are (1) renal agenesis, (2) multicystic kidney, (3) double ureters, and (4) hydronephrosis.[24,28,110,122] These anomalies may exist alone or in combination with other abnormalities such as Potter facies, duodenal atresia, and Meckel's diverticulum.[122]

Skeletal Anomalies

The most frequent types of skeletal anomalies are (1) sacral hypoplasia and agenesis, (2) hypoplastic limbs, and (3) pes equinovarus.[4,23,24,28,35,119,123] Sacral agenesis is a rare condition, first described by Hohl in 1857.[124] This malformation, although occurring at a higher frequency in offspring of diabetic women, does occur in infants of nondiabetic mothers as well.[123] In this light, sacral agenesis cannot be considered pathognomonic for diabetes-induced malformations. Welch and Atterman[123] indicated that confusion exists with regard to the etiology and identity of this well-known syndrome. They concluded that caudal regression syndrome is influence by at least two factors, a maternal tendency toward diabetes and the effect of a specific human leukocyte antigen (HLA) allele. This conclusion was based on the observation of this syndrome occurring in IDMs and also have a familial pattern in nondiabetic pregnancies as well.[123] These skeletal anomalies are often part of a group of defects involving multiple organs.[125]

Other Anomalies

Single umbilical artery occurs in about 6.4 percent of IDMs, representing a fivefold increase over that seen in the general population.[110,126] This malformation, however, occurs in offspring of both diabetic and nondiabetic mothers and is associated with structural anomalies including polydactyly, vertebral anomalies, clubfoot, and multiple anomalies of the heart and great vessels.[106,126]

Polyhydramnios commonly occurs in pregnant women with diabetes. This condition can be associated with central nervous system and gastrointestinal abnormalities.[10,22,110] The etiology of polyhydramnios is unclear. However, suggested pathogenic mechanisms include increased osmolality, decreased fetal swallowing, high gastrointestinal tract obstructions, and fetal polyuria secondary to fetal hyperglycemia. Experimental work, however, has not provided strong evidence for any of these explanations.[110]

Functional Abnormalities

Results of neurologic follow-up studies of IDMs have been controversial.[109,127–138] Altered intellectual or psychomotor behavior in later adult life has been intensely screened for, with very diverging results. Several reports have suggested that IDMs may show signs of impaired intellectual or psychomotor development.[127–131,136,137] Yssing[129] and Hayword et al[130] found a high incidence of cerebral handicap, and Churchill and co-workers[127] reported that in mothers whose pregnancies were complicated by acetonuria, intellectual impairment was observed in the offspring. A prospective study by Stephens et al[131] also found an increase in intellectual delay at 3 and 5 years of age in IDMs whose mothers had acetonuria. Petersen and collaborators[136] examined 4-year-old children of diabetic mothers and found affected development (Denver Developmental Screening Tests) in 11 of 34 children who had experienced growth delay during the first 8 to 14 week of pregnancy. By contrast, only 4 of the 50 children with no history of early growth delay showed affected development.[136]

There are also several negative reports failing to demonstrate any alteration in the psychomotor or intellectual development of the children of diabetic mothers compared with normal mothers.[132–135] Naeye[109] demonstrated no difference in IQ between offspring of diabetic and nondiabetic mothers. A follow-up study by Persson and Gentz[134] conducted from 1969 to 1972 in offspring of type I diabetic and GDM women reported that the neuropsychological development in both groups of infants was within normal limits. Neither group found a correlation between intellectual status and White classification, gestational age, or insulin requirements of the mother during pregnancy.[109,134]

A relationship between the IQ of the child and maternal levels of ketone bodies in the two last trimesters has been demonstrated.[138,139] Rizzo and colleagues[139] investigated the effect of maternal metabolism in pregnancies complicated by diabetes on the cognitive and behavioral function of 223 offspring. They found that the children's mental-developmental indices and Stanford-Binet scores at 2 years of age correlated inversely with third-trimester plasma β-hydroxybutyrate levels, although they were within normal limits. The above differences among investigators may be accounted for,

in part, by the fact that maternal serum ketone concentrations remained below the threshold for ketonuria as reflected in the results of earlier studies. Experimentally, a good model does not exist for assessing fetal behavioral changes in pregnancy. In the only published study to date, there were only marginal and transient signs of disturbed behavior in the offspring of manifestly diabetic rats.[140]

It has been suggested that functional abnormalities may occur even in the absence of structural anomalies. Widness et al[141] found a 30 percent increase in the level of erythropoietin in a fairly large series of IDMs, whereas Perrine et al[142] reported a consistent delay in the switch from μ-globin to β-globin. These latter findings may be related to suppression of γ-globin gene expression.[142] These observations are relatively new and may provide insight into important developmental mechanisms at the molecular level.

From the aforementioned description, several conclusions can be made regarding diabetes-related anomalies: (1) most organ systems are involved structurally or functionally, (2) there are no diabetes-specific malformations, and (3) developmental disturbances occur during organogenesis.

PATHOGENESIS
Clinical and Experimental Observations

Many etiologic factors have been proposed regarding the mechanism of diabetes-related birth defects. This phenomenon is complicated by the fact that diabetes is not a simple disorder of carbohydrate metabolism but, rather, involves the impairment of lipid and protein metabolism as well.

At the present time, the metabolic alterations associated with hyperglycemia and occurring during early embryonic development are considered the primary teratogens.[23,25,33–35,41,42,45,48,49,102,143–147] It has been suggested that in some cases hypoxemia due to vascular disease may exist, further complicating the already present metabolic alterations.[22] The findings of both clinical and experimental studies have led to the current belief that diabetes-related malformations result from a disruption of developmental processes during organogenesis by metabolic perturbations, primarily hyperglycemia.[30,33,43,77,102,103,145,148–154] Mills and collaborators,[38] using a developmental morphologic dating system of each organ primarily involved in the diabetes-related anomalies, demonstrated that these birth defects occur before the seventh week of pregnancy.

Glycosylated hemoglobin (HbA_{1c}) is expressed as the percentage of total hemoglobin A and provides an integrated retrospective index of glycemic status over the 4 to 8 weeks preceding its determination.[155] The introduction of HbA_{1c} has permitted investigators to confirm the presence of hyperglycemia during very early gestation.[39,40] Miller et al[40] and Leslie et al[39] reported a significantly higher incidence of major congenital anomalies occurring in the offspring of diabetic women who had elevated first-trimester HbA_{1c}). These results illustrate that embryos exposed to the metabolic derangements during this period of organogenesis are at increased risk for teratogenic insults. The above finding would imply a possible role of nonenzymatic glycosylation of proteins in the induction of malformations. However, experimental work from Sadler and Horton[156] does not support this hypothesis. They found that hyperglycemia produces no significant increase in nonenzymatic glycosylation of embryonic, visceral yolk sac, or serum proteins during the culture period, suggesting that this mechanism is not responsible for hyperglycemia-induced malformations in culture.[156] Unfortunately, our understanding of the role of glycosylated proteins is cloudy because so few studies are confined to the critical period of organogenesis when embryos are most susceptible to insults.

Studies have examined the relationship of hyperglycemia, duration of diabetes, vascular complications, and the White classifications with the occurrence of anomalies.[5,22,40] Karlsson and Kjellmer,[5] in a 10-year study of diabetic pregnancies, found a higher rate of malformations among patients with hyperglycemia, long-standing diabetes, and diabetic vasculopathy than among those without the above complications. They, along with Mølsted Pedersen et al,[22] found an increased incidence of malformations among White classes D through F as compared with White classes A through C. Using glycosylated hemoglobin at the 14th week of pregnancy, Miller et al[40] found that the frequency of malformations was correlated not with the White classification but with the degree of glucose control: $HbA_{1c} < 6.9$ percent = 0 percent anomalies; 7.0 to 8.5 percent = 5 percent anomalies; >10 percent = 22.4 percent anomalies. These findings are consistent with Greene and colleagues,[47] who reported a risk of malformations of 3.0 percent with $HbA_1 \leq 9.3$ percent and 40 percent with $HbA_1 \geq 14.4$ percent.

Features other than hyperglycemia have been implicated in the teratogenicity of the maternal environment in diabetic pregnancy. In clinical studies, near-normalized glucose levels do not completely protect or predict congenital malformations.[51] Furthermore, recent animal studies have suggested the existence of other maternal teratogens,[52] such as elevated β-hydroxybutyrate, triglycerides, and BCAA concentrations.[53,63]

It has been suggested that hypoglycemia or hypoglycemic reactions of diabetic women may be causative in the induction of congenital malformations. Human data on this subject are fragmentary,[22] because so few controlled studies are available. In a review of the subject, Reece et al[157] analyzed case reports in the psychiatric literature of anomalous offspring in nondiabetic women receiving insulin shock therapy during pregnancy.[118,119] However, later case reports by Impastato and colleagues[158] found no structural anomalies among the offspring of 19 women who received insulin coma therapy before 10 weeks' gestation.

Findings are also inconclusive when the data specific to diabetes in pregnancy are reviewed. Rowland et al[121] reported a fourfold increase in heart disease in IDMs when the pregnancy was complicated by hypoglycemia. In contrast to these findings, Mølsted Pedersen et al[22] reported that only 8 of 65 diabetic mothers with malformed infants had insulin-related hypoglycemic reactions during the first trimester of pregnancy. Mølsted Pedersen's findings are supported by several recent clinical trials that have demonstrated no increase in the incidence of congenital anomalies despite severe and frequent maternal hypoglycemia.[159–161] Furthermore, because frequent hypoglycemic episodes occur in humans rather commonly with tight glucose control and this stringent metabolic control is associated with a decrease in the malformation rate, hypoglycemia is not likely to be a major contributor to the genesis of congenital anomalies in humans.

Hypoglycemia is teratogenic in vitro, as evidenced by the malformed embryos resulting from culture in a medium in which the glucose concentration was reduced to less than 2 to 3 mmol/L.[162–165] Animal in vivo data on hypoglycemia and outcome of pregnancy are relatively rare. Landauer[166] and Zwilling[167] suggested that insulin (rather than hypoglycemia) would be teratogenic, based on studies in which they injected large doses of insulin into eggs and found skeletal malformations in the chickens. Similar findings in the same animal have been reported by others.[168,169] Insulin has also been injected in high doses in pregnant rabbits[170–172] and resulted in congenital malformations. Also, similar experiments have been performed on mice[173] and rats[174–177] with almost identical results. There also exists a negative experimental in vivo study in which no malformations could be demonstrated despite massive insulin doses to the mother.[178] The teratogenic role of insulin in clinical settings is doubtful, as maternal insulin is considered to traverse the placenta very sparingly, and fetal pancreatic β-cells do not elaborate insulin until about 12 weeks of gestation, which is beyond the period of organogenesis.[22,179,180]

The question of a genetic contribution to congenital malformations in IDMs has also been raised. Eriksson et al[181] reported that the frequency of congenital malformations in the offspring of streptozocin-induced diabetic rats differed among Sprague-Dawley substrains. This difference existed despite similar levels of glycemic control. The U substrain showed a 19 percent frequency of skeletal malformations and an increased frequency of resorbed fetuses, whereas the H strain showed no skeletal malformations and few resorbed fetuses. More recently, Eriksson et al[59] studied hybrids from the U and H strains to determine the relatively contributions of maternal and fetal genotypes. Offspring of H female rats showed a low frequency of skeletal malformations and resorptions, regardless of embryonic genotype, whereas fetuses of U/U of H/U female rats demonstrated higher malformation and resorption rates. These rates were further increased if the embryos were more than 75 percent U genotype. In the rat model, teratogenicity in the susceptible mother appears to be potentiated by the presence of genetically predisposed embryos.[59] In a subsequent study, it was shown that the susceptibility to diabetes-induced congenital malformations in the offspring of U, H, and inbred lines of U rats was associated with a specific isoenzyme of catalase,[182] a finding in line with other studies suggesting a role for metabolism of free oxygen radicals in the teratogenicity of diabetic pregnancy. In contrast to these animal data, human studies have not directly supported a genetic influence in the pathogenesis of diabetic embryopathy. Studies by Chung and Myrianthopoulos[25] from the Perinatal Collaborative Study and by Comess et al[23] from the Pima Indian study compared the incidences of congenital malformations in offspring of diabetic and nondiabetic fathers. They did not find a statistically significant difference between these two groups, thus suggesting that genes predisposing to diabetes in the father do not result in excess congenital malformations.[23,25] These results, along with the diversity in the types of malformations and the absence of repetitive and identical anomalies among siblings, do not support, although they do not entirely exclude, some genetic factor as a major determinant for congenital malformations.[23]

Other factors that have been suggested to play a possible role in diabetes-induced teratogenesis include low levels of zinc and other trace metals,[183–186] altered metabolism of glycosaminoglycans,[187] and increased concentration of somatomedin inhibitors.[188–193] Examination of these potential factors is still at the experimental state. Likewise, the importance of changed uterine blood flow to the conceptus in early[194] and late[144] diabetic pregnancy is presently being studied only in experimental models.

From the above discussion, it can be concluded that the metabolic derangements related to hyperglycemia are a major contribution to the genesis of congenital malformations. In fact, Fuhrmann et al[43] studied the effects of strict glucose control before conception and the incidence of neonatal complications. Of 57 infants born to 56 well-controlled mothers, only 1 was born with a fetal cardiac defect, and of 420 diabetic pregnant women (292 received treatment after 8 weeks of gestation and 128 before conception), prepregnancy glucose control resulted in a significant reduction in the rate of birth defects from 7.5 to 0.8 percent.[43] Kitzmiller et al,[21] in a California-based study, confirmed the results of Fuhrmann et al and concluded that the prevention of marked hyperglycemia in the beginning of pregnancy by intensive management before conception reduces the frequency of major congenital anomalies among IDMs to that of the nondiabetic population. Similar findings were reported by several other investigators.[19,20,39,40,46,47,50,51,195,196]

These data support the notion that hyperglycemia is teratogenic. However, the actual mechanism and the target site of hyperglycemia have not been elucidated by these clinical studies. The results of these studies point to (1) the need for detailed investigations to be performed during the critical period when malformations occur and (2) the likelihood that the etiology and pathogenesis of malformation will be best learned from animal experimentation because of the obvious limitations for such studies being performed in humans.

EXPERIMENTAL ETIOLOGIC STUDIES

Experimental teratology dates back to the work of Hale[197] in 1933 in which he used dietary manipulations to induce congenital malformations. This work represents the first controlled and successful induction of congenital malformations in mammals and led to the evolution of a new field. Many investigators using different agents and different species were able to induce malformations similar to those seen in humans.[2,3,198]

Alloxan was the first drug used to chemically induce diabetes in rodents. Fujimoto et al[199] reported a high incidence of congenital anomalies and a high rate of embryo resorption in rabbits with alloxan-induced diabetes. Barashnev[200] demonstrated a time dependency in which malformations of the brain were noted only when alloxan was administered to rabbits between pregnancy days 2 and 9. The brain was reduced in weight and size, the cortex was thinner, and there was underdevelopment of the vascular network. The retarded growth of the brain capillaries was present even when the brain weight, size, and external appearance were not different from controls. He concluded that pregnancies occurring in association with a slight but persistent disturbance in carbohydrate metabolism could lead to either intrauterine fetal death or fetuses with brain maldevelopment.[200] This period of embryonic vulnerability was further confirmed by other investigators.[41,45,48,49] Similar studies in rodents showed high incidences of malformations of the skeletal system, heart, and eyes as well as increased mortality of the offspring.[201–203] Endo et al,[204] using mice with alloxan-induced diabetes, found an increased incidence of polyploidy, aneuploidy, and chromosomal breaks in malformed offspring. They also found similar results in the blastocysts of diabetic mice.[204]

The major criticism with the model of drug-induced diabetes in animals is the possibility that the embryonic malformation may be due either to the drug itself or to the drug-induced diabetic condition.[205] Other investigators consider these agents, which induce diabetes, to be unlikely teratogens because of their short half-life. For example, the half-life of alloxan is about 2 to 5 minutes. Some groups have used streptozocin because it is presumed to have fewer side effects than does alloxan.[55,205–208]

In one study, glucose was infused in rats to stimulate the hyperglycemic state of diabetes. However, these experiments were performed toward the latter part of pregnancy. Because the period of teratogenic vulnerability is in early pregnancy, it was not surprising that these investigators did not find an increased rate of malformations.[209] However, when glucose was infused into the amniotic cavity during early gestation, malformations were observed.[210] Several other hexoses have also been shown to cause malformations, although the teratogenic effects of glucose seem to be specific for the D-form and increased glucose levels. Reece and others[150–154] have shown that the teratogenicity at increased glucose concentration is independent of its osmolality and related to a direct effect of aberrant metabolic fuel. Several other investigators have supported this view.[55,64,145,211–213]

Conversely, Horii et al[214] found a significant reduction in congenital malformations and fetal mortality rate when insulin was used to treat mice with alloxan-induced diabetes. Subsequently, several investigators emphasized the importance of good metabolic control as a method of preventing embryopathy.[34,41,215]

Last, other investigators have examined the potential teratogenic role of insulin, which remains controversial. Landauer[211] reported an increased incidence of "rumplessness," and Duraiswami[216] found a high rate of skeletal abnormalities in chickens treated with insulin therapy. However, they concluded that fetal maldevelopment is probably related to hyperglycemia and not to the ambient insulin concentration. Interestingly, Sadler and Horton[163] used insulin in mouse embryo culture at concentrations 500 times above a physiologic range and found no evidence of teratogenesis. It has also been shown that when rats fasted during organogenesis, fetal resorption and malformation rates increased, but this phenomenon was preventable by the supplementation of glucose and amino acids during this period.[198] Therefore, the association of starvation and teratogenesis may involve deficiency of glucose or other essential substrates, or even conditions involving ketonemia. Although maternal insulin does not gain access to the fetus as it does not cross the fully developed placenta, the influence of circulating maternal insulin on the embryo and other extraembryonic membranes (e.g., through the yolk sac) during organogenesis remains unknown.

More recently, investigators have begun using spontaneously diabetic rodents in their studies of diabetic malformations. In mice, several strains are known to be spontaneously diabetic. However, they are not suitable for this type of study because they are infertile or have a high resorption rate. In 1978, Nakhooda et al[217] first reported a spontaneously diabetic Wistar strain in Canada. Brownscheidle and Davis[218] and Marliss et al[219] studied fetal malformations in the biobreeding (BB) diabetic rat and reported a 2.3 percent incidence of gross malformations, primarily exencephaly, anophthalmia, microphthalmia, and skeletal malformations.[220] Also, they found that malformations occurred only when the mother was diabetic. Funaki and Mikamo[44] reported that in their colony of Chinese hamsters, the frequency of diabetes was 4.1 percent, and diabetes developed in 90 percent of the inbred generations. This group conducted an extensive and sequential study during early development from ovulation, fertilization, cleavage, and implantation to organogenesis and found no decrease in the number of ovulated eggs before implantation. However, there was a significant increase in embryonic death and gross malformations. They concluded that maternal diabetes has a deleterious effect on embryonic development during organogenesis and also causes reduced fetal growth in later developmental stages.[44]

For both ethical and scientific reasons, animal experimentation is the obvious method for studying teratogenesis. However, experimentation performed under in vivo conditions does not permit the evaluation of separate and independent maternal influences, because several alterations in the maternal milieu act simultaneously on the conceptus. Thus, understanding the effect of independent factors is difficult. The reintroduction of the rodent conceptus culture by New[221–225] revolutionized experimental teratology. This novel experimental model eliminates many complicating factors. The experimental conditions during the exposure time are precise, and absence of the maternal milieu makes the conceptus more accessible to direct observation, manipulation, and possible treatment. Currently, rat and mouse embryos can be grown in culture during the period or organogenesis with better success than other mammalian species.[55,56,59,63, 64,74,77,78,85,92,148–151,156,163,202,205–208,221,232]

As early as 1934, embryo culture was successfully conducted. However, it was not until 1967 that this technique was reintroduced, and subsequently it became widely used for studying developmental events during organogenesis.[221] Deuchar,[202] in one of the earliest experiments using in vitro culture, studied the influence of hyperglycemia on embryo development. Serum was obtained from rats made diabetic by streptozocin induction, 10-day-old embryos were cultured on watch glass covers, and no deleterious embryonic developmental effects were observed. In fact, there was "better growth" than was seen in controls.[202]

Sadler[229] used whole mouse embryos at different embryonic stages of development (two to three somites and four to six somites). These embryos are cultured for 24 hours in serum obtained from rats with diabetes induced by streptozocin and from rats with differing severities of diabetes. He found that embryos grown in serum from severely diabetic rats demonstrated a 60 to 90 percent malformation rate, whereas 28 percent of embryos grown in serum from moderately diabetic animals manifested malformations. Greater susceptibility toward malformations was seen in younger embryos of two to three somites.[229] Several investigators studied the effect of hyperglycemia during organogenesis on rodent embryos by the addition of D-glucose to the incubation medium and culture for 48 hours. They found the rate of malformations to be associated with increasingly elevated glucose levels in the culture medium.[55–57,59,63,74,77,85,92,149–151,208]

A variety of other factors shown to be associated with diabetic malformation has also been investigated. The suspected role of ketone bodies in diabetes-related malformations has been tested in embryo culture, where those compounds have been shown to be teratogenic.[59,64,66,67,69,70,72–74] It was also documented that synergism existed between subteratogenic levels of glucose and β-hydroxybutyrate added to the culture medium.[67] Somatomedin inhibitors are found in high concentration in streptozocin-induced diabetic rats and are now being considered also as a possible teratogen.[190] Sadler and colleagues,[193] using a whole-embryo rodent culture model, were able to demonstrate that the presence of the low-molecular-weight fraction of somatomedin inhibitors was associated with an increased incidence of malformations and impaired growth.

A more recent hypothesis for the mechanism of diabetic embryopathy has been put forth by Eriksson and Borg.[63,74] They have postulated that increased free oxygen radical formation is causally related to diabetes-related malformations. The support for this hypothesis comes mainly from evidence that free oxygen radical scavenging enzymes are protective against glucose-induced malformations. They cultured rat embryos in media containing 10 mM glucose to serve as controls, 50 mM glucose (a concentration capable of producing a major malformation rate of 81 percent, or 50 mM glucose plus the oxygen scavenging enzymes superoxide dismutase, catalase, or glutathione peroxidase. The addition of catalase or glutathione peroxidase to the culture media lowered the malformation rates but did not return them to normal, whereas the addition of superoxide dismutase returned the rate of malformations to those of the controls.[63]

Using the postimplantation rat model Eriksson[74] and colleagues demonstrated the protective effect of free oxygen radical scavenging enzymes in regard to malformations produced by hyperglycemia, β-hydroxybutyrate, and α-ketoisocaproate. The addition of superoxide dismutase to the hyperglycemic medium protected against the teratogenic effects of all three agents.[74] The addition of the pyruvate transport inhibitor α-cyano-4-hydroxycinnamic acid, however, provided significant protection only against the malformations induced by glucose and pyruvate, suggesting that free oxygen radicals, considered to be responsible for teratogenesis, are produced in the mitochondria because these hexoses are oxidized in the mitochondria. The authors offered the hypothesis that embryos exposed to a diabetic milieu experience too much oxidative substrate and too little mitochondrial capacity to handle the increased load of free oxygen radicals. Furthermore, the authors believe that increased free oxygen radical activity leads to enhanced lipid peroxidation, and this, in turn, causes an imbalance in prostaglandin synthesis. This concept provides a plausible linkage of excess production of free oxygen radicals with the MI-arachidonic acid (AA)/prostaglandin aberrant fuel phenomenon.

Abnormalities in intracellular mI and phosphoinositide metabolism have also been implicated in the pathogenesis of diabetic embryopathy. Several investigators[80,83,84,86–91] demonstrated in vitro that increasing concentrations of glucose result in a parallel decrease in the MI concentration in embryos. Conversely, supplementation with MI restores the concentrations to normal values and results in a significant decrease in malformations. Furthermore, in the report of Hashimoto and colleagues,[86] malformation rate was reduced from 33 percent in the hyperglycemic medium to 6 percent when the in vitro medium was supplemented with MI. Studies by Baker et al[80] and Hod et al[88] reported similar results.

Khandelwal and colleagues[233] have performed the only in vivo study with myo-inositol to date. They supplemented streptozocin-induced diabetic pregnancy rats with daily oral MI or AA. The rats were sacrificed on day 12, and embryos and yolk sacs were examined for evidence of malformations. They found that malformation rates were reduced from 22 to 7 percent with either MI or AA supplementation. Furthermore, this difference correlated with MI tissue levels in both embryos and yolk sacs. They concluded that supplementation restores the membrane phospholipid integrity that is depleted by hyperglycemia.

A brief summary of neural tube development is presented below, as this is one of the most common forms of malformations, and serves as useful background information before a detailed discussion at the cellular level.

NORMAL DEVELOPMENT OF THE NEURAL TUBE AND YOLK SAC

During organogenesis, when organ primordia are being formed, the conceptus is most susceptible to teratogenic insults. The central nervous system is the first organ primordium formed and one of the most frequently affected by teratogens.

The original description of the nervous system development dates back to the previous century. However, information relative to our understanding of crucial events of neurulation is still not well understood.[234,235] In vertebrates, neural tube development begins by formation of a groove in the endoderm that later widens and thickens to form a neural plate. Subsequently, folding occurs toward the midline with the eventual fusion or closure. Other elements forming neural tissue are neural crest cells and epidermal placodes.[234] The process of neurulation involves changes in cell shape and surface molecules producing cell adhesions.[236,237] There are relatively few mitotic cells in the neural plate at this stage, and proliferation is not a major factor in neurulation. Immediately after closure of the neural tube, rapid and disproportionate cell proliferation occurs, leading to the formation of the forebrain, midbrain, and hindbrain vesicles. The walls of the recently closed neural tube consist of neuroepithelial cells, which are primitive nerve cells or neuroblasts. In a transverse section of the neural tube during organogenesis, three cell layers are present: the innermost layer, close to the lumen, is the matrix or ventricular layer; next is the mantle layer; and the outermost layer is the marginal layer. Mitosis occurs in the matrix layer, with the daughter cells entering into the matrix and mantle layers. The axons of these cells grow into the marginal layer.[238] The cells that make up the neuroepithelium are the epithelial, neuroglia, and nerve cells.

Throughout intrauterine life, the embryo/fetus is dependent on its extraembryonic membranes, which are derivatives of the wall of the blastocyst. Early studies have provided evidence indicating that the rodent yolk sac is an important site of transport of nutrients and gases between mother and embryo during embryogenesis.[239–243] Payne and Deuchar[244] examined the importance of the different yolk sac layers and demonstrated that only the visceral endodermal yolk sac layer was essential for normal growth and development. Also, the in vitro culture system itself proved that an intact visceral yolk sac layer is essential for the success of the culture.[221–225]

Reece et al[153] proposed that before organogenesis, the newly implanted embryo receives its nutrients via a so-called histotrophic route[77,245,246] (Fig. 9-1). During organogenesis, there is a dramatic change in the route of nutrition with the establishment of the first circulation (vitelline circulation) that provides the means for a hemotrophic type of nutrition.[77,153,245,246] Furthermore, in this period of development, the yolk sac provides protection, transport of nutrients, the site of origin of blood cells and vessels, germ cell primordia, and epithelia of the respiratory and digestive tracts.[237,241–252] Ultrastructural studies have shown that the visceral endodermal yolk sac cells are typical absorptive epithelial cells with a brush border on the apical surface.[150,251–254] These cells contain abundant rough endoplasmic reticulum indicative of active protein synthesis for export and possibly for use by the developing embryo.[77,150,247,251–254] The many mitochondria present in these cells suggest that intense

TYPE OF NUTRITION	HISTOTROPHIC NUTRITION	HEMOTROPHIC NUTRITION	PLACENTAL NUTRITION
STAGE OF DEVELOPMENT	PRE-YOLK SAC	YOLK SAC	PLACENTA
GESTATIONAL AGE	<2 WEEKS	2-5 WEEKS	>5 WEEKS
SCHEMATIC REPRESENTATION			

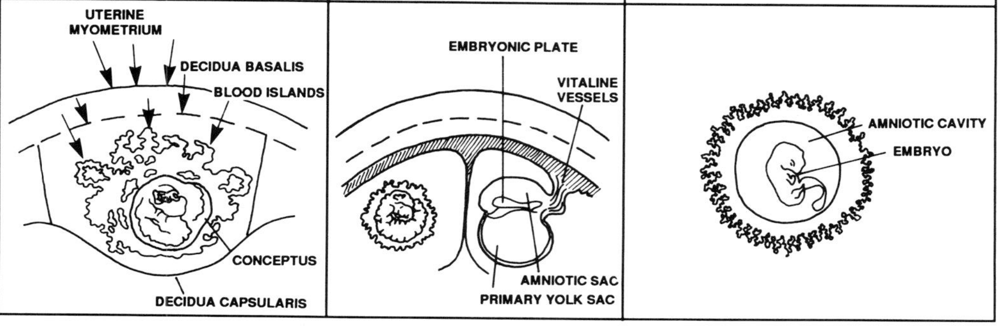

Fig. 9-1. Schematic representation of the stages of yolk sac development and early developmental nutrition. (From Reece et al.,[153] with permission.)

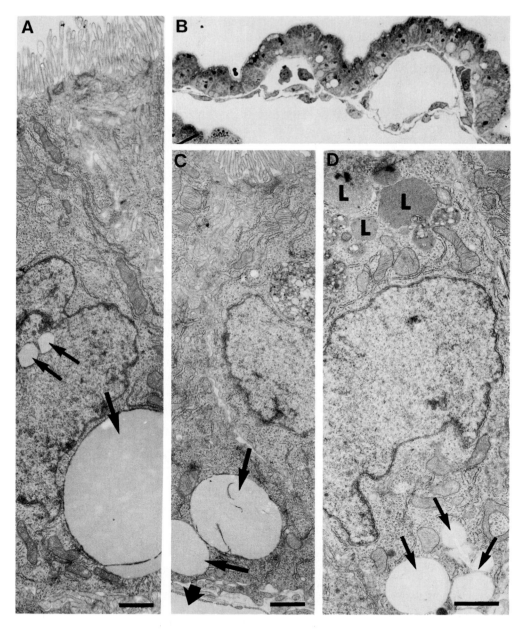

Fig. 9-2. Electron **(A, C, & D)** and light **(B)** micrographs of the visceral endodermal yolk sac layer of conceptuses grown in utero (pregnancy day 12). This layer shows a wave-like surface appearance with underlying vitelline vessels and mesothelium (Fig. B). The apical part of these endodermal cells contain lysosome-like structures, and the basal part contains many lipid droplets (Fig. B). The visceral endodermal cells possess slender microvilli, several mitochondria, free ribosomes, a rich network of rough endoplasmic reticulum (Figs. A, C, & D) and lysosome-like structures (L). *Arrows* (Figs. A, C, & D) point out the lipid droplets in the subnuclear region and in the nucleus. The underlying capillary is shown by a *thick arrowhead* (Fig. C). The basal cell surface has many finger-like projections (Figs. A & C). Bar scale on Figs. A, C, & D: 1 μm. Original magnification of Fig. B: ×40. (From Pinter et al.,[77] with permission.)

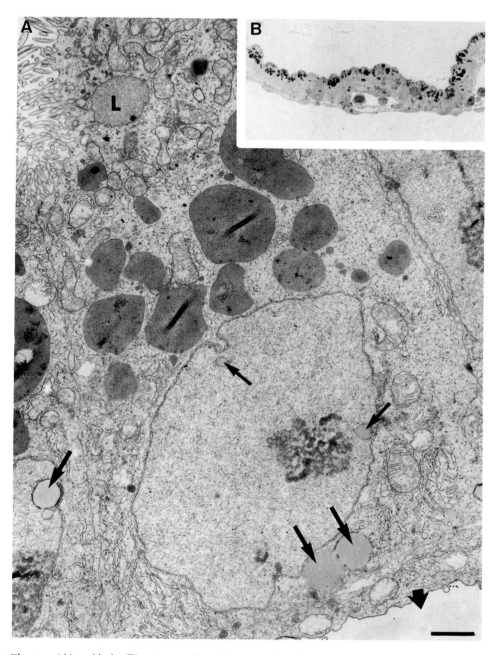

Fig. 9-3. Electron (**A**) and light (**B**) micrographs of the visceral endodermal layer of rat yolk sac from conceptuses cultured from day 10 to 12 in male rat serum. The visceral endodermal layer exhibits a wave-like pattern, with underlying capillaries and mesothelium (Fig. B). The electron micrograph (Fig. A) shows microvilli and several mitochondria, rich endoplasmic reticulum, free ribosomes and many apical lysosome-like (L) structures with varying degrees of electron density. *Arrows* indicate that small lipid droplets at the base of the cell and in the nucleus. An *arrowhead* shows the capillary lumen (Fig. A). Bar scale on Fig. A: 1 μm. Original magnification of Fig. B: ×40. (From Pinter et al.,[77] with permission.)

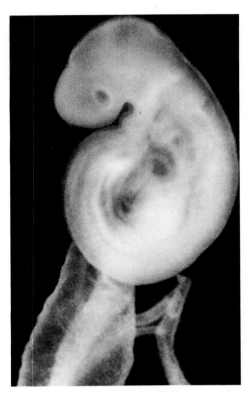

A

Fig. 9-4. (A) A 12-day-old control embryo cultured in male rat serum for 2 days (days 10 to 12). Note the C-shaped form and well-developed structures. (B) A 12-day-old embryo cultured in hyperglycemic medium (750 μg/dl). The embryo is malformed and characterized by incomplete body rotation (*long arrow* indicating tail), heart abnormality with pericardial effusion *(broad arrow)*, and widely open neural tube *(arrowheads)*. The removed yolk sac is seen in Figs. A and B below the embryo. Magnification: ×200.

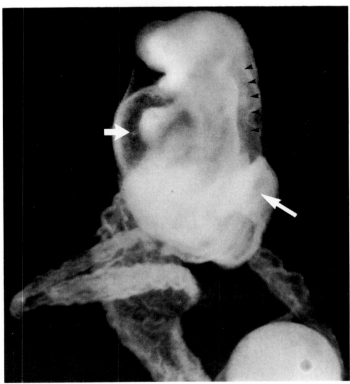

B

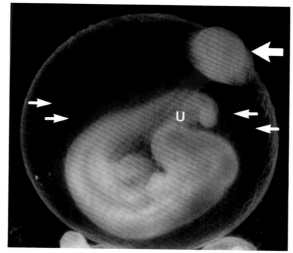

Plate 9-1A

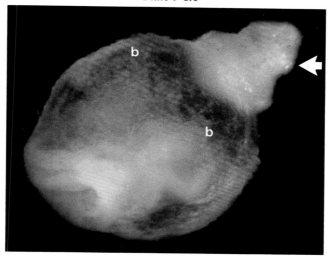

Plate 9-1B

Plate 9-1. Whole mount photographs of conceptuses grown for 2 days in male rat serum, glucose 125 mg/dl **(A),** or in male rat serum with D-glucose added to a final concentration of 750 mg/dl **(B).** Large arrow points to the electoplacental cone. Smaller arrows in **A** point to the normal vitelline vessels that course along the fetal (inner) face of the visceral yolk sac and eventually will form the umbilical vessels **(U).** By contrast, widely dispersed, hypoplastic vitelline vessels and isolated blood islands **(B)** can be seen through the thickened opaque visceral yolk sac of the excess hyperglycemic treated conceptus **(B).** The normal embryo is seen within the visceral yolk sac of the euglycemic treated conceptus **(A).** The deformed embryo in the hyperglycemic treated conceptus is seen as a small dense object within the shaggy yolk sac **(B).** The original magnification of A: ×160; B: ×190. (From Pinter et al.,[151] with permission.)

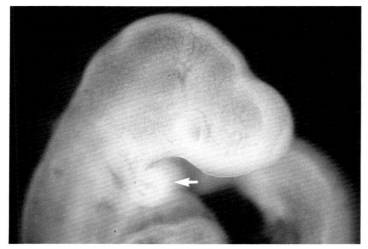

Plate 9-2A

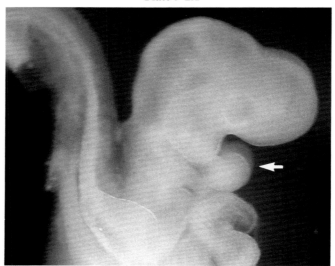

Plate 9-2B

Plate 9-2. Magnification (×400) of head region of 12-day-old embryos cultured in control and hypergly-cemic (750 μg/dl) medium. **(A)** (Control) The well-developed vascular pattern of the head, and the first branchial arch (*arrow*) of a normal embryo. **(B)** (Hyperglycemia exposed) Poorly developed vasculature of the head region in an abnormal embryo with incomplete body rotation.

oxidative phosphorylation occurs, which provides a source of energy.[76,149,246–248] The supranuclear region of these visceral endodermal yolk sac cells contains lysosome-like structures, coated pits, and vesicles, whereas the intranuclear region contains large stored lipid droplets[77,151,253] (Figs. 9-2 and 9-3).

The whole embryo culture system has enabled the study of neural tube and yolk sac development during a time that corresponds to postconception weeks 3 to 5 in human gestation.[255] Rat embryos are explanted on pregnancy day 9.5 and cultured for 48 hours.[77,148–151] Examination of conceptuses is performed at the end of culture. Developmental events during this period include the establishment of the vitelline circulation, development of heart, neural tube, face, optic and otic vesicles, and somites, and body rotation.[256] These events are consistent, reproducible, and similar to conceptuses grown in vivo.[151,223,255,257,258]

The neural tube is normally closed by the end of the culture period, and normal conceptus development can be seen (Plate 9-1 and Fig. 9-4). Light microscopic examination reveals an intact three-layered epithelium with a surrounding mesenchymal layer and ectoderm. The cells of the closed neural tube are arranged in palisades, and many of them are located at the luminal surface and show signs of mitotic activity (Fig. 9-5A). Under electron microscopy, these cells appear immature, spherical, and blast-like with scant cytoplasm, large nuclei, and few cell organelles. No cell processes are found in the neuroepithelium (Fig. 9-6).

From the supportive role of the yolk sac during organogenesis, as well as the ultrastructural features of the visceral endodermal yolk sac cells, it seems evident that the yolk sac is a crucial organ to normal embryogenesis.[226,252,254]

Many major events occur in the fourth week, including formation of the central nervous system, primitive gut, heart, and vascular systems. A portion of the yolk sac becomes incorporated into the embryo to form the primitive gut, which contributes to the epithelial lining of the esophagus, trachea, bronchial tree, and respiratory surface of the lung. Other derivatives of the yolk sac endoderm include the epithelia of the liver, gallbladder, bile duct, pancreas, duodenum, and small and large intestine. The remaining communication is a slender vascularized stalk between the yolk sac and embryo.[245,246] Hasseldahl and Larson[247,250] reported ultrastructural similarities between the liver and the yolk sac. Gitlin and others[259–261] subsequently showed

in humans that the yolk sac has a protein synthetic function before the liver assumes this role. These proteins include an α-fetoprotein, transferrin, $α_1$-antitrypsin, albumin, ferritin, and apolipoproteins A and B. Furthermore, the human yolk sac secretes substantial amounts of apolipoproteins and is a potential major source of a wide variety of apolipoproteins during organogenesis[262] and thus may be considered a site of active and early protein production. Because the visceral endodermal yolk sac cells contain elaborate rough endoplasmic reticulum, it seems reasonable to assume that this is a major site of protein synthesis for embryonic use. Interest has been focused on the protein synthetic function of the conceptus during early development.[263–271] Shi et al[262] found that the visceral endodermal yolk sac cells are the earliest intrinsic source of apolipoproteins in mouse embryos. These apolipoproteins are lipid carrier molecules and are also synthesized by the liver and the gut over the period of embryonic development. The epithelial lining of these organs is a derivative of the endodermal yolk sac cells. The known functions of apolipoproteins include the solubilization of lipids, the recognition and modulation of enzymes involved in lipid metabolism, and the binding of lipoproteins to their cellular receptors. Also, lipoproteins are needed to allow rapid growth of undifferentiated human teratoma cells. This fact raises the possibility that the undifferentiated, rapidly multiplying embryonic cells also have similar requirements.[77,151]

ABNORMAL DEVELOPMENT OF THE NEURAL TUBE AND YOLK SAC

Studies of diabetes-related teratogenesis in the laboratories of Reece et al and Pinter et al, as well as other investigators, focus on the mechanism of teratogenesis and possible target sites of action. The postimplantation whole rat conceptus culture is used.[77,148–151,156, 221–225,228,230,255] A common finding is that conceptuses cultured in hyperglycemic media are growth-retarded with multiple anomalies (Figs. 9-4B and 9-5B and Table 9-3). The frequency of these malformations are related to the glucose concentration (350 mg/dl, 2 times normal concentration = 10 to 20 percent; 750 mg/dl, 4 times normal concentration = 50 percent; 950 mg/dl, 6 times normal concentration = 100 percent). The

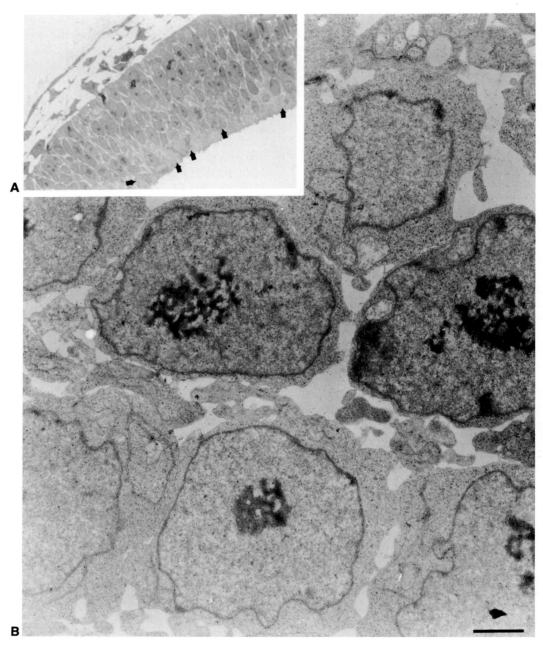

Fig. 9-5. Light **(A)** and electron **(B)** micrographs of the neuroepithelium of a rat embryo cultured in normal male rat serum between days 10 and 12. The three layers of the neuroepithelium (ependymal, mantle, marginal) and the surrounding mesoderm can be seen. *Arrows* indicate the ependymal surface with cells tightly held together in mitosis. The mantle layer shows cells separated from each other by extracellular spaces. The electron micrograph (Fig. B) shows profiles with electron dense nuclei, nucleoli, and cytoplasm. The cell membranes are complex with multiple polypoid folds. Short cytoplasmic processes establish intercellular connections. Bar scale: 1 μm; original magnification of light micrograph: ×40. (From Reece et al,[54] with permission.)

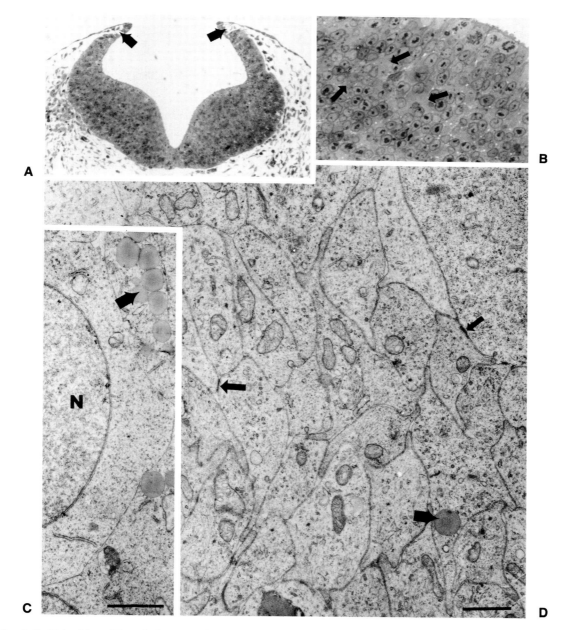

Fig. 9-6. Light **(A & B)** and electron **(C & D)** micrographs of the neuroepithelium of a rat embryo cultured between days 10 and 12 in male rat serum containing added D-glucose (total concentration of 750 mg/dl). (Fig. A) Cross section of an open neural tube. Note that the mesenchymal layer attaches to the neuroepithelial cell layer *(arrows)*. (Fig. B) High-power magnification of the neuroepithelium. The neuroblasts are generally round or cuboidal and closely opposed to each other without intervening spaces. *Arrows* indicate cell-free areas containing homogeneous material. Electron micrograph (Fig. D) demonstrates extensive neuropil formation in the "homogeneous-like" areas indicated with *arrows* on Fig. B. These neural processes contain neurotubules and occasionally some non-membrane-bound apparently lipid droplets *(large arrow)*. Between these neural processes are membrane specializations *(small arrows)*. (Fig. C) A pair of cell bodies in detail, one of which contains a less electron dense nucleus (N) and cytoplasm without projections, as compared with controls. Also, several lipid droplets can be observed in the cytoplasm *(large arrow)*. Bar scale: 1 μm; original magnification of Fig. A: ×10; Fig. B: ×40 (From Reece et al,[54] with permission.)

Table 9-3. Evaluation of Rat Conceptuses in Control and Hyperglycemic Culture Conditions[a]

Culture Conditions	Postincubation Conceptus Size (mm)		Embryos with Malformations
	YSD	CRL	
Control:			
D-glucose = 125 mg/dl	x = 5.56	x = 5.06	None
Osmolality = 280 mOsm/kg	SD = 0.733	SD = 0.266	
D-glucose = 750 mg/dl	x = 4.51	x = 4.31	21 (50%)
Osmolality = 305 mOsm/kg	SD = 0.848	SD = 0.865	
	P < .001	P < .001	
	(A v B)	(A v B)	
L-glucose = 625 mg/dl	x = 5.19	x = 4.21	None
D-glucose = 125 mg/dl (total glucose = 750 mg/dl)	SD = 0.17	SD = 0.79	
Osmolality = 306 mOsm/kg	P = NS	P < .001	
	(A v C)	(A v C)	

Abbreviations: YSD, yolk sac diameter; CRL, crown-rump length.
[a] Preincubation conceptus diameter about 1.00 mm, measured in the midregion between the embryonic and ectoplacental cones.
(Evaluation from Witschi,[256] with permission.)

neural tube demonstrates failure of closure, loss of ordered cellular arrangement, and mitotic cells that are few in number and remote from the luminal surface (Fig. 9-6A). Homogeneous material is present between cells at the site of failed fusion (Fig. 9-2B). Electron microscopic examination of these areas revealed many cell processes containing mitochondria, microtubules, and lipid droplets (Figs. 9-2C and 9-4D). Morphometric analysis demonstrated that the percentage of neural tissue occupied by cell processes (neuropil) is significantly increased and that occupied by the blood vessels was significantly decreased (Table 9-4).[148,272] Warkany and Lemire[273] emphasized the development of abnormal vessel formation occurring as early as the third week of pregnancy. The mitochondria of the neural tube in embryos from high glucose cul-

ture media, corresponding to rat gestational age of day 11, display marked high-amplitude swelling.[64] This swelling is also present to some degree in other types of embryonic cells, as well as in embryos from diabetic rats of gestational days 9 to 12, whereas it is not present in organs from day 15 fetuses of diabetic rats.[64] These results highlight the embryonic mitochondria as an organelle of specific morphologic vulnerability in a diabetic environment.

The findings observed in hyperglycemic conditions are unique, because neuropil formation never occurs before complete neural tube closure. In fact, examination of normal 14-day-old embryos did not reveal the magnitude of neuropil formation that is seen in hyperglycemic conditions.[148] This premature specialization that leads to loss of cellular arrangement has resulted

Table 9-4. Morphometric Analysis of Embryonic Neuroepithelium and Yolk Sac Surface in Control and Experimental Conditions[a]

Experimental Condition	Neural Tube Surface Occupied by		Yolk Sac Surface Occupied by Blood Vessels
	Blood Vessels (%)	Neuropil (%)	
In vivo control	12.1 ± 1.8	1.5 ± 0.6	46.0 ± 5.0
In vitro control	9.7 ± 0.4	1.5 ± 0.8[b]	9.0 ± 0.9[c]
950 mg/ml D-glucose	3.1 ± 0.1[c]	13.3 ± 2.5[c]	3.9 ± 1.4[c]
950 mg/ml D-glucose + 20 μg/ml arachidonic acid	8.2 ± 0.4[b]	1.5 ± 0.4[b]	23.2 ± 8.2[b]

[a] Data are mean ± SEM from 10 semithin sections evaluated from each embryo and yolk sac.
[b] Value is significantly (P < .0001) different from that of experimental group, 950 mg/ml D-glucose.
[c] Value is significantly (P < .001) different from that of in vitro controls.
(Morphometry from Weibel,[272] with permission.)

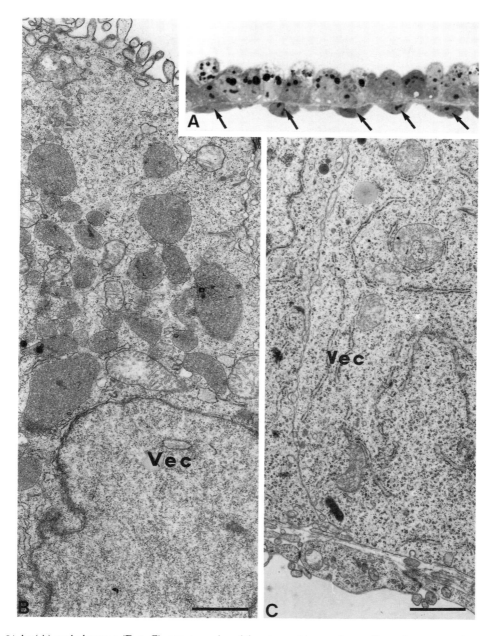

Fig. 9-7. Light **(A)** and electron **(B & C)** micrographs of the visceral layer of rat yolk sac from an embryo cultured in male rat serum containing D-glucose (total concentration, 750 mg/dl) from day 10 to 12. The embryo had an open neural tube. (Fig. A) The visceral endodermal cell layer is flat, and in this area, the mesothelial cells *(arrows)* are closely opposed to the endodermal layer without capillary lumens or blood cells. Electron micrographs (Figs. B & C) show the upper (Fig. B) and basal (Fig. C) part of visceral endodermal cells. These cells contain scant endoplasmic reticulum, few ribosome rosettes, and dilated mitochondria with lucent matrix. The nucleus contains less electron dense chromatin than in controls. Microvilli are short and thick. Bar scale on Figs. B and C: 1 μm. Original magnification of Fig. A: ×40 (From Pinter et al,[151] with permission.)

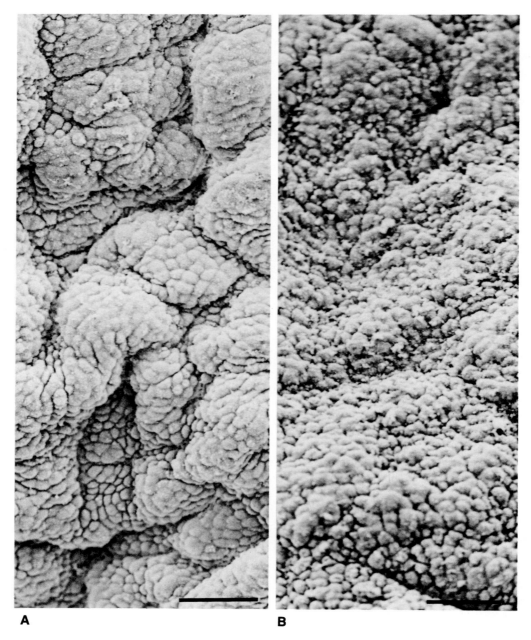

A   **B**

Fig. 9-8. Scanning electron micrographs of the outer surface properties of the visceral endodermal yolk sac layer of 12-day-old conceptuses cultured in control and hyperglycemic sera. **(A)** The yolk sac of controls, with many cells forming groups sitting on underlying blood vessels and giving a wave-like appearance. **(B)** The yolk sac surface of conceptuses cultured in hypoglycemic serum (950 μg/dl). These cells have flattened surfaces, with poorly developed underlying blood vessels. Bar scale: 50 μm.

in early divergence of neuroepithelial cell precursors. This aberration in cell development may be expected to have functional consequences because the accurate location of neurons and their processes is fundamental to the establishment of the correct patterns of neuronal connections.[257,274]

In these experiments, conceptuses grown in hyperglycemic serum are not only decreased in size and malformed but have consistently poor yolk sac and embryonic vessel development[77,148,151] (Figs. 9-4B and 9-5B). The visceral endodermal yolk sac cells show the following ultrastructural alterations: the microvilli are short and broad; the mitochondria are swollen; and there is marked decrease in rough endoplasmic reticulum. Also, a significant reduction in the number and size of lipid droplets, with a parallel increase in the number and size of lysosome-like structures, is also present[77,151] (Fig. 9-7). These alterations are present only when the D-form of glucose is used and absent when L-glucose is added to the culture medium at the same concentration and osmolality.[151] In the presence of hyperglycemia (always referring to D-glucose except when stated otherwise), the yolk sac endoderm demonstrates characteristic ultrastructural features of cell injury. These morphologic changes could have resulted from a variety of factors. Usually, in disease states, the cell injury is mediated via an interference in the energy supply to the cell or by damage to cell membranes.[275] We found severe impairment in the development of the yolk sac and embryonic vasculature, along with the presence of mitochondrial swelling, followed by disaggregation of polyribosomes in the rough endoplasmic reticulum, with the latest change being alterations in the lysosomes.[273] All these changes were observed in the visceral endodermal yolk sac cells[77,151] (Fig. 9-7). Tentatively, the cell injury described above could occur by deprivation of appropriate oxygen supply with rapid and severe impairment in oxidative phosphorylation and a fall in adenosine triphosphate (ATP) level with a parallel rise of inorganic phosphorus level, thus activating the glycolytic pathway and leading to the generation of lactic acid.[275]

To the best of our knowledge, no information is available on alterations in protein synthetic function of the visceral yolk sac cells in hyperglycemic conditions. However, the significant decrease in the quantity of rough endoplasmic reticulum in the yolk sac cells could reflect an alteration in protein synthesis with resultant abnormality in embryonic development.

Using scanning electron microscopy, Pinter et al[150] also found distortion of apical microvilli (Fig. 9-8) and alterations of surface specializations of blood cells (Fig. 9-9). These findings could also reflect altered function of the cytoskeleton associated with an impairment of energy supply, changes in ion movements, and alteration in pH levels.[150,276]

The above finding suggests that the yolk sac is actively involved in abnormal embryogenesis. The abnormal vasculature observed in hyperglycemic conditions is present during a critical phase of development when the mode of nutrition changes from being histotrophic to hemotropic.[150,153] The alterations in vessel development may lead to tissue under perfusion of the embryo with consequent hypoxia, acidosis, and cell injury. The abnormalities in the yolk sac tissue, which is the site of origin of epithelia of many embryonic organs, may result in developmental defects in these organs.

PREVENTION

Several successful attempts to block diabetes-induced embryonic dysmorphogenesis have been reported from in vitro experimentation. Thus, the growth retardation and neural tube defects elicited by high glucose concentration have been diminished by supplementation of MI,[79,86,88,89,91] AA,[76,77] prostaglandins,[81,82] or a series of compounds with antioxidant properties[63,74,92,275] to the culture medium. Embryos cultured in high β-hydroxybutyrate concentration show dysmorphogenesis to a lesser degree if antioxidants are added to the culture medium[74,275]; likewise in a combination of subteratogenic doses of glucose, β-hydroxybutyrate, and α-ketoisocaproate (a metabolite of leucine), the malformations are diminished by the addition of superoxide dismutase.[74]

The multitude of treatments effective in vitro are in contrast to the situation in vivo. Aside from insulin treatment of the pregnant diabetic animal, there are a few therapies reported to offer protection against embryonic dysmorphogenesis in experimental diabetic pregnancy. Goldman and collaborators[76] injected AA into pregnant diabetic mice and were able to diminish the rate of congenital malformations in the offspring. The addition of the antioxidant, butylated hydroxytoluen, to the diet of pregnant diabetic rats is shown to decrease the incidence of skeletal malformations in the offspring.[278]

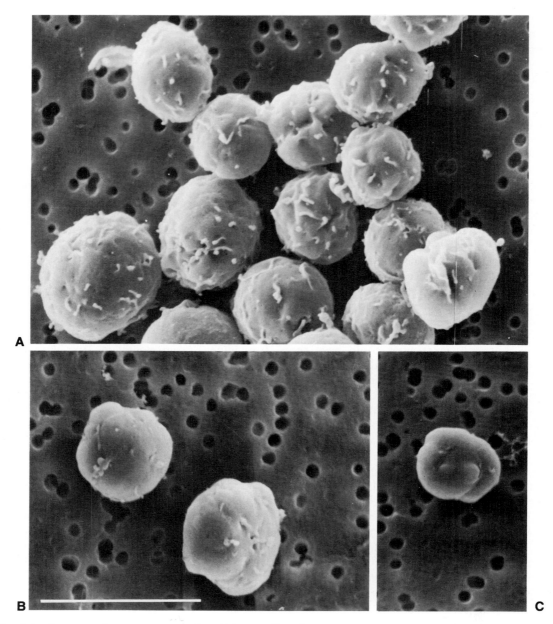

Fig. 9-9. Scanning electron micrographs of blood cells collected from 12-day-old conceptuses and cultured in control and hyperglycemic media. **(A)** (Controls) Many blood cells are seen characterized by enlarged surface area, crater formations, and surface infoldings or pseudopodia. **(B & C)** (Hyperglycemia medium) The blood cells are smooth with less prominent surface infoldings. Bar scale: 10 μm.

Table 9-5. Evaluation of Rat Conceptuses Cultured from Days 10 to 12 in Control and Experimental Conditions[a]

Culture Conditions	After Incubation		Embryonic Malformations (%)
	Yolk Sac Diameter (mm)	Crown-Rump Length (mm)	
In vitro control (n = 19) (mean ± SD)	4.04 ± 0.14	3.78 ± 0.34	0
In vitro control + 20 µg/ml arachidonic acid (n = 18) (mean ± SD)	4.36 ± 0.42 P < .003 (A v B)	3.78 ± 0.40 P < .004 (A v B)	0
In vitro control + 80 µg/ml arachidonic acid (n = 6) (mean ± SD)	4.56 ± 0.3 P < .001 (A v C)	4.44 ± 0.38 P < .001 (A v C)	0
950 mg/dl D-glucose (n = 17) (mean ± SD)	3.36 ± 0.63 P < .001 (A v D)	3.24 ± 0.46 P < .001 (A v D)	100
950 mg/dl D-glucose + 20 µg/ml arachidonic acid (n = 20) (mean ± SD)	4.34 ± 0.57	3.78 ± 0.29	20
950 mg/ml D-glucose + 80 µg/ml arachidonic acid (n = 16) (mean ± SD)	4.58 ± 0.12 P < .001 (D v F and A v F)	P < .001 (D v F and D v F)	0

[a] Preincubation conceptus diameter about 1.00 mm, measured in the midregion between the embryonic pole and ectoplacental cones.

The protection from embryonic dysmorphogenesis by these different agents has been amply documented. Pinter and co-workers[77] showed that AA supplementation to high-glucose culture medium diminished the increased malformation rate and, also, the characteristic cytoarchitectural changes that were observed in diabetic embryopathy were prevented with AA supplementation (Table 9-5 and Fig. 9-6). The conceptuses demonstrated normal embryonic and yolk sac vascularization and development (Fig. 9-9 and Plate 9-2). At the cellular level, the advanced neuropil formation seen in embryos with open neural tubes (Figs. 9-6D and 9-10B) was prevented (Fig. 9-10A). The rough endoplasmic reticulum was normalized by the treatment, as were the number and size of lipid droplets and the lysosome-like structures in the endodermal yolk sac cells[38] (Fig. 9-11 and Table 9-6). Biochemical disturbances are also normalized by antiteratogenic treatment of embryos in vitro, using arachidonic acid supplementation of high-glucose cultured embryos.[149] The fatty acid content of yolk sac triglycerides are found to be similar to those of controls, and an increase in cholesterol esters in both yolk sac and embryo is observed, with a parallel decrease in oleic acid in major lipid groups.[149] The elevated oleic acid content in major lipid groups of these conceptuses indicates a relative deficiency in essential fatty acids. After 48 hours of culture, a high residual fatty acid content remained in the hyperglycemic culture medium. This fact highlights the altered absorptive functions of the yolk sac during organogenesis in the hyperglycemic

conditions. In a later study, we used horseradish peroxidase as a tracer protein to assess the transport function of the visceral endodermal yolk sac, cells of conceptuses cultured in both control and hyperglycemic media. We found that during hyperglycemia-induced embryopathy, there is a concomitant yolk sac failure evidenced by morphologic alterations and impaired endocytosis.[152]

Diabetes mellitus is a complex metabolic disease. Disturbances in lipid metabolism are accompanied by an increase in serum lipoproteins and free fatty acids and a decrease in high-density lipoproteins.[279,280] In poorly controlled diabetic individuals, high levels of serum free fatty acids are present, whereas patients with vascular complications have increased serum palmitic and oleic acids and decreased linoleic acid and AA levels.[281]

Using gas-liquid chromatography, Pinter et al[149] analyzed the fatty acid composition of the major lipid components of rat conceptuses. Analysis demonstrated an increase in triglycerides, an increased AA and oleic acid content in phospholipids and nonesterified fatty acids, and a decrease in cholesterol esters in yolk sacs exposed to hyperglycemia. Normally, the level of free AA in cytoplasm is low and is determined by the balance of hydrolysis and re-esterification of released fatty acids into other lipids.[279] A high turnover of neutral lipid AA in brain has been observed, and this may be indicative of an as-yet-unexplored role of neutral lipids in AA liberation.[277] These considerations suggest that

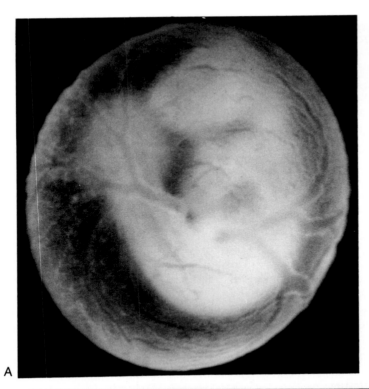

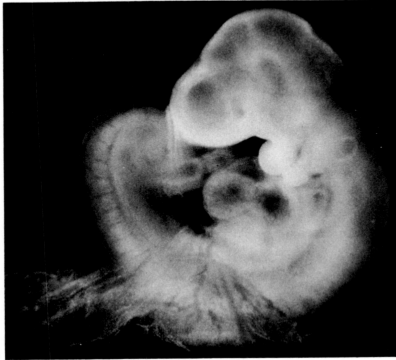

Fig. 9-10. Whole mount photographs of 12-day-old conceptuses cultured for 2 days in male rat serum with added D-glucose (concentration, 950 μg/dl) and arachidonic acid (20 μg/ml). **(A)** A normal well-vascularized yolk sac. **(B)** The normal embryo after removal of the yolk sac.

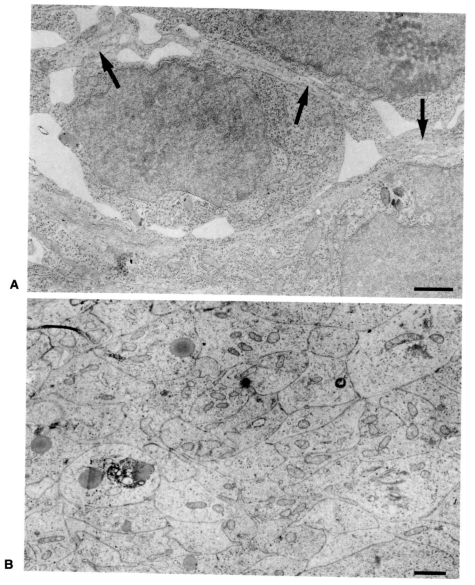

Fig. 9-11. **(A)** The neuroepithelium dissected from the rhombencephalon area of a rat conceptus cultured from days 10 to 12 in hyperglycemic medium with added arachidonic acid (950 mg/dl of D-glucose and 20 μg/ml of arachidonic acid in male rat serum). The neuroepithelial cells show "blast-like" features: large-sized nucleus, less expanded perikaryon, few mitochondria, and free ribosome rosettes. Between the neuroepithelial cells, few cell processes *(arrows)* could be observed. **(B)** An electron micrograph taken from the rhombencephalon area of the open neural tube of a conceptus cultured from days 10 to 12 in hyperglycemic medium (950 mg/dl of D-glucose in male rat serum) without the addition of arachidonic acid. The electron micrograph demonstrates prematurely formed intercellular neuropil, a characteristic feature frequently seen in open neural tube close to the site of failed fusion. The neuropil includes interdigitating cell processes containing neurofilaments and neurotubules, some of which contain free ribosomes, mitochondria, and lipid droplets. Bar scale: 1 μm. (From Pinter et al,[77] with permission.)

Table 9-6. Morphometric Analysis of the Visceral Endodermal Yolk Sac Cells in Control and Experimental Conditions[a]

Experimental Conditions	Cell Volume Occupied By				
	Lysosome-like Vacuoles (%)	Rough Endoplasmic Reticulum (%)	Mitochondria (%)	Golgi Apparatus (%)	Lipid Droplets (%)
In vitro control	7.6 ± 0.5	13.1 ± 0.8	11.5 ± 0.5	1.3 ± 0.2	21.2 ± 1.9[b]
In vitro control	9.5 ± 0.4	9.2 ± 0.9	10.4 ± 0.8	1.8 ± 0.1	6.8 ± 0.6[c]
In vitro control + 20 µg/ml arachidonic acid	10.0 ± 1.2	12.9 ± 1.3	7.0 ± 0.8	2.6 ± 0.8	19.2 ± 2.0[c]
950 mg/ml D-glucose +20 µg/ml arachidonic acid	46.2 ± 4.1[bc] 8.6 ± 0.4	3.4 ± 0.2[bc] 12.5 ± 6	8.2 ± 1.2 10.5 ± 1.0	0.8 ± 0.2 1.8 ± 0.1	1.7 ± 0.2 12.2 ± 1.1[bc]

[a] Data are mean ± SEM from 10 conceptuses in each group. All data are from 12-day-old in vivo and in vitro rat yolk sacs.
[b] Value is significantly different ($P < .001$) from that of in vitro control.
[c] Values is significantly different ($P < .001$) from that of the in vivo control.
[d] (Morphometry from Weibel,[272] with permission.)

dietary supplementation of linoleic acid can have a beneficial effect on the biochemical and morphologic changes.[280,281] In fact, using linoleic acid-rich diets to decrease vascular complications was reported as early as 1941.[281] These findings were confirmed in 1975 by Hoetsmuller,[282,283] who also demonstrated the hypoglycemic and insulin-sparing effect of this fatty acid. In a continuing in vivo study in our laboratory, Reece et al[284] have fed rats safflower oil (high in linoleic acid and AA) and primrose oil (lower in linoleic acid and AA) and were able to demonstrate that both polyunsaturated fatty acids produced a lowering of the malformation rate. However, the diminution with safflower oil was significantly lower than with primrose oil.[284]

Another type of prevention was recently reported by Eriksson and collaborators.[92] They used embryos from a mouse strain with increased endogenous superoxide dismutase activity due to the incorporation of a transgene (hCuZnSOD) into the genome[285] and subjected these to a diabetes-like in vitro environment with high glucose or high β-hydroxybutyrate concentrations. It was found that the transgenic embryos were more resistant to the teratogenic effects of these two compounds than the nontransgenic relatives, thus indicating that the antioxidant defense systems may play an important role in the prevention of congenital malformations. Hagay et al[286] have recently confirmed this in an in vivo superoxide dismutase transgenic diabetic mouse model, demonstrating a lower rate of malformation than in the diabetic nontransgenic animals.

In the light of the number of different therapies available in vitro and in vivo to block embryonic dys-

morphogenesis, it is pertinent to ask if there exists a common pathway between the different possible teratogenic mechanisms in diabetic pregnancy. Evidently, in the hyperglycemic milieu, the intracellular levels of MI and AA decrease, and at the same time, the intracellular sorbitol concentrations increase. These processes have implications for intracellular signaling, prostaglandin biosynthesis, and the levels of intracellular antioxidants, such as nicotinamide-adenine dinucleotide phosphate (NADPH) and (reduced) glutathione (GSH).[275,287-293] The high glucose concentration seems to induce the generation of free oxygen radicals and cause morphologic damage in the mitochondria of the embryo.[64,74] The excess levels of free oxygen radicals and the decreased antioxidant defense status would allow enhanced peroxidation of embryonic lipids.[294] Increased lipid peroxidation can cause a reduction in prostacyclin levels and an imbalance in prostaglandin synthesis,[288] but it has also been shown that the cellular GSH content determines the rate of prostaglandin E$_2$ biosynthesis after oxidant stress.[292] Furthermore, the hyperglycemic condition may effect DNA, either directly[295-300] or by changing the mode of gene expression in the embryo.[301,302] It would seem that the processes are clearly interrelated and that the oxidative metabolism may be of central importance. More work is needed, however, to completely clarify the situation, but it is of interest in this context that antioxidant treatment has been shown to diminish the diabetes-induced complications in experimental animal models.[277,278,301,302]

At the present time, the mechanism of protective

action of AA and MI against embryopathy is evolving. A relative AA-deficiency state seems to exist, which could adversely affect membranogenesis and membrane function.[77,149] Because AA is the precursor of the prostaglandins, which are widely distributed in many cells, the protective mechanism of AA could act through this pathway.[76] Arachidonate in mammalian cells is esterified to glycophospholipids and found as an essential part of membranes.[260,302] Golde and Van Deenen[303] showed that AA at the 2-position of phosphatidylcholine should be accompanied by a saturated fatty acid, such as palmitic or stearic acid, on the first position to maintain proper membrane fluidity. This structural situation is also necessary for normal absorptive functions of the membrane for intact enzyme function.[303] The cell membrane fluidity is also influenced by the intracellular concentrations of cholesterol and phospholipid, which are dependent on intracellular cholesterol esterification and influenced by de novo synthesis of saturated fatty acids. In the diabetic state, a decrease in desaturation of membrane lipids with consequent decrease in membrane fluidity is observed.[304,305]

SUMMARY

Congenital malformations convey a major financial and social burden to society. Epidemiologic, clinical, and animal studies indicate that these malformations occur in early pregnancy, are influenced by the abnormal maternal metabolic milieu, and seem to result from a combination of more than one factor. Unfortunately, during the critical period of organogenesis, the pregnancy is hardly recognizable, making evaluation and study extremely difficult. Also, there are obvious limitations to human study for technical and ethical reasons. Animal experimentation, however, has shown that these malformations can be produced in many vertebrates and are similar to those seen in humans. The mechanism for induction of dysmorphogenesis in experimental diabetic pregnancy has been shown to include generation of free oxygen radicals and to be associated with alterations in the embryonic levels of AA, prostaglandins, and MI. Most of the animal experiments have focused on defects at the embryo level excluding the extraembryonic membranes. Current investigations provide evidence that the yolk sac plays an integral role in diabetic embryopathy. The experimental use of several different compounds such as AA, MI, and antioxidants offer significant promise for the future in serving as a pharmacologic prophylactics against diabetic embryopathy.

REFERENCES

1. Windham GD, Edmonds LD: Current trends in the incidence of neural tube defect. Pediatrics 70:33, 1982
2. Kalter H, Warkany J: Congenital malformations: etiologic factors and their role in prevention. N Engl J Med 308:424, 1983
3. Kalter H, Warkany J: Congenital malformations. N Engl J Med 308:491, 1983
4. Driscoll SG: The pathology of pregnancy complicated by diabetes mellitus. Med Clin North Am 49:1053, 1965
5. Karlsson K, Kjellmer I: The outcome of diabetic pregnancies in relation to the mother's blood sugar level. Am J Obstet Gynecol 112:213, 1972
6. Pedersen J: The Pregnant Diabetic and Her Newborn: Problems and Management. 2nd ed. Williams and Wilkins, Baltimore, 1977
7. Drury MI, Green AT, Stronge JM: Pregnancy complicated by clinical diabetes mellitus: a study of 600 pregnancies. Am J Obstet Gynecol 49:519, 1977
8. Gabbe SG: Congenital malformations in infants of diabetic mothers. Obstet Gynecol Surv 32:125, 1977
9. Gabbe SG, Mestman JH, Freeman RK et al: Management and outcome of pregnancy in diabetes mellitus. Classes B to R. Am J Obstet Gynecol 129:723, 1977
10. Kitzmiller JL, Cloherty JP, Younger MD et al: Diabetic pregnancy and perinatal morbidity. Am J Obstet Gynecol 131:560, 1978
11. Tsang RC, Ballard J, Braun C: The infants of the diabetic mother: today and tomorrow. Clin Obstet Gynecol 24:125, 1981
12. Beard RW, Lowry C: Commentary: the British survey of diabetic pregnancies. Br J Obstet Gynaecol 89:783, 1982
13. Olofsson P, Sjöberg NO, Solum T, Svenningsen NW: Changing panorama of perinatal and infant mortality in diabetic pregnancy. Acta Obstet Gynecol Scand 63:467, 1984
14. Olofsson P, Liedholm H, Sartor G et al: Diabetes and pregnancy: a 21-year Swedish material. Acta Obstet Gynecol Scand, suppl. 122, 63:1, 1984
15. Freinkel N, Metzger BE, Phelps RL et al: Gestational diabetes mellitus: heterogeneity of maternal age, weight, insulin secretion, HLA antigens, and islet cell antibodies and the impact of maternal metabolism on pancreatic β-cell and somatic development in the offspring. Diabetes 34:1, 1985

16. Hadden DR: Diabetes in pregnancy 1985: clinical controversy. Diabetologia 29:1, 1986

17. Mølsted-Pedersen L, Kühl C: Obstetrical management in diabetic pregnancy: the Copenhagen experience. Diabetologia 29:13, 1986

18. Levin ME, Rigg LA, Marshall RE: Pregnancy and diabetes. Arch Intern Med 146:758, 1986

19. Damm P, Mølsted-Pedersen L: Significant decrease in congenital malformations in newborn infants of an selected population of diabetic women. Am J Obstet Gynecol 161:1163, 1989

20. Hanson U, Persson B, Thunell S: Relationship between haemoglobin A1c in early type 1 (insulin-dependent) diabetic pregnancy and the occurrence of spontaneous abortion and fetal malformation in Sweden. Diabetologia 33:100, 1990

21. Kitzmiller JL, Gavin LA, Gin GD et al: Preconception care of diabetes. Glycemic control prevents congenital anomalies. JAMA 265:731, 1991

22. Mølsted Pedersen L, Tygstrups I, Pedersen J: Congenital malformations in newborn infants of diabetic women: correlation with maternal diabetic vascular complications. Lancet 1:1124, 1964

23. Comess LJ, Bennett PH, Burch TA, Miller M: Congenital anomalies and diabetes in the Pima Indians of Arizona. Diabetes 18:471, 1969

24. Kucera J: Rate and type of congenital anomalies among offspring of diabetic women. J Reprod Med 7:61, 1971

25. Chung CS, Myrianthopoulos NC: Factors affecting risks of congenital malformation, II. Effect of maternal diabetes on congenital malformations. Birth Defects 11:23, 1975

26. Soler NG, Walsh CH, Malins JM: Congenital malformations in infants of diabetic mothers. Q J Med 45:303, 1976

27. Ballard JL, Holroyde J, Tsang RC et al: High malformation rates and decreased mortality in infants of diabetic mothers managed after the first trimester of pregnancy (1956–1978). Am J Obstet Gynecol 148:1111, 1979

28. Mills JL: Malformations in infants of diabetic mothers. Teratology 25:385, 1982

29. Sherman JL, Elias S, Martin AO et al: Diabetes in pregnancy. Northwestern University series (1977–1981). I. Prospective study of anomalies in offspring of mothers with diabetes mellitus. Am J Obstet Gynecol 146:263, 1983

30. Goldman A, Dicker D, Feldberg D et al: Pregnancy outcome in patients with insulin-dependent diabetes mellitus with preconceptional diabetic control: a comparative study. Am J Obstet Gynecol 155:293, 1986

31. Miodovnik M, Mimouni F, Dignam PSJ et al: Major malformations in infants of IDDM women. Diabetes Care 11:713, 1988

32. Becerra JE, Khoury MJ, Cordero JF, Erickson JD: Diabetes mellitus during pregnancy and the risks for specific birth defects: a population-based case-control study. Pediatrics 85:1, 1990

33. Freinkel N: Banting Lecture 1980: of pregnancy and progeny. Diabetes 29:1023, 1980

34. Eriksson UJ: Congenital malformations in diabetic animal models—a review. Diabetes Res 1:57, 1984

35. Reece EA, Homko CJ, Wu YK, Wiznitzer A: Metabolic fuel mixtures and diabetic embryopathy. Clin Perinat 20:517, 1993

36. Baker L, Piddington R: Diabetic embryopathy: a selective review of recent trends. J Diab Comp 7:204, 1993

37. Buchanan TA, Kitzmiller JL: Metabolic interactions of diabetes and pregnancy. Annu Rev Med 45:245, 1994

38. Mills JL, Baker L, Goldman AS: Malformations in infants of diabetic mothers occur before the seventh gestational week: implications for treatment. Diabetes 28:292, 1979

39. Leslie RDG, Pyke DA, John PN, White JN: Hemoglobin A1 in diabetic pregnancy. Lancet 2:958, 1978

40. Miller E, Hare JW, Cloherty JP et al: Elevated maternal hemoglobin. A1C in early pregnancy and major congenital anomales in infants of diabetic mothers. N Engl J Med 304:1331, 1981

41. Baker L, Egler JM, Klein SH, Goldman AS: Meticulous control of diabetes during organogenesis prevents congenital lumbosacral defects in rats. Diabetes 30:955, 1981

42. Eriksson EJ, Dahlström E, Larsson KS, Hellerström C: Increased incidence of congenital malformations in the offspring of diabetic rats and their prevention by maternal insulin therapy. Diabetes 31:1, 1982

43. Fuhrmann K, Reiher H, Semmler K et al: Prevention of congenital malformations in infants of insulin-dependent diabetic mothers. Diabetes Care 6:219, 1983

44. Funaki K, Mikamo K: Developmental-stage-dependent teratogenic effects of maternal spontaneous diabetes in the chinese hamster. Diabetes 32:738, 1983

45. Eriksson UJ, Lewis NJ, Freinkel N: Growth retardation during early organogenesis in embryos of experimentally diabetic rats. Diabetes 33:281, 1984

46. Ylinen K, Aula P, Stenman U-H et al: Risk of minor and major fetal malformations in diabetics with high hemoglobin A1c values in early pregnancy. BMJ 289:345, 1984

47. Greene MF, Hare JW, Cloherty JP et al: First-trimester hemoglobin A1 and risk for major malformation and spontaneous abortion in diabetic pregnancy. Teratology 39:225, 1989

48. Eriksson RSM, Thunberg L, Eriksson UJ: Effects of interrupted insulin treatment on fetal outcome of pregnancy diabetic rats. Diabetes 38:764, 1989

49. Eriksson UJ, Bone AJ, Turnbull DM, Baird JD: Timed interruption of insulin therapy in diabetic BB/E rat pregnancy: effects on maternal metabolism and fetal outcome. Acta Endocrinol (Copenh) 120:800, 1989

50. Rosenn B, Miodowvnik M, Coms CA et al: Preconception management of insulin-dependent diabetes: improvement of pregnancy outcome. Obstet Gynecol 77:846, 1991

51. Mills JL, Knopp RH, Simpson JL et al: National Institute of Child Health and Human Development Diabetes in Early Pregnancy Study: lack of relation of increased malformation rates in infants of diabetic mothers to glycemic control during organogenesis. N Engl J Med 318:671, 1988

52. Buchanan TA, Denno KM, Sipos GF, Sadler TW: Diabetic teratogenesis: in vitro evidence for a multifactorial etiology with little contribution from glucose per se. Diabetes 43:656, 1994

53. Styrud J, Thunberg L, Nybacka O, Eriksson UJ: Correlations between maternal metabolism and deranged development in the offspring of normal and diabetic rats. Pediatr Res 37:343, 1995

54. Reece EA, Pinter E, Leranth CZ et al: Ultrastructural analysis of malformations of the embryonic neural axis induced by hyperglycemic conceptus culture. Teratology 32:363, 1985

55. Cockroft DL, Coppola PT: Teratogenic effects of excess glucose on head-fold rat embryos in culture. Teratology 16:141, 1977

56. Sadler TW: Effects of maternal diabetes on early embryogenesis. II. Hyperglycemia-induced exencephaly. Teratology 21:349, 1980

57. Garnham EA, Beck F, Clarke CA et al: Effects of glucose on rat embryos in culture. Diabetologia 25:291, 1983

58. Zusman I, Ornoy A, Yaffe P, Shafrir E: Effects of glucose and serum from streptozotocin-diabetic and non-diabetic rats on the in vitro development of preimplantation mouse embryos. Isr J Med Sci 21:359, 1985

59. Eriksson UJ: Importance of genetic predisposition and maternal environment for the occurrence of congenital malformations in offspring of diabetic rats. Teratology 37:365, 1988

60. Diamond MP, Harbert-Moley K, Logan J et al: Manifestation of diabetes mellitus on mouse follicular and preembryo development: effects of hyperglycemia per se. Metabolism 39:220, 1990

61. Styrud J, Eriksson UJ: Effects of D-glucose and b-hydroxybutyric acid on the in vitro development of (pre)chondrocytes from embryos of normal and diabetic rats. Acta Endocrinol (Copenh) 122:487, 1990

62. De Hertogh R, Vanderheyden I, Pampfer S et al: Stimulatory and inhibitory effects of glucose and insulin on rat blastocyst development in vitro. Diabetes 40:641, 1991

63. Eriksson UJ, Borg LAH: Protection by free oxygen radical scavenging enzymes against glucose-induced embryonic malformations in vitro. Diabetologia 34:325, 1991

64. Yang X, Borg LAH, Eriksson UJ: Altered mitochondrial morphology of rat embryos in diabetic pregnancy. Anat Rec 241:255, 1995

65. Bhasin S, Shambaugh GE III: Fetal fuels. V. Ketone bodies inhibit pyrimidine biosynthesis in fetal rat brain. Am J Physiol 243:E234, 1982

66. Horton WE Jr, Sadler TW: Effects of maternal diabetes on early embryogenesis: alteration in morphogenesis produced by the ketone body. Beta-hydroxybutyrate. Diabetes 32:610, 1983

67. Lewis NJ, Akazawa S, Freinkel N: Teratogenesis from beta-hydroxybutyrate during organogenesis in rat embryo organ culture and enhancement by subteratogenic glucose. Diabetes, suppl. I, 32:11A, 1983

68. Shambaugh GE III, Angulo MC, Koehler RR: Fetal fuels. VII. Ketone bodies inhibit synthesis of purines in fetal rat brain. Am J Physiol 247:E111, 1984

69. Sheehan EA, Beck F, Clarke CA, Stanisstreet M: Effects of β-hydroxybutyrate on rat embryos grown in culture. Experientia 41:273, 1985

70. Horton WE, Sadler TW, Hunter ES: Effects of hyperketonemia on mouse embryonic and fetal glucose metabolism in vitro. Teratology 31:227, 1985

71. Zusman I, Yaffe P, Ornoy A: Effects of metabolic factors in the diabetic state on the in vitro development of preimplantation mouse embryos. Teratology 35:77, 1987

72. Hunter ES, Sadler TW, Wynn RE: A potential mechanism of DL-b-hydroxybutyrate-induced malformations in mouse embryos. Am J Physiol 253:E72, 1987

73. Moore DCP, Stanisstreet M, Clarke CA: Morphological and physiological effects of b-hydroxybutyrate on rat embryos grown in vitro at different stages. Teratology 40:237, 1989

74. Eriksson UJ, Borg LAH: Diabetes and embryonic malformations: role of substrate-induced free oxygen radical production for dysmorphogenesis in cultured rat embryos. Diabetes 42:411, 1993

75. Moley KH, Vaughn WK, Diamond MP: Manifestations of diabetes mellitus on mouse preimplantation development: effect of elevated concentration of metabolic intermediates. Hum Reprod 9:113, 1994

76. Goldman AS, Baker L, Piddington R et al: Hyperglycemia-induced teratogenesis is mediated by a functional deficiency of arachidonic acid. Proc Natl Acad Sci USA 82:8227, 1985

77. Pinter E, Reece EA, Leranth C et al: Arachidonic acid prevents hyperglycemia-associated yolk sac damage and embryopathy. Am J Obstet Gynecol 155:691, 1986

78. Engström E, Haglung Å, Eriksson UJ: Effects of maternal diabetes or in vitro hyperglycemia on uptake of palmitic and arachidonic acid by rat embryos. Pediatr Res 30: 150, 1991

79. Pinter E, Reece EA, Ogburn P et al: Relative essential fatty acid deficiency in hyperglycemia-induced embryopathy. Am J Obstet Gynecol 159:1484, 1988

80. Baker L, Piddington R, Goldman AS et al: Myo-inositol and prostaglandins reverse the glucose inhibition of neural tube fusion in cultured mouse embryos. Diabetologia 33:593, 1990

81. Goto MP, Goldman AS, Uhing MR: PGE2 prevents anomalies induced by hyperglycemia or diabetic serum in mouse embryos. Diabetes 41:1644, 1992

82. Eriksson UJ, Naeser P, Brolin S: Increased accumulation of sorbitol in embryos of manifest diabetic rats. Diabetes 35:1356, 1986

83. Hod M, Star S, Passoneau J et al: Effect of hyperglycemia on sorbital and myo-inositol content of cultured rat conceptus: failure of aldose reductase inhibitors to modify myo-inositol depletion and dysmorphogenesis. Biochem Biophys Res Commun 140:974, 1986

84. Sussman I, Matschinsky FM: Diabetes affects sorbitol and myo-inositol levels of neuroectodermal tissue during embryogenesis in rat. Diabetes 37:974, 1988

85. Eriksson UJ, Naeser P, Brolin SE: Influence of sorbitol accumulation on growth and development of embryos cultured in elevated levels of glucose and fructose. Diabetes Res 11:27, 1989

86. Hashimoto M, Akazawa S, Akazawa M et al: Effects of hyperglycemia on sorbitol and myo-inositol contents of cultured embryos: treatment with aldose reductase inhibitor and myo-inositol supplementation. Diabetologia 33:597, 1990

87. Weigensberg MJ, Garcia-Palmer FJ, Freinkel N: Uptake of myo-inositol by early-somite rat conceptus. Transport kinetics and effects of hyperglycemia. Diabetes 39: 575, 1990

88. Hod M, Star S, Passonneau JV et al: Glucose-induced dysmorphogenesis in the cultured rat conceptus: prevention by supplementation with myo-inositol. Isr J Med Sci 26:541, 1990

89. Akashi M, Akazawa S, Akazawa M et al: Effects of insulin and myo-inositol on embryo growth and development during early organogenesis in streptozotocin-induced diabetic rats. Diabetes 40:1574, 1991

90. Strieleman PJ, Connors MA, Metzger BE: Phosphoinositide metabolism in the developing conceptus. Effects of hyperglycemia and scyllo-inositol in rat embryo culture. Diabetes 41:989, 1992

91. Strieleman PJ, Metzger BE: Glucose and scyllo-inositol impair phosphoinositide hydrolysis in the 10.5 day cultured rat conceptus: a role in dysmorphogenesis? Teratology 48:267, 1993

92. Eriksson UJ, Borg LAH, Hagay Z, Groner Y: Increased superoxide dismutase (SOD) activity in embryos of transgenic mice protects from the teratogenic effects of a diabetic environment. Diabetes, suppl. 1, 42:85A, 1993

93. Duncan JM: On puerperal diabetes. Trans Obstet Soc Lond 24:256, 1882

94. Joslin EP: Treatment of Diabetes Mellitus. 3rd Ed. Lea and Febiger, Philadelphia, 1923

95. Pedersen JF, Mølsted-Pedersen L, Martensen HB: Fetal growth delay and maternal hemoglobin A1C in early diabetic pregnancy. Obstet Gynecol 64:351, 1984

96. Rubin A, Murphy DP: Studies in human reproduction. III. The frequency of congenital malformations in the offspring of nondiabetic individuals. J Pediatr 53:579, 1958

97. LeCorche E: Du Diabetic dans ses rapports avec la vie uterine menstruation et al grusesse. Ann Gynecol 24: 257, 1885

98. White P: Pregnancy complicating diabetes. p. 618. In Joslin EP (ed): The Treatment of Diabetes Mellitus. 6th Ed. Henry Klimpton, London, 1937

99. White P: Diabetes mellitus in pregnancy. Clin Perinatol 1:331, 1974

100. White P: Pregnancy and diabetes medical aspects. Med Clin North Am 49:1015, 1965

101. White P: Pregnancy complicating diabetes. Am J Med 7: 609, 1949

102. Freinkel N, Metzger BE: Pregnancy as a tissue culture experience: the critical implications of maternal metabolism for fetal development. Pregnancy, Metabolism, Diabetes and the Fetus Ciba Foundation Series. Exerpta Medica 63:109, 1979

103. Freinkel N: Fuel-mediated teratogenesis: diabetes in pregnancy as paradigm for evaluating the developmental impact of maternal fuels. p. 563. In Serrano-Rios M, Lefebvre PJ (eds): Diabetes 1985. Elsevier Science Publishers, New York, 1985

104. Adashi EY, Pinto H, Tyson JE: Impact of maternal euglycemia on fetal outcome in diabetic pregnancy. Am J Obstet Gynecol 133:268, 1979

105. Freinkel N: Metabolic implications of mild disturbances in maternal carbohydrate intolerance. Diabetes Care 3: 399, 1980

106. Dignan PSJ: Teratogenic risk and counselling in diabetes. Clin Obstet Gynecol 24:149, 1981

107. Grix A Jr, Curry C, Hall BD: Patterns of multiple malformations in infants of diabetic mothers. Birth Defects 18: 55, 1982

108. Neave C: Congenital malformations in offspring of diabetics. Ph.D. thesis, Harvard University, Boston, 1967

109. Naeye RL: The outcome of diabetic pregnancies. A prospective study. p. 227. In Pregnancy Metabolism, Diabetes and the Fetus, Ciba Foundation Symposium 63. Elsevier/Excerpta Medical, North Holland, Amsterdam, 1979

110. Reece EA, Hobbins JC: Diabetic embryopathy: pathogenesis, prenatal diagnosis and prevention. Obstet Gynecol Surv 41:325, 1986

111. Naftolin F, Diamond M, Pinter E et al: A hypothesis concerning the general basis of organogenetic congenital anomalies. Am J Obstet Gynecol 157:1, 1987

112. Dekaban A, Magee KR: Occurrence of neurologic abnormalities in infants of diabetic mothers. Neurology 8:193, 1958

113. Eunpu DL, Zackai EH: Neural tube defects, diabetes, and serum alpha-fetoprotein screening. Am J Obstet Gynecol 147:729, 1983

114. Farquhar JW: The infant of the diabetic mother. Postgrad Med J 45:806, 1969

115. Milunsky A: A prenatal diagnosis of neural tube defects: the importance of serum alpha fetoprotein screening in diabetic pregnant women. Am J Obstet Gynecol 142:1030, 1982

116. Zacharias JF, Jenkins JH, Marion JP: The incidence of neural tube defects in the fetus and neonate of the insulin-dependent diabetic woman. Am J Obstet Gynecol 150:797, 1984

117. Barr M, Hanson JW, Currey K et al: Holoprosencephaly in infants of diabetic mothers. J Pediatr 102:565, 1983

118. Matsunaga E, Shiota K: Holoprosencephaly in human embryos: epidemiologic studies of 150 cases. Teratology 16:261, 1977

119. Rusnak SL, Driscoll SG: Congenital spinal anomalies in infants of diabetic mothers. Pediatrics 35:989, 1965

120. Herre HD, Horky Z: Die Missbildunsgsfrequenz bei kindern diabetischer Mutter. Zentralbl Gynakol 86:758, 1964

121. Rowland TW, Hubbell JP, Nadas AS: Congenital heart disease in infants of diabetic mothers. J Pediatr 83:815, 1973

122. Crooij MG, Westhuis M, Shoemaker J, Exalto N: Ultrasonographic measurement of the yolk sac. Br J Obstet Gynaecol 89:931, 1983

123. Welch JP, Aterman K: The syndrome of caudal dysplasia: a review, including etiologic considerations and evidence of heterogeneity. Pediatr Pathol 2:313, 1984

124. Hohl AF: Zur Pathologie des Beckens. p. 61 In: Das Schrag-ovale. Leipzig, Wilhelm Ergleman, 1857

125. His W: Die Entwicklung der ersten Nervenbahnon bei menschliche Embryo: Uebersichtliche Darstellung. Arch Anat Physiol Anat Abt 92:368, 1887

126. Froehlich LA, Fugikuta T: Significance of a single umbilical artery. Am J Obstet Gynecol 4:274, 1966

127. Churchill JA, Berendes HW, Nemore J: Neuropsychological deficits in children of diabetic mothers: a report from the collaborative study of cerebral palsy. Am J Obstet Gynecol 105:257, 1969

128. Bibergeil H, Gödel E, Amendt P: Diabetes and pregnancy: early and late prognosis of children of diabetic mothers. p. 427. In Camerini-Davalos RA, Cole HS (eds): Early Diabetes in Early Life. Academic Press, New York, 1975

129. Yssing M: Long term prognosis of children born to mothers diabetic when pregnant. p. 575. In Comerini-Davalos RA, Cole HS (eds): Early Diabetes in Early Life. Academic Press, New York, 1975

130. Hayword JC, McRae KN, Dilling LA: Prognosis of infants of diabetic mothers in relation to neonatal hypoglycemia. Dev Med Child Neurol 18:471, 1976

131. Stephens JA, Baker GL, Kitchell M: Outcome at ages 1, 3 and 5 years of children born to diabetic women. Am J Obstet Gynecol 127:408, 1977

132. Cummins M, Norrish M: Follow-up of children of diabetic mothers. Arch Dis Child 55:259, 1980

133. Hadden DR, Byrne E, Trotter I et al: Physical and psychological health of children of type 1 (insulin-dependent) diabetic mothers. Diabetologia 26:250, 1984

134. Persson B, Gentz J: Follow-up of children of insulin-dependent and gestational diabetic mothers: Neuropsychological outcome. Acta Paediatr Scand 73:349, 1984

135. Persson B: Longterm morbidity in infants of diabetic mothers. Acta Endocrinol (Copenh), 277(suppl.): 156, 1986

136. Petersen MB, Pedersen SA, Greisen G et al: Early growth delay in diabetic pregnancy: relation to psychomotor development at age 4. BMJ 296:598, 1988

137. Rizzo T, Freinkel N, Metzger BE et al: Correlations between antepartum maternal metabolism and newborn behavior. Am J Obstet Gynecol 163:1458, 1990

138. Silverman BL, Rizzo T, Green OC et al: Long-term prospective evaluation of offspring of diabetic mothers. Diabetes, suppl. 2, 40:121, 1991

139. Rizzo T, Metzger BE, Burns WJ, Burns K: Correlations between antepartum maternal metabolism and intelligence of offspring. N Engl J Med 325:911, 1991

140. Johansson B, Meyerson B, Eriksson UJ: Behavioral effects of an intrauterine or neonatal diabetic environment in the rat. Biol Neonate 59:226, 1991

141. Widness JA, Susa JB, Garcia JF: Increased erythropoiesis and elevated erythropoietin in infants of diabetic mothers and in hyperinsulinemic rhesus fetuses. J Clin Invest 67:637, 1982

142. Perrine SP, Greene MF, Faller DV: Delay in fetal globin switch in infants of diabetic mothers. N Engl J Med 312:334, 1985

143. Fulop M: Lactic acidosis in diabetic patients. Arch Intern Med 136:137, 1976
144. Eriksson UJ, Jansson L: Diabetes in pregnancy decreased placental blood flow and disturbed fetal developments in rats. Pediatr Res 18:735, 1984
145. Freinkel N, Lewis N, Akazawa S et al: The honeybee syndrome—implications of the teratogenicity of mannose in rat embryo culture. N Engl J Med 310:223, 1984
146. Kennedy L, Baynes JW: Non-enzymatic glycosylation and the chronic complications of diabetes: an overview. Diabetologia 26:93, 1984
147. Eriksson UJ: Diabetes in pregnancy: retarded fetal growth, congenital malformations and feto-maternal concentrations of zinc, copper and managese in the rat. J Nutr 114:477, 1984
148. Reece EA, Pinter EA, Leranth CZ et al: Malformations of the neural tube induced by in vitro hyperglycemia: an ultrastructural analysis. Teratology 32:363, 1985
149. Pinter E, Reece EA, Leranth CZ et al: Arachidonic acid prevents hyperglycemia associated yolk sac damage and embryopathy: modifications in polyunsaturated fatty acids provide clues for pathogenesis. Am J Obstet Gynecol 155:691, 1986
150. Pinter E, Reece EA, Leranth CZ et al: Surface alterations of the embryonic blood cells and the visceral endodermal yolk sac layer under hyperglycemic conditions revealed by scanning electrons microscopy, abstracted. Proc Soc Perinatal Obstet 25, 1986
151. Pinter E, Reece EA, Leranth CZ et al: Yolk sac failure in embryopathy due to hyperglycemia: ultrastructural analysis of yolk sac differentiation associated with embryopathy in rat conceptuses under hyperglycemic conditions. Teratology 33:73, 1986
152. Reece EA, Pinter E, Leranth CZ et al: Yolk sac failure in embryopathy due to hyperglycemia: horseradish peroxidase uptake in the assessment of yolk sac dysfunction. Obstet Gynecol 74:755, 1989
153. Reece EA, Pinter E, Homko C et al: The yolk sac theory: closing the circle on why diabetes associated malformations occur. J Soc Gynecol Invest 1:3, 1994
154. Reece EA, Wiznitzer A, Homko CJ, WU Y-K: Experimental algorithm of factors critical for diabetic teratogenesis. Submitted for publication
155. Bunn HF, Haney DN, Kamin S et al: The biosynthesis of human hemoglobin A1C: slow glycosylation of hemoglobin in vivo. J Clin Invest 57:1652, 1976
156. Sadler TW, Horton WE: Whole embryo culture. A screening technique for teratogens? Teratogenesis Carcinog Mutagen 2:243, 1982
157. Reece EA, Homko CJ, Wiznitzer A: Hypoglycemia in pregnancies complicated by diabetes mellitus: maternal and fetal considerations. Clin Obstet Gynecol 37:50, 1994
158. Impastato DJ, Gabriel AR, Lardar EH: Electric and insulin shock therapy during pregnancy. Dis Nerv Syst 25:542, 1964
159. Bergman M, Seaton TB, Auerhahn CC et al: The incidence of gestational hypoglycemia in insulin-dependent and non-insulin-dependent diabetic women. NY State J Med 86:174, 1986
160. Rayburn W, Piehl E, Jacober S et al: Severe hypoglycemia during pregnancy: its frequency and predisposing factors in diabetic women. Int J Gynaecol Obstet 24:263, 1986
161. Kimmerle R, Heinemann L, Delecki A, Berger M: Severe hypoglycemia incidence and predisposing factors in 85 pregnancies of type I diabetic women. Diabetes Care 15:1034, 1992
162. Ellington SKL: In vivo and in vitro studies on the effects of maternal fasting during embryonic organogenesis in the rat. Reprod Fertil 60:383, 1980
163. Sadler TW, Horton WE Jr: Effects of maternal diabetes on early embryogenesis: the role of insulin and insulin therapy. Diabetes 32:1070, 1983
164. Akazawa S, Akazawa M, Hashimoto M et al: Effects of hypoglycemia on early embryogenesis in rat embryo organ culture. Diabetologia 30:791, 1987
165. Sadler TW, Hunter ES III: Hypoglycemia: how little is too much for the embryo? Am J Obstet Gynecol 157:190, 1987
166. Landauer W: Rumplessness of chicken embryos produced by the injection of insulin in other chemicals. J Exp Zool 98:65, 1945
167. Zwilling E: Association of hypoglycemia with insulin micromelia in chick embryos. J Exp Zool 109:197, 1948
168. Duraiswami PK: Insulin-induced skeletal abnormalities in developing chickens. BMJ 2:384, 1950
169. Rabinovitch AL, Gibson MA: Skeletogenesis in insulin-treated chick embryos. II. Histochemical observations, with particular reference to the tibiotarsus. Teratology 6:51, 1972
170. Chomette G: Entwicklungsstörungen nach Insulinschock beim trächtigen Kaninchen. Beitr Pathol Anat 115:439, 1955
171. Brinsmade A, Büchner F, Rübsaamen H: Missbildungen am Kaninchen embryo durch Insulininjektion beim Muttertier. Naturwissenschaften 43:259, 1956
172. Brinsmade AB: Entwicklungsstörungen am Kaninchen-embryo nach Glukosemangel beim trächtigen Muttertier. Beitr Pathol Anat 117:140, 1957
173. Smithberg M, Runner MN: Teratogenic effects of hypoglycemic treatments in inbred strains of mice. Am J Anat 113:479, 1963
174. Lichtenstein H, Guest GM, Warkanay J: Abnormalities in offspring of white rats given protamine zinc insulin during pregnancy. Proc Soc Exp Biol Med 78:398, 1951

175. Love EJ, Kinch RAH, Stevenson JAF: The effect of protamine zinc insulin on the outcome of pregnancy in the normal rat. Diabetes 13:44, 1964

176. Hannah RS, Moore KL: Effects of fasting and insulin on skeletal development in rats. Teratology 4:135, 1971

177. Buchanan TA, Schemmer JK, Freinkel N: Embryotoxic effects of brief maternal insulin-hypoglycemia during organogenesis in the rat. J Clin Invest 78:643, 1986

178. Ream JR Jr, Weingarten PL, Pappas AM: Evaluation of the prenatal effects of massive doses of insulin in rats. Teratology 3:29, 1970

179. Steinke J, Driscoll S: The extractable insulin content of pancreas from fetuses and infants of diabetic and control mothers. Diabetes 14:573, 1965

180. Kathan S, Schwartz R, Adam P: Placental barrier to human insulin I125 in insulin-dependent diabetic mothers. J Clin Endocrinol Metab 40:139, 1975

181. Eriksson UJ, Dahlstrom VE, Lithell HO: Diabetes in pregnancy: influence of genetic background and maternal diabetic state on the incidence of skeletal malformations in the fetal rat. Acta Endocrinol 277:66, 1986

182. Eriksson UJ, den Bieman M, Prins JB, van Zutphen LFM: Differences in susceptibility for diabetes induced malformations in separated rat colonies of common origin. p. 53. In Proceedings of the 4th FELASA Symposium, Lyon, France, 1990

183. Hurley LS, Gowan J, Swenerton H: Teratogenic effects of short-term and transitory zinc deficiency in rats. Teratology 4:199, 1971

184. Eriksson UJ: Diabetes in pregnancy: retarded fetal growth, congenital malformations and feto-maternal concentrations of zinc, copper and manganese in the rat. J Nutr 114:477, 1984

185. Uriu-Hare JY, Stern JS, Reaven GM, Keen CL: The effect of maternal diabetes on trace element status and fetal development in the rat. Diabetes 34:1031, 1985

186. Styrud J, Dahlström VE, Eriksson UJ: Induction of skeletal malformations in the offspring of rats fed a zinc-deficient diet. Upsala J Med Sci 91:29, 1986

187. Unger E, Eriksson UJ: Regionally disturbed production of cartilage proteoglycans in malformed fetuses from diabetic rats. Diabetologia 35:517, 1992

188. Yde H: The growth-hormone dependent sulphation factor in serum of untreated diabetics. Lancet 2:626, 1964

189. Winter R, Phillips LS, Klein MN et al: Somatomedin activity and diabetic control in children with insulin dependent diabetes. Diabetes 28:952, 1979

190. Phillips LS, Belosky DC, Reichard LA: Nutrition and somatomedin. V. Action and measurement of somatomedin inhibitor(s) in serum from diabetic rats. Endocrinology 104:1513, 1979

191. D'Ercole JA, Applewhite GT, Underwood LE: Evidence that somatomedin is synthesized by multiple tissues in the fetus. Dev Biol 75:315, 1980

192. Phillips LS, Bajaj VR, Fusco AC, Matheson CK: Nutrition and somatomedin. XI. Studies of somatomedin inhibitors in rats with streptozotocin-induced diabetes. Diabetes 32:1117, 1983

193. Sadler TW, Phillips LS, Balkan W et al: Somatomedin inhibitors from diabetic rat serum alter growth and development of mouse embryos in culture. Diabetes 35: 861, 1986

194. Wentzel P, Jansson L, Eriksson UJ: Diabetes in pregnancy: uterine blood flow and embryonic development in the rat. Submitted for publication

195. Steel JM, Johnstone FD, Johnstone FD et al: Can prepregnancy care of diabetic women reduce the risk of abnormal babies? BMJ 185:353, 1982

196. Elixhauser A, Weschler JM, Kitzmiller JL et al: Cost-benefit analysis of preconception care for women with established diabetes mellitus. Diabetes Care 16:1146, 1993

197. Hale FL: Pigs born without eyeballs. J Hered 24:105, 1933

198. Kalter H, Warkany J: Experimental production of congenital malformations in mammals by metabolic procedure. Physiol Rev 39:69, 1959

199. Fujimoto S, Sumi T, Kwzukawa S et al: The genesis of experimental anomalies—fetal anomalies in reference to experimental diabetes in rabbit. J Osaka City Med Ctr 7:62, 1958

200. Barashnev YI: Malformation of fetal brain resulting from alloxan diabetes in mother. Arkh Patol 26:63, 1964

201. Watanabe G, Ingalls TH: Congenital malformations in the offspring of alloxan-diabetic mice. Diabetes 12:66, 1963

202. Deuchar EM: Embryonic malformations in rats resulting from maternal diabetes: preliminary observations. J Embryol Exp Morphol 41:03, 1977

203. Deuchar EM: Experimental evidence relating fetal anomalies to diabetes. p. 247. In Sutherland HW, Stowers JM (eds): Carbohydrate Metabolism in Pregnancy and the Newborn. Springer Verlag, New York, 1979

204. Endo A: Teratogenesis of diabetic mice treated with alloxan prior to conception. Arch Environ Health 12:492, 1966

205. Deuchar EM: Effects of streptozotocin on early rat embryos grown in culture. Experientia 34:84, 1977

206. Sadler TW: Effects of maternal diabetes on early embryogenesis. I. The teratogenic potential of diabetic serum. Teratology 21:339, 1980

207. Eriksson UJ, Styrud J, Eriksson RSM: Diabetes in pregnancy: genetic and temporal relationships of maldevelopment in the offspring of diabetic rats. p. 51. In Sutherland HW, Stowers JM (eds): 4th International

Colloquium on Carbohydrate Metabolism in Pregnancy and the Newborn. Springer-Verlag, Berlin, 1989

208. Styrud J, Eriksson UJ: Development of rat embryos in culture media containing different concentrations of normal and diabetic rat serum. Teratology 46:473, 1992

209. Asplund K: Effects of intermittent glucose infusion in pregnant rats on the functional development of the foetal pancreatic B-cells. J Endocrinol 59:287, 1973

210. Clavert A, Wolff-Quenot MJ, Buck P: Etude de l'action embryopathigue du glucose en injuction intrammniotique. C R Soc Biol (Paris) 166:1789, 1972

211. Landauer W: Is insulin a teratogen? Teratology 5:129, 1972

212. Cockroft DL, Freinkel N, Phillips LS, Shambaugh GE: Metabolic factors affecting organogenesis in diabetic pregnancy, abstracted. Clin Res 29:577A, 1981

213. Buchanan TA, Freinkel N, Lewis NJ et al: Fuel-mediated teratogenesis. Use of D-mannose to modify organogenesis in the rat embryo in vivo. J Clin Invest 75:1927, 1985

214. Horii K, Watanabe G, Ingalls TH: Experimental diabetes in pregnant mice: prevention of congenital malformations in offspring by insulin. Diabetes 15:194, 1966

215. Brownscheidle CM, Wootten V, Mathieu MH et al: The effects of maternal diabetes on fetal maturation and neonatal health. Metabolism 32:148, 1983

216. Duraiswami P: Insulin-induced skeletal anomalies in developing chickens. BMJ 2:384, 1950

217. Nakhooda AF, Like AA, Chappel CI et al: The spontaneous Wistar rat (The 'BB' rat); studies prior to and during development of the overt syndrome. Diabetologia 14:199, 1978

218. Brownscheidle CM, Davis DL: Diabetes in pregnancy: a preliminary study of the pancreas, placenta and malformations in the BB Wistar rat. Placenta, suppl 203, 19: 203, 1981

219. Marliss EB, Nakhooda AF, Poussier P, Sima AAF: The diabetic syndrome of the "BB" Wistar rat: possible relevance to type I (insulin-dependent) diabetes in man. Diabetologia 22:225, 1982

220. Scott J, Engelhard VH, Curnow RT, Benjamin DC: Prevention of diabetes in BB rats. I. Evidence suggesting a requirement for mature T cells in bone marrow inoculum of neonatally injected rats. Diabetes 35:1034, 1986

221. New DAT: Development of explanted rat embryos in circulating medium. J Embryol Exp Morphol 17:513, 1967

222. New DAT: Methods for culture of post implantation embyros of rodents. p. 305. In Daniel JC (ed): Method in Mammalian Embryology. Freeman, San Francisco, 1971

223. New DAT, Coppola PT, Cockroft DL: Comparison of growth in vitro and in vivo of post-implantation rat embryos. J Embryol Exp Morphol 36:133, 1976

224. New DAT: Techniques for assessment of teratologic effects. Environ Health Perspect 18:105, 1977

225. New DAT: Whole-embryo culture and the study of mammalian embryos during organogenesis. Biol Rev 53:81, 1978

226. Brent LR, Johnson AJ, Jensen M: The production of congenital malformations using tissue antisera. VII. Yolk-sac antiserum. Teratology 4:255, 1971

227. Buckley SK, Steele CE, New CAT: In vitro development of early postimplantation rat embryo. Dev Biol 65:396, 1978

228. Sanyal MK, Wiebke EA: Oxygen requirement for in vitro growth and differentiation of the rat conceptus during organogenesis phase of embryo development. Biol Reprod 20:639, 1979

229. Sadler TW: Culture of early somite mouse embryos during organogenesis. J Embryol Exp Morphol 49:17, 1979

230. Sanyal MK, Naftolin F: In-vitro development of the mammalian embryo. J Exp Zool 228:235, 1986

231. Eriksson UJ: Rat embryos exposed to a teratogenic diabetic environment in vitro are protected by the antioxidant N-acetylcysteine. Eur J Endocrinol, suppl. 1, 130: 20, 1994

232. Eriksson UJ: Antioxidants protect rat embryos from diabetes-induced dysmorphogenesis, abstracted. 15th Int Diab Fed Congr Abstracts 410, 1994

233. Khandelwal M, Wu Y-K, Borenstein M, Reece EA: Dietary phospholipid therapy, hyperglycemia-induced membrane changes and associated diabetic embryopathy. Society of Perinatal Obstetricians, January 23–28, 1995, in Atlanta, Georgia

234. O'Rahilly R, Gardner E: The timing and sequence of events in the development of the human nervous system, during the embryonic period proper. Z Anat Entwick Gesch 134:1, 1971

235. Schroeder TE: Mechanism of morphogenesis: the embryonic neural tube. Br J Neurosci 2:183, 1971

236. Burnside MD, Jacobson AG: Analysis of morphogenetic movements in the neuronal plate of the New Taricha torosa. Dev Biol 18:537, 1968

237. Edeman GM: Cell adhesion molecules. Science 219:450, 1983

238. Purves D, Lichtmann JW: Principles of Neural Development. Sinauer Assoc, Inc., Sunderland, MA, 1985

239. Everett JW: Morphological and physiological studies of the placenta in the albino rat. J Exp Zool 70:243, 1935

240. Brunschwig AE: notes on experiments in placental permeability. Anat Rec 34:237, 1927

241. Leung CCK, Watabe H, Brent RL: The effect of heterologous antisera on embryonic development. Am J Anat 148:457, 1977

242. Freeman SJ, Beck F, Lloyd JB: The role of the visceral

yolk sac in mediating protein utilization by rat embryos cultured in vitro. J Embryol Exp Morphol 66:223, 1981

243. Muglia L, Locker J: Extra pancreatic insulin gene expression in the fetal rat. Proc Natl Acad Sci USA 81:3635, 1984

244. Payne GS, Deuchar EM: An in vitro study of function of embryonic membranes in the rat. J Embryol Exp Morphol 27:533, 1972

245. Moore KL: The Developing Human: Clinically Oriented Embryology. WB Saunders, Philadelphia, 1982

246. Sadler TW: Langman's Medical Embryology. 5th Ed. Williams and Wilkins, Baltimore, 1985

247. Hesseldahl H, Larson JF: Ultrastructure of humans yolk-sac endoderm, mesenchyme, tubules and mesothelium. Am J Anat 126:315, 1969

248. Hoyes AD: The human fetal yolk sac: an ultrastructural study of four specimens. Z Zellforsch Mikrosk Anat 99:469, 1969

249. Moore AS, Metcalf D: Ontogeny of the hemopoietic system: yolk sac original of in vivo and in vitro colony forming cells in the developing mouse embryo. Br J Haematol 18:279, 1970

250. Hesseldahl H, Larson JF: Hemopoiesis and blood vessels in human yolk sac. Acta Anat 78:274, 1971

251. Gonzales-Cruse F: The human yolk sac and yolk sac (endodermal sinus) tremors: a review. Prospect Pediatr Pathol 5:179, 1979

252. Gonzales-Crussi F, Roth LM: The human yolk sac and yolk sac carcinoma. Hum Pathol 7:675, 1976

253. Padykula HA, Deren JJ, Wilson TH: Development of structure and function in the mammalian yolk sac. I. Developmental morphology and vitamin B12 uptake of the rat yolk sac. Dev Biol 13:311, 1966

254. Freeman SJ, Brent RL, Lloyd JB: The effects of teratogenic antiserum on yolk-sac function in rat embryos cultured in vitro. J Embryol Exp Morphol 71:63, 1982

255. Warner CW, Sadler TW, Shockey J, Smith MK: A comparison of the in vivo and in vitro response of mammalian embryos to a teratogenic insult. Toxicology 28:271, 1983

256. Witschi E: Development: prenatal vertebrae development: rat. p. 304. In Altman PL, Dittmer DS (eds): Growth, Biological Handbooks. Federation of American Societies for Experimental Biology, Washington, DC, 1972

257. Lewitt P, Rack P: Immunoperoxidase localization of glial fibrillary acidic protein in radial glial-cells and astrocytes of the developing rhesus monkey brain. J Comp Neurol 193:815, 1980

258. Gupta M, Gulamhusein PA, Beck F: Morphometric analysis of the visceral yolk sac endoderm in the rat in vivo and in vitro. J Reprod Fertil 65:239, 1982

259. Gitlin D, Boseman M: Fetus-specific serum proteins in several mammals and their relation to human alpha-fetoprotein. Biochem Physiol 32:327, 1967

260. Gitlin D, Boseman M: Sites of serum alphafetoprotein synthesis in the human and in the rat. J Clin Invest 46:1010, 1967

261. Gitlin D, Perricelli A, Gitlin GM: Synthesis of alpha-fetoprotein by liver, yolk sac, and gastrointestinal tract of the human conceptus. Cancer Res 32:979, 1972

262. Shi W-K, Hopkin B, Thompson S et al: Synthesis of apolipoproteins, alphafetoprotein, albumin, and transferring by the human foetal yolk sac and other foetal organs. J Embryol Exp Morphol 85:191, 1985

263. Dziadek M, Adamson E: Localization and synthesis of alphafetoprotein in post-implantation mouse embryos. J Embryol Exp Morphol 43:289, 1978

264. Adamson ED: The location and synthesis of transferrin in mouse embryos and teratocarcinoma cells. Dev Biol 91:227, 1982

265. Dziadek MA, Andrews GK: Tissue specificity of alpha-fetoprotein messenger RNA expression during mouse embryogenesis. EMBO J 2:549, 1983

266. Meehan RR, Barlow DP, Hill RE et al: Pattern of serum protein gene expression in mouse visceral yolk sac and fetal liver. EMBO J 3:1881, 1984

267. Driscoll DM, Getz GS: Extrahepatic synthesis of apolipoprotein E. J Lipid Res 25:1368, 1984

268. Meek J, Adamson ED: Transferrin foetal and adult mouse tissues: synthesis, storage and secretion. J Embryol Exp Morphol 86:205, 1985

269. Lovell-Badge RH, Evans MJ, Bellairs R: Protein synthetic patterns of tissues in the early chick embryo. J Embryol Exp Morphol 85:65, 1985

270. Hopkins B, Sharpe CR, Baralle FE, Graham CF: Organ distribution of apolipoprotein gene transcripts in 6–12 weeks post fertilization human embryos. J Embryol Exp Morphol 97:177, 1986

271. Williams CL, Priscott PK, Oliver IT, Yeoh GCT: Albumin and transferrin synthesis in whole rat embryo cultures. J Embryol Exp Morphol 92:33, 1986

272. Weibel RE: Stereological principles for morphometry in electron microscopic cytology. Int Rev Cytol 26:235, 1969

273. Warkany J, Lemire RJ: Arteriovenous malformations of the brain: a teratologic challenge. Teratology 29:333, 1984

274. Lewitt P, Cooper ML, Rakic P: Coexistence of neuronal and glial precursor cells in the cerebral ventricular zone of the fetal monkey: an ultrastructural immunoperoxidase study. J Neurosci 1:27, 1981

275. Slauson DO, Cooper BJ: Mechanisms of Disease. A Textbook of Comparative General Pathology. Williams and Wilkins, Baltimore, 1982

276. Trump BF, Berezesky IK: Cellular ion regulation and disease: a hypothesis. Curr Top Membr Transport 25:279, 1985

277. Eriksson UJ: Rat embryos exposed to a teratogenic diabetic environment in vitro are protected by the antioxidant N-acetylcysteine. Eur J Endocrinol, suppl. 1, 130:20, 1994

278. Eriksson UJ: Antioxidants protect rat embryos from diabetes-induced dysmorphogenesis, abstracted. Int Diab Fed Congr Abstr 15:410, 1994

279. Irvine RF: How is the level of free arachidonic acid controlled in mammalian cells? Biochem J 204:3, 1982

280. Kinsell LW, Michaels GD, Walker G et al: Dietary linoleic acid and linoleate: effects in diabetic and non-diabetic subjects with and without vascular disease. Diabetes 8:179, 1959

281. Snapper I: Chinese Lessons to Western Medicine. Interscience, New York, 1941

282. Houtsmuller AJ: Significance of linoleic acid in the metabolism and therapy of diabetes mellitus. World Rev Nutr Diet 39:85, 1982

283. Houtsmuller AJ: The role of fat in the treatment of diabetes mellitus. p. 231. In Vergrosen X (ed): The Role of Fats in Human Nutrition. Academic Press, London, 1975

284. Reece EA, Wu Y-K, Wiznitzer A et al: Dietary polyunsaturated fatty acids prevent malformations in offspring of diabetic rats. Presented at SPO, San Francisco, CA February 8–13, 1993

285. Epstein CJ, Avraham KB, Lovett S et al: Transgenic mice with increased CuZn-superoxide dismutase activity: an animal model of dosage effects in Down's syndrome. Proc Natl Acad Sci USA 84:8044, 1987

286. Hagay ZJ, Weiss I, Zusman I et al: Prevention of diabetic embryopathy by over expression of the free radical scavenging enzyme superoxide dismutase in transgenic mouse embryos. Am J Obstet Gynecol, in press

287. Lapetina EG: Regulation of arachidonic acid production: role of phospholipases C and A2. Trends Pharmacol Sci 3:115, 1982

288. Warso MA, Lands WEM: Lipid peroxidation in relation to prostacyclin and thromboxane physiology and pathophysiology. Br Med Bull 39:277, 1983

289. Wolff SP: Diabetes mellitus and free radicals. Free radicals, transition metals and oxidative stress in the aetiology of diabetes mellitus and complications. Br Med Bull 49:642, 1993

290. Harris C, Stark KL, Juchau MR: Glutathione status and the incidence of neural tube defects elicited by direct acting teratogens in vitro. Teratology 37:577, 1988

291. Harris C: Glutathione biosynthesis in the post implantation rat conceptus in vitro. Toxicol Appl Pharmacol 120:247, 1993

292. Kashiwagi A, Asahina T, Ikebuchi M et al: Abnormal glutathione metabolism and increased cytotoxicity caused by H202 in human umbilical vein endothelial cells cultured in high glucose medium. Diabetologia 37:264, 1994

293. Hempel SL, Wessels DA: Prostaglandin E2 synthesis after oxidant stress is dependant on cell glutathione content. Am J Physiol 266 (Cell Physiol 35):C 1392, 1994

294. Simán CM, Borg LAH, Eriksson UJ: Disturbed development, low vitamin E concentration, and increased lipid peroxidation in embryos of diabetic rats. Diabetologia, suppl. 1, 37:A171, 1994

295. Bucala R, Model P, Cerami A: Modification of DNA by reducing sugars: a possible mechanism for nucleic acid ageing and age-related dysfunction in gene expression. Proc Natl Acad Sci USA 81:105, 1984

296. Morita J, Ueda K, Nanjo S, Komano T: Sequence specific damage of DNA induced by reducing sugars. Nucleic Acid Res 13:449, 1985

297. Lee A, Plump A, DeSimone C et al: A role for DNA mutations in diabetes-associated teratogenesis in transgenic embryos. Diabetes 44:20, 1995

298. Schreck R, Rieber P, Baeuerle PA: Reactive oxygen intermediates as apparently widely used messengers in the activation of the NF-κB transcription factor and HIV-1. EMBO J 10:2247, 1991

299. Cagliero E, Forsberg H, Sala R et al: Maternal diabetes induces increased expression of extracellular matrix components in rat embryos. Diabetes 42:975, 1993

300. Forsberg H, Cagliero E, Eriksson UJ: Increased superoxide dismutase levels in embryos subjected to a diabetic environment. Submitted for publication

301. Bravenboer B, Kappelle AC, Hamers FPT et al: Potential use of glutathione for the prevention and treatment of diabetic neuropathy in the streptozotocin-induced diabetic rat. Diabetologia 35:813, 1992

302. Cameron NE, Cotter MA, Archibald V et al: Anti-oxidant and pro-oxidant effects on nerve conduction velocity, endoneurial blood flow and oxygen tension in non-diabetic and streptozotocin-diabetic rats. Diabetologia 37:449, 1994

303. Golde LHG, van Deenen LLH: The effect of dietary fat on the molecular species lecithin from rat liver. Biochim Biophys Acta 125:496, 1966

304. Zilversmit DB: A proposal linking atherogenesis to the interaction of endothelial lipoprotein lipase with triglyceride rich lipoprotein. Circ Res 33:633, 1973

305. Goldman AS, Goto MP: Biochemical basis of diabetic embryopathy. Isr J Med Sci 27:469, 1991

10

Glucose Evaluation and Control

E. ALBERT REECE
CAROL J. HOMKO

Diabetes mellitus is a metabolic disorder that can significantly alter the environment in which the fetus develops, leading to complications such as congenital malformations, hyperinsulinism, growth aberrations, stillbirths, delayed pulmonic maturation, and even neonatal death.[1]

Perinatal morbidity and mortality, however, have significantly decreased since the discovery of insulin.[2-8] Before 1922, at a time when metabolic control of diabetic patients was poor, the fetal death rate was about 60 to 70 percent. In fact, the Joslin Clinic reported that no ketosis-prone diabetic woman delivered a live infant. The maternal mortality rate was also high, resulting in death of about 30 percent of those afflicted. After the availability and proper use of insulin, there has been a decreasing incidence of perinatal mortality, such that most centers report rates of 2 to 4 percent.[6,9,10] The critical factor in this improvement has been the awareness that normalization of maternal glucose was essential to maternal and fetal health. Several studies report improved fetal outcome under a stringent program of maternal metabolic control.[5,9-15] Gyves and associates[5] reported a study of 96 diabetic patients in whom the combined perinatal mortality rate was reduced from 13.5 to 4.2 percent. Subsequent observations by Gabbe and associates[9] lend further support to the declining trend in perinatal mortality. The major studies reveal that as the mean maternal blood glucose decreases, the mortality rate also decreases. A linear regression depicting these data suggests that at a mean maternal blood glucose of 84 mg/dl, there will be no increase in infant mortality over the risk in the general population[6] (Fig. 10-1).

Also, several investigators have reported an association between malformations and glucose control early in pregnancy while other studies have demonstrated that strict metabolic control in the periconception period can, in fact, reduce the incidence of these anomalies. Fuhrmann and colleagues[16] compared two groups of women with insulin-dependent diabetes mellitus (IDDM): 128 women who began intensive therapy before conception and 292 women in whom strict metabolic control was begun after 8 weeks' gestation. They found only one malformation (0.8 percent) in the group that received preconception treatment versus 22 infants (7.5 percent) with major congenital anomalies born to the group of late registrants. Kitzmiller and colleagues[17] reported similar results. They prospectively followed 84 women with IDDM who were recruited before conception and compared them with 110 women with IDDM who entered care after 6 weeks' gestation. They found a significant reduction in congenital anomalies between the two groups: 1.2 percent in the group that achieved preconception control versus 10.9 percent in the group that did not. These findings have been replicated by other investigators.[18,19] The dominant philosophy is that preconception glycemic control can reduce the overall incidence of diabetic embryopathy, which has become the leading cause of morbidity and mortality in infants of diabetic mothers (IDMs).

Other significant advances in maternal and neonatal care, fetal surveillance, assessment of lung maturity, and the treatment of fetal and maternal complications have also played a role in the improved perinatal out-

155

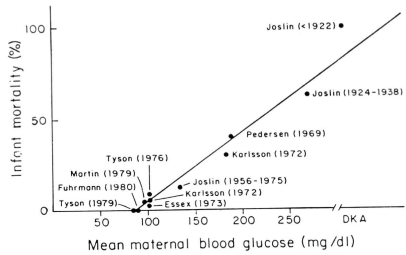

Fig. 10-1. Mean maternal glucose control versus infant mortality rate, demonstrating that at a mean maternal blood glucose of 84 mg/dl, the risk of infant mortality is comparable with that of the general population. (Jovanovic and Peterson,[6] with permission.)

comes seen in pregnancies complicated by diabetes.[20] However, despite the possible roles that these advances have played in lowering perinatal mortality, the evidence provided by several controlled studies supports the current belief that good metabolic control is essential to normal fetal outcome. The aspect of diabetes care that remains debatable is what constitutes the optimal level of metabolic control in diabetic pregnancy. This subject requires the consideration of several interrelated factors, including goals for metabolic control, the definition of maternal euglycemia, and methods of glucose evaluation and control.

GOALS FOR METABOLIC CONTROL

The diabetic state during pregnancy is complicated by perturbations in the hormonal milieu that have an effect on the overall metabolism. During pregnancy, maternal glucose crosses the placenta by facilitated diffusion, whereas amino acids are actively transported. Of particular importance is the transfer to the fetus of gluconeogenic amino acids such as alanine. Maternal loss of glucose and gluconeogenic substrate to the fetus occurs simultaneously with a decrease in mater-

nal fasting blood glucose to about 55 to 65 mg/dl, as well as a decrease in mean blood glucose to 70 to 80 mg/dl.[3,21–24] However, as gestation advances, the diabetogenic effects of pregnancy are brought about by the following factors: (1) the production of increasing amounts of placental hormones that antagonize insulin action, (2) enzymes contained within the placenta itself degrading maternal insulin, and (3) enhanced production of maternal glucose in the fasted state.

Diabetogenic hormones include human placental lactogen (HPL), a polypeptide of placental origin. Circulating levels of this hormone increase progressively with increasing placental size. HPL promotes free fatty acid (FFA) production by stimulating lipolysis. FFAs, in turn, promote peripheral tissue resistance to insulin, leading to downregulation of insulin receptors and compensatory hyperinsulinemia. In addition, insulin turnover is increased during pregnancy because of increased degradation by placental enzymes similar to liver insulinase.[6,17–19]

Despite these perturbations during pregnancy, the maintenance of normal fuel metabolism remains essential to normal embryonal/fetal growth and development. Karlsson and Kjellmer[10] demonstrated the relationship between fetal outcome and glucose control, showing that the third-trimester mean maternal blood glucose was linearly correlated with the perinatal mortality rate. Mean third-trimester plasma glucose values of greater than 150 mg/dl were associated with a perinatal mortality of 23.6 percent, whereas mean plasma glucose concentrations between 100 and 150 mg/dl and less than 100 mg/dl were associated with rates of 15.3 and 3.8 percent, respectively. Similarly, a decrease in certain morbidities was also observed when the mean plasma glucose value was less than 100 mg/dl. Several other authors have further emphasized the beneficial effects of glucose control on diabetic pregnancy outcome.[5,21,25–31] Although perinatal morbidity has also declined with improved metabolic control, some aspects, namely, macrosomia, persist despite these efforts.[15] Hence, the metabolic goal of establishing "euglycemia" during pregnancy is well supported by numerous studies.

The criteria for satisfactory metabolic control vary widely, and even studies showing low perinatal morbidity and mortality differ in their details. For example, the report of Karlsson and Kjellmer[10] reported a low perinatal mortality at a mean third-trimester blood glucose value of less than 100 mg/dl. These mean values were obtained by the averaging of three daily determinations at unspecified times in relation to meals, and these tests were performed between 30 weeks' gestation and term. Other studies have reported a perinatal mortality rate of less than 5 percent associated with a mean blood glucose value below 120 mg/dl. Some of these studies have averaged glucose determinations taken at 7:00 AM, 10:00 AM, noon, 4:00 PM, and 7:00 PM during the last 28 days of pregnancy, whereas others have combined a mixture of gestational and IDDM patients.[4–7,21] It is difficult to interpret whether the good outcomes are attributable to the metabolic control achieved or the mild degree of the diabetes, or both.[21]

Furthermore, studies, notably that of Leveno et al,[32] have questioned the association of stringent glucose control and pregnancy outcome. Leveno et al[32] described successful outcome of diabetic pregnancy with maternal glucose levels significantly higher than that reported by others.[8,10,14,21,27,28] In the study of Leveno et al, 14 percent of patients had a mean preprandial plasma glucose value of 106 mg/dl, 66 percent had levels of 142.7 mg/dl, and 20 percent had a mean value of 197 mg/dl. The overall perinatal death rate was 4.2 percent, without any significant differences in the perinatal mortality or morbidity rate observed between the above groups. However, the observed differences were in the direction supporting tight control. From the aforementioned studies, it is clear that the measures of control used by investigators have been so varied that it is difficult to compare these studies and thus establish optimum criteria for metabolic control. Except for the study of Leveno et al,[32] which is at variance with other reports, most studies found a correlation of lower blood glucose levels, regardless of the criteria used, with improved fetal outcome.

Other investigators, in an attempt to obtain a more comprehensive glucose profile, have conducted 24-

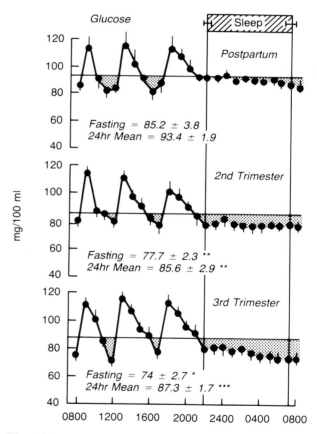

Fig. 10-2. Excursion of plasma glucose during a 24-hour glucose profile in six normal pregnant women during the second and third trimesters of pregnancy and 6 to 11 weeks postpartum. Meals are indicated by ●. Data points reflect ± SEM. Horizontal lines represent the 24-hour mean. *P < .05; ** P < .01; *** P < .005. (From Cousins et al,[26] with permission.)

Table 10-1. Diurnal Plasma Glucose Profile in Normal and Diabetic Women

| | Plasma Glucose (mg/dl) | | |
	Normal	Chemical Diabetes	Insulin-Dependent Diabetes
Mean diurnal	84	101	106
Mean daytime	88	106	117
Maximum diurnal	113	145	179
Minimum diurnal	67	76	53
Diurnal plasma glucose range	46	69	125

(Modified from Gillmer et al,[1] with permission.)

hour metabolic profiles in diabetic and nondiabetic patients and tried to establish achievable goals.[26,33–35] Cousins et al[26] conducted a longitudinal study to quantitate the progressive effects of the second and third trimesters of normal pregnancy on plasma glucose, insulin, and C-peptide. Such studies were conducted in six nonobese women with normal 3-hour glucose tolerance tests and without prenatal or postpartum complications. Hourly plasma samples were obtained throughout a 24-hour period in the second (22 to 26 weeks) and third (35 to 37 weeks) trimesters of pregnancy and again at 6 to 11 weeks after delivery. A diurnal rhythm of plasma glucose, insulin, and C-peptide was demonstrated in all study periods (Fig. 10-2). During meals, increases in plasma glucose and insulin above the 24-hour mean were small and not significantly modified by pregnancy. During the third trimester only, the peak values for both plasma glucose and insulin were significantly increased. There was also nocturnal hypoglycemia. The authors concluded that the observation of a marked diurnal rhythm of plasma glucose and the relative nocturnal hypoglycemia in normal pregnancy provide some guidelines for the metabolic management of diabetic pregnancies. Gillmer et al[1,33] also studied the diurnal metabolic profile of diabetic and nondiabetic pregnant women in the third trimester of pregnancy. Patients were hospitalized during the third trimester for at least 2 weeks, and "optimal" diabetic control was achieved (Table 10-1 and Fig. 10-3). The results of their study illustrate that by using stringent metabolic control, levels of glucose control can be achieved in women with diabetes that are comparable with normal control subjects. For example, the mean daytime plasma glucose value in the diabetic subject was 117 mg/dl versus 88 mg/dl in the normal group. The glycemic excursions were greater in the women with diabetes, with lower minimal plasma glucose levels at night and higher maximum plasma glucose values in the daytime (Table 10-1). From these diurnal profiles, normative data were ascertained regarding achievable glycemic control in the third trimester of pregnancy. Furthermore, these data also serve as a working definition of euglycemia in pregnancy as described in Figure 10-3, with a range from 70 to 120 mg/dl throughout the 24-hour period, with a lower level during the sleep period.

The feasibility of maintaining normal glucose pro-

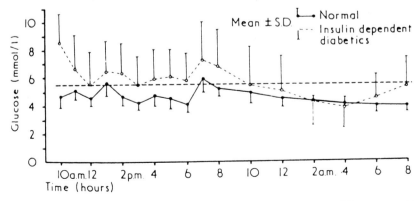

Fig. 10-3. Diurnal glucose profiles in 13 insulin-dependent diabetic patients and 9 women with normal glucose tolerance studied between 32 and 35 weeks of pregnancy. (From Gillmer et al.,[1] with permission.)

files in IDDM women has been studied by several investigators.[11,28,36–38] Jovanovic et al[37] reported a small series of 10 patients who were in the first trimester of their pregnancy and were maintained in tight glucose control using intensive conventional insulin therapy. These patients performed five to eight blood glucose determinations per day, and their average hemoglobin A_{1c} (HbA$_{1c}$) fell from 9.4 percent to about 5 percent. The infants were described as showing no signs of macrosomia, hypoglycemia, hyperbilirubinemia, hypocalcemia, or respiratory distress. In this study, the authors concluded that normal glycemia not only could be achieved in early pregnancy but could be maintained for prolonged periods in the outpatient setting. Normal plasma glucose levels were achieved after only 1 week of treatment. This finding greatly reduced the length of hospitalization reported in previous studies,[6] in which 1 month of strict diabetic control in a hospital was required for normalization of glucose. Kitzmiller et al,[38] using continuous subcutaneous insulin therapy, also demonstrated that good diabetic control was achievable during early pregnancy. With 24 IDDM patients, reasonable control was achieved in the fasting blood glucose (119 ± 30 mg/dl) and postprandial blood glucose (133 ± 34 mg/dl) levels. This was accompanied by an average of 2.2 ± 1.5 symptomatic hypoglycemic episodes per week. We and others have also confirmed the feasibility of stringent metabolic control throughout pregnancy and reported perinatal mortality rates less than 5 percent.[7,9,25,36,39,40]

The various studies discussed clearly indicate the benefit of normal glucose control throughout pregnancy, and the feasibility of tight glucose control has been demonstrated even in early pregnancy. Other questions that arise include, Does tight glucose control lead to aberrations in other metabolic fuels? Do we normalize other metabolic fuels simply by controlling glucose? Should we be measuring and controlling other metabolites as well?

Reece and associates conducted third-trimester meal studies in 22 pregnant diabetic women and 7 pregnant nondiabetic women to address the above questions. Determinations of FFAs, branched chain amino acid, alanine, ketones, triglycerides, cholesterol, and insulin were obtained before a standardized mixed-meal breakfast and repeated every 15 to 30 minutes for 150 minutes after the meal. Except for insulin, no significant differences between diabetic individuals and controls were observed for all metabolites assayed. This finding suggests that normalization of glucose results in normalizations of other metabolic fuels. Therefore, the assessment of glucose control reflects the metabolic profile of other insulin-sensitive fuels, which need not be measured independently. However, to achieve normalization of these metabolic fuels, increased exogenous insulin was required.[41]

The results of the many aforementioned studies provide justification for stringent metabolic control during pregnancy and evidence for its feasibility. The goal of normal glycemic control throughout pregnancy has been generally adopted as part of the standard care for pregnancies complicated by diabetes.

HISTORY OF GLUCOSE EVALUATION

After the discovery and availability of insulin, it was recognized that therapy could be based on some measure of glucose levels. Repeated blood glucose measurements were feasible for hospitalized patients. However, continuous outpatient evaluation posed a problem. Urine testing for glucose was introduced, using a color change with Fehling's solution (copper sulfate). This was a cumbersome process involving the boiling of urine with the solution in a test tube, as well as the use of a color change that acted as an index for the glucose content.[42–44] Despite the laborious nature of this task, such a technique allowed patients an opportunity to regulate their glucose levels as outpatients. It eventually became clear that urine testing provided very limited information. This was especially true for pregnant diabetic patients in whom the renal threshold is lowered because the increase in glomerular filtration rate is not accompanied by an equivalent increase in tubular reabsorption of glucose.[45] This alteration leads to glucosuria even at fairly low blood glucose levels. In light of the above, improved glucose control could only be accomplished by the ascertainment of circulating blood glucose levels.

The achievement of euglycemia requires frequent daily blood glucose determinations. The introduction of portable blood glucose meters made it possible for individuals with diabetes to evaluate blood glucose with ease several times per day. The initial reports of self-monitoring of blood glucose (SMBG) appeared in early 1978.[42,44,46,47] Subsequent studies with larger numbers of subjects confirmed the initial reports that SMBG is feasible, practical, and acceptable to patients; that blood glucose determinations are sufficiently accurate for clinical use; and that glycemic control may be improved if SMBG is used as a part of a treatment program[46,48–50]

This continued SMBG at home produced greater understanding and motivation among patients, led to shorter hospital stays, and improved glucose control. Also, patients found SMBG more informative than urine tests. Peacock et al[51] found that patients who performed SMBG achieved better glucose control than patients who were hospitalized.

In another study by Hanson et al,[52] the authors compared the value of SMBG with hospital care in the 32nd to 36th week of pregnancy. This was a prospective randomized study of 100 pregnancies, of which 54 were in the home group and 46 in the hospital group. There were no significant differences either in blood glucose control achieved or in pregnancy complications between the two groups. However, 10 of the 54 patients had to interrupt home monitoring because of pregnancy complications. The perinatal mortality rates were not significantly different in the two treatment groups. This prospective randomized study demonstrated that it is possible to achieve a similar degree of blood glucose control with either SMBG or hospital care in diabetic patients during the last trimester of pregnancy. In addition, this form of glucose control can be achieved without any significant increase in perinatal morbidity or mortality.

These and other studies have demonstrated that the use of SMBG permits the attainment of euglycemia throughout gestation. Some studies have shown that SMBG achieves better control than monitoring in the hospital, whereas others have shown that equivalent control is achieved. In any event, the use of SMBG has significantly improved the overall care of outpatient diabetes management.[6,22,28,31,46–48,53,54]

However, certain metabolic and physiologic changes of pregnancy may interfere with the accuracy of reflectance meters. In pregnancy, glucose levels and hematocrit values are lower than in the nonpregnant state whereas triglyceride and cholesterol levels are increased. These changes could affect meter accuracy. Harkness and colleagues[55] compared four commonly used reflectance meters against the Beckman ASTRA

in 17 gravid IDDM women. All the instruments tested showed unacceptable combinations of proportional and constant bias based on laboratory standards. The use of reflectance meters for metabolic regulation during pregnancy should be monitored carefully for accuracy by obtaining monthly glycosylated hemoglobin levels and by periodically checking the machine against standard values.

Home blood glucose monitoring has become the mainstay of outpatient management of pregnancies complicated by diabetes mellitus. Although reports have shown that patients sometimes falsely report blood glucose values, it has been shown that, in general, SMBG data correlate very well with automated laboratories. Jovanovic et al[37] reported correlation coefficients as high as 0.91 when the patients' technique was compared with a trained technician using an autoanalyzer. Finally, the introduction of stringent metabolic control on an outpatient basis became possible with the use of SMBG.

MONITORING FREQUENCY AND GLYCEMIC STANDARDS

The frequency of SMBG depends on the severity of the diabetes. However, in general, blood glucose determinations should be obtained four to eight times per day every day in patients with IDDM. Glucose control in patients with type 1 diabetes (IDDM) may deteriorate if SMBG is reduced to less than four determinations per day.[46] Because 18 to 20 percent of women with gestational diabetes will require insulin therapy during the course of the pregnancy, it is necessary to obtain one set of blood glucose values at fasting, 2 hours after breakfast, and a predinner determination at least once per week.[27]

Although it is widely accepted that the level of metabolic control achieved in the pregnancy complicated by diabetes significantly affects perinatal outcome, what constitutes optimal control is not exactly known. Landon, Gabbe and colleagues[56] assessed the relationship between glycemic control and perinatal outcome in 75 women with class B through D diabetes. They divided their population into two groups: women who achieved mean fasting and preprandial capillary blood glucose values of less than 110 mg/dl and those whose mean blood glucose values were greater than 110 mg/

dl. They found that better blood glucose control (<110 mg/dl) significantly reduced the incidence of macrosomia, as well as several other neonatal complications. The authors concluded that maintaining mean capillary blood glucose values of less than 110 mg/dl may reduce several major forms of morbidity in the IDM.

Combs and colleagues[57] undertook a study to determine the gestational ages at which maternal hyperglycemia is most closely related to macrosomia, as well as to determine whether fetal macrosomia is associated with elevations of fasting glucose or postprandial glucose levels, or both. The investigators examined perinatal outcomes in 111 consecutive pregnancies of women with class B through RF diabetes. Of the women in their sample, 29 percent delivered macrosomic infants and were compared with those without macrosomic infants. The authors found that the incidence of macrosomia rose progressively with increasing postprandial glucose levels. Postprandial glucose levels of less than 130 mg/dl reduced the incidence of macrosomia, but levels of less than 120 mg/dl eliminated this complication. They therefore recommended a glucose level of 130 mg/dl as a reasonable target for the 1-hour postprandial glucose. These data are supported by the Diabetes in Early Pregnancy Study,[58] which demonstrated that third-trimester nonfasting glucose levels are the strongest predictors of percentile birthweight in IDMs.

Furthermore, the Diabetes in Early Pregnancy Study also found no relationship between fasting or postprandial glucose levels and macrosomia after 32 weeks' gestation, as in the study reported by Lin and colleagues.[59] It would, therefore, appear that good glycemic control must be instituted by the early third trimester to prevent macrosomia. However, conversely they found that postprandial glucose values of less than 130 mg/dl were associated with increasing numbers of small-for-gestational-age (SGA) infants. Other investigators have also found a similar association between low maternal glucose levels and SGA infants in both nondiabetic women[60] and women with gestational diabetes.[61]

In theory, the standard for glycemic control during pregnancy is normalcy. It is a logical approach to achieve as near-normal glucose levels as possible without undue hypoglycemia; attempts to determine blood glucose targets will need to be individualized for each woman. Based on the above data, blood glucose targets of less than 95 to 100 but greater than 60 mg/dl fasting and 1-hour postprandial levels of less than 140 or 2-hour levels of less than 120 mg/dl but greater than 80 mg/dl would appear to be both reasonable and achievable goals.

METHODS OF SELF-MONITORING OF BLOOD GLUCOSE

Currently, several methods are available for testing blood glucose. All use reagent strips on which a drop of blood is placed to be read either by visual comparison with a color chart or by a reflectance meter. The patient's finger is pricked using a sharp 21- to 25-gauge lancet. A variety of lancets and lancing devices is now available. Table 10-2 summarizes the important features of most of the available finger-sticking devices.

An adequate drop of blood can be enhanced by placing the hand in warm water before pricking. The thumb and fourth finger have better blood supply than the remaining digits and may be preferred sites for pricking. Also, the peripheral aspects of the finger are less sensitive that the ball of the finger and may be considered preferred areas.[46]

Glucose Oxidase-Impregnated Reagent Strips

The drop of blood is placed on a glucose oxidase-impregnated reagent strip. These strips contain a buffered mixture of glucose oxidase, peroxidase, and a chromogen system. The glucose oxidase catalyzes the oxidation of glucose to gluconic acid and hydrogen peroxide. Peroxidase then catalyzes the reaction of hydrogen peroxide with the chromogen system, producing a color that varies with the concentration of glucose originally present.[40,62] The reaction on the reagent strip must be carefully timed, then interpreted either by visual comparison with a color chart or by a glucose meter.

Although most reagent strips can be read by visual inspection, they are more accurate when read by a meter. Test strips designed to be read by visual inspection are listed in Table 10-3.

Visual interpretation has an element of subjectivity. Not all patients can distinguish the color gradations

Table 10-2. Summary of Important Features of the Available Finger-Sticking Devices

Name (Manufacturer/Distributor)	Features and Supplies
Auto-Lancet (Palco)	Comes with 1 regular, 1 deep tip (guard), 2 lancets, case; guard screws on; 5-year warranty
Autolet (Owen Mumford/Ulster Scientific)	3 platform depths
Autolet Lite (Owen Mumford/Ulster Scientific)	3 platform depths; self-arming; lancet ejection for safety
Autolet II Clinisafe (Ulster Scientific)	Comes with 20 platforms (10 each of 2 different depths), 10 Unilets, and vinyl wallet
B-D Autolance (Becton Dickinson)	One-piece construction; automatic, for use only with 23-gauge B-D Micro-Fine Lancets (5 starter B-D Micro-Fine Lancets included)
Dialet (Home Diagnostics, Inc.)	Pen-shaped; comes with one regular, one deep tip; for safety, blue dot appears when device is armed
Glucolet Automatic Lancing Device (Miles Inc. [Ames])	Comes with 10 Gluco System lancets, one opaque regular puncture endcap, multilingual instruction insert
Hypolet Auto Lancet Device (Supreme Medical)	Pen-shaped; clear guard for adults; colored guard for children
Medi-Let (Medicore)	Kit includes device; comes with 20 platforms, two depths, and 10 lancets; patented lancet ejector arm; uses all lancets except B-D Autolance; made in United States
MediSense Lancing Device (MediSense)	Lightweight, ultra TLC lancets; provides controlled depth penetration and 5-year warranty; pen-shaped
Penlet II Automatic Blood Sampling Device (LifeScan)	Pen-shaped; hands-off lancet removal system to minimize possibility of sticks; comes with LifeScan lancets and two different caps to control the depth of penetration
Unistik II (Owen Mumford, Inc.)	Single use for safety and disposability; device and lancet are one; punctures and retracts automatically; 50/box
Unistik I (Owen Mumford, Inc.)	Same as above; available in two puncture depths

(Modified from American Diabetes Association,[115] with permission.)

with sufficient accuracy; thus many patients express their blood glucose readings as a range between values. Because of these limitations, meters are very useful for most patients and are particularly necessary during pregnancy when the precise ascertainment of glucose level is needed.

Reflectance Meters

Several battery-powered portable glucose reflectance meters are available. These devices determine the glucose concentration by transforming a signal that is dependent on the amount of light reflected from the test

Table 10-3. Test Strips Intended for Visual Reading

Name (Manufacturer)	Color Chart Increments (mg/dl)	Instructions for Use
Chemstrip bG (Boehringer Mannheim)	20, 40, 80, 120, 180, 240	Wipe after 1 minute; read after 2
Diascan (Home Diagnostics, Inc.)	20, 40, 80, 120, 180, 300, 500, 800	Wipe after 30 seconds; wait an additional 60 seconds; read
Glucostix Reagent Strips (Miles Inc. [Ames])	20, 40, 70, 110, 140, 180, 250, 400, 800	Blot after 30 seconds; wait an additional 90 seconds; read
Supreme Strips (Supreme Medical)	low, 20, 40, 70, 120, 180, 240, 400, high	Apply blood to test areas; wait 60 seconds and turn strip over; compare color of reverse side with color chart
TrendStrips (Supreme Medical)	0, 20, 40, 80, 120, 180, 240, 400, 800	Wipe after 1 minute; read after 2 minutes. If >240, wait an additional minute; read

(Modified from American Diabetes Association,[115] with permission.)

Table 10-4. Summary of Important Features of Most of the Available Glucose Meters

Name (Manufacturer)	Test Strip Used	Range (mg/dl)	Test Time	Memory Capacity
Accu-Chek III (Boehringer Mannheim)	Chemstrip bG	20–500	120	20-value memory
CheckMate (Cascade Medical)	CheckMate or CheckMate Plus	40–400	60–90	Stores up to 40 results
CheckMate Plus (Cascade Medical)	CheckMate Plus	25–500	15–70	Stores up to 255 results with time and date and insulin type and dosage
Companion 2 Sensor (MediSense, Inc.)	Pen 2/Companion 2	20–600	20	
Diascan-S (Home Diagnostics, Inc.)	Diascan	10–600	90	Automatic memory of last 10 readings
ExacTech Companion Sensor (MediSense, Inc.)	ExacTech	40–450	30	
ExacTech Pen Sensor (MediSense, Inc.)	ExacTech	40–450	30	Last reading recall
Glucometer Elite Diabetes Care System (Miles Inc. [Ames])	Glucometer Elite	40–500	60	One test memory
Glucometer M+ (Miles Inc. [Ames])	Glucofilm	20–500	60	300 entries of blood glucose results, insulin, diet, exercise, and special events by date and time
Glucometer 3 Diabetes Care System (Miles Inc. [Ames])	Glucofilm	20–500	60	Stores up to 10 results
Glucose Alert (Polymer Technology)	Glucose Alert	30–400	50	Can display up to 100 previous results
One Touch BASIC (LifeScan)	One Touch	0–600	45	Stores last test result
One Touch II (LifeScan)	One Touch	0–600	45	250 results with date and time
Pen 2 Sensor (MediSense, Inc.)	Pen 2/Companion 2	20–600	20	Extended memory
Supreme bG Meter (Supreme Medical)	Supreme bG	40–400	55	Memory for the significant glucose values
Accu-Chek Easy (Boehringer Mannheim Corp.)	Easy Test Strips	20–500	15–60	30-value memory
Tracer II (Boehringer Mannheim Corp.)	Tracer bG	40–400	120	
ULTRA (Home Diagnostics, Inc.)	ULTRA +	0–600	45	

(Modified from American Diabetes Association,[115] with permission.)

strip. These meters have also been shown to have a close correlation with automated laboratory methods.[37,42,44,45,63] The magnitude of differences is small (± 10 percent) when the blood glucose level is less than 300 mg/dl.

Table 10-4 summarizes the important features of most of the glucose meters currently available. The latest models use simplified user techniques that have eliminated the need for timing and blood removal from the test strips. Most of these second-generation glucose meters are also available with memory capacity. Studies with these meters suggest that the memory capacity improves accurate reporting and thus has an effect on the overall achievement of euglycemia. Initial work by Mazze et al[64] reported on 19 clinic patients who used a glucometer (Ames, Elkhart, Indiana) with a memory capacity (M-Glucometer) for 2 weeks. Ap-

proximately 26 percent of the logbook entries were different from capillary blood glucose results recorded by the M-Glucometer. The main source of error was omitting high glucose results and substituting lower values. In a subsequent study, patients were made aware of the memory capacity of these glucose meters, and patient performance improved significantly.

In another study by Moses[65] conducted in 18 patients using M-Glucometers, the findings were somewhat different. These patients were advised that the M-Glucometer had a memory capacity of storing all their results, and if there were any recording errors, the data could be excluded by pressing a button. These patients were not informed that an attempted erasure would be displayed on subsequent printouts. In this study, erasure was attempted in a maximum of 1.2 percent of the total, significantly less that was found by Mazze et al.[64] Although the above studies are admittedly not comparable in design, significant differences in reporting errors did exist. It is possible that these differences may be due to inherent disparities in the population studied and may not reflect a general orientation of diabetic patients to misrepresent their blood glucose values. Accurate information is essential for optimal diabetes care. However, we need to exercise extreme care and sensitivity as we introduce these new devices with their potential for "double-checking" the blood glucose determinations obtained and reported by patients. As mentioned previously, SMBG allows patients to be more involved in their care, giving them a sense of responsibility for their health. We hope that these new memory glucometers do not destroy that sense of participation, causing patients to become less motivated and more noncompliant. Obviously, the full effects of these new devices will not be known for some time.

Other Forms of Glucose Determination

Other methods of glucose evaluation are directed toward the overall assessment of glycemic control. Some of these methods include glycosylated hemoglobin or proteins. More information is available on glycosylated hemoglobin, because it has been available for a fairly long time and has been studied in individuals with and without diabetes. Fructosamine, a different form of protein glycosylation, is fairly new, and few data are available on its use and accuracy.

Glycosylated Hemoglobins

In 1958, Allen and co-workers[66] identified three small fractions of HbA (HbA$_{1a}$, HbA$_{1b}$, HbA$_{1c}$) that had a faster chromatographic mobility than the remainder of the HbA. These small fractions or glycoproteins have been subsequently referred to as glycosylated hemoglobin, glycohemoglobin, or generically HbA$_1$. It was not until these glycohemoglobins were found to be increased in diabetic patients that their clinical usefulness was realized.[67-76]

The glycosylation reaction is a slow nonenzymatic irreversible covalent bonding of glucose to various amino acids. HbA$_{1c}$ is the largest of these minor hemoglobins and has glucose attached to the N-terminal va-

line amino acid of the β-chains of HbA. HbA$_{1c}$ is structurally identical to HbA except for the presence of a glucose moiety attached to the N-terminal valine amino acid of the β-chains via a Schiff base.[70,77] Bunn et al[78] showed that the Schiff base undergoes an Amadori rearrangement (i.e., a shift from an α-hydroxyaldimine [Schiff base] to a β-ketamine) to form a stable and relatively irreversible ketamine linkage. In vivo studies showed that glycosylation of HbA to form HbA$_{1c}$ is a post-translational modification of HbA$_1$, occurring as a slow nonenzymatic process in the circulating red blood cells.[70,77] The level of glycohemoglobin represents a retrospective integration of the overall glycemic control during the 4 to 6 weeks preceding the glucose determination. This glycemic level is proportional to the time-averaged blood glucose to which the red blood cells were exposed during their lifetime.[70,78-83]

The use of HbA$_1$ has been investigated in numerous studies. O'Shaughnessy et al[73] measured HbA$_1$ in the blood of 50 normal nonpregnant women, 29 normal pregnant women, and 21 pregnant diabetic patients. In normal pregnancy, HbA$_1$ did not differ significantly from values in nonpregnancy nor vary with the gestational age. It was also found that marked elevations in HbA$_1$ (elevations >10 percent) reliably predict poor diabetic control; that HbA$_1$ is neither useful for fine glucose control nor useful as a screen for gestational diabetes; and that HbA$_1$ is not predictive of newborn birthweights. Not all studies have confirmed these results.[79,84-86]

Miller et al[8] did not find HbA$_{1c}$ values to be predictive of abnormal maternal glucose tolerance, infant birthweight, or long-term glucose control in diabetic patients. There is general agreement, however, that HbA$_1$ is a "rough gauge" of overall glycemic control. The correlation may not be precise and may not accurately reflect fluctuations in glucose levels, but it does provide a crude index of glucose control for the 4 to 8 weeks preceding HbA$_1$ determination.

Both clinical and laboratory studies have shown a relationship between glycemic status during organogenesis, as reflected by glycohemoglobins and the incidence of birth defects.[87-89] Leslie et al[87] conducted serial studies in 25 pregnant diabetic women at 4-week intervals and at 6 weeks postpartum and found that HbA$_1$ decreased from the first to the third trimester, most probably as a function of glucose control. HbA$_1$ also increased postpartum as control was lessened.

More important, however, was the observation that three of five pregnant diabetic women whose initial HbA[1] was above normal gave birth to children with fatal congenital anomalies. Subsequent work by Miller et al,[88] Ylinen et al,[89] and Green et al,[90] demonstrated that HbA[1] was correlated with the malformation rate. HbA[1] therefore becomes a useful clinical tool for grossly assessing a patient's risk of diabetes-related malformations. Most patients present to the physician in the late first or second trimester of pregnancy, beyond the time when any therapeutic intervention may be used to decrease the risk of major malformations. However, HbA[1] may be used to assess this risk as a basis for further studies, namely, α-fetoprotein or ultrasound (or both) and as a guide for counseling.

There are limitations to the use of HbA[1] such as with the hemoglobinopathies and many other medical conditions.[91] HbA[1] is determined by the use of cation exchange column chromatography. This method of analysis is related to the electrophoretic mobility of the molecule. In the case of sickle hemoglobinopathy, there is a substitution of the number 6 amino acid on the β-chain, thus altering the electrophoretic mobility of the molecule. Although the total molecular glycosylation does not change, the change in electrophoretic mobility causes HbA[1c] to elute into a smaller fraction, giving a spuriously low level of glycosylated hemoglobin.[92,93] In patients with thalassemia, HbF and HbA[1c] elute at almost the same sites, resulting in a spurious increase in HbA[1c].[94] Similarly, patients with both conditions tend to have normal values due to a lowering effect of the sickle component and an elevating effect of the thalassemia component. Besides the above conditions, which can spuriously alter the HbA[1] reading, other conditions can affect the HbA[1] level, including alcoholism and anemia.[94,95] In this light, caution has to be exercised when HbA[1] is used to evaluate glucose control.

The advent of glycosylated hemoglobin was initially met with warm welcome and excitement. A single test was finally here that would provide overall glucose control and might convey prognostic significance to pregnancy outcome and long-term diabetes. As stated previously, many studies have investigated this problem, and except for the correlation between glycemic control as measured by HbA and birth defects, other claims of HbA being correlated with birthweight, placental size, long-term glucose control, or mild glucose intolerance remain unsettled.

Fructosamine

Major criticisms of glycosylated hemoglobin include its long "memory," low sensitivity for mild glucose intolerance, and potential confounding factors. Therefore, several investigators have examined the use of the fructosamine assay to screen reliably for gestational diabetes and as an index of short-term control.

Fructosamine is a marker for glycosylated serum protein. This test measures the serum glycosyl protein by recognizing the Amadori rearrangement product formed by the reaction of glucose and protein molecules. The potential advantages of fructosamine include decreased day-to-day variation and apparently a shorter "memory," so re-equilibration to a new level requires a shorter time.[96,97]

In a study by Roberts et al,[96] fructosamine was measured in 79 diabetic pregnant women and 20 women with gestational diabetes. The test detected 17 (85 percent) of the women with gestational diabetes and gave only (45 percent) false-positive results. However, several other investigators have reported a lower sensitivity for the fructosamine assay in the detection of gestational diabetes mellitus.

Cefalu and colleagues[98] found no difference in baseline serum glycosylated protein levels between women with and without gestational diabetes. However, in women with pregestational diabetes followed at 2-week intervals, they found serum glycosylated protein correlated significantly with fasting blood glucose ($r = .81; P < .001$) and mean outpatient blood glucose levels ($r = .62; P < .001$). No correlation was found between HbA[1c] and either fasting blood glucose or mean outpatient glucose level. The authors concluded that although the serum fructosamine is not a useful screening test for gestational diabetes, it does show potential as an objective marker of short-term glycemic control.

Parfitt and colleagues[99] also found that fructosamine predicted levels of mean blood glucose more precisely than HbA[1] in pregnancies complicated by diabetes. However, others[100] have found serum fructosamine and HbA[1] to give comparable information regarding short-term glycemic control while still others have found the assay to have limited use in the management of diabetic pregnancies.[101,102] At this time, the fructosamine test has not been evaluated sufficiently to support routine clinical use.

ACHIEVEMENT OF BLOOD GLUCOSE CONTROL

As stated earlier, intensive therapy regimens and the establishment of maternal euglycemia have dramatically improved fetal outcomes in pregnancies complicated by diabetes. In fact, normalization of maternal glucose control has been accepted as the main therapeutic goal of these pregnancies for several years. However, the benefits of strict metabolic control go far beyond pregnancy. Evidence from the recently completed multicenter Diabetes Control and Complications Trial (DCCT) suggests that tight glycemic control should be maintained for life.[103] This landmark trial conclusively demonstrated that intensive diabetes therapy effectively delays the onset and slows the progression of microvascular complications in patients with IDDM. Two groups of patients were followed for 9 years; one group was treated conventionally, and the other group was treated intensively (with multiple insulin injections and frequent blood glucose monitoring). Previous trials[104,105] of intensive versus conventional therapy for IDDM had demonstrated a transient worsening of retinopathy during the first year of therapy. However, in the DCCT, this early worsening disappeared by 18 months in most cases, and by the study termination, these patients with early worsening had a 74 percent reduction in the risk of subsequent progression as compared with patients who received conventional therapy. For women who have not previously been maintained on intensive therapy regimens, pregnancy may provide the impetus and the opportunity to initiate such therapy.

The achievement of optimal glucose control is primarily by a combination of diet, exercise, and insulin therapy.[6,22,27,37,106] Each mode of therapy is covered elsewhere in this text. However, a brief discussion is presented on insulin and its method of administration.

The ultimate goal of any insulin delivery system is to simulate the pattern of normal insulin secretion. It has been shown that normal subjects secrete 24 to 37 units of insulin daily, primarily at mealtimes. In addition, nondiabetic individuals have a preprandial portal insulin level of 29 μU/ml, with a simultaneous peripheral insulin level of 9 μU/ml. Fifteen minutes after starting a meal, the insulin levels increase and reach a maximum within 1 hour. The peripheral insulin level will always remain approximately one-third of the portal insulin concentration.[107] Although it probably will never be possible to achieve identical insulin profiles with peripheral insulin therapy (conventional or pump treatment), we can attempt to achieve normalization of basal and postprandial plasma glucose levels.

Many centers have found that the therapeutic insulin regimen that best achieves euglycemia is a combination of intermediate-acting and short-acting insulin in split dosage. At our institution, we have found that euglycemia can be maintained in about 80 percent of our patients receiving mixed insulin injections twice each day. About 15 percent will require three injections, and the remainder will require an injection before each meal.

The advent of the insulin pump is another advance in diabetes care that was greeted with enthusiasm. The pump has theoretical advantages compared with conventional insulin therapy, namely, delivering a continuous basal level of insulin subcutaneously and a bolus at each meal. Such a system simulates the natural state more closely than does conventional therapy with intermittent insulin injections. Many series have demonstrated that the continuous subcutaneous insulin infusion (CSII) can be a safe and effective means of glucose control in both pregnant and nonpregnant diabetic patients.[38,108–110] In fact, few uncontrolled studies have suggested that the use of CSII may achieve better than conventional therapy.

A randomized clinical trial by Coustan et al[36] was conducted among 22 IDDM patients, in which one group of 11 patients received intensive conventional therapy and the other 11 patients received CSII therapy. No significant difference between the two forms of insulin administration was observed with regard to glucose control, assessed by mean blood glucose, HbA$_1$, or mean amplitude of glycemic excursions or with regard to the severity and frequency of hypoglycemia and fetal outcome. These results were obtained from both the patient's home blood glucose recordings and 24-hour inpatient glucose profiles conducted once during each trimester.

The above study should not be interpreted to suggest that CSII is without value. On the contrary, CSII remains a valuable means of achieving euglycemia, especially in patients with very erratic eating schedules or patients who require several daily insulin injections. This study demonstrates that equivalent glucose control and fetal outcome can be achieved with either

Table 10-5. Features of Insulin Pumps

| Pump Model (Manu-facturer) | Weight (oz) | Battery (type/life/cost) | Basals | | | Alarms | | | Features |
			No.	Range (U/h)	Smallest Bolus	Occlu-sion	Run-away	Near Empty	
MiniMed 506 (MiniMed Technologies)	3.6	Three 1.5-volt Eveready; 2–3-mo life; available in drugstores	6 profiles, advanced temporary basal rate (can deliver more or less insulin for a set duration of 30 minutes to 16 hours)	0.0–25.0	0.1 U	Yes	Yes	Yes	Toll-free 24-hour service and support; memory recall (up to 7 days); pump conducts a safety check every minute, every programming change, and before each motor stroke; free video on pump therapy; waterproof, floatable, and impact-resistant protective case available
H-Tron V100 (Disetronic Medical Systems)	Less than 3.5	2–3-volt silver oxide; 2–4-mo life	24 profiles plus temporary, 20 deliveries per hour at any programmed rate	0.0–10.0	0.1U	Yes	Yes	Yes	Patient receives two pumps and free safety inspections; the pump is waterproof without an additional case; video and manual available; toll-free 24-hour support service; the pump is compatible with all infusion sets

(Modified from American Diabetes Association,[115] with permission.)

intensive conventional therapy or CSII. However, the physician will need to determine which patients will benefit from either form of therapy.

Table 10-5 outlines two of the available insulin pumps, with descriptions of many of the features associated with each. In general, these newer generation pumps are smaller and simpler to use.

The insulin pumps discussed above are all the open-loop type in which an insulin-dosage schedule is programmed into the machine to be delivered to the patient throughout the day. Obviously, a perfected closed-loop insulin pump system that is capable of detecting the blood glucose level and delivering an appropriate amount of insulin would be ideal for the treatment of diabetes. There are a few studies of closed-loop systems tested in animals and in a limited number of diabetic volunteers using a needle-type glucose sensor and a computer calculation of infusion rates of insulin or glucagon, or both.[111–114] Despite encouraging preliminary work, an ideal system has not yet been achieved.

SUMMARY

The foregoing discussion has described the evolution of glucose evaluation and control as a standard form of diabetes care. Although randomized prospective studies have not proved that the reduced perinatal mortality rate was caused by the overall improvement in glycemic control, this relationship is well documented by numerous uncontrolled studies, the results are reproducible, and the concept is very well accepted, precluding a randomized study in the future. With the establishment of such a premise, a variety of methods for both glucose evaluation and control has been introduced.

The recent advances with regard to glucose monitoring have been formidable. Improved techniques and further modifications of present devices, and possibly even the introduction of newer ones such as a perfected closed-loop insulin pump, will enhance current methods of glucose evaluation and control. Such improvement in devices and techniques would be expected to advance the treatment of diabetes mellitus in pregnancy closer toward levels of morbidity and mortality seen in the general population.

REFERENCES

1. Gillmer MDG, Beard RW, Brooke FM et al: Carbohydrate metabolism in pregnancy. I. Diurnal plasma glucose profile in normal and diabetic women. BMJ 3:399, 1975
2. Freinkel N, Dooley SL, Metzger BE: Care of the pregnant woman with insulin-dependent diabetes mellitus. N Engl J Med 313:96, 1985
3. Freinkel N: Pregnancy metabolism, diabetes and the fetus. p. 124. Ciba Foundation Symposium 63 (new series). Excerpta Medica, Amsterdam, 1979
4. Gabbe SG: Medical complications of pregnancy management of diabetes in pregnancy: six decades of experience. p. 37. In Pitkin RM, Zlatnik FJ (eds): Year Book of Obstetrics and Gynecology. Part I: Obstetrics. Year Book Medical Publishers, Chicago, 1980
5. Gyves MT, Rodman HM, Little AB et al: A modern approach to management of pregnant diabetics: a two-year analysis of perinatal outcomes. Am J Obstet Gynecol 128:606, 1977
6. Jovanovic L, Peterson CM: Management of the pregnant, insulin-dependent diabetic woman. Diabetes Care 3:63, 1980
7. Kitzmiller JL, Cloherty JP, Younger MD et al: Diabetic pregnancy and perinatal morbidity. Am J Obstet Gynecol 131:560, 1978
8. Miller JM Jr, Crenshaw MC Jr, Welt SI: Hemoglobin A_{1c} in normal and diabetic pregnancy. JAMA 242:2785, 1979
9. Gabbe SG, Mestman JH, Freeman RK et al: Management and outcome of pregnancy in diabetes mellitus, classes B to R. Am J Obstet Gynecol 129:723, 1977
10. Karlsson K, Kjellmer I: The outcome of diabetic pregnancies in relation to the mother's blood sugar level. Am J Obstet Gynecol 112:213, 1972
11. Jovanovic L, Druzin M, Peterson CM: Effect of euglycemia on the outcome of pregnancy in insulin-dependent diabetic women as compared with normal control subjects. Am J Med 71:921, 1981
12. Landon MB: Diabetes mellitus and other endocrine diseases. p. 1097. In Gabbe SG, Niebyl JR, Simpson JL (eds): Obstetrics. Churchill Livingstone, New York, 1991
13. Skyler JS, O'Sullivan MJ: Diabetes and pregnancy. p. 603. In Kohler PO (ed): Clinical Endocrinology. John Wiley & Sons, New York, 1986
14. Adashi EY, Pinto H, Tyson JE: Impact of maternal euglycemia on fetal outcome in diabetic pregnancy. Am J Obstet Gynecol 133:268, 1979
15. Sack RA: The large infant. Am J Obstet Gynecol 104:195, 1969
16. Fuhrmann K, Reiher H, Semmler K et al: Prevention of congenital malformations in infants of insulin-dependent diabetic mothers. Diabetes Care 6:219, 1983
17. Kitzmiller JL, Gavin LA, Gin GD et al: Preconception management of diabetes continued through early pregnancy prevents the excess frequency of major congenital anomalies in infants of diabetic mothers. JAMA 265: 731, 1991
18. Goldman JA, Dicker D, Feldberg et al: Pregnancy outcome in patients with insulin-dependent diabetes mellitus with preconceptional diabetic control: a comparative study. Am J Obstet Gynecol 155:293, 1986
19. Steel JM, Johnstone FD, Smith AF: Five years experience of a "prepregnancy" clinic for insulin-dependent diabetics. BMJ 285:353, 1982
20. Steel JM, Johnstone FD, Hepburn DA, Smith AF: Can prepregnancy care of diabetic women reduce the risk of abnormal babies? BMJ 301:1070, 1990
21. Seeds AE, Knowles HC: Metabolic control of diabetic pregnancy. Clin Obstet Gynecol 24:51, 1981
22. Jovanovic L, Peterson CM: Optimal insulin delivery for the pregnant diabetic patient. Diabetes Care 5:24, 1982
23. Kitzmiller JL: The endocrine pancreas and maternal metabolism. p. 26. In Tulchinsky D, Ryan KJ (eds): Maternal-Fetal Endocrinology. WB Saunders, Philadelphia, 1980
24. Knopp RH, Montes A, Childs M et al: Metabolic adjustments in normal and diabetic pregnancy. Clin Obstet Gynecol 24:21, 1981
25. Artal R, Golde SH, Dorey F et al: The effect of plasma glucose variability on neonatal outcome in the pregnant diabetic patient. Am J Obstet Gynecol 147:537, 1983
26. Cousins L, Rigg L, Hollingsworth D et al: The 24-hour excursion and diurnal rhythm of glucose, insulin, and

C-peptide in normal pregnancy. Am J Obstet Gynecol 136:483, 1980

27. Coustan DR: Recent advances in the management of diabetic pregnant women. Clin Perinatol 7:299, 1980

28. Coustan DR, Berkowitz RL, Hobbins JC: Tight metabolic control of overt diabetes in pregnancy. Am J Med 68:845, 1980

29. Felig P, Bergman M: Intensive ambulatory treatment of insulin-dependent diabetes. Ann Intern Med 97:225, 1982

30. Siperstein MD, Foster DW, Knowles HC et al: Control of glucose and diabetic vascular disease. N Engl J Med 296:1060, 1977

31. Weiss PAM, Hofmann H: Intensified conventional insulin therapy for the pregnant diabetic patient. Obstet Gynecol 64:629, 1984

32. Leveno KJ, Hauth JC, Gilstrap LC III et al: Appraisal of "rigid" blood glucose control during pregnancy in the overtly diabetic woman. Am J Obstet Gynecol 135:853, 1979

33. Gillmer MDG, Beard RW, Oakley NW et al: Diurnal plasma free fatty acid profiles in normal and diabetic pregnancies. BMJ 2:670, 1977

34. Lewis SB, Wallen JD, Kuzuya H et al: Circadian variation of serum glucose, C-peptide immunoreactivity and free insulin in normal and insulin-treated diabetic pregnant subjects. Diabetologia 12:343, 1970

35. Rizvi J, Gillmer MDG, Oakley NW et al: Evaluation of plasma glucose control in pregnancy complicated by chemical diabetes. Br J Obstet Gynaecol 87:383, 1980

36. Coustan DR, Reece RA, Sherwin R et al: A randomized clinical trial of insulin pump vs. intensive conventional therapy in diabetic pregnancies. JAMA 255:631, 1986

37. Jovanovic L, Peterson CM, Saxena BB et al: Feasibility of maintaining normal glucose profiles in insulin-dependent pregnant diabetic women. Am J Med 68:105, 1980

38. Kitzmiller JL, Younger MD, Hare JW et al: Continuous subcutaneous insulin therapy during early pregnancy. Obstet Gynecol 66:606, 1985

39. Gabbe SG, Mestman JH, Freeman RK et al: Management and outcome of class A diabetes mellitus. Am J Obstet Gynecol 127:465, 1977

40. Martin TR, Allen AC, Stinson D: Overt diabetes in pregnancy. Am J Obstet Gynecol 133:275, 1979

41. Reece EA, Coustan D, Sherwin R et al: Does intensive glycemic control in diabetic pregnancies result in normalization of other metabolic fuels. Am J Obstet Gynecol 165:126, 1991

42. Sonksen PH: Home monitoring of blood glucose by diabetic patients. Acta Endocrinol (Copenh) 94:145, 1980

43. Sonksen PH, Judd SL, Lowy C: Home monitoring of blood glucose: method for improving diabetic control. Lancet 1:729, 1978

44. Sonksen PH, Judd S, Lowy C: Home monitoring of blood glucose: new approach to management of insulin-dependent diabetic patients in Great Britain. Diabetes Care 3:100, 1980

45. Landon MB, Gabbe SG: Glucose monitoring and insulin administration in the pregnant diabetic patient. Clin Obstet Gynecol 28:496, 1985

46. Skyler JS: Self-monitoring of blood glucose. Med Clin North Am 66:1227, 1982

47. Walford S, Gale EAM, Allison SP et al: Self-monitoring of blood glucose. Lancet 1:732, 1978

48. Espersen T, Klebe JG: Self-monitoring of blood glucose in pregnant diabetics. Acta Obstet Gynecol Scand 64:11, 1985

49. Skyler JS, Robertson EG, Lasky IA et al: Blood glucose control during pregnancy. Diabetes Care 3:69, 1980

50. Soeldner JS: Treatment of diabetes mellitus by devices. Am J Med 70:183, 1981

51. Peacock I, Hunter JC, Walford S et al: Self-monitoring of blood glucose in diabetic pregnancy. BMJ 2:1333, 1979

52. Hanson U, Persson B, Ericksson E et al: Self-monitoring of blood glucose by diabetic women during the third trimester of pregnancy. Am J Obstet Gynecol 150:817, 1984

53. Varner MW: Efficacy of home glucose monitoring in diabetic pregnancy. Am J Med 75:592, 1983

54. Lewis SB, Murray WK, Wallen JD et al: Improved glucose control in nonhospitalized pregnant diabetic patients. diabetologia 48:260, 1576

55. Harkness LJ, Ashwood ER, Parsons S, Lenke RR: Comparison of the accuracy of glucose reflectance meters in pregnant insulin-dependent diabetics. Obstet Gynecol 77:181, 1991

56. Landon MB, Gabbe SG, Piana R et al: Neonatal morbidity in pregnancy complicated by diabetes mellitus: predictive value of maternal glycemic profiles. Am J Obstet Gynecol 156:1089, 1987

57. Combs AC, Gunderson E, Kitzmiller JL et al: Relationship of fetal macrosomia to maternal postprandial glucose control during pregnancy. Diabetes Care 15:1251, 1992

58. Jovanovic-Peterson L, Peterson CM, Reed GF et al: Maternal postprandial glucose levels and infant birth weight: the diabetes in early pregnancy study. Am J Obstet Gynecol 164:103, 1991

59. Lin CC, River J, River P et al: Good diabetic control early in pregnancy and favorable fetal outcome. Obstet Gynecol 67:51, 1986

60. Abell DA: The significance of abnormal glucose tolerance (hyperglycemia and hypoglycemia) in pregnancy. Br J Obstet Gynaecol 86:214, 1979

61. Langer A, Levy J, Brustman L et al: Glycemic control in gestational diabetes mellitus—how tight is tight enough: small for gestational age versus large for gestational age? Am J Obstet Gynecol 161:646, 1989

62. Stubbs SM, Pyke DA, Brudenell JM et al: Management of the pregnant diabetic: home or hospital, with or without glucose meters? Lancet 2:1122, 1980

63. Shapiro B, Savage PJ, Lomatch D et al: A comparison of accuracy and estimated cost of methods for home blood glucose monitoring. Diabetes Care 4:396, 1981

64. Mazze RS, Shamson H, Pasmantier R et al: Reliability of blood–glucose monitoring by patients with diabetes mellitus. Am J Med 77:211, 1984

65. Moses RG: Assessment of reliability of patients performing SMBG with a portable reflectance meter with memory capacity (M-glucometer). Diabetes Care 9:670, 1986

66. Allen DW, Schroder WA, Balog J: Observations on the chromatographic heterogeneity of normal adults and fetal hemoglobin: a study of the effects of crystallization and chromatography on the heterogeneity and isoleucine content. J Am Chem Soc 80:1628, 1958

67. Bookchin RM, Gallop PM: Structure of hemoglobin A_{1c}. Nature of the N-terminal β chain blocking group. Biochem Biophys Res Commun 32:86, 1968

68. Ditzel J, Kjaergaard JJ: Hemoglobin A_{1c} concentrations after initial treatment for newly discovered diabetes. BMJ 1:741, 1978

69. Dunn PJ, Cole RA, Soeldner JS et al: Temporal relationship of glycosylated haemoglobin concentrations to glucose control in diabetics. Diabetologia 17:213, 1979

70. Gabbay KH: Glycosylated hemoglobin and diabetic control. N Engl J Med 295:443, 1976

71. Koenig RJ, Peterson CM, Jones RL et al: Correlation of glucose regulation and hemoglobin A_{1c} in diabetes mellitus. N Engl J Med 295:417, 1976

72. Lapp CA, Huff TA, Bransome ED Jr: Detection of abnormal hemoglobin variants during glycohemoglobin analysis. Clin Chem 26:355, 1980

73. O'Shaughnessy R, Russ J, Zuspan FP: Glycosylated hemoglobins and diabetes mellitus in pregnancy. Am J Obstet Gynecol 135:783, 1979

74. Schwartz HC, King KC, Schwartz AL et al: Effects of pregnancy on hemoglobin A_{1c} in normal, gestational diabetic and diabetic women. Diabetes 25:1118, 1976

75. Tahbar S: An abnormal hemoglobin in red cells of diabetics. Clin Chim Acta 22:296, 1968

76. Trivelli LA, Ranney HM, Lai HT: Hemoglobin components in patients with diabetes mellitus. N Engl J Med 284:353, 1971

77. Gabbay KH, Hasty K, Breslow JL et al: Glycosylated hemoglobins and long-term blood glucose control in diabetes mellitus. J Clin Endocrinol Metab 44:859, 1977

78. Bunn HF, Haney DN, Gabbay KH et al: Further identification of the nature and linkage of the carbohydrate in hemoglobin A_{1c}. Biochem Biophys Res Commun 67:103, 1975

79. Bunn HF, Haney DN, Kamin S et al: The biosynthesis of human hemoglobin A_{1c}: slow glycosylation of hemoglobin in vivo. J Clin Invest 57:1652, 1976

80. Haney DN, Bunn HF: Glycosylation of hemoglobin in vitro: affinity labeling of hemoglobin by glucose-6-phosphate. Proc Natl Acad Sci USA 73:3534, 1976

81. Huisman RG, Dozy AM: Studies on the heterogeneity of hemoglobin. V. Binding of hemoglobin with oxidized glutathione. J Lab Clin Med 60:302, 1962

82. Karamanos B, Christacopoulos P, Zacharious N et al: Rapid changes of the hemoglobin A_{1c} (HbA_{1c}) fraction following alterations of diabetic control. Diabetologia 13:406, 1977

83. Leslie RDG, Pyke DA, John PN et al: How quickly can haemoglobin A_1 increase? BMJ 2:19, 1979

84. Gonen B, Rochman H, Rubenstein AH et al: Haemoglobin A1: an indicator of the metabolic control of diabetic patients. Lancet 2:734, 1977

85. Vintzileos AM, Thompson JP: Glycohemoglobin determinations in normal pregnancy and in insulin-dependent diabetics. Obstet Gynecol 56:435, 1980

86. Widness JA, Schwartz HC, Thompson D et al: Glycohemoglobin (HbA_{1c}): a predictor of birth weight in infants of diabetic mothers. J Pediatr 92:8, 1978

87. Leslie RDG, Pyke DA, John PN: Hemoglobin A_1 in diabetic pregnancy. Lancet 2:958, 1978

88. Miller E, Hare JW, Cloherty JP et al: Elevated maternal hemoglobin A_{1c} in early pregnancy and major congenital anomalies in infants of diabetic mothers. N Engl J Med 304:1331, 1981

89. Ylinen K, Raivio K, Teramo K: Haemoglobin A_{1c} predicts the perinatal outcome in insulin-dependent diabetic pregnancies. Br J Obstet Gynaecol 38:961, 1981

90. Greene MF, Have JW, Cloherty JP et al: First trimester hemoglobin A_1 and risk for major malformations and spontaneous abortion in diabetic pregnancy. Tertology 39:225, 1989

91. Fitzgerald MD, Cauchi MN: Glycosylated hemoglobins in patients with a hemoglobinopathy. Clin Chem 26:360, 1980

92. Aleyassine H: Glycosylation of hemoglobin S and hemoglobin C. Clin Chem 25:526, 1980

93. Aleyassine H: Low proportions of glycosylated hemoglobin associated with hemoglobin S and hemoglobin C. Clin Chem 25:1484, 1979

94. Baxi L, Barad D, Reece EA et al: Use of glycosylated hemoglobin as a screen for macrosomia in gestational diabetes. Obstet Gynecol 64:347, 1984

95. Mitchell TR, Anderson D, Shepperd J: Iron deficiency, hemachromatosis, and glycosylated hemoglobin. Lancet 2:747, 1980

96. Roberts AB, Court DJ, Henley P et al: Fructosamine in diabetic pregnancy. Lancet 2:998, 1983

97. Baker JR, O'Connor JP, Metcalf PA et al: The clinical utility of serum fructosamine estimation, a possible screening test for diabetes mellitus. BMJ 287:863, 1983

98. Cefalu WT, Prather KL, Chester DL et al: Total serum glycosylated proteins in detection and monitoring of gestational diabetes. Diabetes Care 13:872, 1990

99. Parfitt VJ, Clark JD, Turner GM, Hartog M: Use of fructosamine and glycated hemoglobin to verify self blood glucose monitoring data in diabetic pregnancy. Diabetic Med 10:162, 1993

100. Thai AC, Lui KF, Lowes NY et al: Serial measurements of serum fructosamine and glycosylated haemoglobin as indices of glycemic control in diabetic pregnancy. Ann Acad Med Singapore 20:732, 1991

101. Watson WJ, Herbert WA, Prior TW, Chapman JF: Glycosylated hemoglobin and fructosamine: indicators of glycemic control in pregnancies complicated by diabetic mellitus. J Reprod Med 36:731, 1991

102. Windeler J, Kobberling J: The fructosamine assay in diagnosis and control of diabetes mellitus: scientific evidence for its clinical usefulness? J Clin Chem Clin Biochem 28:129, 1990

103. DCCT Research: The effect of intensive treatment of diabetes on the development and progression of long-term, complications in insulin-dependent diabetes mellitus. N Engl J Med 329:997, 1993

104. Kroc Collaborative Study Group: Blood glucose control and the evolution of diabetic retinopathy and albuminuria: a preliminary multicenter trial. N Engl J Med 311:365, 1984

105. Dahl-Jorgensen K, Brinchmann-Hansen O, Hanssen KF et al: Rapid tightening of blood glucose control leads to transient deterioration of retinopathy in insulin dependent diabetes mellitus: the Oslo study. BMJ 290:811, 1990

106. Faiman G, Topper E, Goldman J et al: Dietary adjustment during self-blood-glucose monitoring in pregnant women with insulin-dependent diabetes mellitus. J Am Diet Assoc 84:816, 1984

107. Tattersall R, Gale E: Patient self-monitoring of blood glucose and refinements of conventional insulin treatment. Am J Med 70:177, 1981

108. Pickup JC, Keen H, Parsons JA, Alberti KGMM: Continuous subcutaneous insulin infusion: an approach to achieving normoglycemia. BMJ 1:204, 1978

109. Potter JM, Reckless JPD, Cullen DR: Subcutaneous continuous insulin infusion and control of blood glucose concentration in diabetics in third trimester of pregnancy. BMJ 28:1099, 1980

110. Rudolf MCJ, Coustan DR, Sherwin RS et al: Efficacy of the insulin pump in the home treatment of pregnant diabetics. Diabetes 30:891, 1981

111. Rupp MCJ, Barbosa JJ, Blackshear PJ et al: The use of an implantable insulin pump in the treatment of type II diabetics. N Engl J Med 307:265, 1982

112. Shichiri M, Kawamori R, Hakui N et al: Closed-loop glycemic control with a wearable artificial endocrine pancreas. Diabetes 33:1200, 1984

113. Shichiri M, Asakawa N, Yamasaki Y et al: Telemetry glucose monitoring device with needle-type glucose sensor: a useful tool for blood glucose monitoring in diabetic individuals. Diabetes Care 9:298, 1986

114. Shichiri M, Yamasaki Y, Kawamori R et al: Wearable artificial endocrine pancreas with needle-type glucose sensor. Lancet 2:1129, 1982

115. American Diabetes Association: Buyer's Guide to Diabetes supplies. Diabetes Forecast, ADA, Alexandria, VA, 1993

11

Insulin Treatment

MARK B. LANDON
STEVEN G. GABBE

The introduction of insulin into clinical practice in 1922 remains the most significant advancement in the treatment of pregnancy complicated by diabetes mellitus. Before that time, pregnancy in the diabetic women was uncommon and was accompanied by high maternal and fetal mortality rates.[1] Despite White's admonition that the early use of insulin during pregnancy appeared to have its greatest impact in reducing maternal mortality and morbidity, adequate techniques were not available for many years to monitor blood glucose closely throughout gestation.[2] Over the past 20 years, self-blood glucose monitoring and intensive insulin therapy have combined to make achievement of near-physiologic euglycemia a therapeutic reality for many pregnant diabetic women. The result of such efforts has been a steady decline in fetal and neonatal mortality rates, which, excluding major congenital malformations, are now nearly equivalent to those observed in normal pregnancy.[3]

Several techniques for insulin administration have been used to achieve optimum glucose control during pregnancy (Table 11-1). The efficacy of these regimens depends on frequent glucose determinations. Self-monitoring systems provide the best means by which patients can determine their glucose control. This advancement in the therapy of diabetes has enabled women of reproductive age to assume a greater role in the treatment of their disease both before conception and during pregnancy. Adjustments in insulin dosage, diet, and exercise based on frequent monitoring of glucose levels is especially important during pregnancy when normal physiologic changes occur that can alter insulin requirements dramatically.

NORMAL INSULIN SECRETION

Insulin is required for normal carbohydrate, protein, and lipid metabolism. Individuals with type I or insulin-dependent diabetes mellitus (IDDM) do not produce sufficient quantities of this hormone and require exogenous insulin to prevent fatal ketoacidosis. By contrast, individuals with non-insulin-dependent (type II) diabetes mellitus (NIDDM) do not require endogenous insulin for survival. However, during pregnancy, many of these individuals will demonstrate marked insulin resistance, requiring supplemental insulin for adequate blood glucose control. Similarly, women with gestational diabetes mellitus, may be unable to regulate glycemia with dietary manipulation alone and may require multiple injections of insulin for this purpose.

In nondiabetic individuals, basal insulin secretion into the portal system takes place at a rate of approximately 1 U/h. Food intake results in a stimulated release of 5 to 10 U of insulin from the pancreatic β-cells, such that the total daily insulin secretion in a normal individual is approximately 40 U/d.[4] Basal insulin secretion seems to limit hepatic glucose production in the postabsorptive state. Fasting blood glucose levels correlate well with hepatic glucose production and measures of long-term glycemic control such as glycosylated hemoglobin levels.[4] Long-acting insulin preparations are prescribed to simulate basal insulin production. The endogenous insulin secretion stimulated by meals promotes disposal of ingested nutrients, primarily glucose, into peripheral tissues. This phase of insulin secretion is synchronized with the rise in blood glucose in response to feeding. Once surges in post-meal glucose levels subside, there is a prompt diminu-

Table 11-1. Target Glucose Levels During Pregnancy

Time	mg/dl
Before breakfast	60–90
Before lunch, dinner, bedtime snack	60–105
After meals (2 hours)	≤120
2:00 AM to 6:00 AM	>60

tion in insulin secretion and a return to basal or post-absorptive levels. Premeal insulin administration of short-acting or regular insulin preparations is thus physiologically important in replacement regimens designed for the pregnant woman with diabetes.

As with any hormone replacement, the primary goal is to achieve physiologic hormone levels at the site of hormone action. The objective of insulin replacement regimens in both the pregnant and nonpregnant states is further complicated by the need to simulate normal secretion patterns despite rapid changes in response to nutrient intake and physiologic stimuli such as exercise. Unfortunately, available insulin preparations and regimens are clearly less than physiologic. For example, the peak effects of subcutaneously administered human regular insulin are delayed until 3 to 4 hours after injection and may be present as long as 8 hours. Similarly, intermediate-acting and long-acting preparations such as Ultralente insulin, designed to mimic basal secretion, have demonstrable peaks in their action. The administration of regular insulin by continuous subcutaneous (insulin) infusion (CSII) or pump therapy has been hailed as the most suitable method to mimic normal basal insulin secretion. Yet, individuals treated with this regimen, which includes both basal infusions and mealtime boluses, can demonstrate significantly elevated serum insulin levels.[4]

INSULIN PREPARATIONS

Great advances have been made in the production of highly purified insulins for patient use. Today, clinicians can choose from a variety of preparations emphasizing species specificity and improved purity. Despite the production of highly purified preparations from animal sources in the form of beef or pork insulin,

these types of insulin have now been largely replaced by the manufacture of human insulin by recombinant DNA technology, as well as the introduction of several genetically engineered insulin analogs. Insulin is available in short-, intermediate-, and long-acting forms that may be administered separately or mixed in the same syringe. Short-acting insulins include regular and Semilente; the intermediate-acting preparations are Lente and NPH (Table 11-2). Human insulin preparations are also marketed as mixtures of short- and intermediate-acting varieties in 10 percent steps ranging from 10:90 percent to 50:50 percent. Predetermined mixtures of 70 percent NPH and 30 percent regular have gained popularity but may be of limited value in pregnancy regimens when a single component in the dosage must be changed or if intermediate-acting insulin only is to be given at bedtime. The only long-acting insulin preparation is Ultralente. Ultralente mimics basal insulin secretion and is administered either before breakfast or dinner. Many physicians have been reluctant to use Ultralente insulin during pregnancy because of its long duration of action (≤36 hours), which, when coupled with next-day administration of mealtime regular insulin, might increase the risk of hypoglycemia.

Animal insulin has minor structural differences from the human hormone. Porcine insulin contains an alanine residue instead of threonine at the carboxyl-terminal of the β-chain, whereas beef insulin substitutes alanine and valine at positions 8 and 10 on the α-chain (for threonine and isoleucine).[5] Thus, there is remarkable homology of sequences between human and commercially available animal insulin preparations. Because bovine insulin is less similar to human insulin than is porcine, bovine insulin is more immunogenic.[5] These minor differences in structure do not appear to be crucial to the binding or action of insulin. Receptor binding and cellular interactions of human insulin, in fact, do not differ significantly from those of beef or pork insulin.[6] Amino acid substitutions may, however, influence the tendency for dimer formation.[7] Similarly, the physiochemical properties of human and animal insulins differ because of their various amino acid sequences. The addition of one extra hydroxyl group due to threonine in human insulin increases its hydrophilic and decreases its lipophilic properties compared with porcine insulin. It follows that human insulin is more soluble in aqueous solution than is porcine insulin.

Table 11-2. Types of Insulin

	Source	Onset (h)	Peak (h)	Duration (h)
Short-Acting				
Humulin R (Lilly)	Human	0.5	2–4	5–7
Velosulin-H (Novo Nordisk)	Human	0.5	1–3	8
Novolin R (Novo Nordisk)	Human	0.5	2.5–5	6–8
Iletin I (Lilly) regular	Beef/pork	0.5	2–4	5–7
Iletin II (Lilly) regular	Pork	0.5	2–4	5–7
Regular Standard (Novo Nordisk)	Pork	0.5	2.5–5	8
Regular Purified (Novo Nordisk)	Pork	0.5	2.5–5	8
Velosulin (Novo Nordisk)	Purified	0.5	1–3	8
Intermediate-Acting				
Humulin Lente (Lilly)	Human	1–3	6–12	18–24
Humulin NPH (Lilly)	Human	1–2	6–12	18–24
Novolin L (Novo Nordisk)	Human	2.5	7–15	22
Novolin N (Novo Nordisk)	Human	1.5	4–12	24
Semi Lente (Novo Nordisk)	Beef	1.5	5–10	16
Lente (Novo Nordisk)	Beef	2.5	7–15	24
NPH (Novo Nordisk)	Beef	1.5	4–12	24
Lente Purified (Novo Nordisk)	Pork	2.5	7–15	22
NPH Purified (Novo Nordisk)	Pork	1.5	4–12	24
Insulated Purified NPH (Novo Nordisk)	Pork	1.5	4–12	24
Iletin I (Lilly) Lente	Beef/pork	1–3	6–12	>24
Iletin I (Lilly) NPH	Beef/pork	1–2	6–12	>24
Iletin II (Lilly) Lente	Pork	1–3	6–12	>24
Iletin II (Lilly) NPH	Pork	1–2	6–12	>24
Long-Acting				
Humulin Ultralente (Lilly)	Human	4–6	8–20	24–28
Ultralente (Novo Nordisk)	Beef	4	10–30	36
Ultralenta (Lilly) Iletin II	Beef/pork	4–6	14–24	28–36

INSULIN PRODUCTION

The introduction of methods to mass produce human insulin over the past decades has been a by-product of advances in molecular genetic technology, most importantly, recombinant DNA techniques. Originally, human insulin was produced by exchanging alanine in position β30 of porcine insulin with threonine, using an enzymatic method or semisynthetic technique. Subsequently, the semisynthetic production of insulin has given way to biosynthetic production. Originally, the α- and β-chains were produced separately and required combination. At present, biosynthetic human proinsulin, with a three-dimensional structure identical to the natural hormone can be produced by bacterial cells. The correct three-dimensional or spherical structure is essential for receptor binding and thus biologic action. The three-dimensional structure of human insulin does differ slightly from porcine insulin. In practice, human proinsulin is produced and is then enzymatically cleaved to insulin and C-peptide.

Further purification results in biosynthetic human insulin (Fig. 11-1).

INSULIN IMMUNOGENICITY

The introduction of human insulin has permitted investigation of the role of antibodies to animal-derived insulin preparations in relation to pregnancy outcome. Almost all patients treated with animal-derived insulin for more than 10 years will have detectable anti-insulin antibodies.[5] The presence of these antibodies can significantly affect the pharmacokinetics of insulin. Normally, the plasma concentration of insulin will depend on four variables: absorption rate, endogenous insulin secretion, distribution volume, and catabolism.[8] Rarely, the affinity of antibodies for insulin as well as their binding capacity may be so high that little free insulin is present. In most individuals, circulating IgG anti-insulin antibodies are basically carrier proteins with varying degrees of affinity for insulin. Biologic

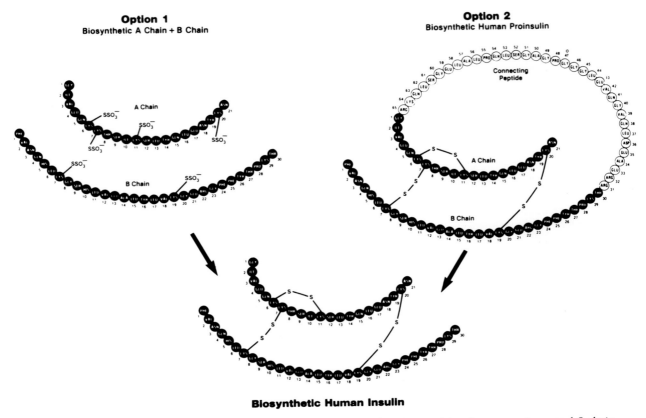

Fig. 11-1. Two pathways for producing biosynthetic human insulin. Option 1 involves separate α- and β-chain production and subsequent combination. Option 2 involves the production of proinsulin from which C-peptide is cleaved enzymatically, resulting in insulin formation. (From Frank and Chance,[69] with permission.)

activity is affected by this process, which results in the release of bound insulin at unpredictable times and may produce unexplained episodes of hypoglycemia. In early pregnancy, insulin antibody titers do not appear to alter insulin requirements or the ability to achieve normoglycemia.[9] Whereas mean levels of antibodies fall after a patient has been changed to a highly purified or human insulin preparation,[10] that benefit alone may not justify this therapeutic maneuver. Nevertheless, the American Diabetes Association suggests that human insulin is preferred for use in pregnant women and in women considering pregnancy.[11] Changing insulin species may affect blood glucose control and often requires a 10 to 20 percent reduction in dose when switching from animal to human preparations. Human insulin is also recommended for the treatment of newly diagnosed diabetes or women with gestational diabetes.

Although insulin antibodies do cross the placenta, they are cleared within the first year of life.[12] There does not appear to be a correlation between cord C-peptide levels and cord insulin antibody levels, suggesting that insulin antibodies do not contribute to hyperinsulinism in the fetus. The clinical significance of maternal insulin antibody levels continues to be debated, although the data of Mylvaganam et al[12] indicate that neonatal morbidity may be increased in the offspring of mothers with higher insulin antibody titers. Following the observation that maternal IgG insulin antibodies can transport insulin across the placenta, Menon and colleagues[13] reported that IDDM women with demonstrable insulin antibodies were at increased risk of producing macrosomic infants. Unfortunately, maternal glycemic control was not analyzed in this report. Subsequently, Rosenn and co-workers[14] from the same institution found no difference in fetal growth characteristics in women treated with human versus animal insulin, suggesting lower antibody production alone did not prevent fetal macrosomia. Jovanovic-Peterson and colleagues[15] conducted the only prospective controlled trial of human versus animal insulin during gestation. These investigators reported that neither maternal or infant antibody levels could be related to the type of insulin used. Of significance, type I diabetic women randomized to human insulin in early pregnancy manifested improved glycemic control, fewer large-for-gestational-age infants, and lower childhood C-peptide response to both glucose and amino acid challenge at 3 months of age in the offspring.[15]

Extremely low immunogenicity is a property of human insulin preparations and, in part, reflects the purification process. The production of semisynthetic insulin preparations has used well established methods in the preparation of porcine insulin. Monocomponent porcine insulin serves as a substrate, thereby avoiding contamination with proinsulin, glucagon, pancreatic polypeptide, somatostatin, and vasoactive intestinal peptides. Recombinant DNA technology, used in the production of biosynthetic human insulin, presents a risk of contamination of the insulin product with various bacterial or yeast polypeptides. The obstacle to achieving purity has largely been overcome with intact proinsulin production in place of α- and β-chain extraction and recombination. This sophisticated purification process has resulted in human insulin preparations that are pure and free of significant contamination. Antibodies to *Escherichia coli*-derived peptides are thus uncommon in subjects treated with human insulin for several months.[16] However, human insulin use is associated with immunogenic potential, albeit lower than that of animal-derived insulin preparations.[17] IgG insulin antibodies at very low levels can be found in approximately 50 percent of diabetic patients after exclusive treatment with biosynthetic or semisynthetic human insulin for 2 years.[5] Relatively high levels of IgG insulin antibody are present in most patients who have a history of pretreatment with impure insulin preparations. Studies performed on newly diagnosed type I patients have surprisingly demonstrated that only two-thirds remain IgG insulin antibody-free; whereas one-third produce low levels of antibody after treatment with semisynthetic preparations.[18] A comparison between this treatment and purified porcine monocomponent insulin revealed higher antibody levels with the latter agent. A further comparison of the immunogenicity of biosynthetic insulin and purified pork insulin documented identical frequencies of antibody production in both groups during the initial 3 months; however, levels were lower in follow-up in the human insulin-treated group.[19] The clinical relevance of the slightly lower immunogenic potential of human insulin compared with highly purified porcine insulin is debatable. Although some have suggested that even low levels of insulin antibodies can adversely affect β-cell function, a large randomized controlled study failed to demonstrate any difference in β-cell function between human monocomponent- and porcine monocomponent-treated individuals.[20] The mechanism by which human insulin induces antibody formation is unknown. Intravenously administered insulin is essentially nonimmunogenic. Deamidation of insulin, as well as additives, could play a role in eliciting an immune response. Transformation products such as covalently aggregated dimers, common in commercial preparations, have a slower metabolism and are highly immunogenic. Degradation products found in subcutaneous depots likely play a role as well.

PHARMACOLOGIC CONSIDERATIONS

Studies investigating insulin absorption or insulin action (or both) are plentiful but may be difficult to compare due to methodologic differences, dosing variation, and the use of different sites of administration. As previously mentioned, prior use of animal insulin and subsequent antibody formation may lead to variable dissociation rates of insulin from circulating antibody complexes, which can affect the bioavailability of exogenous insulin. Pharmacodynamic properties of insulin are studied by following the hypoglycemic effect of subcutaneous-administered insulin over a specified time period. Because hypoglycemia may trigger a counterregulatory response, blood glucose is best kept constant by intravenous infusion to maintain normoglycemia using euglycemic clamp techniques. Glucose requirement is thus a measure of the biologic activity and potency of insulin. A recent survey indicates poor definition of the time-action profiles of many insulin preparations due to methodologic flaws in these studies.[21] An analysis of 22 studies revealed a range of onset of action of 8 to 30 minutes for human regular insulin. Peak action varied from 45 minutes to 4 hours. Within each study, subject variation was considerable and likely reflects differences in insulin transport to target tissues.[21]

Pharmacokinetic studies investigating the absorption of short-acting human versus porcine insulin have produced conflicting results with either similar absorption rates or more rapid absorption of human insulin demonstrated.[22,23] Euglycemic clamp studies reveal that both insulins have similar biologic activities that are dose-dependent.[24] The mechanism of faster absorption of human insulin in comparison with porcine regular insulin may be explained by the greater hydrophilic nature of human insulin. Alternatively, the $\beta30$ amino acid differences may affect dimer association and the tendency to dissociate.

Studies of short-acting human insulin in different concentrations report the onset of action between 15 and 30 minutes, with peak action between 150 and 180 minutes after subcutaneous injection. A slightly faster absorption was found with the U40 formulation compared with the commonly used U100 formulation.[25] Glucose infusion rates were similar with both preparations and remained greater than 50 percent maximal at 6 hours, indicating the longer duration of action of exogenous insulin compared with an endogenous response.

As the rapid initial delivery of insulin is vital in reducing meal-related glycemic excursions, the faster onset of action observed with human insulin might be preferable to short-acting animal preparations. Despite this, postprandial glycemic excursions have not consistently been reduced in studies comparing human and porcine insulin.[26]

Intermediate-acting human insulin preparations also show variable results in pharmacologic studies when compared with animal preparations. In an early pharmacodynamic trial, no difference in the decline of blood glucose levels could be demonstrated with human compared with animal NPH preparations.[27] More recent observations support a more rapid onset and shorter duration of action than with corresponding animal insulins.[28,29] However, disappearance rates of iodine 125 (^{125}I)-labeled human or porcine NPH insulin do not differ significantly when administered to diabetic individuals.[30] Again, differences in absorption cited above may reflect the relative hydrophilic nature of human insulin, whereas other pharmacodynamic differences might be explained by interaction of the various species products with protamine.

In an early double-blind crossover trial in nonpregnant established diabetic individuals, significantly higher blood glucose levels were observed in the fasting and early evening periods in patients receiving human insulin versus animal insulin.[31] The authors attributed this finding to more rapid absorption of human NPH insulin. Subsequently, a study of 96 insulin-treated patients revealed a modest elevation in fasting glucose levels (11.1 versus 9.3 mmol/l) and glycosylated hemoglobin A (HbA$_1$) (11.7 versus 11.0 percent) in human insulin-treated patients.[32] Finally, the question as to whether human NPH might be less clinically effective was tested in a long-term double-blind crossover study of 22 patients. No significant differences were observed in glucose profiles, HbA$_{1c}$ levels, hypoglycemia, and dose requirements in patients receiving semisynthetic NPH insulin compared with porcine insulin.[33]

NPH insulin appears to be absorbed at a faster rate than zinc insulin (Lente insulin). A euglycemic clamp study comparing human Lente demonstrated an increased metabolic effect within the first several hours after injection.[34] The onset of action (half-maximal action) of four commonly prescribed human NPH preparations is within 2.5 to 3 hours, with peak action at 5 to 7 hours and duration of action (defined as >25 percent maximal action) between 13 and 16 hours.

More rapid absorption and shorter duration of action of intermediate-acting human insulins may have particular clinical importance in pregnant women. The administration of human NPH insulin before the evening meal might increase the likelihood of nocturnal hypoglycemia. Elevated fasting blood glucose concentrations might also result from diminished insulin action by the following morning. Fasting glucose concentrations can be significantly lowered when the evening dose of human NPH insulin is given at bedtime instead of before supper.[35] Human NPH insulin appears to have a distinct advantage over human Lente in that it can be premixed with short-acting insulin in one syringe without a considerable change in time-action profiles. The principal effect of Lente is to retard the onset of action of short-acting insulin. The delay is a result of binding of regular insulin to zinc, which results in amorphous precipitation of zinc insulin. This phenomenon does not occur with mixing of human regular and NPH insulins.

Ultralente insulin preparations manufactured with bovine and porcine insulin have different pharmacokinetic characteristics from human Ultralente insulin.[36] Human zinc insulin binds water more avidly than pork insulin, leading to better solubility of human Ultralente preparations and faster absorption. The Ultralente formulation with bovine insulin has a very long duration ($\leq$32 hours) and demonstrates no peak affect.[36] By contrast, human Ultralente insulin's effect peaks after 8 to 9 hours, and its duration of action is shorter than that of bovine Ultralente. A study comparing time-action profiles of human Ultralente and human NPH revealed a peak action of 10 hours, which was two-thirds that of NPH.[37] Plasma insulin levels returned to baseline at 20 hours for both groups, indicating that the duration of action of human ultralente is not considerably longer than that of NPH insulin. This observation would suggest that a single daily injection of human Ultralente insulin is insufficient to provide for basal need and that twice daily injections are necessary. The high variability of insulin bioavailability of Ultralente insulin preparations has discouraged the use of these preparations during pregnancy. However, limited data are available concerning human Ultralente administration to pregnant women.

METHODS OF INSULIN ADMINISTRATION

During pregnancy, conventional insulin therapy often needs to be abandoned in favor of intensive therapy to achieve the best glycemic control possible for each patient. Conventional insulin regimens have classically included one to two injections of insulin, usually before breakfast and the evening meal, complemented by self-blood glucose monitoring and adjustment of insulin dose according to glucose profiles. Patients are instructed on dietary composition, insulin action, recognition and treatment of hypoglycemia, adjusting insulin dosage for exercise and sick days, and monitoring for hyperglycemia and potential ketosis. These princi-

ples form the foundation for intensive insulin therapy in which an attempt is made to simulate physiologic insulin requirements. Insulin administration is provided for both basal needs and meals, and rapid adjustments are made in response to glucose measurements. The treatment regimen often involves three to four daily injections or the use of CSII devices. With either approach, frequent self-blood glucose monitoring is fundamental to achieve the therapeutic objective of physiologic glucose control. Patients are instructed on an insulin dose for each meal and at bedtime if necessary. Mealtime insulin needs are determined by the composition of the meal, the premeal glucose measurement, and the level of activity anticipated after the meal. Basal or intermediate-acting insulin requirements are determined by periodic 2:00 AM to 4:00 AM glucose measurements as well as late-afternoon values that reflect morning NPH or Lente action. During pregnancy, many diabetic women develop the self-management skills essential to an intensive insulin therapy regimen.

In patients who are not well controlled, a brief period of hospitalization is often necessary for the initiation of therapy. Individual adjustments to the regimens implemented can then be made. It is gratifying for many patients to believe they can take charge of their own diabetic control. In our experience, patients who have previously followed a prescribed dosage regimen for years gain confidence in making adjustments in their insulin dosage after a short time. Patients are encouraged to contact their physician at any time if questions should arise concerning the management of their diabetes. During early pregnancy, patients are instructed to report their glucose values by telephone at least weekly.

MULTIPLE INJECTION REGIMENS

Insulin is generally administered in two to three injections. We prefer a three-injection regimen, although most patients present taking a combination of intermediate-acting and regular insulin before dinner and breakfast (Fig. 11-2). As a general rule, the amount of intermediate-acting insulin will exceed the regular component by a 2:1 ratio. Patients usually receive two-thirds of their total dose with breakfast and the remaining one-third in the evening as a combined dose with dinner or split into components with regular insulin

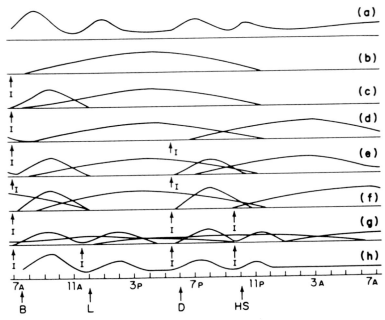

Fig. 11-2. Action curves of various insulin administration schemes as they compare with normal insulin secretion: *(a)* normal insulin secretion; *(b)* AM: NPH; *(c)* AM: NPH and regular; *(d)* AM: NPH, PM: NPH; *(e)* AM: NPH and regular, PM: NPH and regular; *(f)* AM: NPH and regular PM: regular, HS: NPH; *(g)* AM: Ultralente and regular, L: Regular, PM: Ultralente and regular, HS: regular; *(h)* CSII pump. Note that only panel *(h)* mimics panel *(a)*. I, injection; B, breakfast; L, lunch; D, dinner; HS, bedtime snack. (From Jovanovic et al,[70] with permission.)

at dinnertime and intermediate-acting insulin at bedtime in an effort to minimize periods of nocturnal hypoglycemia. These episodes frequently occur when the mother is in a relative fasting state while placental and fetal glucose consumption continue. Finally, some women may require a small dose of regular insulin before lunch, thus constituting a four-injection daily regimen.

Subcutaneous injection of insulin introduces numerous variables that can affect insulin absorption and, in turn, circulating insulin levels. Insulin absorption is clearly affected by injection site selection, with absorption being diminished in the lower extremity compared with the abdominal wall. It has been demonstrated that ^{125}I-labeled rapid-acting insulin disappears 86 percent faster from the abdomen than from the leg.[38] Thus, to maintain consistency, the type of injection site should not be changed frequently. The large abdominal surface area provides for adequate rotation while minimizing the variability associated with mov-

ing the injection from abdomen to extremity. After proper counseling, most pregnant women will accept abdominal injection. Remarkably, absorption variation still approaches as much as 30 percent when the identical site and dose of insulin is administered to the same individual.[39]

The depth of injection and skin temperature can also affect insulin absorption. Local heat produced by exercise can accelerate absorption and consequently elevate circulating insulin levels.[40] Despite efforts to achieve excellent glycemic control, variable absorption of injected insulin remains an elusive problem that can no doubt influence postmeal glucose excursions.

CONTINUOUS SUBCUTANEOUS INSULIN INFUSION

In the late-1970s, insulin delivery systems were developed that could mimic the pattern of secretion of the normal pancreas. These systems adjusted for minute-to-minute changes in blood glucose concentration. One of the first such devices, the Biostator (Miles Laboratory), is a computerized closed-loop autoanalyzer that withdraws small amounts of venous blood through a double-lumen catheter. A glucose sensor measures the glucose concentration and its rate of change over the previous 4 minutes. The amount of insulin or dextrose to be infused is determined by these data. This unit, which is the size of a microwave oven, has been used successfully for acute blood glucose regulation in small numbers of obstetric patients during the third trimester and at the time of cesarean delivery.[41] Natrass et al[42] used a glucose-controlled insulin infusion system during labor in a few IDDM patients. Mean glucose concentrations ranging from 83 to 94 mg/dl were achieved without any reported complications.[42] Such closed-loop systems remain primarily research tools because of their cost and need for an indwelling venous catheter. Also, their large size has prevented them from being suitable for ambulatory use. However, research continues on implantable insulin pumps with glucose monitoring, providing for an internal closed-loop system. The primary obstacle to development of such systems has been in vivo glucose sensing capability. In addition, concerns regarding calibration requirements over time, occlusion of sensor tips, and selection of an optimal method for glucose measurement (glucose oxidase versus spectroscopy) need to be addressed in future research.

Although implantable open-loop insulin pumps were first used in the early 1980s, these devices have experienced relatively little clinical use. The pumps are implanted subcutaneously, usually on the left side of the abdomen with the catheter tip being placed within the peritoneum. Clinical experience demonstrates a remarkably low incidence of electronic device failure or infection. Catheter obstruction is the most significant complication and may require a laparoscopic procedure to relieve. The main advantage of an implantable open-loop system is the precision of insulin dosage and greater initial absorption of insulin into the portal system. Currently a research tool, these devices require surgical placement and are expensive. Whether an advantage over subcutaneous delivery systems exists awaits further study.

There has now been considerable experience with open-loop CSII during pregnancy (Table 11-3). The pump is a battery-powered unit that is usually attached

Table 11-3. Advantages and Disadvantages of Continuous Subcutaneous Insulin Infusion in Pregnancy

Advantages
- Continuous basal rate delivery of insulin decreases mean glucose excursions
- Portable size allows for ambulatory use
- Eliminates the need for multiple daily injections
- May increase patient enthusiasm and encourage contact with health care team

Disadvantages
- Requires excellent patient compliance
- May require more intensive glucose monitoring
- Mechanical problems can produce hypo- and hyperglycemia
- Increased potential for ketoacidosis with pump failure
- Potential infection at insertion site
- May be uncomfortable to wear in late pregnancy

to the anterior abdominal wall and may be worn during most daily activities. These systems provide continuous short-acting insulin therapy via a subcutaneous infusion. The basal infusion rate and bolus doses to cover meals are determined by frequent self-monitoring of blood glucose. A basal infusion rate is generally close to 1 U/h.

Pregnant patients will often require hospitalization before initiation of pump therapy. Women must be educated regarding the strategy of continuous infusion and have their glucose stabilized over several days. This requires that multiple blood glucose determinations be made for the prevention of periods of hyper- and hypoglycemia. Glucose values may become normalized with minimal amplitude of daily excursions in most patients.

Episodes of hypoglycemia are not uncommon with pump therapy. These are usually secondary to errors in dose selection or failure to adhere to the required diet.[43] The risk of nocturnal hypoglycemia, which is increased in the pregnant state, necessitates that great care be undertaken in selecting patients for CSII. Patients who fail to exhibit normal counterregulatory responses to hypoglycemia should probably be discouraged from using an insulin pump.

The mechanics of the CSII systems are relatively simple. A fine-gauge butterfly needle device is attached by connecting tubing to the pump. This cannula is reimplanted every 2 to 3 days at a different site in the anterior abdominal wall. Short-acting (regular) insulin is stored in the pump syringe. Infusion occurs at a basal rate, which can be fixed or altered for specific time of day by a computer program. For example, the basal rate can be programmed for a lower dose at night. Similarly, prandial boluses can be delivered manually or by computer preset. Half the total daily insulin is usually given as the basal rate and the remainder as premeal boluses infused 15 to 45 minutes before each meal. The largest bolus (30 to 35 percent) is administered with breakfast, followed by 25 percent before dinner and 15 to 20 percent before snacks.

Patients without any pancreatic reserve may have rapid elevations of blood glucose if there is pump failure or intercurrent infection. Since the advent of buffered insulin, insulin aggregation leading to occlusion of the silastic infusion tubing is uncommon. Initial experience with insulin pumps suggested a high risk of ketoacidosis with pump failure or intercurrent infection. Failure of the pump is associated with a steady rise in ketonemia in the nonpregnant patient. In a series of 1,880 patient-months of treatment with CSII in 101 patients, 29 episodes of ketoacidosis were encountered.[44] Fifteen episodes were judged to be secondary to pump failure. Such mechanical problems, including needle dislodgment, are less common today. However, episodes of ketoacidosis often reflect inadequate training of the patient in dealing with pump failure, such as the need for conventional insulin injection in such situations.

Rudolf et al[43] reported a trial of pump therapy in seven class D, F, and R diabetic patients treated from 10 to 29 weeks' gestation until delivery. Mean blood glucose values fell slightly while HbA$_{1c}$ was reduced to the normal range. More significant, the mean amplitude of glycemic excursions fell. There were few mechanical complications of therapy, most notably episodes of hypoglycemia related to dose selection error. Neonatal outcome was excellent, all infants being delivered at term without macrosomia or significant morbidity.

Cohen and colleagues[45] reported five women receiving CSII therapy during the third trimester after having achieved optimal glycemic control with a multiple injection regimen. Pump therapy did not improve glycemic control in these patients, as determined by mean glucose or glycemic excretions. There did appear to be a trend toward decreased periods of significant hyperglycemia. Frequent early-morning hypoglycemia was observed and corrected by decreasing the basal infusion rate during the late-evening and early-morning hours.

The necessity of using continuous infusion pumps to achieve glycemic control has been challenged. Schiffrin and Belmonte[46] studied 20 nonpregnant diabetic patients in a prospective randomized crossover study that compared multiple subcutaneous injections with continuous insulin infusion therapy. Sixteen patients completed the study, which revealed no significant difference in the degree of metabolic control. Mean fasting capillary glucose was lower in seven pump therapy patients, supporting the hypothesis that continuous basal infusion may optimize control at night.

In the largest reported studies of pregnant women, Coustan and colleagues[47] randomized 22 patients to intensive conventional therapy with multiple injections versus pump therapy. There were no differences between the two treatment groups with respect to outpatient mean glucose levels, glycosylated hemoglobin levels, or glycemic excursions.

To summarize, the limitations of pump therapy outlined above as well as the complications of this method have decreased enthusiasm for its use during pregnancy. Also, serious concern exists regarding abrupt initiation of tight glycemic control in nonpregnant patients beginning pump therapy, which may adversely affect established diabetic retinopathy.[48] In our practice over the past 15 years, we have found it necessary to institute pump therapy to achieve good glycemic control in only one patient. It must be appreciated that CSII does not guarantee improved glucoregulation. However, we do recommend that women who have demonstrated good glycemic control using continuous infusion devices before pregnancy be maintained on this therapy throughout gestation.

INSULIN REQUIREMENTS

It is well appreciated that insulin requirements rise during pregnancy, largely because of the increased concentration of circulating contrainsulin hormones. Several studies have attempted to document the change in insulin dosage required to maintain tight metabolic control throughout gestation. Although these reports provide insight into the characteristics of each given population, management must clearly be individualized because algorithms for insulin dosage should be based on self-reported glucose data.

More than a decade ago, Jovanovic and colleagues[49]

reported that constant insulin adjustment was necessary to keep up with the increasing insulin requirements of pregnancy. In a study of 40 IDDM women within 15 percent ideal body weight maintained on a 30-kcal/kg diet, the total insulin dose was raised from 0.7 U/kg/d in the first trimester to 0.8 U/kg/d at week 18, 0.9 U/kg/d at week 26, and 1.0 U/kg/d at week 36. An increasing standard deviation was noted with advancing gestation, as the dose was more uniform at the beginning of gestation than toward the end. In this series, 11 patients were markedly obese at the start of pregnancy; 6 required 1.2 U/kg/d at term; 3 required 2 U/kg/d at term, and 2 required 3 U/kg/d at term.

Langer and co-workers[50] also evaluated insulin requirements in pregestational diabetic subjects. Their investigation had two unique features previously not reported: (1) patients with type I and type II diabetes were analyzed separately and (2) all patients used a memory-based reflectance meter to ensure a means of obtaining verified self-monitored glucose values. A total of 103 patients (63 with type I and 40 with type II diabetes) were enrolled in this study. Both type I and type II patients demonstrated a triphasic insulin pattern, with type II diabetic women requiring significantly higher doses of insulin during each trimester (Fig. 11-3). During the first trimester, no difference was found between type I and type II subjects. During the second trimester, a significant increase in insulin requirement emerged (10 percent for patients with type I diabetes compared with 33 percent for those with type II diabetes). In the third trimester, a 40 percent increase was found for those women with type II diabetes. These authors speculated that increased body mass and heightened insulin resistance in type II patients contributed to this large adjustment in insulin requirement.

Controversy has surrounded the clinical finding of diminished or falling insulin requirements in late pregnancy. Malins[51] reported a 4.5 percent fetal loss rate in 67 women with no increase in insulin requirement in late pregnancy. Actual falls in insulin requirements are less common and have been associated with fetal death if substantial. Before the advent of fetal monitoring, some declines in insulin requirement may have occurred because of fetal death, thus making the observation a result of the demise rather than the cause. McManus and Ryan[52] described 20 of 32 (62 percent) IDDM women with a decline in insulin dose (12 ± 2 percent) after 36 weeks' gestation, which was associated with a longer duration of diabetes but not with age, prepregnancy body mass index, weight gain, or maternal or fetal complications. More recently, Steel

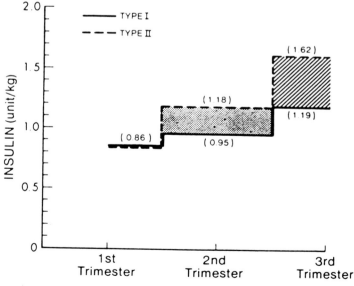

Fig. 11-3. Triphasic pattern of insulin requirements by trimester of pregnancy for both type I and type II diabetes when corrected for weight. (From Langer et al,[50] with permission.)

and colleagues[53] reported much greater decreases (>30 percent) in insulin requirements, often occurring before 36 weeks in 18 of 237 type I patients. In these cases, no abnormal fetal outcomes were observed. As reported by others, Steel found a substantial rise in insulin dose for most type I pregnant women. The dose rose from a mean of 0.83 ± 0.39 U/kg before pregnancy to a peak of 1.63 ± 0.65 U/kg. The mean absolute increase in insulin requirement was 52 U, with a greater incremental increase in the daytime insulin dose than at night. The degree of rise was significantly related to maternal weight gain between 20 and 29 weeks and initial maternal weight and was inversely related to the duration of diabetes. Insulin dose was also unrelated to the degree of control, complications of pregnancy, White class, or perinatal outcome. This study, as well as our own experience, suggests that current algorithms for insulin therapy based on body weight and gestational age are inappropriate, as wide variations in insulin requirements are observed in women with pregestational diabetes. An increase in insulin dosage can generally be anticipated by the second trimester, which can be related in part to weight gain and prepregnancy weight. Large falls in insulin requirement remain unexplained and may not be associated with placental failure.[53]

INSULIN-INDUCED HYPOGLYCEMIA

Hypoglycemia represents the limiting factor in regimens emphasizing intensive insulin therapy for patients with IDDM. Most individuals with IDDM for more than a few years have no β-cell reserve as well as deficient α-cell (glucagon) response to hypoglycemia, thus placing them at increased risk of severe hypoglycemic reactions. Women with long-standing diabetes may also demonstrate deficient epinephrine, cortisol, and growth hormone responses to insulin-induced hypoglycemia. Such individuals commonly suffer an average of one to two symptomatic episodes of hypoglycemia each week. Temporarily disabling hypoglycemia with coma or seizure occurs in as many as 25 percent of IDDM individuals in the course of 1 year and causes 4 percent of deaths due to IDDM.[54] The fear of severe hypoglycemia can be psychologically disabling for some patients and frightening for health care providers who must guide patients seeking improved glycemic control with intensified insulin regimens.

Cryer and Gerich[54] categorized three pathophysiologic conditions that compromise defenses against hyperinsulinemia and are associated with a high frequency of iatrogenic hypoglycemia in individuals with IDDM: (1) hypoglycemia unawareness—the loss of neurogenic (autonomic) warning symptoms of developing hypoglycemia; (2) defective glucose counterregulation attributable to the combined deficiencies of the glucagon and epinephrine secretory responses to falling blood glucose concentrations; and (3) altered glycemic thresholds (lower plasma glucose concentrations required) for symptoms and for activation of glucose counterregulatory systems during intensive therapy that effectively lowers overall plasma glucose concentrations. The above hypoglycemia-associated syndromes share pathophysiologic features, including reduced autonomic response to hypoglycemia, yet are considered a separate entity from diabetic autonomic neuropathy.

Hypoglycemia may occur when excessive insulin is administered or not timed well in relation to meals or exercise. Less common etiologies include diminished endogenous production or reduced clearance of exogenous insulin as occurs in renal insufficiency. A recent review of the Diabetes Control and Complications Trial (DCCT) Research Group indicates that many severe hypoglycemic episodes are not related to the above events.[55] Thus, clinical research efforts have centered on the glucose counterregulatory systems, which are defective when mild or moderate hyperinsulinemia results in clinical hypoglycemia. It has also been hypothesized that recent antecedent hypoglycemia may play a role in the pathogenesis of hypoglycemia-associated autonomic insufficiency. Apparently, recent antecedent hypoglycemia results in substantially lower glucose levels required to produce both symptomatic and autonomic responses to subsequent hypoglycemia in nondiabetic individuals.[56] If confirmed in patients with IDDM, this observation might explain how recurrent severe hypoglycemia can result in a "vicious cycle" as previous hypoglycemic episodes could reduce both hypoglycemia awareness and autonomic responses to the event.[56]

It has also been postulated that human insulin treatment compared with that of animal insulin may produce relative hypoglycemia unawareness. Heine et al,[57] using a hyperinsulinemic-hypoglycemic clamp technique, reported reduced autonomic symptoms and lower plasma norepinephrine levels to hypoglycemia produced by human insulin infusion compared with animal species. Other investigators have failed to confirm these results.[58] One neuroglycopenic symptom, lack of concentration, may be more common during treatment with human insulin.[59] Aside from this observation and with recent metabolic studies demonstrating comparable counterregulatory responses to hypoglycemia induced by various insulin species, it is unlikely that severe hypoglycemia is a major concern when changing pregnant women from animal insulins to human preparations.

The risk of hypoglycemia during pregnancy is likely to be increased as fetoplacental glucose consumption continues in the fasting state and exogenous insulin can limit other substrate availability. The effect of maternal hypoglycemia on early embryonic development has been studied by Sadler and Hunter.[60] Using mouse embryos, these investigators demonstrated that glucose levels approximately 50 percent of normal were teratogenic and lower glucose concentrations were lethal to the developing embryo. The dysmophogenic effects of hypoglycemia in rodent models may be observed with brief episodes of hypoglycemia (1 hour) during intervals coincident with the stages of neurulation. Freinkel[61] hypothesized that this period of sensitivity to hypoglycemia represented early embryonic dependence on glycolysis for metabolic energy. During late neurulation, brief periods of hypoglycemia did not produce a teratogenic effect. Freinkel[61] hypothesized that later in organogenesis, the embryo could use oxidative metabolism and alternative fuel sources.

The human fetus seems to be protected from hypoglycemia. There is no convincing evidence that brief episodes of hypoglycemia are associated with teratogenesis in human pregnancy, although caution is advised, since study of subtle effects on neurobehavioral development would be difficult to execute and interpret. Of significance, however, is that both the Diabetes in Early Pregnancy Study and the California Diabetes in Pregnancy Project have failed to show an association between maternal hypoglycemic events and an increased risk for malformations in the offspring.[62,63] In addition, fetal death has not been associated with significant hypoglycemic reactions.

Our experience and that of others suggest that significant hypoglycemic episodes are more frequent during

pregnancy. Much of this disparity, no doubt, stems from more stringent attempts at glucose regulation after conception. Hypoglycemia unawareness, which is associated with a reduced adrenomedullary epinephrine response to hypoglycemia, is more pronounced during gestation. Pregnant women will frequently report that hypoglycemia "sneaks up" on them faster and without warning when compared with their prepregnancy experience. Diamond and colleagues[64] confirmed that growth hormone response to hypoglycemia is impaired in pregnant women with IDDM. Using a hypoglycemic clamp technique to lower glucose from 5.8 mM (105 mg/dl) to 2.5 mmol (45 mg/dl) over 200 minutes in nine well-controlled patients, these investigators demonstrated a reduction in basal growth hormone levels and stimulated glucagon, cortisol, and epinephrine levels when compared with nondiabetic controls. These data suggest that pregnant iabetic women do manifest a defective counterregulatory response to hypoglycemia, which may be exacerbated by improved glucose control. Increasing insulin requirements and dosage may further impair this response by suppression of glucagon levels.[65]

In contrast to the Diamond study, Nisell and colleagues[66] recently reported that both hormonal and circulatory responses to acute hypoglycemia are not altered in diabetic women during pregnancy. These authors noted similar increases in epinephrine and norepinephrine as well as diminished cortisol and glucagon responses to the same degree in the group of nine diabetic women studied both during the third trimester and postpartum. Placental scintigraphy studies revealed no consistent changes in placental blood flow, which was unrelated to glucose and catecholamine responses. The hormonal findings in this study might be explained in part by relatively high baseline cortisol levels during pregnancy, which could prevent a further increase with hypoglycemia. However, the disparity between catecholamine responses in this study and that of Diamond's study cannot be fully explained. Nisell et al[66] suggest that although the clamp technique allows a more precise definition of the hypoglycemic stimulus than the intravenous insulin tolerance testing used in his study, Diamond's conclusions could be questioned because nondiabetic control subjects were not studied during pregnancy.

Despite the above considerations, clinical efforts to improve glycemia during pregnancy have met with success and relatively little morbidity from insulin-induced hypoglycemia. The practitioner should carefully select those patients for whom some relaxation in glycemic control may be reasonable. With this consideration of safety in mind, patients must also be instructed to test glucose levels frequently, and family members should be educated about the treatment of hypoglycemia, including glucagon injections.

MANAGEMENT DURING LABOR AND DELIVERY

The goal of maintaining euglycemia during pregnancy is also important during labor and delivery. Prolonged hyperglycemia, which produces mean glucose values exceeding 90 mg/dl, significantly increases the frequency of neonatal hypoglycemia.[67] Such morbidity may occur despite the presence of excellent control before the onset of labor. The intrapartum management of the diabetic patient, therefore, requires that careful attention be given to maternal glucose values, the glucose infusion rate, and insulin dosage. In general, glucose determinations are made every 1 to 2 hours with a portable glucose reflectance meter at the bedside. A flow sheet to summarize these data is helpful.

Several approaches have been used to maintain maternal euglycemia during labor and delivery. Most investigators have used a continuous infusion combining both insulin and glucose. Five units of regular insulin are added to 500 ml of a 5 percent dextrose solution. An infusion rate of 100 to 125 ml/h usually results in good glucose control. Insulin may also be infused from a syringe pump and adjusted to maintain normal glucose values.

Jovanovic and Peterson[68] confirmed both the decreased need for insulin and the constant glucose requirement during the first stage of labor in a series of well-controlled patients.[66] Using a glucose-controlled insulin infusion system, the Biostator, they demonstrated that insulin requirements fell to zero during the active first stage of labor while glucose infusion rates were maintained at 2.55 mg/kg/min to achieve blood glucose levels of 70 to 90 mg/dl. Oxytocin infusion did not appear to influence glucose control. Why insulin requirements fall during labor is poorly understood. This fall may reflect decreasing maternal levels of anti-insulin hormones produced by the placenta.

A simplified regimen has been devised by Jovanovic

Table 11-4. Insulin Management During Labor and Delivery

Usual dose of intermediate-acting insulin is given at bedtime

Morning dose of insulin is withheld

Intravenous infusion of normal saline is begun

Once active labor begins or glucose levels fall to <70 mg/dl, the infusion is changed from saline to 5% dextrose and delivered at a rate of 2.5 mg/kg/min

Glucose levels are checked hourly using a portable reflectance meter, allowing for adjustment in the infusion rate

Regular (short-acting) insulin is administered by intravenous infusion if glucose levels are >140 mg/dl

(Adapted from Jovanovic and Peterson,[68] with permission.)

based on these data[68] (Table 11-4). In well-controlled patients, the usual dose of NPH insulin is given at bedtime and the morning insulin dose is withheld. Once active labor begins or glucose levels fall below 68 mg/dl, the infusion is changed from saline to 5 percent dextrose and delivered at a rate of 2.5 mg/kg/min. Glucose values are recorded, and the infusion rate is adjusted accordingly. Regular insulin is administered if glucose values exceed 140 mg/dl. In general, the starting dose is 1 U/h. Insulin is often required during the second stage of labor as catecholamine levels rise.

In patients who undergo elective cesarean section, the procedure is scheduled for the early morning to simplify glucose control and maximize resources for neonatal care (Table 11-5). Patients are instructed to take their usual evening insulin dose on the day before delivery. The patient is given nothing by mouth, and the usual morning insulin dose is withheld. Before epidural anesthesia, patients should receive a "load" of a

Table 11-5. Insulin Management for Elective Cesarean Delivery

Schedule for early morning to simplify glycemic control

Administer usual evening insulin dose on the day before delivery; patient is NPO after midnight

Usual morning insulin dose is withheld and glucose level is assessed at the bedside before surgery and hourly thereafter

Dextrose is administered intravenously if glucose level is <70 mg/dl

Glycemic control is achieved and intravenous infusion of short-acting insulin

Before epidural anesthesia, patients should receive an intravenous load of a non-glucose-containing solution to reduce maternal hypotension non-glucose-containing solution intravenously to reduce maternal hypotension. Epidural anesthesia is preferred because it enables the anesthesiologist to evaluate the mental state of the patient and detect potential hypoglycemia. After surgery, glucose levels are monitored every 2 hours, and an intravenous solution of 5 percent dextrose is administered.

After delivery, insulin requirements are usually significantly reduced. Because of the changing hormonal milieu, multiple subcutaneous injection regimens are the preferred form of therapy. The objective of strict control used in the antepartum period is relaxed. Patients who deliver vaginally and who are able to eat a regular diet are given one-half their prepregnancy dose of NPH insulin on the morning of the first postpartum day. If the prepregnancy dose is unknown, we often prescribe one-third to one-half the end-of-pregnancy dose. Frequently, capillary glucose determinations help guide the insulin dosage. Sliding scale insulin management is discouraged. Insulin should be prescribed based on careful review of previous and current glucose measurement as well as diet. If a patient has been given supplemental regular insulin in addition to the morning NPH dose, the amount of NPH insulin given on the following morning is increased by an amount equal to two-thirds the additional regular insulin. With this method, most patients are stabilized within a few days of delivery.

Patients who undergo a cesarean delivery receive regular insulin during the first 24 to 48 hours postoperatively to maintain glucose values of less than 200 mg/dl. As their diet is advanced, NPH insulin is administered based on the regular insulin requirement of the preceding day. All postpartum patients are encouraged to breast-feed. Insulin requirements may be somewhat lower in lactating women (see Ch. 29).

Most patients can be discharged from the hospital between 2 and 4 days postpartum, depending on the mode of delivery. Patients are encouraged to continue with self-glucose monitoring techniques and to make additional adjustments in their daily insulin needs.

CONCLUSIONS

Glucose control and thus insulin therapy are the cornerstone for success in the pregnancy complicated by IDDM. Frequent assessment of glycemic status with in-

dividual tailoring of insulin dosage is required. Although not relaxing the objective of near-physiologic control, the limitations of insulin replacement must be appreciated, as well as the potential dangers of this important drug.

REFERENCES

1. Gabbe SG: Pregnancy in women with diabetes mellitus: the beginning. Clin Perinatol 20:507, 1993
2. White P: Diabetes in pregnancy. In Joslin EP (ed): The Treatment of Diabetes Mellitus. 4th Ed. Lea & Febiger, Philadelphia, 1928
3. Landon MB, Gabbe SG: Diabetes and pregnancy. Med Clin North Am 72:6, 1988
4. Galloway JA, Chance RE: Insulin agonist therapy: a challenge for the 1990s. Clin Ther 12:460, 1990
5. Schernthaner G: Immunogenecity and allergenic potential of animal and human insulins. Diabetes Care 16:155, 1993
6. Home PD, Massi-Benedetti M, Shepherd GAA et al: A comparison of the activity and disposal of semi-synthetic human insulin and porcine insulin in normal man by the glucose clamp technique. Diabetologia 22:41, 1982
7. Gregory R, Edwards S, Yakman NA: Demonstration of insulin transformation products in insulin vials by high performance liquid chromatography. Diabetes Care 14:42, 1991
8. Binder C, Lawritzen T, Faber O, Pramming S: Insulin pharmacokinetics. Diabetes Care 7:188, 1984
9. Jovanovic L, Mills JL, Peterson CM: Anti-insulin antibody titers do not influence control or insulin requirements in early pregnancy. Diabetes Care 7:68, 1984
10. Heding LG, Larsson Y, Luduigsson J: The immunogenicity of insulin preparation: antibody levels before and after transfer to highly purified porcine insulin. Diabetologia 19:511, 1980
11. American Diabetes Association: Position statement: insulin administration. Diabetes Care, suppl. 2, 16:31, 1994
12. Mylvaganam R, Stowers JM, Steel JM et al: Insulin immunogenicity in pregnancy: maternal and fetal studies. Diabetologia 24:19, 1983
13. Menon RK, Cohen RM, Sperling MA et al: Transplacental passage of insulin in pregnant women with IDDM: its role in fetal macrosomia. N Engl J Med 323:309, 1990
14. Rosenn B, Miodovnik M, Coombs CA, et al: Human versus animal insulin in the management of insulin-dependent diabetes: lack of effect on fetal growth. Obstet Gynecol 78:590, 1991
15. Jovanovic-Peterson L, Kitzmiller JL, Peterson CM: Ran-

domized trial of human versus animal species insulin in the diabetic pregnant women: improved glycemic control, not fewer antibodies to insulin, influences birthweight. Am J Obstet Gynecol 16:1325, 1992

16. Baker RS, Ross JW, Schmidtke JR, Smith WC: Preliminary studies on the immunogenicity and amount of Escherichuman insulina coli polypeptides in biosynthetic human insulin produced by recombinant DNA technology. Lancet 2:1139, 1981

17. Grammer LC, Roberts M, Patterson R: IgE and IgG antibody against human (rDNA) insulin in patients with systemic insulin allergy. J Lab Clin Med 105:108, 1985

18. Schernthaner G, Borkenstein M, Fink M et al: Immunogenicity of human insulin (Novo) or pork monocomponent insulin in HLA-DR-typed insulin dependent diabetic individuals. Diabetes Care, suppl. 1, 6:43, 1983

19. Fineberg SE, Galloway JA, Fineberg NS et al: Immunogenicity of human insulin of recombinant DNA origin. Diabetologia 25:465, 1983

20. Marshall MO, Heding LG, Villumsen J et al: Development of insulin antibodies, metabolic control and B-cell function in newly diagnosed insulin dependent diabetic children treated with monocomponent human insulin or monocomponent porcine insulin. Diabetes Res 9:169, 1988

21. Frohnauer MK, Anderson JH: Lack of consistent definitions of the pharmacokinetics of human insulin, abstracted. Diabetes, suppl. 1, 40:460A, 1991

22. Sestoft L, Volund A, Gammeltoft S: The biological properties of human insulin. J Intern Med 212:21, 1982

23. Pramming S, Lauritzen T, Thorsteinsson B et al: Absorption of soluble and isophane semi-synthetic human and porcine insulin in insulin-dependent diabetic subjects. Acta Endocrinol 105:215, 1984

24. Botterman P, Gyaram H, Wahl K et al: Pharmacokinetics of biosynthetic human insulin and characteristics of its effect. Diabetes Care 4:168, 1981

25. Heinemann L, Chantelan EA, Starke AAR: Pharmacokinetics and pharmacodynamics of subcutaneously administered U40 and U100 formulation of regular human insulin. Diabetic Metab 18:21, 1992

26. Scott R, Smith J: Insulin delivery with meals: plasma insulin profiles after bolus injection of human or porcine, neutral insulin. Diabetic Metab 9:95, 1983

27. Galloway JA, Spradlin CT, Root MA, Fineberg SE: The plasma glucose response of normal fasting subjects to neutral regular and NPH biosynthetic human and purified pork insulins. Diabetes Care 4:183, 1981

28. Owens DR, Jones IR, Birtwell AJ et al: Study of porcine and human isophane (NPH) insulins in normal subjects. Diabetologia 26:261, 1984

29. Massi-Bendetti M, Bueti A, Mannino D et al: Kinetics and metabolic activity of biosynthetic NPH insulin evaluated by the glucose clamp technique. Diabetes Care 7:132, 1984

30. Hilderbrandt P, Birch K, Sestoft L, Volund A: Dose dependent subcutaneous absorption of porcine, bovine, and human NPH insulins. J Intern Med 215:69, 1984

31. Clark AJL, Knight G, Wiles PG et al: Biosynthetic human insulin in the treatment of diabetes: a double-blind crossover trial in established diabetic patients. Lancet 2:354, 1982

32. Home PD, Mann NP, Hotchinson AS et al: A fifteen-month double-blind crossover study of the efficacy and antigenicity of human and pork insulins. Diabetic Med 1:93, 1984

33. Pedersen C, Hoegholm A: A comparison of semisynthetic human NPH insulin and porcine NPH insulin in the treatment of insulin dependent diabetes mellitus. Diabetic Med 4:304, 1987

34. Francis AJ, Home PD, Hanning I et al: Intermediate acting insulin given at bedtime: effect on blood glucose concentrations before and after breakfast. BMJ 286:173, 1983

35. Landon MB, Gabbe SG: Glucose monitoring and insulin administration in the pregnant diabetic patient. Clin Obstet Gynecol 28:496, 1985

36. Seigler DE, Olssen GM, Agramonte RF et al: Pharmacokinetics of long acting (Ultralente) insulin preparations. Diab Nutr Metab 4:267, 1991

37. Holman RR, Steemson J, Darling P et al: Human Ultralente insulin. BMJ 288:665, 1984

38. Koivisto VA, Felig P: Alterations in insulin absorption in diabetic patients. N Engl J Med 92:59, 1989

39. Galloway JA, Spradlin CT, Howey DC, Dupre J: Intrasubject differences in pharmacokinetic and pharmacodynamic responses: the immutable problem of present-day treatment? p. 23. In Serrano-Rios M, Leferbre PJ (eds): Diabetes 1985: Proceedings of the 12th Congress of the International Diabetes Federation, Madrid, September 1985. International Congress Series no. 700. Excerpta Medico, Amsterdam, 1986

40. Zinman B, Vranic M, Albisser AM et al: The role of insulin in the metabolic response to exercise in diabetic man. Diabetes, suppl. 1, 28:76, 1979

41. Santiago JV, Clarke WL, Arios F: Studies with a pancreatic beta cell simulator in the third trimester of pregnancies complicated by diabetes. Am J Obstet Gynecol 132:455, 1978

42. Natrass M, Alberti KGMM, Dennis JK et al: A glucose controlled insulin infusion system for diabetic women during labor. BMJ 2:599, 1978

43. Rudolf MCJ, Coustan DR, Sherwin RS et al: Efficacy of the insulin pump in the home treatment of pregnant diabetics. Diabetes 30:891, 1981

44. Peden NR, Braaten JT, McKendry JBR: Diabetic ketoacidosis during long term treatment with continuous subcutaneous insulin infusion. Diabetes Care 7:1, 1984

45. Cohen AW, Liston RM, Mennuti MT, Gabbe SG: Glycemic control in pregnant diabetic women using a continuous subcutaneous insulin infusion pump. J Reprod Med 27: 651, 1982

46. Schiffrin A, Belmonte MM: Comparison between continuous subcutaneous insulin infusion and multiple injections of insulin. Diabetes 32:255, 1982

47. Coustan DR, Reece EA, Sherwin RS et al: A randomized clinical trial of the insulin pump vs. intensive conventional therapy in diabetic pregnancies. JAMA 255:631, 1986

48. Brinchmann-Hansen O, Dahl-Jorgensen K, Hanssen KF, Sandvik L: The response of diabetic retinopathy to 41 months of multiple insulin injection, insulin pumps, and conventional insulin therapy. Arch Ophthalmol 106: 1242, 1988

49. Jovanovic L, Druzin M, Peterson CM: Effect of euglycemia on the outcome of pregnancy in insulin-dependent diabetic women as compared with normal control subjects. Am J Med 7:921, 1981

50. Langer O, Anyaegbunam A, Brustman L et al: Pregestational diabetes: insulin requirements throughout pregnancy. Am J Obstet Gynecol 159:616, 1988

51. Malins J: Clinical Diabetes Mellitus. Eyre & Spottiswoode, London, 1968

52. McManus R, Ryan EA: Insulin requirements in insulin-dependent and insulin requiring gestational diabetic women during the final month of pregnancy. Diabetes Care 15:1323, 1992

53. Steel JM, Johnstone FD, Hume R, Mao JH: Insulin requirements during pregnancy in women with type I diabetes. Obstet Gynecol 83:253, 1994

54. Cryer PE, Gerich JE: Hypoglycemia in insulin dependent diabetes mellitus: insulin excess and defective glucose counterregulation. p. 526. In Rufkin H, Porte D (eds): Ellenberg and Rifkin's Diabetes Mellitus: Theory and Practice. 4th Ed. Elsevier, New York, 1990

55. Diabetes Control and Complications Trial Research Group: Epidemiology of severe hypoglycemia in the Diabetes Control and Complications Trial. Am J Med 90:450, 1991

56. Cryer PE; Iatrogenic hypoglycemia as a cause of hypoglycemia-associated autonomic failure in IDDM: a vicious cycle. Diabetes 41:255, 1992

57. Heine RJ, VanderHyden EAP, VanderVeen EA: Responses to human and porcine insulin in healthy subjects. Lancet 2:946, 1989

58. Kern W, Lieb K, Kerner W et al: Differential effects of human and pork insulin induced hypoglycemia on neuronal function in humans. Diabetes 39:1091, 1990

59. Berger W, Keller U, Honegger B, Jaeggi G: Warning symptoms of hypoglycemia during treatment with human and porcine insulin in diabetes mellitus. Lancet 1:1041, 1989

60. Sadler TW, Hunter ES III: Hypoglycemia: how little is too much for the embryo? Am J Obstet Gynecol 157:190, 1993

61. Freinkel N: Diabetic embryopathy and fuel-mediated organ teratogenesis: lessons from animal models. Horm Metab Res 20:463, 1988

62. Mills JL, Knopp RH, Simpson JP et al: Lack of relations of increased malformation rates in infants of diabetic mothers to glycemic control during organogenesis. N Engl J Med 318:671, 1988

63. Kitzmiller JL, Gavin LA, Gin GD et al: Preconception management of diabetes continued through early pregnancy prevents the excess frequency of major congenital anomalies in infants of diabetic mothers. JAMA 265:731, 1991

64. Diamond MP, Reece EA, Caprio S et al: Impairment of counterregulatory hormone responses to hypoglycemia in pregnant women with insulin-dependent diabetes mellitus. Am J Obstet Gynecol 166:70, 1992

65. Liu D, Adamson U, Lins P et al: Inhibitory effect of circulating insulin of glucagon secretion during hypoglycemia in type I diabetic patients. Diabetes Care 15:59, 1992

66. Nisel H, Persson B, Hanson V et al: Hormonal, metabolic, and circulatory response to insulin-induced hypoglycemia in pregnant and nonpregnant women with insulin-dependent diabetes. Am J Perinatol 11:231, 1994

67. Soler NG, Soler SM, Malino JM: Neonatal morbidity among infants of diabetic mothers. Diabetes Care 1:340, 1978

68. Jovanovic L, Peterson CM: Insulin and glucose requirements during the first stage of labor in insulin dependent diabetic women. Am J Med 75:607, 1983

69. Frank BH, Chance RE: Two routes for producing human insulin utilizing recombinant DNA technology. Munch Med Wochenschr, suppl. 1, 125:S14, 1983

70. Jovanovic L, Peterson CM, Fuhrmann K: Diabetes and Pregnancy: Teratology, Toxicity and Treatment. p. 305. Praeger, New York, 1986.

12
Dietary Management

BARBARA LUKE
MAUREEN A. MURTAUGH

HISTORICAL PERSPECTIVE

Before the discovery of insulin by Banting and Best in 1921, the association between diabetes mellitus and pregnancy was almost nonexistent: women with diabetes had irregular ovulatory cycles and rarely conceived. Among the few who did become pregnant, the perinatal mortality rate for their infants was greater than 42 percent.[1] Before insulin therapy, diabetic diets included regimens with as much as 85 to 90 percent of calories from fat, alternating with days restricted to only vegetables, fasting, or severe caloric restriction. The first physician of the preinsulin era who focused specifically on the diets of pregnant women with diabetes was Joslin.[2] He recommended a low-carbohydrate and moderate fat and protein diet; fasting was advised when excessive glycosuria was present.

The use of starvation therapy during the early years of insulin availability resulted in general malnutrition, delayed puberty, anovulation, and reduced fertility in many women with diabetes.[3] When insulin therapy was combined with a more liberal diet, fertility rose dramatically. The publication of exchange lists by the American Diabetes Association (ADA) in 1950 simplified the calculation and planning of diabetic diets, although the prevailing philosophy for pregnant women with diabetes limited sodium intake and restricted weight gain to 12 lb or less.[4,5]

As a result of improved metabolic and dietary management of pregnant women with diabetes during recent years, perinatal mortality rates are now comparable with those of the nondiabetic general population.[6] During recent years, diet therapy for diabetes has grown to include such areas as glycemic responses of various foods, soluble versus insoluble fibers, the role of monounsaturated fats, and the use of artificial sweeteners. This chapter discusses the nutritional requirements during pregnancy and the special considerations when pregnancy is complicated by diabetes.

NUTRITIONAL NEEDS DURING PREGNANCY
Metabolic Alterations of Pregnancy and Diabetes

Pregnancy itself results in alterations in metabolism, including reductions in fasting blood glucose and plasma insulin, and elevations in postprandial glucose, free fatty acids (FFAs), plasma ketones, insulin resistance, and plasma cholesterol and triglycerides. Insulin requirements during pregnancy increase two- to three-fold as a result of the rise in estrogen, progesterone, human placental lactogen, and possibly placental insulinase. Diabetes further potentiates the metabolic alterations of pregnancy. There is a relative deficiency of insulin, due to tissue resistance, decreased production, and increased degradation. Elevations in plasma glucose, FFAs, triglycerides, and branched chain amino acids result from this insulin deficiency (see Ch. 5 for more detail).

Pregestational versus Gestational Diabetes

During pregnancy, the nutritional management of pregestational and gestational diabetes differs, depending only on whether insulin is used. With insulin therapy, meal timing and the inclusion of snacks must be matched to the insulin schedule. The nutritional re-

191

quirements for women with diabetes during pregnancy are the same regardless of whether they are receiving insulin therapy.

Recommended Dietary Allowances

In the United States, the recommended dietary allowances (RDAs) of the Food and Nutrition Board of the National Academy of Sciences provide the foundation for dietary recommendations, including during pregnancy.[7] The most current edition of the RDAs includes recommendations for 19 nutrients, as well as estimated minimum requirements (EMRs) of sodium, chloride, and potassium, and the estimated safe and adequate daily dietary intakes (ESADDIs) of biotin, pantothenic acid, copper, manganese, fluoride, chromium, and molybdenum. A summary of the 1989 RDAs, ESADDIs, and EMRs for adult women before and during pregnancy is given in Table 12-1. Only the requirements for iron, folic acid, and vitamin D double during pregnancy. The requirements for calcium, phosphorus, thiamin, and vitamin B_6 increase by 33 to 50 percent; protein, zinc, and riboflavin increase by 20 to 25 percent; and vitamins A, B_{12}, C, and calories, selenium, magnesium, iodine, and niacin increase by 18 percent or less.

According to national survey data, most women of childbearing age consume diets that meet or exceed the RDAs for most nutrients.[8] Nutrients most likely to be present at 80 percent or less of the RDA in women's diets include vitamin B_6, calcium, magnesium, iron, zinc, and copper.[8] Food sources rich in these nutrients (meats, poultry, fish, and dairy products) are all recommended in additional amounts during pregnancy.

The diet prescribed for pregestational or gestational diabetes has changed dramatically in recent decades and is much more like the diet of the general, nondiabetic population. The challenge is to meet the nutritional requirements of pregnancy while maintaining good metabolic control of the diabetes. The current dietary prescription for patients with diabetes includes 10 to 20 percent of calories as protein and the remainder of calories divided between carbohydrate and fat according to the individual's glucose, lipid, and weight profile.[9]

Caloric Requirement

As recommended in the National Academy of Sciences' 1990 report on nutrition during pregnancy,[10] the caloric intake during pregnancy should be based on the

Table 12-1. Summary of the 1989 RDAs, ESADDIs, and EMRs for Adult Women Aged 25–50 Years, Nonpregnant and Pregnant

Nutrient	Nonpregnant Levels	Pregnant Levels
RDAs		
Folic acid	180 µg	400 µg
Vitamin D	5 µg	10 µg
Iron	15 mg	30 mg
Calcium	800 mg	1,200 mg
Phosphorus	800 mg	1,200 mg
Vitamin B_6	1.6 mg	2.2 mg
Thiamin	1.1 mg	1.5 mg
Zinc	12 mg	15 mg
Vitamin E	8 mg	10 mg
Riboflavin	1.3 mg	1.6 mg
Protein	50 mg	60 mg
Selenium	55 µg	65 µg·
Iodine	150 µg	175 µg
Vitamin C	60 mg	70 mg
Energy	2,200 kcal	2,500 kcal
Magnesium	280 mg	320 mg
Niacin	15 mg	17 mg
Vitamin B_{12}	2.0 µg	2.2 µg
Vitamin A	800 µg RE[a]	800 µg RE
Vitamin K	65 µg	65 µg
ESADDIs		
Biotin	30–100 µg	
Pantothenic acid	4–7 mg	
Copper	1.5–3.0 mg	
Manganese	2.0–5.0 mg	
Fluoride	1.5–4.0 mg	
Chromium	50–200 µg	
Molybdenum	75–250 µg	
EMRs		
Sodium	500 mg	
Chloride	750 mg	
Potassium	2,000 mg	

Abbreviations: RDAs, recommended dietary allowances; ESADDIs, estimated safe and adequate daily dietary intakes; EMR, estimated minimum requirements; RE, retinal equivalent; —, no additional recommendations during pregnancy.

[a] 1 RE = 1 µ retinol or 6 µg B-carotene.

pregnant woman's pregravid weight and appropriate rate of weight gain to achieve the optimal total gestational weight gain. For the normal weight woman, the caloric requirement during pregnancy is calculated as 36 kcal/kg/d (2,200 kcal/d) for the first trimester, increasing to 40 kcal/kg/d (2,500 kcal/d) during the second and third trimesters.[7] Jovanovic-Peterson and Peterson[11] recommend 30 kcal/kg/d for normal weight women (80 to 120 percent of ideal body weight), 40 kcal/kg/d for underweight women (<80 percent ideal body weight), and 24 kcal/kg/d for overweight women (>120 percent ideal body weight), based on the concept of sustaining women above the ketonuric threshold while preventing postprandial hyperglycemia. These daily caloric allowances translate into weight gains of about 25 to 35 lb, as 3.5 lb during the first trimester and about 1 lb/wk during the second and third trimesters for normal weight women; 28 to 40 lb for underweight women, as 5 lb during the first trimester and slightly more than 1 lb/wk during the second and third trimesters; and 15 to 25 lb for overweight women, as 2 lb during the first trimester and about 0.67 lb/wk during the second and third trimesters.[10]

The caloric requirement and subsequent weight gain in overweight women with and without diabetes during pregnancy is controversial. Although there is concern regarding the potential adverse fetal effect of maternal ketonuria with insufficient caloric intake, studies of overweight pregnant women with diabetes have shown improved pregnancy outcomes with moderate caloric restriction (25 kcal/kg/d or 1,800 to 2,000 kcal/d).[12,13] Severe maternal ketosis, which would affect maternal acid-base balance, should be avoided because it would adversely affect both the mother and her fetus. With severe caloric restriction (<1,200 kcal/d), ketonuria may occur, and prolonged in utero exposure may be associated with neurodevelopmental problems.[14]

Carbohydrates

Types and Percentage of Calories

The recommended carbohydrate content of the diabetic diet has risen steadily from 20 percent in 1921 to 55 to 60 percent in 1986. Higher carbohydrate recommendations have been used by various investigators, including 60, 65, and 85 percent, resulting in improved glycemic control and lowered exogenous insulin requirements.[15–19] The most current ADA guidelines suggest individualization of the percentage of calories from carbohydrate,[9] but levels of 40 to 50 percent may be more appropriate during pregnancy to maintain euglycemia.[20] A euglycemic diet, designed to blunt postprandial hyperglycemia, has been shown to be effective. The postpradial blood glucose level is influenced by the carbohydrate content of the meal.[21] In pregnancies complicated by diabetes, the postprandial blood glucose level is a major factor in the development of neonatal macrosomia.[22] Women who are

insulin resistant may need to reduce the carbohydrate content of their diets to 40 percent of calories.

Traditionally, diet therapy for diabetes has been based on the concept that there are two main classes of carbohydrates: *simple* or *refined* (glucose, sucrose, and fructose), which are rapidly absorbed and cause a relatively large rise in blood glucose, and *complex* or *starches* (such as rice, potatoes, and legumes), which are digested and absorbed more slowly and result in a smaller rise in blood glucose. Complex carbohydrates with fiber, such as whole-grain breads and cereals, brown rice, and fresh fruits and vegetables, should be substituted for simple or refined carbohydrates whenever possible. Sucrose may be used in modest amounts, depending on the degree of metabolic control. If used, it should be included in meals with other foods and preferably additional fiber.

Glycemic Index

Individuals with diabetes have traditionally been counseled to avoid simple sugars in the belief that these specific carbohydrates would result in hyperglycemia and poor metabolic control of the disease. Recent studies, however, have shown that the glycemic response of a specific carbohydrate food, whether simple or complex, is influenced by three factors: (1) the amount of processing and preparation (cooked or uncooked); (2) the amount and type of dietary fiber also in the food and other foods ingested at the same meal; and (3) the nature of the carbohydrate itself, including ripeness and digestability of the starch component. For example, studies have shown that glucose, potatoes, and honey produce similar postprandial glucose responses, whereas rice, beans, and fructose yield a similar but lower glycemic response.[23,24] Different glycemic responses have been observed even when a single food is prepared in different ways: whole rice results in a flatter glycemic response curve than does the ingestion of rice flour, and wheat in pasta produces a lower blood glucose than does wheat in bread.[25,26] Jenkins and co-workers[23] suggested the use of a glycemic index to characterize foods, based on the blood glucose response to a food in comparison with the response to an equivalent amount of glucose (Table 12-2). Using this standard of evaluation, legumes, peas, and soya beans produce the lowest glycemic response, whereas potatoes and carrots elicit the highest. Also,

Table 12-2. Glycemic Index of Selected Foods[a]

100%	40–49%
Glucose	Porridge oats
80–99%	Sweet potato
Cornflakes	Oranges
Carrots	Sponge cake
Potatoes (instant)	Peach
Maltose	Pear
Honey	**30–39%**
70–79%	Butter beans
Bread (whole grain)	Blackeye peas
Rice (white)	Chick peas
New Potatoes	Apples (Golden Delicious)
	Ice cream
60–69%	Milk (skim or whole)
Bread (white)	Yogurt
Brown rice	Tomato soup
Shredded wheat	**20–29%**
Bananas	Kidney beans
Raisins	Lentils
50–59%	Fructose
Buckwheat	**10–19%**
Spaghetti	Soya beans
Sweet corn	Peanuts
All-Bran cereal	
Frozen peas	
Yams	
Sucrose	
Potato chips	

[a] The glycemic index is the area under the blood glucose response curve for each food, expressed as the area, after taking the same amount of carbohydrate as glucose.

the incorporation of simple sugars into processed foods[27] or meals[28] does not aggravate postprandial hyperglycemia. To date, the glycemic index and the effect of incorporating simple sugars into the diet has been evaluated only in nonpregnant individuals with diabetes; their use in pregnancies complicated by diabetes remains to be determined.

Artificial Sweeteners

The use of sugar substitutes or artifical sweeteners is neither needed nor necessary for individuals with diabetes. They may be helpful, though, in complying with the recommendation to avoid simple sugars. Currently, three sugar substitutes or artifical sweeteners are on the market: saccharin, aspartame, and acesulfame-K. These last two sweeteners were approved in the 1980s, and three other artifical sweeteners (Sucralose, Alitame, and Cyclamate) are currently pending approval by the Food and Drug Administration (FDA). Saccharin, a petroleum derivative, is not metabolized by the body and is excreted unchanged by the kidneys. Stable in heat and in solution, saccharin has a relative sweetness 300 times that of sucrose. In 1977, the FDA proposed a ban on saccharin because it had been shown to be a weak carcinogen in animals. Because of public opposition to the ban, Congress passed the Saccharin Study and Labeling Act, which permitted continued use of the sweeteners pending further studies. Presently, the saccharin moratorium has been extended six times, with the lastest extention in 1992 due to expire in May of 1997. The consumption of saccharin has dropped dramatically since the introduction of aspartame in 1981. Saccharin can cross the placenta, although there is no evidence that it is harmful to the fetus.

Aspartame (NutraSweet), is a dipeptide of L-aspartic acid and L-phenylalanine methyl ester, which is metabolized in the intestine to aspartate, phenylalanine, and methanol. Aspartame was approved by the FDA as a tabletop sweetener and for several dry product applications in 1981 and for carbonated beverages in 1983. Aspartame is 180 to 200 times sweeter than sugar, and its use is estimated to be equal to 25 percent of the total sugar intake in the United States. The primary limitation of this sweetener is its susceptability to hydrolysis and loss of sweetness at high temperatures and alkaline or neutral pH values. An encapsulated form of aspartame may soon permit the use of this sweetener in baked products, although FDA approval is still pending. The use of aspartame during pregnancy has been investigated. Aspartic acid does not readily cross the placenta, and methanol levels are only minimally elevated. Phenylalanine, the third breakdown product of aspartame, does cross the placenta, and fetal levels can be 1.3 times higher than maternal levels.[29] Maternal phenylalanine levels have been found to be consistently below toxic levels, even at twice the FDA acceptable daily intake of this sweetener.[29,30]

Acesulfame-K, a potassium salt of a cyclic sulfonamide, is 200 times sweeter than sugar. It is marketed under the brand names of Sunette, Sweet One, and Swiss Sweet. It has a synergistic sweetening effect with other sweeteners and an excellent shelf life and is heatstable. Like saccharin, it is not metabolized by the body and is excreted unchanged by the kidneys. In high concentrations, acesulfame-K has a bitter aftertaste. Extensive testing has not demonstrated the use of acesulfame-K to be harmful during pregnancy.

Fiber

Dietary fiber is defined as all components of food that are resistant to hydrolysis by digestion. Dietary fiber is found exclusively in plant foods, including cereal grains, legumes, and fruits and vegetables. Dietary fiber is of two types: water-soluble or water-insoluble. Water-soluble fiber, such as pectins, gums, and polysaccharides, influence glucose and insulin levels by delaying the intestinal absorption of nutrients, resulting in a more gradual rise in blood glucose. Foods high in water-soluble fibers include fruits (especially citrus and apples), oats, barley, and legumes. Water-insoluble fiber, such as cellulose, lignin, and most hemicelluloses, have a greater effect on increasing gastrointestinal transit times and fecal bulk and less effect on plasma glucose and insulin levels. Foods high in water-insoluble fiber include wheat flour, cereals, and bran.

Although dietary fiber was effectively used to control hyperglycemia with the inclusion of oatmeal in the diabetic diet by von Noorden in 1903,[31] not until 1976 were the therapeutic effects of dietary fiber on postprandial glycemic and serum insulin responses in people with diabetes clinically demonstrated.[32,33] Studies of nonpregnant patients with diabetes show beneficial effects of high-carbohydrate, high-fiber, low-fat diets, including decreased postprandial hyperglycemia, mean plasma glucose, glycosuria, and insulin requirement.[34–37] Recent studies in pregnancy using high-carbohydrate, high-fiber diets are not in total agreement. Ney et al[18] reported that such diets result in lower insulin requirements and better glycemic control of diabetes during pregnancy, whereas Reece et al[38,39] did not find a significant difference between glycemic control and insulin requirements when these diets were used in pregnant patients with diabetes.

Protein

The recommended dietary allowance for protein is 60 g/d, or about 1 g/kg body weight.[7] The optimal percentage of calories from protein has not been determined, although most diets range from 12 to 20 percent. This allowance must provide for both the maternal physiologic adjustments and the growth and development of the fetus and placenta. The RDA for protein is generous because of uncertainties regarding the efficiency of protein storage and use during pregnancy, as well as potential adverse effects from an inadequate intake.

Because most amino acids are gluconeogenic, it has traditionally been believed that high-protein diets for individuals with diabetes help stabilize glucose levels by providing a substrate for glucose production when needed. Because of the interrelationship between glucose, protein, and fatty acid metabolism, dietary protein in excess of needs will result in a compensatory increase in blood levels of glucose and fatty acids.

Fat

To achieve normoglycemia, dietary fat can be liberalized up to 40 percent of calories.[20] Saturated fat, found mainly in animal fats, meats, hydrogenated shortenings, palm oil, coconut oil, cocoa butter, whole milk dairy products, and commercial baked goods, should be limited to one-third of fat calories or less. Monounsaturated fat, found mainly in canola oil, olive oil, and peanut oil, should account for one-third or more of calories from fat. The remaining calories from fat should come from polyunsaturated fats, as found in vegetable oils and fish oils.

MEAL PLANNING APPROACHES
General Considerations

Although the nutritional needs of women with gestational diabetes and pregestational diabetes are similar, some differences do exist in approaches to meal planning. In all cases, however, food, and particularly carbohydrate, must be balanced with insulin (either exogenous or endogenous production) to achieve appropriate glycemia. Individual adjustments in meal planning according to a patient's life-style, exercise, and cultural habits or preferences are the cornerstone of successful nutrition counseling for diabetes.

Recommended distribution of calories among meals (Table 12-3) is similar between gestational and pregestational diabetes. However, controversy does exist over the number of snacks for women with gestational diabetes.[40] Some recommend three meals with only a bedtime snack for obese women with gestational diabetes.[41,42] Others have advised smaller meals with appropriate between-meal snacks.

Restriction of calories at breakfast to 10 to 15 percent

Table 12-3. Calorie and Carbohydrate Distribution to Maintain Normoglycemia

Meal	Calories (%)
Breakfast	10–15
Snack	5–10
Lunch	20–30
Snack	5–10
Dinner	20–30
Snack	5–10

(Adapted from American Diabetes Association,[40] with permission.)

of total is promoted by some to maintain acceptable glycemic profiles despite morning insulin resistance, particularly in gestational diabetes.[40] Others[43] allow breakfast to consist of 20 to 25 percent of total daily calories. Avoiding fruit, fruit juices, and highly refined and processed cereals at breakfast is often necessary to maintain acceptable glycemia.[40] Addition of a mid-morning snack including both protein and carbohydrate is sometimes useful to prevent excessive hunger at lunch, particularly for those with a breakfast planned as 10 percent of total calories.

The composition of calories within a meal may also be important for maintaining postprandial glycemic control in gestational diabetes. Peterson and Jovanovic-Peterson[21] demonstrated that restricting carbohydrate content within a meal to 33, 45, and 40 percent for breakfast, lunch, and dinner, respectively, was needed to maintain glycemic control. Including sufficient carbohydrate in snacks enables total carbohydrate to reach 40 to 50 percent of total calories. No studies are available to address the specific types of carbohydrates or fats with regard to glycemia or pregnancy outcome. Therefore, the general guidelines for diabetes such as including high-fiber choices when possible and limiting saturated fats to 10 percent of calories should be followed.[44]

For lean women with gestational diabetes (within 10 percent of ideal body weight before pregnancy), the approach is more similar to the approach for women with pregestational diabetes. Three meals and three snacks are considered optimal (ADA). Frequent meals and snacks are appropriate for both early pregnancy nausea and vomiting and third-trimester abdominal crowding, which can lead to early satiety. Snacks are used to reduce the risks of rapid decreases of blood glucose due to insulin action.

Exchange Lists

The exchange list is the most commonly used meal planning strategy.[4] This approach is useful for developing consistency and promoting appropriate balance of carbohydrates and calories throughout the day. Meal portions, appropriate low-fat choices, and high-fiber choices are specified in the educational materials. However, some patients find that using the exchange lists for meal planning is too restrictive, particularly when eating out or on special occasions.

Carbohydrate Counting and Total Available Glucose

Other approaches such as carbohydrate counting and total available glucose (TAG) are becoming more common[45,46] (Table 12-4). These methods match insulin with the amount of carbohydrate or available glucose,[47] respectively, in the diet and are compatible with achieving the tight metabolic control desired during pregnancy. These approaches provide many patients with an increased sense of flexibility. Carbohydrate counting and TAG approaches are observed to

Table 12-4. Meal Planning Approaches

	Emphasis on Glucose Control	Easy to Learn	Easy to Follow
Exchange lists	Moderate	No	No
Healthy food choices (appropriate for GDM or low education level)	Low	Yes	Yes
Carbohydrate counting	Yes	Yes	Moderately
TAG (suitable for IDDM)	Yes	No	No
Point system	Moderate	Moderately	Moderately
Month of meals (suitable for GDM with adjustment for appropriate calories)	Moderate	Yes	Yes

Abbreviations: GDM, gestational diabetes mellitus; TAG, total available glucose; IDDM, insulin-dependent diabetes mellitus.
(Adapted from Pastors,[52] with permission.)

result in fat intakes above the recommended levels.[46,47] Appropriate education regarding fat with carbohydrate counting or TAG can result in appropriate nutrient intakes.[47]

The choice of meal planning strategy depends on the patient's type of diabetes, educational level, lifestyle habits, motivation, and economic restraints. Many approaches are used successfully. Therefore, the important factor is application of meal planning strategies to fit an individual. Pregnant patients are often more motivated than others. Taking advantage of teachable moments is important in achieving optimal coordination of diet, insulin, and exercise regimes and ultimately positive pregnancy and other health outcomes.

DIETARY BEHAVIOR

General Considerations

Persons with insulin-dependent diabetes mellitus (IDDM) often find following their diet the most difficult component of their diabetes treatment.[48,49] Several specific dietary behaviors are associated with the ability to achieve lower hemoglobin A_{1c} (HbA_{1c}) levels in the Diabetes Control and Complications Trial.[50] Adhering to the prescribed meal plan and making adjustments in food or insulin in response to elevated blood sugars helped to reduce HbA_{1c}. In addition, those who consistently ate their bedtime snack and followed specific guidelines to treat hypoglycemia were able to achieve slightly lower HbA_{1c} levels than those who ate extra snacks (who had higher levels of HbA_{1c}).

The approaches to individualized meal planning discussed above are important to the patients' ability to adhere. In addition, all patients, but particularly patients with gestational diabetes who require insulin and women with pregestational diabetes, require continuing education to address sick day management, holidays, baby showers, and dining out. Patients using almost any meal planning strategy can be taught to adjust the insulin according to carbohydrate intake (Table 12-5). Using these methods, blood sugar levels are maintained proactively rather than responsively, and patients can enjoy special meals while maintaining appropriate postprandial glycemia. We find that helping patients manage special occasions not only results in adequate glycemia but in a stronger patient–health care team alliance.

Table 12-5. Adjusting Insulin According to Carbohydrate Intake

Weight	Insulin/ Carbohydrate	Adjustments for Diet	
		Blood Glucose	Insulin
100–109 lb	1 U:16 g CHO*	<70 mg/dl	X–2 U
109 + X lb	1 U:16 − (X/ 10) g CHO	70–100 mg/dl	X U
		100–140 mg/dl	X + 2 U
		>140 mg/dl	X + 4 U

X, 1.5 U regular insulin for every 10 g carbohydrate at breakfast or 1 U regular insulin for every 10 g carbohydrate at lunch or dinner; CHO, carbohydrate.
(Data from American Diabetes Association[40] and Choppin and Jovanovic-Peterson.[43])

Treatment of Hypoglycemia

Overtreatment of hypoglycemia causes rebound hyperglycemia and may contribute to poor glycemic control. Patients who eat until they feel better have higher levels of HbA_{1c} than those who eat a specific amount and then wait 15 minutes before eating more.[50] Glucose tablets or gels work more quickly than milk or orange juice and result in a more similar and consistent glycemic response without rebound hyperglycemia.[51] Patients should be encouraged to use glucose tablets or another specific source of 15 g carbohydrate such as 1 cup low-fat milk. Patients learn how much their blood sugar will rise with their specific treatment and become less likely to overtreat.

Food diaries or records periodically kept by patients are useful in identifying food choices and behaviors that affect blood glucose. Together, patients and dietitians can develop strategies to prevent hyper- and hypoglycemia by discussing more appropriate food choices, food portions, or mealtimes. More important, patients are involved in the process of determining better ways of managing particular dietary situations. Food records draw both the dietitians and the patients' attention to the usual patterns and life-styles and their effects on blood glucose control.

LIFE-STYLE CONSIDERATIONS

Although most of our patients' life-styles are amenable to the three-meal-and-three-snack pattern, some are not. Women who work nights and sleep until early afternoon are challenging. Careful coordination of in-

Table 12-6. Food Adjustments for Exercise

Blood Glucose Level	Moderate (30–60 min)
100–160 mg/dl	Increase intake by 15 g carbohydrate
160–250 mg/dl	Do not increase food intake
>250 mg/dl (with positive urine ketones)	Do not exercise until glucose control improves

(Adapted from Pastors,[52] with permission)

sulin peaks and mealtimes allows patients to continue their present life-style while achieving acceptable glycemia. Women whose work does not allow consistent mealtimes may be adequately managed using regular insulin when meals are eaten. Women who use continuous subcutaneous insulin pumps can match their insulin to their food intake and have tremendous flexibility with mealtimes. Extensive individualization and continuing education coordinated among the dietitian, nurse, and perinatologist are the keys to successful management of patients with special life-style considerations.

Women may be encouraged to continue sensible exercise programs with the perinatologist's approval. The optimal time for exercise is 60 to 90 minutes after meals for both patients having either gestational or pregestational diabetes.[40] Regularly scheduled exercise can be planned as part of the overall treatment and may not require alterations, but additional or occasional exercise may require additional food intake[52] (Table 12-6) (see Ch. 13).

CONCLUSIONS

Dietary management must be individualized. Cultural, life-style, economic, and educational factors influence the approach to education and the composition of the diet. Resources for customizing the diabetic diet are given in Table 12-7. Methods range from emphasizing general guidelines for good nutrition[41] to structured meal planning strategies.[46,47] Regardless of approach, the common goals for women with gestational and pregestational diabetes are to meet the maternal and fetal nutritional needs while optimizing health and glycemia. Educating or empowering patients to manage situations can result in good glycemic control.

Table 12-7. Dietary Management Resources

Exchange lists for meal planning
Healthy food choices
Month of Meals and *Month of Meals 2*
   American Diabetes Association, Inc.
   Diabetes Information Center
   1600 Duke Street
   Alexandria, VA 22314
   800/ADA-DISC

Franz MF: Exchanges for All Occasions. Chronimed Publishing, Minnetonka, MN 1993

Total available glucose (TAG) approach
   General Clinical Research Center
   Medical University of South Carolina
   171 Ashley Avenue
   Charleston, SC 29401

Point system approach
   Diet Teach Programs, Inc.
   P.O. Box 1832
   Sun City, AZ 85372

Carbohydrate counting approach
   The Complete Calorie and Carbohydrate Counter for Dining Out. Simon and Schuster, New York, 1987
   Kraus B: Calories and Carbohydrates. 10th Ed. New American Library, New York, 1990
   Netzer C: Complete Book of Food Counts. Bantam Doubleday Dell, New York, 1988

REFERENCES

1. Williams JW: The clinical significance of glycosuria in pregnant women. Am J Med Sci 137:1, 1909
2. Joslin EP: The Treatment of Diabetes Mellitus with Observations upon the Disease Based upon One Thousand Cases. 1st ed. Lea & Febiger, Philadelphia, 1916
3. Parson E, Randall LM, Wilder RM: Pregnancy and diabetes. Med Clin North Am 10:679, 1926
4. Meal Planning with Exchange Lists. American Diabetes Association, Inc., and the American Dietetic Association, New York, 1949
5. Ney D, Hollingsworth DR: Nutritional management of pregnancy complicated by diabetes: historical perspective. Diabetes Care 4:647, 1981
6. Freinkel N, Dooley SL, Metzger BE: Care of the pregnant woman with insulin-dependent diabetes mellitus. N Engl J Med 313:96, 1985
7. National Academy of Sciences: Recommended Dietary Allowances. 10th Ed. National Academy Press, Washington, D.C., 1989
8. U.S. Department of Agriculture, Human Nutrition Information Service, Nutrition Monitoring Division: Nationwide Food Consumption Survey, Continuing Survey of Food Intakes by Individuals. Report no. 85-4. U.S. Government Printing Office, Hyattsville, Md., 1987

9. American Diabetes Association: Nutritional recommendations and principles for individuals with diabetes mellitus. Diabetes Care 10:126, 1987

10. National Academy of Sciences: Nutrition during Pregnancy. National Academy Press, Washington, D.C., 1990

11. Jovanovic-Peterson L, Peterson CM: Dietary manipulation as a primary treatment strategy for pregnancies complicated by diabetes. J Am Coll Nutr 9:320, 1990

12. Algert S, Shragg P, Hollingsworth DR: Moderate caloric restriction in obese women with gestational diabetes. Obstet Gynecol 65:487, 1985

13. Boberg C, Gillmer MDG, Brunner EJ et al: Obesity in pregnancy: the effect of dietary advice. Diabetes Care 3: 476, 1980

14. Rizzo T, Metzger BE, Burns WJ: Correlations between antepartum maternal metabolism and intelligence of offspring. N Engl J Med 325:911, 1991

15. Weinsier RL, Seeman A, Herrera G et al: High-and low-carbohydrate diets in diabetes mellitus. Ann Intern Med 80:332, 1974

16. Stone DB, Connor WE: The prolonged effects of a low cholesterol, high carbohydrate diet on the serum lipids in diabetic patients. Diabetes 12:127, 1963

17. Brunzell JD, Lerner RL, Hazzard WR et al: Improved glucose tolerance with high carbohydrate feeding in mild diabetes. N Engl J Med 284:521, 1971

18. Ney D, Hollingsworth DR, Cousins L: Decreased insulin requirement and improved control of diabetes in pregnant women given a high-carbohydrate, high-fiber, low-fat diet. Diabetes Care 5:529, 1982

19. Garg A, Bonanome A, Grundy SM et al: Comparison of a high-carbohydrate diet with a high-monounsaturated-fat diet in patients with non-insulin-dependent diabetes mellitus. N Engl J Med 319:829, 1988

20. Jovanovic-Peterson L, Peterson CM: Dietary manipulation as a primary treatment strategy for pregnancies complicated by diabetes. J Am Coll Nutr 9:320, 1990

21. Peterson CM, Jovanovic-Peterson L: Percentage of carbohydrate and glycemic response to breakfast, lunch, and dinner in women with gestational diabetes. Diabetes, suppl. 2, 40:172, 1991

22. Jovanovic-Peterson L, Peterson CM, Reed G, NICHD-DIEP: Maternal postprandial glucose levels predict birth weight. Am J Obstet Gynecol 164:103, 1991

23. Jenkins DJA, Wolever TMS, Taylor RH et al: Glycemic index of foods: a physiological basis for carbohydrate exchange. Am J Clin Nutr 34:362, 1981

24. Crapo PA, Insel J, Sperling M, Kolterman OG: Comparison of serum glucose, insulin, and glucagon responses to different types of complex carbohydrate in noninsulin-dependent diabetic patients. Am J Clin Nutr 34:184, 1981

25. O'Dea K, Nestel PJ, Antonoff L: Physical factors influencing postprandial glucose and insulin responses to starch. Am J Clin Nutr 33:760, 1980

26. Jenkins DJA, Wolever TMS, Jenkins AL et al: Glycemic response to wheat products: reduced response to pasta but no effect of fiber. Diabetes Care 6:155, 1983

27. Crapo PA, Scarlett JA, Kolterman OG: Comparison of the metabolic responses to fructose and sucrose sweetened foods. Am J Clin Nutr 36:256, 1982

28. Bantle JP, Laine DC, Castle GW et al: Postprandial glucose and insulin responses to meals containing different carbohydrates in normal and diabetic subjects. N Engl J Med 309:7, 1983

29. Horwitz DL, Bauer-Nehrling JK: Can aspartame meet our expectations? J Am Diet Assoc 83:142, 1983

30. Sturtevant FM: Use of aspartame during pregnancy. Int J Fertil 30:85, 1985

31. von Noorden C: Veber Hafercuren ber schwerem diabetes mellitus Ber Klin Wochenschr 40:817, 1903

32. Jenkins DJA, Leeds AR, Gassull MA et al: Unabsorbable carbohydrate and diabetes: decreased postprandial hyperglycemia. Lancet 2:172, 1976

33. Kiehm TG, Anderson JW, Ward K: Beneficial effects of a high carbohydrate, high fiber diet on hyperglycemic diabetic men. Am J Clin Nutr 29:895, 1976

34. Miranda PM, Horwitz DL: High-fiber diets in the treatment of diabetes mellitus. Ann Intern Med 88:482, 1978

35. Jenkins DJA, Leeds AR, Gassull MA et al: Decrease in postprandial insulin and glucose concentrations by guar and pectin. Ann Intern Med 86:20, 1977

36. Anderson JW, Ward K: High-carbohydrate, high-fiber diets for insulin treated men with diabetes mellitus. Am J Clin Nutr 32:2312, 1979

37. Christiansen JS, Bonnevie-Nielsen V, Svendsen PA et al: Effect of guar gum on 24-hour insulin requirements of insulin-dependent diabetic subjects as assessed by an artificial pancreas. Diabetes Care 3:659, 1980

38. Reece EA, Hagay Z, Gay LJ et al: A randomized clinical trial of a fiber-enriched diabetic diet vs the standard ADA-recommended diet in the management of diabetes mellitus in pregnancy. J Maternal-Fetal Med (in press)

39. Reece EA, Hagay Z, Caseria D et al: Do fiber-enriched diabetic diets have glucose lowering effects in pregnancy? Am J Perinatol 10:272, 1993

40. American Diabetes Association: Medical Management of Pregnancy Complicated by Diabetes. American Diabetes Association, Alexandria, VA, 1993

41. Abrams RS, Coustan DR: Gestational diabetes update. Clin Diabetes 8:1, 1990

42. Ney DM: Nutritional management of diabetes during pregnancy. Diabetology 7:1, 1988

43. Ney DM: Maternal nutrition and diet. In Hollingsworth

DR (ed): Pregnancy, Diabetes, and Birth, A Management Guide. 2nd Ed. Williams & Wilkins, Baltimore, 1992

44. American Diabetes Association: Nutritional recommendations and principles for individuals with diabetes mellitus: 1986. Diabetes Care 10:126, 1987

45. Pastors JG: Alternatives to the exchanges system for teaching meal planning to persons with diabetes. Diabetes Educ 18:57, 1992

46. DCCT Research Group: Nutrition interventions for intensive therapy in the Diabetes Control and Complications Trial. J Am Diet Assoc 93:768, 1993

47. Chanteleau E, Sonnenberg GE, Stanitzek-Schmidt I et al: Diet liberalization and metabolic control in type I diabetic outpatients treated by continuous subcutaneous insulin infusion. Diabetes Care 5:612, 1982

48. Lockwood D, Frey ML, Gladish NA, Hiss R: The biggest problem in diabetes. Diabetes Educ 12:30, 1986

49. House WC, Pendleton L, Parker L: Patients' versus physicians attribution of reasons for non-compliance with diet. Diabetes Care 9:434, 1986

50. Delahanty LM, Halford BN: The role of diet behaviors in achieving improved glycemic control in intensively treated patients in the Diabetes Control and Complications Trial. Diabetes Care 16:1453, 1993

51. Brodows RG, Williams C, Amatruda JM: Treatment of insulin reactions in diabetics. JAMA 252:3378, 1984

52. Pastors JG: Nutritional Care of Diabetes. Joyce Green Pastors/Nutritional Dimension, Inc., San Marcos, Calif., 1992

53. Choppin J, Jovanovic-Peterson L: Matching food with insulin. Diabetes Prof 1, Spring 1991

13

Exercise in Normal and Diabetic Pregnancies

MARSHALL W. CARPENTER

The cardiovascular, metabolic, and endocrine responses that characterize exertion have two effects. Nutrients and oxygen are delivered to exercising muscle to sustain exertional activity, and blood flow is maintained to nonexercising tissue at sufficient levels to preserve tissue integrity and the internal environment of the exercising individual. Pregnancy also profoundly affects cardiovascular and endocrine functions. Its effects on the normal response to exercise and the effect of acute and chronic exercise on pregnancy have been examined in animal and human investigations. Diabetes mellitus alters fuel availability and, in the case of type I diabetes, the ability of the animal to adapt to exertion. Both may adversely affect maternal and fetal homeostasis during exercise.

For purposes of addressing the clinical issues of exercise during pregnancy, diabetes may be divided into types I and II and gestational diabetes mellitus (GDM). The diagnostic criteria are explained elsewhere in this text. Type I diabetes has two characteristics that influence the physiologic response to exertion. First, there is no endogenous insulin production. Consequently, the metabolic requirements of a planned exercise bout need to be anticipated by modification of exogenous insulin dose and diet before exertion. Second, type I diabetes is often complicated by deficits in counter-regulatory endocrine responses and other end organ damage, both of which may limit homeostasis during and after exercise. Type II diabetes mellitus is often complicated by obesity, hypertension, hyperlipidemia, and varying combinations of insulin resistance and inadequate insulin release. Particularly in the older gravida, cardiovascular disease may be present as a result of these factors. Each of these characteristics may influ-

ence the risks and use of exercise in pregnancies complicated by type II diabetes mellitus. GDM is defined as glucose intolerance first identified during pregnancy.[1] Consequently, individuals with GDM can differ with respect to abnormalities in insulin release or sensitivity and the degree of metabolic derangement. The effect of exercise on glucose homeostasis in these patients, therefore, may vary and, in small study sample sizes, may be difficult to reproduce. Few studies have addressed the use of exercise in maintaining maternal glycemic control during pregnancy. Regardless of the pathogenesis of maternal hyperglycemia, the goal of therapy in pregnancy complicated by diabetes remains the preservation of normal fetal environment by maintaining "normal" metabolic control and by identifying or preventing altered perfusion of the fetoplacental unit. Little is known about the effect of maternal exercise on fetal environment. Accordingly, present recommendations regarding exercise in normal and diabetic pregnancy will likely undergo substantial modification in the future.

NONPREGNANT, NONDIABETIC PEOPLE

Acute Cardiovascular Effects

Exertion elicits changes in cardiorespiratory function that provide increased perfusion of and delivery of oxygen and fuel to exercising muscle. Oxygen uptake ($\dot{V}O_2$) increases immediately with exertion. It is the product of oxygen delivery (expressed as cardiac output) and oxygen extraction expressed as the arteriovenous oxygen difference (avDO$_2$). The rearranged Fick equation ($\dot{V}O_2$ = heart rate × stroke volume × avDO$_2$) describes the central role of these two processes in determining exercise capacity. $\dot{V}O_2$ increases to 10 to 20 times that at rest as maximal exercise intensity is reached. Maximal $\dot{V}O_2$ ($\dot{V}O_2$ max) is reached when further increases in exercise intensity (power) elicit no further increase in whole-body $\dot{V}O_2$. At this point, further increases in exercise intensity are achieved by anaerobic glycolysis. Blood lactate levels, which begin to rise when approximately 60 percent $\dot{V}O_2$max is reached, rise in an accelerated fashion as $\dot{V}O_2$max is reached (Fig. 13-1). This "plateau" of $\dot{V}O_2$, which defines $\dot{V}O_2$max (or maximal aerobic power), provides a benchmark against which relative intensities of physical exertion can be compared among individuals with differing aerobic capacities. For example, regardless of the level of aerobic capacity, all individuals will be found to have increasing plasma lactate at exercise intensity of greater than 60 percent $\dot{V}O_2$max. In most clinical circumstances, $\dot{V}O_2$max is limited by cardiac output and not by $\dot{V}O_2$ by the lung.

Cardiac output increases nearly linearly with $\dot{V}O_2$ at a ratio of 6:1. Likewise, heart rate increases linearly with rising exercise intensity to two to three times resting values at $\dot{V}O_2$max. Stroke volume increases to near-peak values at approximately 40 to 50 percent $\dot{V}O_2$max and increases minimally at higher exertional intensities.[2,3] The proportionate distribution of cardiac output during exercise changes dramatically. This is accomplished by vasoconstriction of vascular beds not serving exercising muscle. This is associated with production of norepinephrine by the peripheral vasculature. Accordingly, splanchnic and renal perfusion decrease in absolute values even with mild exercise and fall with increasing exercise intensity. Skin perfusion is increased with moderate exercise but falls as maximal aerobic capacity is approached.[4,5] The proportion of cardiac output perfusing exercising muscle at $\dot{V}O_2$max approaches 90 percent in trained individuals compared with sedentary controls.[6] As $\dot{V}O_2$max is reached, avDO$_2$ increases due to increased peripheral oxygen extraction. In highly trained athletes, hemoglobin desaturation may occur at maximal exertion. Ventilation increases linearly with exertional intensity until approximately 50 percent $\dot{V}O_2$max, at which point, the ratio of ventilation to $\dot{V}O_2$ almost doubles, going from 20 to 25 L to as much as 40 L for every 1-L increase in $\dot{V}O_2$.

Chronic Cardiovascular Effects

Aerobic exercise training occurs when repeated exertion is performed "of sufficient intensity, duration and frequency to ... improve maximal aerobic power."[6] Aerobic power is measured by observations of the body's ability to transport oxygen from the atmosphere to exercising muscle. $\dot{V}O_2$ depends on multiple cardiovascular factors, including body size, maximal heart rate (which decreases with age), stroke volume, the muscle mass used in each exercise, and the antecedent level of activity of the individual.

Cross-sectional studies of endurance athletes have commonly noted higher left ventricular end-diastolic volume without change in left ventricular wall thickness compared with sedentary controls. A review of longitudinal studies of endurance (aerobic) training of sedentary subjects indicates only a modest 2.4 percent increase in end-diastolic volume.[7] However, aerobic training produces an increase in $\dot{V}O_2$max up to 33 percent by both central and peripheral effects, depending on the duration and intensity of the training program.[8]

Exertional training produces increases in aerobic capacity by modifying cardiac and peripheral vascular physiology. Cardiac changes induced by chronic exertion include increased vascularization of the myocardium, slowing of resting heart rate (secondary to increased resting stroke volume and increased resting vagal tone), and increased contribution of stroke vol-

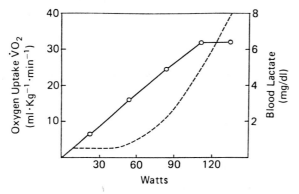

Fig. 13-1. Characteristic oxygen uptake ($\dot{V}O_2$) and blood lactate response to incremental power output (workload). (From Carpenter and Sady,[112] with permission.)

ume to cardiac output at high exertional intensity. The peripheral effects of exercise training that result in increased aerobic capacity include increased capillary density, local avDO$_2$, and maximal blood flow rate through the trained muscle. Physiologic measurements used to identify increased aerobic power include resting pulse, stroke volume, $\dot{V}O_2$ per cardiac cycle (oxygen pulse), and observed or estimated $\dot{V}O_2$max.

Acute Endocrine Effects

Exercise activates the sympathoadrenal system, which increases glucose production directly by stimulating glycogenolysis and gluconeogenesis. Increased glucose production is stimulated indirectly by inhibiting insulin secretion via α-adrenergic receptor stimulation and by stimulating glucagon secretion through activation of β-adrenergic receptors. Moderate exertion for 40 to 45 minutes produces a 50 percent fall in plasma insulin and a one-third rise in plasma glucagon while plasma glucose is rising.[9] The fall in circulating insulin does not affect glucose uptake in the exercising dog. Thus, the effect of reduced insulin concentration appears to promote glucose production. Complete suppression of glucagon release is associated with exercise-induced hypoglycemia, but increased hepatic glucose production with exercise appears to require only basal glucagon concentrations.[10]

Insulin suppression occurs with both intermittent or sustained exertion. Glucagon release is highly dependent on sustained exertion, rising 35 percent after 30 minutes of intense interrupted exertion and 300 percent after 81 minutes of intense interrupted exercise. Norepinephrine concentration rises with moderate exertional intensity, whereas epinephrine rises only with intense exertion. However, duration of exhaustive exercise does not appear to further augment the release of either hormone.[11]

Acute Metabolic Effects

The relative contribution of various fuels to sustain muscular activity is a function of prior training, nutritional status, exercise type and duration, and especially, exercise intensity. Fat is the primary fuel for exercising muscle. It is found in roughly 100-fold abundance in the body (6×10^5 kJ) compared with muscle (5×10^3 kJ) and hepatic (1.5×10^3 kJ) glycogen stores. It is oxidized preferentially at submaximal exertion. This is demonstrated by changes in the respiratory exchange ratio, which is defined as the ratio of carbon dioxide production to $\dot{V}O_2$ ($\dot{V}CO_2/\dot{V}O_2$) and is an approximation, under steady-state conditions, of the ratio of carbon dioxide production to oxygen consumption in the whole animal, the respiratory quotient (RQ). As exertional intensity is increased, the respiratory exchange ratio approaches unity. Because the RQ of fat is 0.7 and that of carbohydrate is 1.0, this indicates that increased exercise intensity produces a shift from fatty acid oxidation to glycolytic oxidation. This shift appears to be a result of decreased oxygen availability, as indicated by a concomitant rise in muscle reduced nicotinamide adenine dinucleotide.[12] This is further supported by observing a rise in respiratory exchange ratio when inspired oxygen concentration is reduced from 21 percent to 14 percent during conditions of fixed moderate exertion.[13] Consequently, the duration at which near-maximal exertion can be maintained is limited by the carbohydrate stores in liver and muscle.

Net arteriovenous lactate differences in exercising muscle are noted even with mild exercise. Thus, increased plasma lactate levels noted at exercise intensity approaching maximal aerobic power indicate that muscle production of lactate exceeds lactate clearance by other muscles and liver. This may result from hormonally mediated increases in glycogenolysis and glycolysis, recruitment of fast-twitch glycolytic muscle fibers, and a redistribution of blood flow from tissues that clear lactate from circulating blood (liver) to exercising muscle. Increased lactate in tissues may suppress lipolysis, further increasing demand for carbohydrate by exercising muscle under these conditions.[14] The exercise intensity at which increased lactate in plasma is measured is reproducible when measured repeatedly within individuals and is increased by endurance training.

When exercise commences, muscle adenosine triphosphate and phosphocreatine may provide enough stored energy for 6 to 8 seconds of intense muscular activity. Nonoxidative energy from glycogenolysis and glycolysis in the muscle can provide the requisite energy for 1 to 3 minutes of maximal exercise. Intense exertion, lasting more than 4 to 5 minutes, depends on blood glucose, glycerol, and free fatty acid, which diffuse from capillary to muscle mitochondria. The splanchnic production of glucose rises fourfold by 40 minutes in moderate exercise.[9] Exertion lasting more than 2 hours depends on free fatty acid production. These conditions increase lipolysis and may produce a fall in blood glucose, perhaps due to exhaustion of hepatic glycogen stores.

Plasma Glucose and Glucose Uptake During and After Acute Exercise

Plasma glucose remains unchanged during brief, moderate exertion, rises 15 to 20 percent during intense exertion, and falls gradually during prolonged, moderate work. Plasma glucose is maintained by a two- to fivefold increase in hepatic glucose production, which is increasingly derived from gluconeogenic activity as duration of exertion increases.[15,16] After exhaustive exercise, glucose concentration continues to rise transiently, remaining elevated up to 30 minutes later.[17]

During exercise, glucose uptake by muscle increases linearly with exercise duration and with exercise intensity, reaching values 50 times resting values at maximal aerobic effort.[18] This increase in muscle glucose uptake occurs even at very low insulin concentrations of 0.2 to 1.2 μU/ml but not in the absence of circulating insulin.[19]

After exertion, insulin-mediated glucose uptake is increased in exercised muscle compared with nonexercised muscle measured 4 hours after single leg exercise in sedentary men.[20] Both submaximal and maximal insulin-mediated glucose uptake is increased, suggesting that both receptor (insulin sensitivity) and postreceptor (insulin responsiveness) changes occur after exertion. However, this effect cannot be demonstrated in endurance-trained athletes after a single exercise bout.[21] These observations have not been attempted in insulin-resistant women with glucose intolerance in pregnancy.

Obese individuals demonstrate the same postexercise proportionate increase in submaximal insulin-mediated glucose uptake (about 25 percent) as lean individuals compared with baseline values.[22] However, obese individuals demonstrate no increase in maximal insulin-mediated glucose uptake after exertion. These data suggest that some postreceptor defects in obesity may not respond to the acute effects of exertion.

Lipid Effects

Acute exertion has a variable effect on total plasma cholesterol (T-C). The most reproducible effect is at 4 to 72 hours after intense and prolonged exercise, when a lowering of T-C is observed. Plasma triglyceride concentration falls acutely after isolated exertion. This is probably due to an increase in lipoprotein lipase activity with secondary catabolism of triglycerides. This effect is marginal in individuals with low baseline plasma triglyceride levels but may be more marked in those with hypertriglyceridemia.[23]

Metabolic Effects of Exercise Training

During the 24-hour cycle of daily activity, approximately 10 percent of caloric consumption is used for the thermic effect of feeding, the oxidation of ingested food, and energy requirements of digestion. Physical activity can account for 15 to 30 percent or more of daily energy expenditure. Sixty to seventy-five percent of total caloric expenditure is resting metabolic rate (RMR). Consequently, changes in RMR of relatively minor proportions may have a significant effect on total caloric requirements. The acute effect of a single bout of exertion on RMR is in doubt, although very intense and prolonged exertion may be followed by a measurable increase.[24] Cohort studies describe a reproducible increase in RMR in sedentary individuals subjected to training programs of weeks' duration.[25,26] The reported increases of approximately 8 percent are much less than the 50 percent higher values observed in cross-sectional studies of individuals with high compared with those with low $\dot{V}O_2max$.[27] This suggests that level of activity alone explains only a portion of the discrepancy. Genetic factors, the intensity of the exertional training, and caloric restriction but probably not degree of obesity influence the effect of exercise training on RMR. Nevertheless, an RMR increase of 8 percent, attributable to exertional training, may be sufficient to induce euglycemia in pregnancy complicated with mild glucose intolerance, commonly found in GDM, even when glucose intolerance is the result of combined defects in insulin release and action.

Insulin sensitivity, measured as submaximal insulin-mediated glucose uptake during a hyperinsulinemic, euglycemic clamp, returns to values found in sedentary individuals after 5 to 7 days of detraining.[21,28] This is reflected in a contemporaneous fall in percentage-specific insulin binding to erythrocytes, suggesting that a reduction in insulin receptors may cause this effect. However, maximal insulin-mediated glucose uptake (insulin responsiveness) remains unchanged in the days after detraining. This suggests that an isolated exercise bout changes insulin receptor number or function but that exercise training also affects postreceptor events in muscle that are not the product of a single exercise stress.

Six-week training in obese sedentary subjects, who initially demonstrated increased fasting and glucose-stimulated plasma insulin concentrations, resulted in a 26 percent decrease in both variables. Exercise-trained subjects also demonstrated a significant increase in total-body glucose uptake during the hyperinsulinemic, euglycemic clamp due to both increased peripheral uptake of glucose and greater suppression of hepatic glucose production.[29]

Lipid Effects

Chronic exertion may decrease very low-density lipoprotein triglyceride (VLDL-T) synthesis as a result of increased insulin sensitivity and a reduction in percentage of body fat. Exercise training is more effective in triglyceride lowering in those patients whose values are elevated before physical training. Chronic effects may result from increased skeletal muscle or adipose tissue lipoprotein lipase activity, a reduction in hepatic triglyceride synthesis, and a reduction in adiposity.

In men, the most reproducible effect of chronic exertion on plasma cholesterol concentration is a rise in high-density lipoprotein cholesterol (HDL-C), particularly in the HDL_2 subfraction. A dose-response effect of the intensity of exertional training and increase in HDL-C has been demonstrated.[30] This also correlates with exercise-related increases in insulin sensitivity and reductions in adiposity. Small decreases in low-density lipoprotein cholesterol (LDL-C) occur with moderate exercise training.

However, exercise training has demonstrated little or no effect on plasma lipids in nondiabetic sedentary women. This may be due to the lower plasma T-C and LDL-C and higher HDL-C concentrations found in sedentary women before menopause compared with men. Women also have higher lipoprotein lipase activity than men. These sex differences may limit the observed effect of chronic exertion on lipoprotein metabolism.[31,32]

Endocrine Effects of Exercise Training

The direct effect of chronic exercise on the hypothalamic-pituitary-ovarian axis and its indirect nutritional effects are beyond the scope of this chapter. Chronic exertion probably affects the acute hormonal response to individual exercise bouts. For example, the epinephrine response usually attending intense exertion may have a different effect on fuel metabolism in chronically exercised animals than in those that are sedentary. Normal rats subjected to 10 weeks of treadmill training showed a reduced glycemic response to epinephrine and diminished insulin suppression by epinephrine. Training produced no change in glucagon response to epinephrine in these rats. By contrast, training in streptozocin-induced diabetic rats produced a similar reduction in epinephrine-induced hyperglycemia but no effect on epinephrine-induced suppression of insulin release and a reduction of the twofold increased glucagon response to epinephrine to normal.[33] The changes in exercise-induced hormonal response and changes in the effects of these hormonal responses that may be caused by chronic exercise training have not been explored in pregnancy.

PREGNANT, NONDIABETIC WOMEN

Cardiovascular Function at Rest

The endocrinologic and metabolic effects of pregnancy have been reviewed in Chapter 5. The cardiovascular effects of pregnancy are summarized here as a necessary foundation to understanding the potential benefits and risks of acute exertion and physical training in normal and diabetic pregnancies.

Second only to the effects of acute exertion, pregnancy produces the most profound nonpathologic change in mammalian cardiovascular physiology. Cardiovascular changes have been measured as early as 6 weeks after conception in the human, when cardiac output increases by 23 percent and stroke volume by 20 percent.[34,36] This may be a result of a primary reduction in peripheral vascular resistance, which has been linked to the effects of estrogen and progesterone.[37] Plasma volume increases by 45 percent by the third trimester and red blood cell volume increases by more than 20 percent by mid-pregnancy,[38,39] resulting in a dilutional anemia. Cardiac output increases by approximately 35 percent and resting $\dot{V}O_2$ increases by 13 to 30 percent, whereas weight increases by an average of only 13 percent during pregnancy. This is reflected, in part, in a decreased avDO$_2$ during pregnancy. The increase in resting $\dot{V}O_2$ during pregnancy also begins early; half of the increase observed may occur in the first trimester.[40] Others have found, however, that resting $\dot{V}O_2$ increases in proportion to increased body weight; that is, $\dot{V}O_2$ per kilogram is unchanged from pregnancy to postpartum.[41] End-diastolic volume and stroke volume[34,35,42] appear to increase during pregnancy. Consequently, both cardiac and hematologic changes of pregnancy may serve to increase aerobic power during pregnancy, independent of exertional training.

Acute Cardiovascular Response to Isolated Exertion

An augmentation of exercise-induced increases in $\dot{V}O_2$ has been observed inconsistently during pregnancy.[42–47] Identical submaximal treadmill and cycle exercise tests performed in late pregnancy and postpartum identified a 9 percent increase in absolute (liters per minute) $\dot{V}O_2$ with weight-supported exertion and a 12 percent higher $\dot{V}O_2$ during treadmill (weight-bearing) exertion during pregnancy compared with the exercise-produced $\dot{V}O_2$ increment measured in the postpartum state. Most (75 percent) of these differences were accounted for by pregnancy-related weight changes.[41] The increased resting $\dot{V}O_2$ during pregnancy and the increased absolute increment in $\dot{V}O_2$ with any submaximal workload results in most exertional tasks being carried out at a higher percentage of $\dot{V}O_2$max. As noted above, the identical "external" workload during pregnancy will require a higher respiratory exchange ratio with a higher relative oxidation of glucose relative to fatty acids and a higher sympathoadrenal response. This means that maternal exertion at an identical workload will result in a metabolic response that elicits a higher lactate plasma concentration. Also, maternal exertion during pregnancy

will cause an augmentation of the normal redistribution of cardiac output to exercising muscle because the exertion is taking place at a higher percentage of $\dot{V}O_2$max.

Pregnancy does not alter the 5:1 to 6:1 ratio between cardiac output and $\dot{V}O_2$ observed in the nonpregnant state.[44] Pregnancy may alter the relative contribution of stroke volume and heart rate to increased cardiac output during high-intensity exertion. Increases in stroke volume may continue to contribute to increased cardiac output during incremental exertion at higher percentages of $\dot{V}O_2$max in pregnancy compared with the nonpregnant state.[44] This appears to alter the predictive heart rate–$\dot{V}O_2$ formula for $\dot{V}O_2$max during pregnancy.[48] $\dot{V}O_2$max does not appear to be altered by pregnancy.[48,49] However, peak age-specific pulse may be somewhat lower during pregnancy by 4 beats/min.[49]

Recovery from exertion may be impeded by pregnancy. Stroke volume falls after completion of moderate exertion to a greater degree in late pregnancy (23 percent) than postpartum (11 percent).[50] This may be due to increased venous pooling in the legs during pregnancy secondary to increased venous compliance and from partial caval obstruction from the late gravid uterus.

Acute Endocrine Response to Exertion

Little has been published about pregnancy-induced changes in endocrine response to exertion. There may be a reduced norepinephrine response to rising to a standing position during pregnancy.[51] This suggests a blunted baroreceptor response. Insulin concentrations may not fall during exercise in pregnancy as much as in the nonpregnant state.[52] Glucagon response to exertion may be augmented by pregnancy,[53] although this finding has not been confirmed. However, these studies were carried out with only very mild maternal exertion, which may not have provided a satisfactory stimulus for differential endocrine effects.

Acute Effect of Maternal Exertion on Fetal Homeostasis

Acute exertion induces a rapid increase in cardiac output and increased perfusion of exercising muscle. The control of exercise-induced altered organ perfusion is not well understood. Studies of norepinephrine arteriovenous gradients across various vascular beds have suggested that, in response to exercise, plasma norepinephrine is derived from inactive muscles, abdominal organs, fat, and myocardium, as well as exercising striated muscle, and results in vasoconstriction and reduced perfusion of nonexercising tissue.[54] However, others have found that exercising muscle makes the largest absolute contribution of norepinephrine to the circulation during exertion, and have suggested that the capacity of tissues to simultaneously release and take up norepinephrine and the marked changes in relative perfusion of organs induced by exertion may invalidate earlier models based only on arteriovenous differences.[55] Despite this uncertainty, reduction of flow to nonexercising tissues probably occurs within 1 to 2 minutes of the start of exertion, even at moderate intensities.

During brief exertion, the reduction of splanchnic perfusion is directly proportional to duration of exertion and the exercise-induced increase in $\dot{V}O_2$.[56] In the pregnant sheep, 10 minutes of exertion at 70 percent $\dot{V}O_2$max reduced uterine blood flow by 8 percent, whereas 40 minutes of exertion at the same intensity reduced uterine blood flow 27 percent. Exercise for 10 minutes at 100 percent $\dot{V}O_2$max resulted in an 11 percent reduction in uterine blood flow. Fetal arterial oxygen tension, oxygen content, and carbon dioxide tension decreased with increasing intensity and was most marked in the 40-minute exercise protocol. Yet, under these conditions, total uterine oxygen consumption was maintained.[49] A more prolonged (1 to 3 hour) treadmill exercise protocol in near-term pregnant sheep compared ewes who completed the protocol with those whose "staggering gait required assistance." There was no appreciable change in uterine blood flow in "nonexhausted" ewes. The exhausted group demonstrated a 28 percent decrease in uterine blood flow and a 29 percent reduction in fetal oxygen tension. Fetal umbilical artery oxygen content decreased 37 percent in this group, but this was associated with an increase in fetal oxygen extraction. Net lactate uptake by the fetus was demonstrated even in the "exhausted" ewes, indicating that fetoplacental oxygen uptake was still maintained in this extreme condition.[57] These observations found significant alterations in fetal environment caused by maternal exertion, which, in other species or in other exercise conditions, might be associated with compromised fetal oxygenation and fuel supply.

Fetal bradycardia may be induced neurogenically by direct baroreceptor stimulation of the vagus nerve from increased fetal blood pressure or by chemoreceptor stimulation by hypoxemia and acidemia, producing increased fetal blood pressure. Fetal hypoxemia may directly depress fetal heart rate. Consequently, because of concerns regarding the effects of human maternal exertion on fetal gas exchange, initial studies of human fetal response used clinical Doppler fetal heart rate monitors during and after maternal exertion. In these studies, fetal bradycardia was noted shortly after the initiation of even mild and moderately intense maternal exertion.[58–60] These observations were probably obscured by maternal motion artifact. Subsequent studies, using continuous two-dimensional sonographic imaging, have examined fetal heart rate response to exertion in mid- and late gestation under conditions of moderate exertion and maximal voluntary effort.[61,62]

In the first study, an 18-minute incremental submaximal exertion peaking at approximately 60 percent $\dot{V}O_2$max was associated with only one fetal bradycardia (<110 beats per minute for ≥10 seconds) in 85 tests. This occurred approximately 1 minute after maternal hypotension during a vasovagal episode. Only one of these tests was followed by a fetal bradycardia. The same subjects then performed a 6- to 10-minute incremental maximal exertion and demonstrated no fetal bradycardia during exertion. However, despite a gradual decrease in exertion after peak effort, 15 episodes of fetal bradycardia were observed after 79 peak exertion sessions. All bradycardia was abrupt in onset, variable in resolution, and unassociated with maternal blood pressure or gestational age (20 to 34 weeks). There was no protective effect of prior maternal exertional history or increased maternal aerobic capacity. All fetuses in this study demonstrated normal fetal heart rate tracings, with fetal heart rate accelerations associated with fetal movement within 30 minutes of maternal exercise cessation. Fetal bradycardia was not associated with subsequent untoward perinatal events.[61] Baseline fetal heart rate appears to increase after moderate maternal exercise.[63,64] Maternal exertion of at least 20 minutes' duration and intensity of 50 to 60 percent $\dot{V}O_2$max appears to be required to elicit this response, which appears to be more pronounced in late pregnancy. This response does not appear to be mediated by increased maternal core temperature, which was increased by only 0.3°C under the conditions of these studies.

Effects of Exercise Training

Limited information is available on the effect of chronic maternal exercise on fetal homeostasis and perinatal outcome. Most prospective studies are not randomized and are, thereby, subject to biased subject selection. Some studies used a detraining protocol rather than the training of sedentary subjects and may have introduced nutritional and body composition-related factors that could have influenced outcome. These observational cohort studies[65–71] have observed an 11 to 24 percent reduction in the absolute weight gain in pregnancy associated with exercise training. Most studies identified a lower birthweight among exercising subjects of 62 to 623 g. However, no studies have identified a significantly earlier gestational age at birth nor a higher incidence of prematurity among offspring of women undergoing chronic exercise training. One study showed an inverse association between exercise frequency and cesarean delivery rate.[70] A nonrandomized detraining study noted a 6 percent cesarean rate among runners and dancers who continued to exercise compared with a rate of 30 percent among 44 subjects who discontinued exercise during pregnancy despite a higher birthweight in this latter group of only 407 g.[67] Neither study offered information regarding the clinical decision for cesarean section. Two randomized trials examined the association of maternal exercise with pregnancy and labor complications.[65,71] No differences in gestational age, fetal growth, cesarean section rates, or fetal compromise at birth were noted. However, subject numbers of 40 and 85 in these studies were insufficient to identify many differences that may be of clinical importance.

These studies suggests that, in normal human pregnancy, moderate exertion, sufficient to induce cardiovascular training effects in sedentary individuals, is not associated with evidence of acute fetal compromise. By their nature, direct measurement of fetal metabolic conditions and cardiovascular response cannot be made in human studies, however. Consequently, fetal effects of maternal exertion sufficient to influence fetal growth, body composition, or development cannot be identified with these studies. Limited observations of perinatal outcome have been largely compromised by inappropriate protocol design or by inadequate subject numbers. Despite these limitations, however, maternal exertion at an intensity and duration shown to produce both cardiovascular and metabolic training effects is probably unassociated with untoward fetal or maternal effects. This suggests that exercise may be investigated as a therapeutic tool in the antenatal care of women with non-insulin-dependent diabetes mellitus (NIDDM) and those with GDM. Whether the reduction in birthweight of offspring of active atheletes compared with sedentary controls can be replicated among sedentary women with glucose intolerance and obesity subjected to exercise training has not been explored as yet. The therapeutic use of exercise in insulin-dependent diabetes mellitus (IDDM) is also in question. The apparent fetal safety of brief maternal exertion described in normal pregnancy has not been examined in pregnancy complicated by IDDM.

PHYSIOLOGIC AND CLINICAL CONSIDERATIONS IN NONPREGNANT AND PREGNANT DIABETIC PATIENTS

Exercise was reportedly prescribed as a treatment for diabetes in the first century BC by the Roman physician Celsus.[72] In the modern era, before insulin treatment, exercise was known to lower blood glucose and improve glucose tolerance.[73,74] Although there has been a commonly held enthusiasm for exercise in IDDM based on early observations of the augmentation of the effects of exogenous insulin by exercise,[75–77] evidence to support exercise as a therapeutic tool to improve overall glycemic control in type I diabetes mellitus (IDDM) is limited.[72] The powerful effects of an obligate exogenous insulin load, variable diet and absorption of food, defective counterregulation, and sympathetic neuropathy render the simple application of exertion in this disorder problematic. For example, two case series cite improved physiologic measures after an exercise training program in IDDM patients.[78,79] Exercise training, producing improved aerobic power, resulted in normalization of hyperglycemia and reduction of plasma ketone concentration. Well-trained men with IDDM demonstrated normal exertional effects on fuel metabolism. However, the logistical demands of a consistent daily exercise program and the lack of effect of these programs beyond the duration of the research intervention have caused some authors to recommend dietary modification and careful glucose surveillance as more realistic long-term methods to effect euglycemia.[80] Yet, despite the lack of data supporting its therapeutic efficacy, exercise is an important recreational feature in the lives of many diabetic patients and may serve to secure a sense of well-being and physical competence. Accordingly, many patients with IDDM may present the physician with the challenge of a continuing exercise training program in the context of pregnancy, with its dietary variability and fetal imperative for near-euglycemia.

The role of exercise in the prevention and treatment of NIDDM (type II) is much more complex. The pathogenesis of type II diabetes is only partly understood but is believed to be the result of a genetic–environmental interaction that may begin in the fetal period.[81] Obesity may characterize up to 90 percent of NIDDM and is more commonly that of central distribution (an increased waist/hip ratio).[82,83] Weight loss, especially when associated with diet and exercise intervention, has been associated with remission of hyperglycemia[84] and prevention of progression of impaired glucose tolerance (IGT) to NIDDM.[85] NIDDM is associated with impaired hepatic sensitivity to glucose, insulin, and glucagon, with associated increased fasting hepatic glucose production and hyperglycemia.[86,87] In addition, insulin-mediated peripheral disposal of glucose is reduced by as much as one-half at euglycemia, although the diabetic subject probably has normal total peripheral glucose disposal at hyperglycemic levels.[88,89] This effect may be related to reduced insulin receptor number, reduced receptor signaling, faulty glucose transport, or impaired enzymatic metabolism of glucose.

Exercise may modify this complex interaction of diet, obesity, hyperlipidemia, central and peripheral insulin resistance, defective insulin release, and postreceptor cellular defects in several ways. Scheduled exercise may reinforce behavior modification to ensure better compliance with diet and medication. Exercise training has been associated with weight reduction, improved lipid profile, and increased aerobic power, itself associated with improved perfusion of chronically exercised muscle.

Nonpregnant Patients with IDDM

The effect of exertion on metabolic control in IDDM is variable. It can be described as the product of the metabolic state at the initiation of exercise, means of delivery of exogenous insulin, recent exertion and diet, impairment of counterregulatory hormone responses, sympathetic autonomic dysfunction, potential cardiac dysfunction, and finally, the social and psychological context in which exercise is undertaken.

The metabolic response to exertion in IDDM is predicated on the metabolic state at the time of exercise. Exercise increases hyperglycemia and accelerates ketone formation when performed during marked insulin deficiency and ketosis. This is probably due to exercise augmentation of hepatic glucose production and fatty acid mobilization.[90] Moderately well-controlled and poorly controlled ketotic IDDM subjects were compared with nondiabetic controls in a 3-hour mild-intensity cycle exercise.[91] Both diabetic groups demonstrated higher lactate, free fatty acid, ketone, and glucagon plasma concentrations than controls. Moderately well-controlled diabetic subjects experienced a fall in glucose concentration despite a rise in plasma glucagon. In ketotic, poorly controlled diabetic subjects, exercise produced a marked rise in glucose concentration and a higher level of ketone bodies and glucagon than in the moderately controlled diabetic group. This experience suggests that exercise should be avoided under conditions of poor metabolic control. This is especially true in pregnancy, in which the fetus is uniquely susceptible to the effects of maternal ketosis. Ketonemia in both nondiabetic and diabetic mothers has been associated with lower intellectual function in offspring. Maternal ketoacidosis has been associated with a high perinatal mortality rate[92] and has been documented to result in fetal heart rate patterns, suggesting fetal hypoxemia that resolves with maternal treatment.[93] Patients who are nonketotic need not avoid exertion but should not withhold insulin before exertion.

Continuous subcutaneous insulin infusion (CSII) became popular in the 1980s. These "open-loop" systems require continued independent surveillance of blood glucose and must be adjusted accordingly. Initial optimism that these devices would improve metabolic control prompted studies of the effect of method of exogenous insulin delivery on metabolic response to exertion in IDDM patients. One study observed the expected exertion-induced fall in plasma glucose from 230 to 160 mg/dl in subjects treated with multiple subcutaneous injections of insulin (MSI).[94] Of interest, subjects treated with CSII who had pre-exertion glucose concentration of 110 mg/dl, demonstrated no change in glucose concentration during or after exertion, similar to nondiabetic controls. The differences may have had more to do with pre-exertion euglycemia rather than CSII, however. In another study, euglycemic IDDM subjects with each type of insulin delivery were subjected to 45 minutes of exertion at 55 percent $\dot{V}O_2$max 2 hours after morning insulin and a standardized breakfast.[95] In a randomized crossover design, subjects were studied at rest after usual morning insulin dose, during exercise after usual morning insulin dose, and after the same protocol after two-

thirds or one-half the usual morning insulin dose and after no morning insulin. Figure 13-2 depicts the varying glucose and free insulin values in each protocol using subcutaneous insulin injection or CSII delivery. Both groups experienced a significant fall in plasma glucose during and after exertion with four of seven CSII subjects and three of six MSI subjects having clinical hypoglycemia. Exercise without preceding prebreakfast insulin was associated with similar hyperglycemia in both groups, whereas that after a 33 or 50 percent reduction in prebreakfast insulin produced little disturbance in glucose concentrations. These studies suggest that, in the context of euglycemia, premeal insulin dose can be safely reduced before anticipated exertion within 2 hours after eating. However, CSII per se does not appear to ensure euglycemia during and after exertion in IDDM.

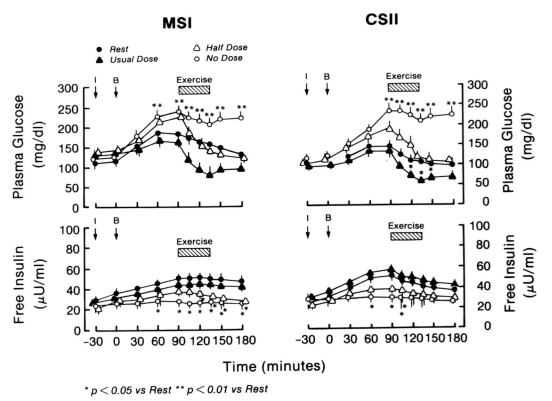

Fig. 13-2. (Left) Plasma glucose and free insulin concentrations in patients treated with multiple subcutaneous injections of insulin (MSI) during rest and exercise studies (mean ± SEM). I, insulin administration; B, start of breakfast. **(Right)** Plasma glucose and free insulin concentration in patients treated with continuous subcutaneous infusion of insulin (CSII) during rest and exercise. (From Schiffrin and Parikh,[95] with permission.)

Pregnant Patients with IDDM

Little has been published regarding exercise during pregnancy complicated by IDDM. One observational study examined two cohorts of sedentary gravidas: normal controls and subjects with IDDM assigned in a nonrandom manner to 20 minutes of "leisurely" walking three times each day or to usual activity.[96] All subjects wore pedometers, and the exercisers did experience more walking. Prescribed walking was not associated with improved metabolic control in diabetic subjects, but these patients had relatively poor metabolic control on study entry, having mean 24-hour glucose values of 174 ± 59 and 165 ± 55 mg/dl in exercisers and controls, which were 103 ± 36 and 111 ± 33, respectively, at end of protocol. This suggests that other treatments exerted more powerful effects on metabolic control than the exercise prescription. Exercise prescription did produce lower fasting cholesterol and triglyceride concentrations in both groups than in their nonexercising controls. Comparison of efficacy of CSII compared with MSI injections for metabolic control during pregnancy suggests that CSII does not reduce glycemic variability nor improve the level of glycemia during pregnancy.[97]

Table 13-1 lists guidelines for exercise in women with IDDM espoused by some authors that have applicability during pregnancy as well.[90] Nondiabetic sedentary women appear to be able to initiate an exercise training program during pregnancy with the same fetal safety as active women who continue their usual exercise during pregnancy.[61] Sedentary women with IDDM, however, may have undiagnosed retinopathy, nephropathy, and myocardial ischemia. We inform our patients with untreated proliferative retinopathy to delay exercise until retinal laser therapy is completed.

The effect of exercise during pregnancy on the progression of diabetic nephropathy is unknown. Although angiotensin-converting enzyme inhibitors have been shown to retard the progression of albuminuria without worsening azotemia in patients with early diabetic nephropathy, these drugs are contraindicated in pregnancy because of their association with fetal growth restriction, fetal loss, and neonatal hypotension. Consequently, pregnancy may result in increased glomerular hydraulic pressure that is untreated because of the above fetal considerations. In theory, therefore, exercise by diabetic patients with albuminuria may thereby exacerbate the progression of nephropathy. Patients with nephropathy and an interest in exercise training in pregnancy should be informed of the uncertain effects of exercise on renal function in their pregnancies.

There is no consensus regarding the appropriate method of screening for silent myocardial ischemia in gravid women with IDDM. Those gravid women with long-standing IDDM who are inclined to perform exercise training during pregnancy may be advised to undergo step or treadmill exertional testing with cardiac monitoring both during and after exertion. Especially in late pregnancy, venous return and cardiac preload may be reduced after exertion, leading to reduced stroke volume and, in the context of sympathetic neuropathy, reduced cardiac output.[50] It may be useful to screen for sympathetic autonomic neuropathy. However, the effect of autonomic neuropathy on exercise safety is uncertain, particularly at modest exercise intensities.

Patients with IDDM are vulnerable to exercise-related hypoglycemia primarily because of the uncertain effects of previously injected insulin. Exogenous insulin plasma concentration does not fall during exertion and the usual increase in hepatic glucose production does not occur. In patients with abnormal glucagon and epinephrine counterregulatory responses, this may produce hypoglycemia. IDDM patients who are

---

Table 13-1. Exercise Guidelines for Women with Type I Diabetes in the Reproductive Age Group (15–40 Years)

Complete history, physical examination, and screening for proliferative retinopathy, nephropathy, and cardiovascular disease

Screen for postural hypotension tachycardia and history of hypoglycemia without autonomic symptoms

Establish diabetic control by MSI or CSII, self-glucose monitoring, and dietary modifications

Initiate a gradual program of postprandial exercise on a regular basis in conjunction with self-glucose monitoring

Adjust pre-exercise insulin dose, food intake, and postexercise carbohydrate supplement

Avoid exercise during peak insulin action

Do not use exercising extremities as insulin injection sites

Alert patients to possibility of exercise-induced hypoglycemia, which may occur several hours after the completion of exercise

Abbreviations: MSI, multiple subcutaneous injections of insulin; CSII, continuous subcutaneous insulin infusion.
(From Zinman and Vranic,[90] with permission.)

pregnant are further prone to exercise-associated hypoglycemia for several reasons. Because of nausea or other discomforts of pregnancy, the patient's diet may be inadequate before exertion. Patients who have been successful in maintaining euglycemia during pregnancy are more vulnerable to delayed postexertional hypoglycemia, which may occur several hours after completion of exertion. Exercise training also increases insulin sensitivity in previously sedentary individuals. This may further increase the risk of unexpected hypoglycemia. Accordingly, patients should be advised to have a glucose monitor and source of glucose available to them in case of late postexertional hypoglycemia. Because of these considerations, we recommend that IDDM patients wishing to begin a new exertional program increase exercise duration and intensity gradually to allow incremental adaptations of diet and insulin dose to the exercise program.

Despite the best efforts on the part of physician and patient in avoiding hypoglycemia in pregnancy, efforts to maintain euglycemia to preserve normal embryonic and fetal development are often complicated by symptomatic neuroglycopenia, requiring support from another individual. Because hypoglycemia may occur even during exertion, we recommend that gravid women who suffer neuroglycopenia, unheralded by sympathetic symptoms, always be accompanied by a person competent to administer subcutaneous glucagon. This is particularly true of such patients engaging in exercise. We recommend that all patients have available, on their person, a source of readily absorbable glucose. Some patients may prefer also to carry a reflectance meter. Some of our patients who prefer to run outdoors have a suitably equipped partner accompany them by bicycle.

Nonpregnant Patients with NIDDM

The therapeutic potential for exercise in NIDDM is supported by both epidemiologic and experimental evidence. The efficacy of chronic exercise training has been more satisfactorily demonstrated in the prevention of NIDDM. There is less evidence that chronic exercise ameliorates established NIDDM.

Epidemiologic studies have suggested that chronic exercise training in individuals with IGT or otherwise at high risk of developing NIDDM reduces the probability of developing diabetes mellitus. A 14-year cohort study of University of Pennsylvania graduates demonstrated development of NIDDM in 202 (3.4 percent) of 5,990 men.[98] Risk of NIDDM was reduced 6 percent for every 500-kcal increment in weekly energy expenditure, independent of obesity and family history of NIDDM. In addition, weight gain since college and hypertension were independent risk factors for NIDDM. The effect of energy expenditure was greater in those at highest risk of NIDDM. Another 8-year cohort study of 87,253 34- to 59-year-old female nurses[99] noted 1,303 new cases (1.5 percent) of NIDDM. Among those who exercised at least weekly, the risk ratio for NIDDM was 0.84 ($P < .005$) after adjusting for obesity. But no dose-response relationship could be demonstrated between frequency of exercise and the development of NIDDM. These studies suggest that either exertional training is protective against NIDDM, as demonstrated by a dose-response relationship in the men's cohort, or that individuals that develop NIDDM do not exercise regularly because of obesity or other reasons, as suggested by the nurse study.

Exercise trials more directly assess the effect of exertion on NIDDM. In a study of 48 men with IGT, subjects were randomized to performing twice-weekly exercise and diet modification, diet alone, or exercise alone. Weight reduction was noted among those randomized to diet alone, but improved glucose tolerance was noted only in those performing the diet/exercise protocol.[84] This study suggests that an intervention combining diet and exercise is more effective in improving glycemia in those with abnormal glucose tolerance.

In a nonrandom controlled trial of dietary and exercise intervention in IGT and diabetes,[85] subjects with mild NIDDM and IGT who were able to complete a 5-year protocol of dietary modification and weight loss and exercise training were examined. Only those with IGT were able to maintain postprandial glycemia of less than 7 mmol, whereas those with NIDDM demonstrated a gradual rise in glycemia despite comparable reductions in postprandial hyperinsulinemia to those found in the IGT group. In the IGT group, improved glucose tolerance was associated with weight reduction and increased $\dot{V}O_2$ max. Another study of men with IGT examined the effect of dietary modification, diet plus placebo, and diet plus tolbutamide in a randomized trial.[100] Among those completing the 10- to 12-year observation period, progression to sustained hyperglycemia (all oral glucose tolerance test values greater than two standard deviations higher than mean values) occurred in 29 percent of observed controls, in 13 percent of those undergoing some dietary intervention without tolbutamide, and in none who continued treatment with tolbutamide. Although none of these subjects was enlisted to perform exercise, data from this and the preceding study suggest that subjects who complete protocols combining multiple interventions show therapeutic effect. It may be that the multi-interventional approach results in one intervention reinforcing compliance with others. Exercise may only reinforce dietary compliance with resulting weight loss and prevention of progressive glucose intolerance.

Studies of exercise intervention in established NIDDM are less encouraging. Several investigations note an improvement in insulin sensitivity after exercise training, as demonstrated by reduced insulin and glucose concentrations after an oral glucose challenge,[101] increased insulin sensitivity during an euglycemic hyperinsulinemic clamp,[102] and a reduction in fasting hepatic glucose production.[103,104] However, these findings are not consistently found. In particular, improvement in fasting glucose, glucose tolerance after an oral load, and glycated hemoglobin levels often cannot be demonstrated after exertional training protocols.[105–107]

Pregnant Patients with NIDDM

A literature search identified no recent published trials of exercise training during pregnancy complicated by NIDDM in the English language literature. However, several conclusions may reasonably be inferred from studies of exercise intervention in IGT and NIDDM in nonpregnant individuals. First, exercise appears to confer its effects only so long as training is continued. This may preclude effective compliance among patients who have substantial obesity or are in late pregnancy. Second, the metabolic effects of training reported among nonpregnant individuals may be less likely during gestation when the glucose intolerance of NIDDM is reinforced by the diabetogenic effects of pregnancy. Third, effective reduction of fasting or postprandial glycemia has not been consistently demonstrated despite findings that exercise training improves several of the component metabolic defects known to contribute to NIDDM. This is especially important during pregnancy, when effective prevention

of macrosomia and other perinatal morbidities requires a much greater reduction of glucose (90 to 106 mg/dl) than that required in the nonpregnant patient. Consequently, exercise training in pregnancy complicated by NIDDM may serve more to reinforce compliance with diet and insulin therapy than to provide a direct effect on glycemic control or fetal growth.

Pregnant Patients with Gestational Diabetes

GDM has been defined as "carbohydrate intolerance of variable severity with onset or first recognition during pregnancy."[1] The hyperglycemia that identifies GDM usually remits during the puerperium. Despite the transient and less-marked hyperglycemia noted in GDM, abnormalities of insulin secretion and action that characterize NIDDM have also been identified in patients with GDM, including obesity, insulin resistance, and abnormal first-phase insulin release.[108] In addition, GDM is a strong predictor for later IGT or NIDDM, with the probability of subsequent development of clinical glucose intolerance within the next two decades in the range of 50 percent.[109] Consequently, GDM may be considered as an early clinical manifestation of NIDDM or IGT.

The therapeutic role of exercise in this disorder may be examined in two ways. First, exercise (along with dietary and pharmacologic intervention) may be effective in preventing progressive obesity and progressive IGT and NIDDM in the same way it has been applied in other clinical trials.[87] Because clinical studies have suggested greater therapeutic effect of exercise and diet modification in IGT than in NIDDM, intervention even earlier in the "natural history" of NIDDM may be hypothesized to be more efficacious. More relevant to the immediate clinical circumstances of the pregnancy complicated by glucose intolerance, the effect of exercise or dietary modification (or both) on maternal glucose (and other nutrient) homeostasis and the effect of combined diet and exercise intervention on the prevention of diabetic fetopathy have had only limited examination.

At least two randomized trials of exercise training in GDM have been published. The first included 41 subjects who, despite dietary therapy, had persistent fasting hyperglycemia of 105 to 140 mg/dl.[110] Enrollment occurred at 28 to 33 weeks' gestational age. Patients were stratified by age and obesity status before randomization. Control subjects were treated with insulin, and the exercise patients performed moderate, laboratory-observed cycle exercise three times weekly for the duration of pregnancy. Four of 21 exercise patients and 3 of 20 controls dropped out of the study and were not analyzed. Of the remainder, no differences in mean blood glucose values (94 ± 5 versus 19 ± 6 mg/dl, respectively) or birthweight (3,369 ± 534 versus 3,482 ± 502 g, respectively) were noted.

The second randomized trial compared 6 weeks of arm crank exercise ($n = 10$) to dietary therapy ($n = 9$) in previously untrained women with GDM, having fasting plasma glucose concentrations of 84 to 106 mg/dl.[111] Exertional heart rate was kept at less than 140 beats per minute, and exercise occurred three times weekly for approximately 20 minutes. In controls, fasting plasma glucose fell during the 6-week trial from 98 ± 13 to 88 ± 6 and the 1-hour post-50-g glucose challenge value fell from 226 ± 33 to 188 ± 13 mg/dl. A markedly improved glycemia occurred in the exercise group. Fasting plasma glucose fell during the 6-week trial from 100 ± 9 to 70 ± 7 and the 1-hour post-50-g glucose challenge value fell from 231 ± 29 to 106 ± 19 mg/dl. Because the exertional intensity and duration were relatively modest and the hand crank exertion did not require weight-bearing, the protocol might have applicability even among obese, sedentary women who characteristically have GDM. Significant effects of exercise on fasting glucose concentrations were noted after only 4 weeks of exercise, suggesting that if diagnostic testing and therapeutic intervention were to be started by 24 to 28 weeks, therapeutic effects of maternal exercise on fetal macrosomia might be found.

Exercise as a therapeutic intervention for fetal indications in GDM remains problematic, however. The preceding study enrolled only 19 subjects, whose motivation may have been uncharacteristic of most women with GDM. Laboratory-observed exercise is expensive and unwieldy for patients. Maintaining exercise compliance in home surroundings for sedentary, obese patients without prior exposure to exercise training for short-term protocols has not been shown to be successful in this type of patient as yet. Despite these concerns, introduction of these patients to dietary and exertional interventions during pregnancy, when health-directed motivation is high, may lay the foundation for later, chronic intervention to prevent subsequent IGT or NIDDM.

REFERENCES

1. Anonymous: Summary and recommendations of the Second International Workshop-Conference on Gestational Diabetes Mellitus. Diabetes, suppl. 2, 34:123, 1985
2. Astrand PO, Cuddy TE, Saltin B, Stenberg J: Cardiac output during submaximal and maximal work. J Appl Physiol 19:268, 1964
3. Karpman VL: Pumping function of the heart and blood flow in great vessels. p. 138. In: Cardiovascular System and Physical Exercise. CRC Press, Boca Raton, Fla. 1987
4. Horvath ES: Exercise in the treatment of NIDDM. Applications for GDM? Diabetes, suppl. 1, 40:33, 1979
5. Hohimer AR, Smith OA: Decreased renal blood flow in baboon during mild dynamic leg exercise. Am J Physiol 236:H141, 1979
6. Astrand PO, Rodahl K: Physical training. p. 420. In: Textbook of Work Physiology. 3rd Ed. McGraw Hill, New York, 1986
7. Peronnet F, Ferguson RI, Perrault H et al: Echocardiography and the athlete's heart. Phys Sport Med 9:102, 1981
8. Saltin B, Blomqvist B, Mitchell JH et al: Response to submaximal and maximal exercise after bed rest and training. Circulation, suppl. 5, 38:1, 1968
9. Felig P, Wahren J: Role of insulin and glucagon in the regulation of hepatic glucose production during exercise. Diabetes, suppl. 28:17, 1979
10. Vranic M, Kawamori R: Essential roles of insulin and glucagon in regulating glucose fluxes during exercise in dogs. Diabetes, suppl. 1, 28:45, 1978
11. Galbo H, Holst JJ, Christensen NJ: Glucagon and plasma catecholamine responses to graded and prolonged exercise in man. J Appl Physiol 38:70, 1975
12. Sahlin K, Katz A, Henriksson J: Redox state and lactate accumulation in human skeletal muscle during dynamic exercise. Biochem J 245:551, 1987
13. Linnarsson D: Dynamics of pulmonary gas exchange and heart rate changes at start and end of exercise. Acta Physiol Scand, suppl. 415:24, 1974
14. Fredholm BB: Inhibition of fatty acid release from adipose tissue by high arterial lactate concentration. Acta Physiol Scand, suppl. 330, 77A, 1969
15. Wahren J, Felig P, Ahlborg G, Jorfeldt L: Glucose metabolism during leg exercise in man. J Clin Invest 50:2715, 1971
16. Wahren J: Glucose turnover during exercise in healthy

men and in patients with diabetes mellitus. Diabetes 28:82, 1979

17. Calles J, Conningham JJ, Nelson L et al: Glucose turnover during recovery from intensive exercise. Diabetes 32:734, 1983

18. Katz A, Groberg S, Sahlin K, Wahren J: Leg glucose uptake during dynamic exercise in man. Am J Physiol 151: E65, 1986

19. Berger M, Hagg S, Ruderman NB: Glucose metabolism in perfused skeletal muscle. Interaction of insulin and exercise on glucose uptake. Biochem J 146:231, 1975

20. Richter EA, Mikines KJ, Galbo H, Kiens B: Effect of exercise in insulin action human skeletal muscle. J Appl Physiol 66:876, 1989

21. Mikines KJ, Sonne B, Tronier B, Galbo H: Effects of acute exercise and detraining on insulin action in trained men. J Appl Physiol 66:704, 1989

22. Devlin JT, Horton ES: Effects of prior high-intensity exercise on glucose metabolism in normal and insulin-resistant men. Diabetes 34:973, 1985

23. Oscai LB, Patterson JA, Bogard DL et al: Normalization of serum triglycerides and lipoprotein electrophoretic patterns by exercise. Am J Cardiol 30:775, 1981

24. Poehlman ET: A review: exercise and its influence on resting energy metabolism in man. Med Sci Sports Exerc 21:515, 1989

25. Tremblay A, Fontain E, Poehlman ET et al: The effect of exercise-training on resting metabolic rate in lean and moderately obese individuals. Int J Obes 10:511, 1986

26. Lennon D, Nagle F, Stratman F et al: Diet and exercise training effects on resting metabolic rate. Int J Obes 9: 39, 1984

27. Poehlman ET, Melby CL, Badylak SF, Calles J: Aerobic fitness and resting energy expenditure in young adult males. Metabolism 38:85, 1989

28. Burstein R, Polychronakos C, Toews CJ et al: Acute reversal of the enhanced insulin action in trained athletes. Diabetes 34:756, 1985

29. DeFronzo RA, Sherwin RS, Kraemer N: Effect of physical training on insulin action in obesity. Diabetes 36:1379, 1987

30. Wood D, Haskell WL, Plair SN et al: Increased exercise level and plasma lipoprotein concentrations: a one year randomized, controlled study in sedentary middle-aged men. Metabolism 32:31, 1983

31. Allison TH, Iammarino RM, Metz KF et al: Failure of exercise to increase high density lipoprotein cholesterol. J Cardiac Rehabil 1:257, 1981

32. Wynne TP, Frey MA, Laubach LL, Glueck CJ: Effect of a controlled exercise program on serum lipoprotein levels in women on oral contraceptives. Metabolism 29: 1267, 1980

33. Nadeay A, Rousseau-Migneron S, Tancrede G et al: Diminished glucagon response to epinephrine in physically trained diabetic rats. Diabetes 34:1278, 1985

34. Rubler S, Damani PM, Pinto ERL: Cardiac size and performance during pregnancy estimated with echocardiography. Am J Cardiol 40:534, 1977

35. Laird-Meeter K, van de Lay G, Bom TH et al: Cardiocirculatory adjustments during pregnancy: an echocardiographic study. Clin Cardiol 2:328, 1979

36. Capeless EL, Clapp JF: Cardiovascular change in early phase of pregnancy. Am J Obstet Gynecol 161:1449, 1989

37. Longo LD: Maternal blood volume and cardiac output during pregnancy: a hypothesis of endocrinologic control. Am J Physiol 245:R720, 1983

38. Hytten FE, Paintin DB: Increase in plasma volume during normal pregnancy. J Obstet Gynaecol Br Cp 70:402, 1963

39. Lund CJ, Donovan JC: Blood volume during pregnancy. Am J Obstet Gynecol 98:393, 1967

40. Clapp JF: Cardiac output and uterine blood flow in the pregnant ewe. Am J Obstet Gynecol 130:419, 1978

41. Carpenter MW, Sady SP, Sady MA et al: Effect of maternal weight gain during pregnancy on exercise performance. J Appl Physiol 68:1173, 1990

42. Ueland K, Novy MJ, Peterson EN, Metcalfe J: Maternal cardiovascular dynamics. Am J Obstet Gynecol 104:856, 1969

43. Knuttgen HG, Emerson K: Physiological response to pregnancy at rest and during exercise. J Appl Physiol 36:549, 1974

44. Sady SA, Carpenter MW, Thompson PD et al: Cardiovascular response to cycle exercise during and after pregnancy. J Appl Physiol 65:336, 1989

45. Pernoll ML, Metcalfe J, Schlenker TT et al: Oxygen consumption at rest and during exercise in pregnancy. Respir Physiol 25:285, 1975

46. Lehmann V, Regnat K: Untersuchung sur korperlighen Belastungsfahigkeit schwangeren Frauen. Der Einfluss standardisierter arbeit aur Herzkreislaumsystem, Ventilation, Gasaustausch, Kohlenhydratstoffwechsel und Saure-Basenhaushalt. Z Geburtshilfe Perinatol 180:279, 1976

47. Blackburn MW, Calloway DH: Heart rate and energy expenditure of pregnant and lactating women. Am J Clin Nutr 42:1161, 1985

48. Sady SA, Carpenter MW, Sady MA et al: Prediction of $\dot{V}O_2$max during cycle exercise in pregnant women. J Appl Physiol 65:657, 1988

49. Lotgering FK, Van Doorn MB, Struijk PC et al: Exercise responses in pregnant sheep: blood gases temperatures and fetal cardiovascular system. J Appl Physiol 55:834, 1983

50. Morton MJ, Paul MS, Campos GR et al: Exercise dynamics in late gestation. Effects of physical training. Am J Obstet Gynecol 159:91, 1985

51. Barron WM, Mujais SK, Zinaman M et al: Plasma catecholamine responses to physiologic stimuli in normal human pregnancy. Am J Obstet Gynecol 154:80, 1986

52. Artal R, Platt LD, Sperling M et al: Exercise in pregnancy. I. Maternal cardiovascular and metabolic responses in normal pregnancy. Am J Obstet Gynecol 140:123, 1981

53. Artal R, Wiswell R, Romeo Y: Hormonal responses to exercise in diabetic and nondiabetic pregnancy patients. Diabetes, suppl. 2, 34:7880, 1985

54. Christensen NJ, Garbo H, Hansen JF et al: Catecholamines and exercise. Diabetes suppl. 1, 28:58, 1979

55. Peronnet F, Beliveau L, Boudreau G et al: Regional plasma catecholamine removal and release at rest and exercise in dogs. Am J Physiol 254:R663, 1988

56. Rowell LB: Human Circulation. Regulation during Physical Stress. Oxford University Press, New York, 1986

57. Clapp JF: Acute exercise stress in the pregnant ewe. Am J Obstet Gynecol 136:489, 1980

58. Artal R, Paul RH, Romeo Y, Wiswel R: Fetal bradycardia induced by maternal exercise. Lancet 2:258, 1984

59. Jovanovic L, Kessler A, Peterson CM: Human maternal and fetal response to graded exercise. J Appl Physiol 58:1719, 1985

60. Artal R, Rutherford S, Romeo Y et al: Fetal heart rate responses to maternal exercise. Diabetes, suppl. 2, 34:78, 1985

61. Carpenter MW, Sady SP, Hoegsberg B et al: Fetal heart rate response to maternal exertion. JAMA 259:20, 1988

62. Lotgering FK, Van Doorn MB, Struijk PC et al: Maximal aerobic exercise in pregnant women: heart rate, O_2 consumption, CO_2 production and ventilation. J Appl Physiol 70:1016, 1991

63. Carpenter MW, Sady S, Haydon B et al: Maternal exercise duration and intensity affect fetal heart rate. American College of Sports Medicine annual meeting, Baltimore, 1989

64. Collings CMS, Curet LB: Fetal heart rate response to maternal exercise. Am J Obstet Gynecol 151:498, 1985

65. Carr SR, Carpenter MW, Terry R et al: Obstetrical Outcome in Aerobically Trained Women. Society for Perinatal Obstetricians, Orlando, FL, 1992

66. Clapp JF, Dickstein S: Endurance exercise and pregnancy outcome. Med Sci Sports Exerc 16:556, 1984

67. Clapp JF, Capeless EL: Neonatal morphometrics after endurance exercise during pregnancy. Am J Obstet Gynecol 163:1805, 1990

68. Clapp JF: The course of labor after endurance exercise during pregnancy. Am J Obstet Gynecol 163:1799, 1990

69. Dale E, Mullinax KM, Bryan D: Exercise during pregnancy: effects on the fetus. Can J Appl Sport Sci 7:98, 1982

70. Hall DC, Kaufmann DA: Effects of aerobic and strength conditioning on pregnancy outcomes. Am J Obstet Gynecol 157:1199, 1987

71. Kulpa PJ, White BM, Visscher R: Aerobic exercise in pregnancy. Am J Obstet Gynecol 156:1395, 1987

72. Vranic M, Horvath S, Wahren J: Exercise and diabetes: an overview. Diabetes, suppl. 1, 28:107, 1978

73. Allen FM, Stillman E, Fritz R: Total dietary regulation in the treatment of diabetes. p. 486. In: Exercise Monograph 11. Rockefeller Institute of Medical Research, New York, 1919

74. Hetzel KL, Long CNH: Metabolism of the diabetic individual during and after muscular exercise. Proc R Soc Lond [Biol] 99:279, 1926

75. Lawrence RD: The effects of exercise on insulin action in diabetes. BMJ 1:648, 1926

76. Joslin EP, Root HF, White P, Marble A: The Treatment of Diabetes Mellitus. 5th Ed. Lea & Febiger, Philadelphia, 1936

77. Marble A, Smith RM: Exercise in diabetes mellitus. Arch Intern Med 58:577, 1936

78. Baevre J, Sovik O, Wisness A et al: Metabolic responses to physical training in young insulin-dependent diabetics. Scand J Clin Lab Invest 45:109, 1985

79. Pruett EDR, Machlum S: Muscular exercise and metabolism in male juvenile diabetics. Scand J Clin Lab Invest 32:139, 1973

80. Kemmer FW, Berger M: Exercise in therapy and the life of diabetic patients. Clin Sci 67:279, 1984

81. Pettit DJ, Aleck KA, Baird RJ et al: Congenital susceptibility to NIDDM. Diabetes 37:622, 1988

82. Kissebah AH, Vydelingum N, Murray R et al: Relation of body fat distribution to metabolic complications of obesity. J Clin Endocrinol Metab 54:254, 1983

83. Ohlson LO, Larsson B, Svardsudd K et al: The influence of body fat distribution on the incidence of diabetes mellitus. Diabetes 34:1055, 1985

84. Saltin B, Lindegrade F, Houston R et al: Physical training and glucose tolerance in middle aged men with chemical diabetes. Diabetes, suppl. 1, 28:30, 1979

85. Eriksson KF, Lindgarde F: Prevention of type 2 (non-insulin-dependent) diabetes mellitus by diet and physical exercise. Diabetologia 34:891, 1991

86. Liljenquist JE, Mueller GL, Cherrington AD et al: Hyperglycemia per se (insulin and glucagon withdrawn) can inhibit hepatic glucose production in man. J Clin Endocrinol Metab 48:171, 1979

87. Sacca L, Hendler R, Sherwin RS: Hyperglycemia inhibits glucose production in man independent of changes in glucoregulatory hormones. J Clin Endocrinol Metab 47:1160, 1978

88. Kolterman OG, Gray RS, Grifin J et al: Receptor and postreceptor defects contribute to the insulin resistance in non-insulin-dependent diabetes mellitus. J Clin Invest 68:957, 1981

89. Revers RR, Fink R, Griffin J et al: Influence of hyperglycemia on insulin's in vivo effects in type II diabetes. J Clin Invest 73:664, 1984

90. Zinman B, Vranic M: Diabetes and exercise. Med Clin North Am 69:145, 1985

91. Berger M, Berchtold P, Cupper JH et al: Metabolic and hormonal effects of muscular exercise in juvenile type diabetics. Diabetologia 13:355, 1977

92. Lufkin G, Nelson R, Hill L et al: An analysis of diabetic pregnancies at Mayo Clinic, 1950–79. Diabetes Care 7:539, 1984

93. Lobue C, Goodin RC: Treatment of fetal distress during diabetic ketoacidosis. J Reprod Med 20:101, 1978

94. Zinman B, Murray FT, Vranic M et al: Glucoregulation during moderate exercise in insulin treated diabetes. J Clin Endocrinol Metab 45:641, 1977

95. Schiffrin A, Parikh S: Accommodating planned exercise in type I diabetic patients on intensive treatment. Diabetes Care 8:337, 1985

96. Hollingsworth DR, Moore TR: Postprandial walking exercise in pregnant insulin-dependent (type 1) diabetic women: reduction of plasma lipid levels but absence of a significant effect on glucemic control. Am J Obstet Gynecol 157:1359, 1987

97. Coustan DR, Reece EA, Sherwin RS et al: A randomized clinical trial of the insulin pump vs intensive conventional therapy in diabetic pregnancies. JAMA 255:631, 1986

98. Helmrich SP, Ragland DR, Leung RW, Paffenbarger RS: Physical activity and reduced occurrence of non-insulin dependent diabetes mellitus. N Engl J Med 325:147, 1991

99. Manson JE, Rimm EB, Stampfer MJ et al: Physical activity and incidence of non-insulin dependent diabetes mellitus in women. Lancet 338:774, 1991

100. Sartor G, Schersten B, Carlstrom S et al: Ten year follow-up of subjects with impaired glucose tolerance: prevention of diabetes by tolbutamide and diet regulation. Diabetes 29:41, 1980

101. Holloszy JO, Schultz J, Kusnierkiewicz H et al: Effects of exercise on glucose tolerance and insulin resistance. Acta Med Scand, suppl., 711:55, 1985

102. Reitman JS, Vasquez B, Klimes I, Nagulesparan M: Improvement of glucose of homeostasis after exercise training in non-insulin-dependent diabetes. Diabetes Care 7:434, 1984

103. Jenkins AB, Furler SM, Bruce DG, Chisholm DJ: Regulation of hepatic glucose output during moderate exercise in non-insulin-dependent diabetes. Metabolism 37:966, 1988

104. Segal KR, Edano A, Albu A et al: Effect of exercise training on insulin sensitivity and glucose metabolism in lean, obese and diabetic men. J App Physiol 71:2402, 1991

105. Kaplan RM, Hartwell SL, Wilson DK, Wallace JP: Effects of diet and exercise interventions on control and quality of life in non-insulin-dependent diabetes mellitus. Gen Intern Med 2:220, 1987

106. Ronemaa T, Mattila K, Lehtonen A, Kallio V: A controlled randomised study on the effect of long term physical exercise on the metabolic control in type 2 diabetic patients. Acta Med Scand 220:219, 1986

107. Wing RR, Epstein LH, Paternostro-Bayles M et al: Exercise in a behavioural weight control programme for obese patients with type 2 (non-insulin-dependent) diabetes. Diabetologia 31:902, 1988

108. Horton ES: Exercise in the treatment of NIDDM. Applications for GDM? Diabetes, suppl. 2, 40:175, 1991

109. O'Sullivan JB: Subsequent morbidity among gestational diabetic women. p. 174. In Sutherland HW, Stowers JM (eds): Carbohydrate Metabolism in Pregnancy and the Newborn. Churchill Livingstone, Edinburgh, 1984

110. Bung P, Artal R, Khodiguian N, Kjos S: Exercise in gestational diabetes: an optional therapeutic approach. Diabetes, suppl. 2, 40:182, 1991

111. Jovanovic-Peterson L, Durak EP, Peterson CM: Randomized trial of diet versus diet plus cardiovascular conditioning on glucose levels in gestational diabetes. Am J Obstet Gynecol 161:415, 1989

112. Carpenter MW, Sady SA: Exercise in pregnancy: effects on metabolism. p. 237. In Kowett RM (ed): Principles of Perinatal-Neonatal Metabolism. Springer-Verlag, New York, 1991

14

Prenatal Diagnosis and Management of Deviant Fetal Growth and Congenital Malformations

E. ALBERT REECE
ALAN M. FRIEDMAN
JOSHUA COPEL
CHARLES S. KLEINMAN

Despite improvement in perinatal morbidity and mortality in well-controlled diabetic pregnancies, problems related to abnormal fetal growth and congenital malformations persist. Most of the perinatal mortality in infants of diabetic mothers (IDM) is now attributed to congenital anomalies, whereas most of the perinatal morbidity is related to growth aberrations.

Ultrasound represents the only viable method that permits the identification of anomalies and the detection of aberrations in fetal growth. It is for this reason that the sonographic assessment of fetal development is so fundamental to the management of diabetic pregnancies.

NORMAL FETAL GROWTH ASSESSMENT

The need for early gestational dating in pregnancies complicated by diabetes is obvious because alterations in fetal growth are related to fetal age, and women with advanced diabetes are rarely permitted to go postterm. It has been demonstrated that 15 percent of patients with good clinical dates are more than 4 weeks

discrepant with ultrasound evaluation.[1] This problem is compounded in women with diabetes who tend to have oligoovulatory cycles, emphasizing the need for ultrasound validation of gestational age early in pregnancy when the technique is most accurate.

FIRST-TRIMESTER BIOMETRY

Traditionally, measurements of the crown-rump length (CRL) have been considered the most accurate method of gestational age estimation. As a single measurement, the CRL is one of the most precise dating methods (±4 to 7 days) until the 12th week of gestation, after which the measurement becomes less accurate because of variable degrees of fetal flexion. The CRL is obtained by measuring the long axis of the embryo (Fig. 14-1).

Pedersen and Molsted-Pederson[2] reported evidence that challenges the accuracy of CRL in dating diabetic pregnancies. Of 99 women with diabetes, 38 had embryos whose CRLs at 7 to 14 weeks were more than 6 days below the mean for gestation. Seven of these fetuses (27 percent) with "early growth delay" were later diagnosed as being anomalous. Although this observa-

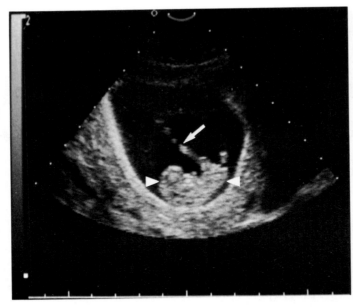

Fig. 14-1. Ultrasound scan of embryo demonstrating measurement of the crown-rump length (arrowheads). Note the umbilical cord (arrow).

tion is of significant interest in the understanding and, perhaps, identification of diabetes-related anomalies, it casts doubt on the accuracy of CRL in diabetic patients, because almost one in three nonanomalous embryos of women with diabetes had early growth delay. The patients in the Pedersen and Molsted-Pederson study had 28- to 30-day cycles before becoming pregnant; nevertheless, this did not preclude them from ovulating late in the conception cycle.

A subsequent study was reported by Keys et al[3] in patients whose date of conception was established either by basal body temperature chart or ovulation induction drugs. These authors found no evidence of growth delay. Cousins and colleagues[4] also performed longitudinal CRL measurements in 20 control pregnancies and 20 pregnancies complicated by diabetes. Like Keys et al, they found no differences between the two groups, including the growth of the two anomalous fetuses in the study. However, the Diabetes in Early Pregnancy Study[5] found small differences between fetuses with malformations as compared with those without malformations, but these differences did not attain statistical significance. Therefore, although a fetus growing in an abnormal metabolic milieu may be at increased risk of growth delay as well as malformation, based on current evidence the sonographic differences are unlikely to be clinically useful as a predictor of congenital malformations. Although this phenomenon is unresolved and controversial, early growth delay should be kept in mind when dating diabetic pregnancies in the first trimester.

SECOND-TRIMESTER BIOMETRY

Biparietal Diameter

When ultrasound was first used in obstetrics, one of the only fetal parameters that could be measured was the biparietal diameter (BPD) (Fig. 14-2). In fact, even after static B-mode images became possible to interpret, many authors thought that the BPD was the gold standard for gestational age estimation and should be measured from an A-mode image. Therefore, many nomograms of the BPD appeared in the literature. They are all reasonably accurate (± 7 to 10 days) through the 26th week of gestation. With the improvement of ultrasound imaging, many other measurements of fetal

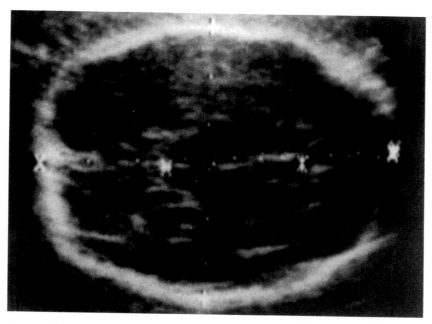

Fig. 14-2. Axial scan of the fetal head at the level of the thalami. This plane is used for obtaining the biparietal diameter, which is shown by the vertical calipers (**x**). (From Reece et al,[125] with permission.)

dimensions have been conducted, and nomograms of other fetal biometric parameters have been introduced.

Occipitofrontal Diameter

The occipitofrontal diameter (OFD) should be obtained in the same plane used for the BPD (Fig. 14-3). An axial plane of the head is obtained at 15 to 20 degrees from the horizontal plane. The thalami, septum cavum pellucidum, and the third ventricle are identifiable at that level. The distance from the mid-echogenic plane of the occipital bone to the mid-echogenic plane of the frontal bone is then measured. Although most ultrasound units have similar axial resolutions, they may vary in their lateral resolutions. The anteroposterior resolution is less than 2 mm in most ultrasound machines, whereas the degree of lateral resolution is generally greater and ranges from 3 to 5 mm.

The head circumference measurement can be calculated using both the short diameter (BPD) and the long diameter (OFD): (BPD + OFD)/2 × 3.14. It can also

be measured by tracing the sonographic image directly on the screen.

Transverse Cerebellar Diameter

Transverse cerebellar diameter (TCD) has become a standard measurement for evaluating the fetal head and somatic growth. The cerebellum is an intracranial structure located in the posterior fossa of the fetal head. Morphologically, it has a butterfly-like shape and is easy to identify sonographically.

Measurements of the TCD are independent of the fetal head and thus remain an accurate method of estimating gestational age. Because the posterior fossa is not affected by external pressure, measurements of the TCD should provide more precise information about fetal growth than other measurements of the bony fetal head. Furthermore, Reece et al[6] have reported that the TCD is not significantly affected by intrauterine growth retardation (IUGR), whereas Hill et al[7] found the TCD to remain relatively unchanged in macrosomic fetuses, and thus it is a useful marker of gestational age in pregnancies complicated by diabetes.

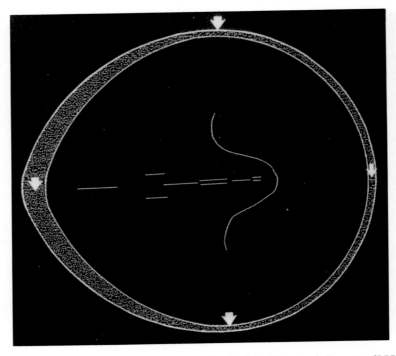

Fig. 14-3. Schematic representation of fetal head at the level of the biparietal diameter (BPD). Measurement of the BPD is performed by placing calipers at the leading edges of the skull table as shown by arrows at the top and bottom of diagram. Occipitofrontal diameter is measured by placing calipers as shown by the laterally placed arrows. (From Reece et al,[125] with permission.)

Abdominal Circumference

The abdominal circumference (AC) is a useful parameter with which to predict birthweight and for assessing fetal growth in the pregnancy complicated by diabetes (Fig. 14-4). Diabetes seems to preferentially affect the AC more than the BPD or long bone length, thus this measurement is particularly useful in identifying either macrosomic or growth-retarded fetuses. The fetal liver is the organ most affected by variations in fetal nutrition; thus, the level of the fetal liver should be chosen as the plane for the AC measurement.

Long Bones

Gestational age can also be estimated from measurements of the fetal long bones such as femur, humerus, tibia, and ulna. Length of the femur and other long bones show a correlation with gestational age approximating that obtained from the BPD. Hadlock et al[8] have

shown that combining biometric data results in a more accurate prediction of gestational age than using one measurement alone, provided outliers are excluded from this average.

Also, when dating pregnancies one must be aware of an occasional familial tendency toward large heads or short limbs that may alter the mean biometric estimate of gestational age. For example, if the BPD or femur length is out of synchrony with every other variable, it would be better to delete this outlier and average the clustered biometric data than to include all measurements in an overall estimation of gestational age.

DEVIANT FETAL GROWTH

The pregnancy complicated by diabetes is at significant risk of growth aberrations. Macrosomia is reported in approximately one-fourth of the offspring born to

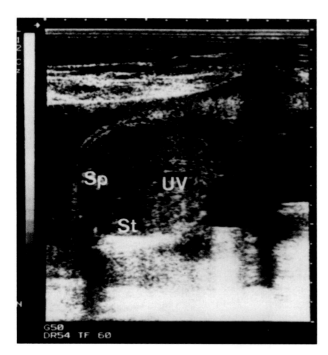

Fig. 14-4. Ultrasound scan showing fetal abdominal circumference. SP, spine; UV, umbilical vein; ST, stomach. (From Reece et al,[126] with permission.)

women with diabetes. Fetal macrosomia is believed to be related to maternal hyperglycemia, which induces fetal hyperglycemia and hyperinsulinemia. These infants are at greater risk of several perinatal complications. Conversely, it has also been demonstrated that women with diabetes are at increased risk of delivering a small-for-gestational-age infant. This form of deviant fetal growth has also been related to disturbances in maternal fuel metabolism. The risk of growth retardation increases with the severity of the mother's diabetic vascular state, and an association has been demonstrated between growth restriction and poor maternal renal function and hypertension.

Macrosomia

Macrosomia is generally defined as a fetal weight in excess of 4,000 g or a birthweight above the 90th percentile for gestational age. Fetuses weighing more than 4,000 g account for 10 percent of all deliveries, whereas fetal weight in excess of 4,500 g occurs in approximately 1 percent of pregnancies.[9,10] In pregnancies complicated by diabetes, the incidence of macrosomia has been reported to be in the range of 20 to 32 percent.[11,12]

The perinatal mortality rate is 0.49 percent and the perinatal morbidity rate is 11.4 percent in infants weighing more than 4,000 g.[12,13] Perinatal mortality rate, when birthweight exceeds 4,500 g, is five times that of nonmacrosomic pregnancies. In fact, most of the severe neonatal morbidity in IDMs results from the traumatic delivery of a macrosomic fetus. The principal causes of injury include shoulder dystocia, fractures, and neurologic damage.

The etiology of macrosomia is thought to be secondary to fetal hyperinsulinemia resulting from maternal hyperglycemia. The fetal pancreas is stimulated by elevated blood glucose to increase production of insulin. Pedersen et al[14] proposed that the concomitant presence of excessive substrate and insulin enhance fetal glycogen synthesis, lipogenesis, and protein synthesis. There are experimental data supporting insulin as the primary growth hormone. The etiopathology of macrosomia is discussed in detail in Chapter 5.

Fetuses of women with diabetes are at high risk of birth trauma not only because of their tendency toward macrosomia but also because of their disproportionately greater growth of the body compared with the head. In fact, increased weight of the insulin-sensitive tissues, including liver, pancreas, heart, lungs, and adrenals has been demonstrated in IDMs. Although patients delivering macrosomic babies often have a protracted labor, this is certainly not an invariable finding in diabetes. Progress in labor is more dependent on the size of the fetal head and the maternal pelvis and less on the size of the fetal body, assuming, of course, that the fetus is in a vertex presentation. Therefore, the diabetic woman whose fetus has head-to-body disproportion can have an apparently normal labor curve before presenting the physician with an impaired shoulder at delivery.

Prenatal Diagnosis

The only way to avoid the unenviable clinical dilemma of macrosomia is to be forewarned. Today with ultrasound, one can estimate fetal weight and, in a variety of ways, assess the relative size of the fetal body compared with the head. Investigators have attempted to identify the infant at risk of macrosomia by using a variety of sonographic parameters. Wladimiroff and associates[15] found that head/chest ratios predicted accelerated growth in 47 percent of large-for-gestational-age (LGA) infants. However, they found no difference between the nondiabetic and diabetic pregnancy. Other investigators have demonstrated greater sensitivity using the abdominal girth rather than the chest size for the prediction of the fetus with accelerated growth.

Tamura and colleagues[16] correlated BPD, head circumference, and AC percentile ranks to birthweight percentiles during the third trimester of pregnancy. Estimated fetal weights (EFW) calculated using Shepard's method[17] were also compared with actual birthweights. The authors found that AC values at the 90th percentile correctly predicted macrosomia in 78 percent of cases, whereas EFW above the 90th percentile predicted macrosomia in 74 percent of cases. However, the head circumference and BPD measurements were significantly less predictive of macrosomia.

Although no approach to the antenatal diagnosis of macrosomia has been 100 percent effective, it behooves the obstetrician to continue to attempt to identify at-risk infants because of the potential for trauma and other related morbidities. Serial ultrasound for EFW and AC should be performed every 4 to 6 weeks. Other biometric parameters useful in the evaluation of fetuses at risk for macrosomia are shown below.

Biparietal Diameter Versus Abdominal Circumference

Ogata and co-workers[18] found that the serial growth of the BPD in fetuses of diabetic women followed the mean for gestation. Not surprisingly, the AC followed two patterns: one conformed to the mean, and the other followed a pattern of "somatic growth acceleration." Those exhibiting accelerated AC growth had substantially more subcutaneous fat as demonstrated by skin fold measurements at birth.

It is clear that BPD alone is a poor predictor of macrosomia, with a sensitivity rate of 47 percent. However, when combined with abdominal circumference and other parameters, the sensitivity increases as demonstrated in Table 14-1.

Head Versus Chest Dimensions

Elliott et al[19] developed a "macrosomic index" based on BPD and an average chest diameter taken at a level just below the heart. The BPD was subtracted from the average of the anteroposterior and transverse diameters of the chest. Eighty-seven percent of macrosomic fetuses had a difference in diameters of greater than 1.4 cm. Conversely, 92 percent of those weighing less than 4,000 g had a macrosomic index of 1.3 cm or less.

This technique represents a very clever way to identify head-to-body disproportion. The chest diameters, however, can be deceptively difficult to measure because the thoracic margins are often not discrete.

Wladimiroff et al[15] used only a minor modification of the above principle in evaluating 30 macrosomic fetuses and 43 fetuses of appropriate weight. Instead of reducing the two diameters of the chest to an average diameter, they calculated this area by adding an additional transverse thoracic plane. To compare chest area to a similar value derived from the cranium, the authors elected to use the square of the BPD. Even though this measurement is not precisely predictive of the head area because the fetal head is elliptic, the results were strikingly similar to those of others. In 93 percent of macrosomic cases, the BPD was greater than the 95th percentile, compared with the expected 5 percent for normal fetuses.

Another variation on the head-to-body disproportion theme is the use of a diameter or circumference measurement made at the level of the umbilical portion of the portal vein. We are more predisposed to this measurement because

1. The edges of the abdomen are more easily identified than the chest
2. The bifurcation of the portal vein is an easily reproducible landmark
3. The measurement is made at the level of the liver, an organ that is particularly insulin-sensitive and, therefore, the most dramatically affected by diabetes-related macrosomia

Yarkoni and colleagues[20] positively correlated abnormal glucose tolerance tests with abnormal BPD/abdominal diameter (AD) ratio. The Campbell and Thoms[21] head circumference (BPD + OFD × 1.57) to AC (AD_1 + AD_2 × 1.57) ratio may be extremely

Table 14-1. Diagnosis of Macrosomia by Ultrasound

Investigations	No. of Patients	Parameters Measured	Criteria	Sensitivity (%)	Specificity (%)	PV + (%)	PV − (%)
Wladimiroff, 1978	30	BPD Fetal chart area	>90 percentile BW	47	95		
Elliott, 1982	23	Chest diameter-BPD	>4,000 g	87		61	
Bracero, 1985	50	BPD, AD, FL AD/FL AD/BPD	>90 percentile BW	79 83	80 60	83 71	76 75
Tamura, 1986	67	AC, EFW	>90 percentile BW	71	71	88	89
Rossavik, 1986	21	Multiple	>90 percentile BW	81	85		
Benson, 1987	20	BPD, FL, AD, AC	>4,000 g	77	84		
Bochner, 1987	41	AC (30–33 wk)	>90th percentile BW	88	83	56	96
Miller, 1988	58	BPD, FL, AC, EFW	≥4,000 g	24–53	94–98	52–71	88–92
Benacerraf, 1988	324	BPD, OFD, AD, EFW	≥4,000 g	65	90		
Landon, 1989	32	BPD, HC, AC, FL, EFW	≥90th percentile	58–84	75–85	68–79	75–89
Chervenak, 1989	81	BPD, FL, AC, EFW	>4,000 g	61	91	70	87

Abbreviations: PV +, predictive value, positive; PV −, predictive value, negative; BPD, biparietal diameter; AD, abdominal diameter; FL, femur length; AC, abdominal circumference; EFW, estimated fetal weight; OFD, occipitofrontal diameter; BW, birthweight. (From Tamura,[122] with permission.)

useful in identifying fetal macrosomia. This is a very promising method for prenatal assessment of fetal macrosomia and potential obstructed labor.

Other Useful Biometric Measurements

In a previous report,[22] the clavicular length was found to be highly correlated with gestational age in the second trimester. The enthusiasm regarding the potential of the clavicular length measurement being more accurate in predicting shoulder dystocia was dampened by our inability to consistently image the clavicle at term because of acoustic shadowing by other structures. Nevertheless, the measurement may be worth attempting in fetuses who are in optimal positions such as the occiput posterior position.

Management and Outcome

Obviously, the optimal management approach for macrosomia is prevention. Indeed, studies have demonstrated a direct relationship between blood glucose levels and birthweights. Therefore, the management goal of all pregnancies complicated by diabetes is maternal euglycemia. However, exactly what threshold of glycemia should be targeted to prevent macrosomia is uncertain. Langer et al[23] found that the incidence of LGA was reduced to a range of 1.4 to 9 percent when

normoglycemia was achieved. Several recent studies[24–26] indicate fetal macrosomia is related to elevated postprandial glucose levels but not to the fasting blood glucose level. Therefore, it is recommended that postprandial blood glucose levels be routinely measured and used as the "yardstick" by which to base therapy and insulin adjustments. For women with gestational diabetes, some investigators have studied the use of prophylactic insulin to prevent macrosomia.[27–29] Most of these trials have demonstrated that prophylactic insulin therapy can, in fact, reduce the incidence of macrosomia as well as other associated perinatal morbidities.

Because maternal glucose levels do not discriminate well between pregnancies at high and low risk of excessive fetal growth, Buchanan and colleagues[30] used ultrasound measurements of the fetal AC to identify infants at high risk of macrosomia. They demonstrated that maternal insulin therapy reduced the excessive fetal growth and adiposity. Their findings support the hypothesis that insulin-treatable factors other than maternal glycemia are important determinants of the risk of aberrant growth in pregnancies complicated by diabetes.

However, if severe macrosomia (>4,500 g) develops, it would seem judicious that a cesarean section should be performed to prevent shoulder dystocia and birth trauma. Management should be individualized for patients with EFWs between 4,000 and 4,500 g. The decision regarding delivery mode should be based on the size of the woman's pelvis, the progress of labor, and the woman's obstetric history. There are also long-term risks associated with macrosomia. There is mounting evidence to suggest that macrosomic infants are more prone to become or remain obese as they age.[31,32] In addition, IDMs are also at a far greater risk of developing diabetes than the general population.[32] It is worth noting that data on adverse outcomes relate to actual birthweight rather than estimated weight and that actual birthweight is always a retrospective diagnosis.

INTRAUTERINE GROWTH RETARDATION

Some women with class F-R diabetes having "end organ" disease that involves the placenta will deliver infants whose birthweights are less than the 10th percentile of mean weight for gestations. These infants are subject to the same increase in perinatal morbidity and mortality as growth-retarded infants of nondiabetic mothers.

Prenatal Diagnosis

A myriad of papers and chapters have been devoted to the diagnosis of IUGR, and therefore, it is not the aim of this chapter to discuss these methods in detail. The BPD and the AC obtained at the level of the umbilical vein can be used to estimate and to diagnose IUGR if such measurements are less than the 10th percentile or more than 2 standard deviations (SD) below the mean. Other sonographic methods include the trunk circumference at the level of the portal branch of the ductus venosus, head/body ratio, hourly fetal urine production rate, and semiquantitative estimation of amniotic fluid volume. All these parameters have been used as diagnostic indices for IUGR with varying degrees of accuracy[33] (Table 14-2).

Head/body ratios are useful in distinguishing symmetric from asymmetric IUGR.[21] Measurements of thigh circumference are useful in indirectly evaluating the degree of deprivation in small-for-dates fetuses.[34] With some ultrasound equipment, it is even possible

Table 14-2. Identification of Small- and Appropriate-for-Gestational-Age Fetuses ($n = 292$) With Ultrasound Within 10 Days of Delivery[a]

Statistics	Parameter (%)					
	BPD	AC	FL	FL/AC	PI	EFW
Sensitivity	73	97	45	55	53	66
Specificity	70	60	98	74	70	94
Predictive value of						
Positive results[b]	51 (21)	51 (21)	89 (64)	48 (20)	44 (18)	88 (65)
Negative results[b]	86 (96)	97 (99)	81 (94)	79 (94)	78 (92)	87 (96)
Prevalence	43	43	43	43	43	43

Abbreviations: BPD, biparietal diameter; AC, abdominal circumference; FL, femur length; PI, ponderal index; EFW, estimated fetal weight.
[a] Prenatal intrauterine growth retardation (IUGR): BPD, AC, FL, and EFW <10th percentile; FL/AC <0.24; PI <2.2; postnatal IUGR: birthweight <10th percentile.
[b] Values in parentheses are those calculated assuming a prevalence of 10 percent.
(From Deter and Harrist,[123] with permission.)

to delineate a diminished layer of subcutaneous abdominal fat in small-for-dates fetuses. A major source of frustration, however, has been the lack of precise gestational age data and, thus, one's inability to differentiate between fetuses who are truly growth retarded from those who are constitutionally small or appropriately grown with inaccurate dates.

Goldstein et al[35] have shown that the TCD is correlated with gestational age. Furthermore, Reece et al[6] reported that in a group of growth-retarded fetuses, the TCD was normal, correlating with the gestational age and, thus, not significantly affected by the growth retardation process. This biometric parameter may prove to be a useful standard against which deviation in growth may be compared.

Doppler

Pulsed Doppler is now being investigated as a means to assess blood flow in the uterine artery and in various parts of the fetal circulatory system. The early results have strongly supported the potential of this method being able to identify the small-for-dates fetus who is hypoxic or nutritionally deprived.[36] Doppler studies attempting to identify fetuses affected by IUGR have

Table 14-3. Comparison of Standard Diagnostic Tests in Prediction of Small-for-Gestational-Age Neonates (Prevalence: 50.0%)

	MCA (%)	UA (%)	Cerebral/Umbilical Ratio (%)
Sensitivity	11.1	40.0	40.0
Specificity	97.7	91.1	100.0
Positive predictive value	83.3	81.8	100.0
Negative predictive value	52.3	60.2	62.5
Accuracy	54.4	65.5	70.0

Abbreviations: MCA, middle cerebral artery; UA, umbilical artery. (From Gramellini et al,[124] with permission.)

not been shown to significantly improve the positive and negative predictive values obtained by standard biometric parameters[37] (Table 14-3).

In IUGR fetuses, there is a decrease in resistance in the cerebral vessels, resulting in an increase in the diastolic component of the middle cerebral artery waveform. This causes a decrease in the pulsatility index (PI), systolic/diastolic (S/D) ratio, and the resistance index (RI). The umbilical artery, which indirectly reflects the status of the placental circulation, will initially display an increased PI, S/D ratio, and RI in the face of fetal compromise followed by an absent or reverse end-diastolic flow. It appears that in the sequence of progressive hypoxia in growth-retarded fetuses, the umbilical artery waveform indices rise to greater than the 95th confidence levels before fetal heart rate monitoring, fetal movement, and breathing are affected. Usually by the time there is absent diastolic flow, other clinical parameters become abnormal. Therefore, Doppler ultrasound is useful as a means of corroborating other diagnostic tests but does not appear superior to current biometric parameters in predicting or detecting growth restrictions.

Management and Outcome

The prognosis for future growth and development for any neonate whose birthweight is less than the 10th percentile for gestational age depends on the physiologic significance of the associated cause. Infants who are small-for-gestational age on a constitutional basis enjoy a good prognosis, although there appears to be an increase in perinatal mortality, even in this group.

The long-term outcome is most significantly influenced by the etiologic basis for the IUGR. An infant whose birthweight is less than the 10th percentile for gestational age on a deprivational basis should also enjoy a good prognosis if delivery occurs without perinatal asphyxia.

In general, symmetric IUGR is likely to be followed by slow growth after birth, whereas infants with asymmetric IUGR are more likely to achieve normal growth patterns after birth. However, if the length of the fetus is also affected, the infant is likely to remain small.[38]

CONGENITAL MALFORMATIONS

The frequency of congenital anomalies among diabetic offspring at birth is estimated at 3 to 6 percent. If one assumes a 27 per 1,000 incidence of major anomalies in the overall population,[39] this represents at least a doubling of the risk of anomalies. Women with gestational diabetes do not seem to have the same tendency for anomalous offspring as women with insulin-dependent diabetes. This is not surprising because the poorer the diabetic control during organogenesis, the greater the chance of congenital anomalies. This concept has been supported by both clinical and laboratory studies. In one study,[40] if hemoglobin A_{1c} (HbA_{1c}) levels were greater than 8.5 percent, there was a 22.5 percent incidence of fetal anomalies; between 7.0 and 8.5 percent, anomalies occurred in 5.1 percent of pregnancies; and less than 6.9 percent, no anomalies were observed. The concept of high blood glucose in the first trimester being teratogenic is further supported by experimental evidence in the in vitro rat model and in vivo animal data.[41] Furthermore, there is encouraging information emanating from several large clinical studies that suggests that strict glucose control before and immediately after conception will decrease the incidence of congenital anomalies[42-45] (Table 14-4).

Obviously, prenatal diagnosis by ultrasound will have no effect on the incidence of anomalies in the offspring of women with diabetes, but it can appreciably affect how a pregnancy is managed. Women with diabetes are generally aware of their increased likelihood to deliver anomalous infants, and a normal ultrasound examination often allays their fear. Furthermore, the ability to perform prenatal diagnosis early in the pregnancy provides the option for early termina-

Table 14-4. Clinical Studies Showing Correlation Between Maternal Glycemic Control and Malformation Rate

Investigator	Control Group			Study Group		
	No. of Patients	Malformation Rate (%)	Glucose Control	No. of Patients	Malformation Rate (%)	Glucose Control
Pedersen and Pederson-Molsted[118] (1979)	284	14.1	Inadequate	363	7.4	Improved
Miller et al[40] (1981)	58	22.4	HbA$_{1c}$ ≥8.5%	58	3.4	HbA$_{1c}$ <8.5%
Fuhrmann et al[42] (1983)	128	7.5	Mean daily plasma glucose ≤110 mg/dl in 20.7% of the patients	292	0.8	Mean daily plasma glucose ≤110 mg/dl in 88.3% of patients
Fuhrmann et al[119] (1984)	144	6.2	87.1% blood glucose reading between 2.3–7.7 mmol/L achieved by only 9.79 of the patients	56	1.7	87% blood glucose reading between 2.3–7.7 mmol/L achieved in patients
Goldman et al[44] (1986)	31	9.6	HbA$_{1c}$ ≥10.4 ± 0.471	44	0	HbA$_{1c}$ ≤7.39 ± 0.49
Kitzmiller et al[120] (1986)	53	15.1	HbA$_{1c}$ <9% in 47% of patients	46	2.2	HbA$_{1c}$ <9% in 87% of patients
Steel[121] (1988)	65	9.2		78	3.9	
Kitzmiller et al[43] (1991)	110	25	HbA$_{1c}$ >10.6	84	1.69	HbA$_{1c}$ <7.9

Abbreviation: HbA$_{1c}$, hemoglobin A$_{1c}$.

tion of pregnancy. Last, some fetuses with spina bifida, gastrointestinal anomalies, cardiac defects, or obstructive uropathy can benefit greatly from information provided by ultrasound that will allow alteration in obstetric management to optimize the fetal outcome.

CENTRAL NERVOUS SYSTEM ANOMALIES

Anencephaly

Anencephaly is the most common anomaly affecting the central nervous system. Its incidence is increased by 0.57 percent in the diabetic pregnancy, which represents a threefold increase over the general population.[46,47]

Anencephaly results from a failure of the neural tube to close completely at the cranial pole during fusion of the neural folds to form the forebrain. This occurs between the second and third week of development. The cerebral hemispheres are usually absent, whereas the brain stem and portions of the midbrain are usually present. Absence of the cranial vault is a constant finding, although portions of cranial bones may be present (Figs. 14-5 and 14-6).

Associated anomalies include spina bifida, cleft lip or palate, clubfoot, and omphalocele. Other characteristic features are a short neck, large tongue, and bulging eyes.

Prenatal Diagnosis

The sonographic diagnosis is usually possible by the 15th week of gestation because of the presence of poorly formed cranial bones and the symmetric absence of the calvarium.[48] Polyhydramnios is frequently associated with anencephaly occurring in approximately 40 to 50 percent of cases.[49] Sonographic evaluation is often elected because of an elevated α-fetoprotein.

Management and Outcome

Termination of pregnancy should be offered to patients carrying anencephalic fetuses, as this condition is unequivocally incomparable with life.

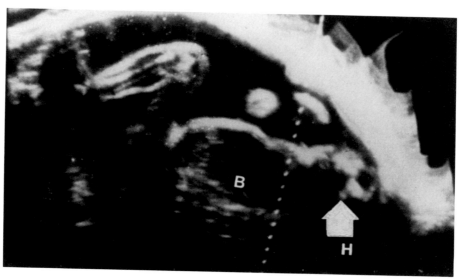

Fig. 14-5. Anencephalic fetus. Poorly visualized cranial bones (arrow) are diagnostic of this condition. B, body; H, head. (From Reece and Hobbins,[112] with permission.)

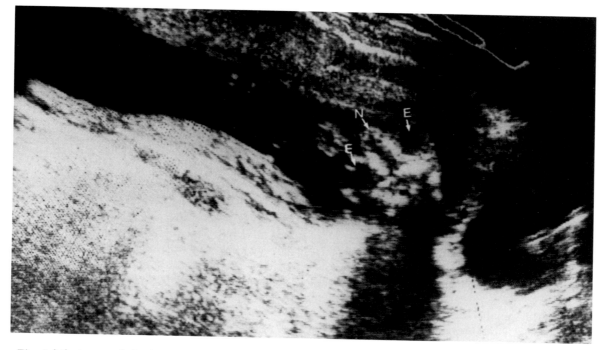

Fig. 14-6. Anencephalic fetus. Facial structures can be seen (arrows), but calvarium is absent. N, nose; E, eyes. (From Reece and Hobbins,[112] with permission.)

Spina Bifida

Fetuses of women with diabetes have been reported to have an impressively higher incidence of neural tube defects (NTD) than the general population (19.5 per 1,000 versus 1 to 2 per 1,000).[50] In view of this tendency, all women with diabetes should be offered maternal serum α-fetoprotein (MSAFP) screening and careful ultrasound examination of the fetal head and spine. Two studies have shown that median MSAFP levels are lower per gestational age in women with diabetes than in women without.[50,51] Although this has been attributed to a greater tendency toward the early growth delay mentioned previously, fetal size in the second trimester (when MSAFP screening is now advocated) has been demonstrated to be different in women with diabetes compared with women without diabetes.

Prenatal Diagnosis

Our ability to diagnose NTD in the antenatal period has dramatically improved as a result of the use of MSAFP screening, amniotic fluid α-fetoprotein, and N-acetylcholinesterase determination combined with ultrasound imaging.

An elevated level of MSAFP is usually the first clue alerting the obstetrician to the possibility of a NTD. A thorough ultrasound examination of the spine is best performed in these circumstances by an operator who has considerable experience in this type of evaluation. Although the positive predictive accuracy of the ultrasound diagnosis of a NTD is high, the negative predictive accuracy is not as reliable. Therefore, management of women with an elevated MSAFP and normal ultrasound should include amniocentesis for amniotic fluid α-fetoprotein and N-acetylcholinesterase determinations for a definitive diagnosis.

A detailed examination of the spine can often prove a formidable task when the fetus is very active or in a less than suitable position. In the coronal plane, the fetal spine appears as three parallel lines, with the additional third line representing the body of the vertebrae. In the transverse plane, the neural canal appears as a closed circle. This canal is lined anteriorly by the ossified vertebral body and posteriorly by the ossified vertebral laminae. Both pedicles and the spinal body comprise the only three ossification centers of the vertebra present in the second trimester, and all three can be easily visualized on ultrasound examination. In the vast majority of cases of open spina bifida, there is "splaying" of the laminae (Fig. 14-7), which creates a picture of a V-shaped spinal configuration on transverse scan or of a divergence in the normally parallel echogenic lines on longitudinal scan in the area of the defect (Fig. 14-8). Perhaps the most important step in the evaluation of the trunk is to demonstrate the integrity of the skin over the spine with a series of transverse and longitudinal scans. If the fetus is against the uterine wall, the sonologist should maneuver the fetus in such a way as to create a pocket of fluid next to the fetal spine to enhance visualization. The fetal cranium can also provide useful indirect information about the spine. In Arnold-Chiari malformations accompanying spina bifida, there is downward traction of the lower midbrain toward or through the foramen magnum. This phenomenon affects the intracranial architecture in a variety of ways:

1. The cerebellar hemispheres become deviated caudally to a point that the transcerebellar diameter is markedly reduced or not measurable at the usual level[52,53]
2. The cisterna magna is obliterated by the herniated brain structures[52] (Fig. 14-9)
3. The lateral ventricles will generally become dilated[52,53]
4. There is a subtle indentation in the frontal skull outline, probably produced by alterations in intracranial pressures. Because this "lemon-like" configuration has only recently been described, it is yet unclear whether this is only a second-trimester phenomenon[53] (Fig. 14-10)

Management and Outcome

If the diagnosis of spina bifida is made before the period of viability, the parents should be offered the option of terminating the pregnancy. In continuing pregnancies, the ideal route of delivery has never been scientifically proved, but because vaginal delivery might cause trauma to the exposed neural elements, it is often avoided.

Parents need to be counseled that the recurrence risk of spina bifida is about 2 percent with one affected sibling and increases to 5.7 to 12 percent if there are two affected siblings.[54]

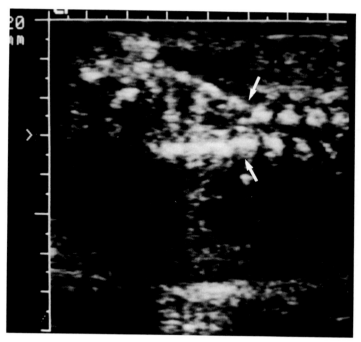

Fig. 14-7. Longitudinal scan of the fetal spinal column depicting the "splaying" or divergence of the vertebral (arrows) suggestive of a neural tube defect.

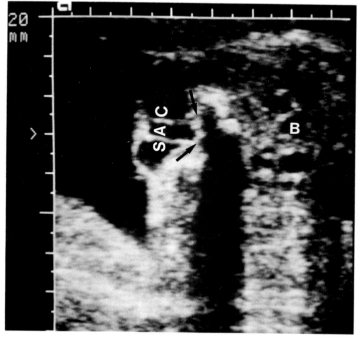

Fig. 14-8. Transverse scan of the fetal spinal column depicting the open neural tube defects (arrows) with a herniated sac (SAC). Dilated loops of bowel can be seen inferior to the defect (B).

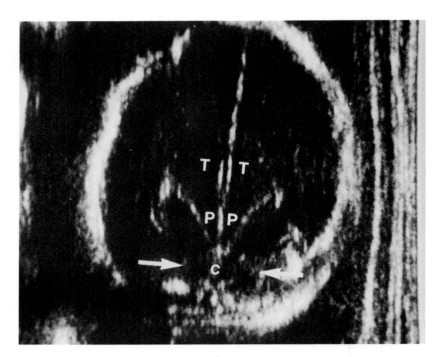

Fig. 14-9. Transverse section of the fetal head at a level slightly below the thalami (T). At this level, the cerebellar peduncles (P) and the cerebellum (C) can be seen. Note the small cerebellum (C) in a fetus with spina bifida and the obliteration of the cisterna magna, which would be seen as an echolucent area inferior to the cerebellum.

Microcephaly

Naeye[55] has reported an increased incidence in IDMs of this relatively rare problem, which ordinarily affects only 1 in 6,200 infants. Microcephaly is defined in the pediatric literature as a head circumference that is more than 3 SD less than the mean for gestation.

Prenatal Diagnosis

The diagnosis can be suspected in utero when the BPD is discrepant by more than 5 weeks from dates. A series by Chervenak et al[56] found that a BPD smaller than 3 SD below the mean was normal in 44 percent of cases. The authors attributed the high incidence of false-positive results to normal variations in fetal head width. Therefore, to diagnose microcephaly, it is necessary to measure the head circumference in relation to other biometric parameters such as fetal bone length and head/body ratio.

Goldstein et al[35] recently assessed the predictive value of a measurement of the frontal portion of the cranium between the cavum septum pellucidum and the inner table of the skull (along the midline) in the diagnosis of microcephaly. In fetuses who are truly microcephalic, the frontal portion of the brain is affected most. These authors developed normative data for the anterior cranial fossa and the frontal lobe of the fetal brain against which fetuses suspected of having microcephaly or any other lesion affecting the anterior fossa could be evaluated. Their preliminary findings indicate that the use of frontal lobe measurements may be more precise than conventional measurements for diagnosing microcephaly.

Management and Outcome

Fetal karyotype and a detailed ultrasound evaluation should be performed if microcephaly is noted. Although the option of termination of pregnancy can be offered if the diagnosis is made before viability, one has to be exceedingly cautious due to the high false-

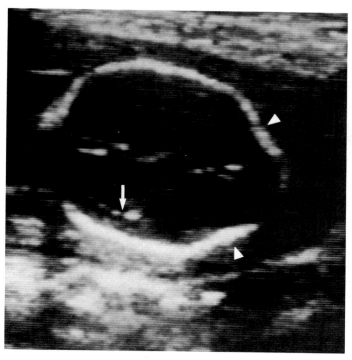

Fig. 14-10. Transverse section of the fetal head at the level of the lateral ventricle. Note the dilated ventricle with the lateral wall of the lateral ventricle approaching the skull table (arrow). The indentation of the skull outline depicts the so-called lemon sign (arrowheads).

positive rate. If the head circumference is between 2 and 3 SD below the mean, most fetuses will be normal; between 3 and 5 SD, the false-positive rate can still be high; beyond 5 SD, the diagnostic accuracy increases. Expectant management is the recommended approach if the diagnosis is made after viability.

Microcephaly is an untreatable condition with a high risk of significant retardation.

CARDIAC ABNORMALITIES

Defects of the cardiovascular system are among the most commonly encountered malformations in the IDM and occur much more frequently in these patients than in infants born to women with normal carbohydrate metabolism.[57,58] Congenital heart disease occurs in approximately 8 in 1,000 births in the general population.[59,60] The frequency with which cardiac anomalies are found among IDMs (1 of 25),[61] coupled with

the relative frequency with which diabetes is encountered in the gravid population, accounts for the interest that fetal cardiologists have had in the pregnant diabetic woman.

Over the past two decades, we have developed an aggressive detection program for fetal cardiovascular disease, largely based on the use of fetal echocardiographic screening of pregnancies particularly "at risk" of fetal congenital heart disease. The goal of our program is the detection and management of structural and functional heart disease in this population. Risk factors for fetal heart disease can be stratified based on fetal, maternal, or familial factors. Among the most prominent maternal risk factors is pre-existing diabetes mellitus.[62,63]

Fetal echocardiography is the primary diagnostic tool used to assess fetal cardiac structure. We believe that there is great practical application for such studies in the evaluation of the fetus of the woman with diabetes mellitus. With current technology, accurate assessment of cardiovascular structure can be obtained with two-dimensional real-time analysis. Pulsed- and continuous-wave Doppler can be used to evaluate intra- and extracardiac flow qualitatively and quantitatively. Qualitative evaluation of diastolic ventricular filling waveforms, for example, may provide important insights into diastolic ventricular compliance. The advent of Doppler color flow mapping has provided information for the qualitative assessment of cardiovascular flow patterns in both the normal and malformed heart.

Two distinct abnormalities of cardiovascular growth and development have been described, based on the timing of abnormal maternal glucose metabolism and fetal endocrine pancreatic activity. When maternal and embryonic/fetal hyperglycemia exist during first-trimester organogenesis, such may be associated with embryopathy resulting in complex structural cardiac malformations. These abnormalities often affect the formation of the cardiac loop, ventricular septation, and migration of the conotruncus and imply a teratogenic exposure between the 21st and 45th days after conception. Alternatively, when maternal hyperglycemia occurs during the third trimester, long after cardiovascular structural formation is complete, there is an increased risk of myocardial hypertrophy related to fetal hyperinsulinemia, which, when severe, can result in diminished cardiac output.

Diabetic Control and Structural Malformation of the Heart

The relationship between maternal metabolic control and an associated cardiac embryopathy has been well described. In general, it is agreed that the more normal the maternal metabolic environment, the lower the incidence of all congenital malformations, including those of the cardiovascular system.[64] By contrast, poor maternal glycemic control has been strongly associated with structural malformations of IDMs.[65–68] Mills et al[69] followed 626 pregnant diabetic women, prospectively dividing them into groups according to the time of entry into the study. There were 347 pregnant diabetic and 389 control nondiabetic women who entered the study within 21 days of conception, and 279 diabetic women who entered later than 21 days after conception. There was an increased fetal malformation rate among the early entry group when compared with the controls, and a significantly higher malformation rate among the late entry group when compared with the early entry group. There was no significant difference in mean blood glucose and glycosylated hemoglobin levels during organogenesis between women whose infants were malformed and those whose infants were not.[69] Their findings suggest the importance of good metabolic control before and immediately after conception, although the optimal level of control necessary to prevent malformations is not yet clear.

Miller et al[65] reported a significant increase in the frequency of congenital malformations in IDM whose first-trimester HbA$_{1c}$ level was in excess of 8.5 percent. Shields et al[70] evaluated diabetic pregnant women who had initial HbA$_{1c}$ levels at 8.5 percent or more and found that there was no critical level that optimally screened for congenital heart disease. However, no cases of congenital heart disease were found in patients with normal first-trimester HbA$_{1c}$ values, leading the authors to conclude that all patients with an initial HbA$_{1c}$ greater than the normal upper limit of 6.1 percent should undergo a complete and thorough fetal echocardiographic examination.[70] Our policy at the Yale Fetal Cardiovascular Center is to recommend fetal echocardiography to all gravid diabetic women regardless of the degree of metabolic control achieved in the first trimester.

Abnormalities of Cardiac Structure

Many different forms of structural cardiac abnormalities have been reported in IDMs. White[71] reported a 1 percent incidence of congenital anomalies, the most common of which were ventricular septal defects (VSD), in a population of 2,147 diabetic pregnancies followed at the Joslin Clinic during the 50 years from 1924 to 1974. Rowland et al[61] found congenital heart disease in 19 of 470 IDMs, an incidence of 4 percent, five times that of the general population.[60] Approximately one-half of these cases consisted of either transposition of the great arteries, VSD, or aortic coarctation.[61]

More recently, Ferencz et al[57] retrospectively evaluated the prevalence of congenital heart disease in IDMs from the Baltimore-Washington Infant Study, a population-based, case-control investigation of cardiovascular malformations. Their database consisted of 2,259 mothers of infants born with congenital heart disease. Diabetes mellitus was present before pregnancy in 1.5

percent, and among these women, there was an association with the occurrence of double-outlet right ventricle (DORV), truncus arteriosus, tetralogy of Fallot (TOF), and VSD.[57] These results differ somewhat from those reported in earlier work, where VSD and transposition of the great arteries (TGA) were associated with maternal diabetes mellitus.[61] Interestingly, TGA was seen in the Ferencz study[57] but in numbers just below what was considered significant. As Ferencz discussed,[57] earlier studies may have classified hearts with DORV and d-malposition of the aorta, as in the Taussig-Bing malformation, as "transposition" hearts, thereby falsely increasing the apparent prevalence of transposition, while underestimating the prevalence of DORV in the fetus of the diabetic gravid woman.

Perhaps the most cogent theory put forward to explain the increased prevalence of DORV, truncus arteriosus, and TOF in the fetus of the diabetic mother focuses on the formation of the conotruncus. Truncus arteriosis, DORV, and TOF result from abnormalities of conotruncal formation (Fig. 14-11). These malformations of the cardiac outflow tract have been shown to occur in chick embryos that have undergone experimental neural crest ablation.[72] For the ventricular outflow tracts to develop normally, neural crest cells, derived from extracardiac ectomesenchymal tissue, must migrate into the conotruncus, where they participate in the formation of the aortopulmonary septum.[72,73] Leatherbury et al[74] demonstrated that ablation of the neural crest in the chick embryo leads to subsequent development of conotruncal malformations and decreased myocardial contractility. Furthermore, these hearts demonstrated ventricular dilation, which appeared to compensate for the decreased contractility by maintaining stroke volume.[74]

Goldmuntz et al[75] suggested that abnormalities of chromosome 22, such as the translocation 22q11 frequently found in patients with DiGeorge syndrome, may contribute to the development of some conotruncal cardiac malformations. Two cases of infants born with DiGeorge syndrome to insulin-dependent mothers have been reported, suggesting that maternal diabetes may be a pathogenic factor in this anomaly.[76] Hyperglycemia or other metabolic derangements during organogenesis may produce some abnormal maternal or embryonic factor(s) that variably affects the formation or migration of normal neural crest cells in the conotruncus. It seems likely that this abnormality occurs at the molecular level, thereby altering the chromosomal expression of the message for conotruncal development with resulting abnormal cardiac morphogenesis.

It is important to recall that gestational diabetic (White's class A) patients, who do not have carbohydrate intolerance and hyperglycemia during embryogenesis, do not have a higher incidence of congenital heart disease or other congenital anomalies than nondiabetic women. Soler et al,[77] in a study conducted in Birmingham, England, found no higher incidence of congenital cardiac malformations among 701 infants born to women with gestational diabetes when compared with nondiabetic women.

Abnormalities of Cardiac Function

The increased cardiac size of IDMs was first reported in 1943 by Miller and Wilson,[78] who noted cardiomegaly by chest radiography in these neonates, together with respiratory distress, cyanosis, and congestive heart failure. Driscoll et al[79] reported an increase in cardiac weight at postmortem examination to 174 percent above control values in IDMs, thought to result from excessive protein, glycogen, and fat synthesis, leading to both myocardial hyperplasia and hypertrophy. Although acknowledging the propensity of IDMs to develop macrosomia, it should be noted that the degree of cardiomegaly was disproportionate to the enlargement of other organs.[79] In 1965, Naeye[80] reported cardiac hyperplasia and hypertrophy in IDMs. However, the cardiac fetopathy associated with abnormal carbohydrate metabolism in the third trimester of pregnancy was initially described by Gutgesell et al.[81] The descriptions of this disorder are of an abnormal and postnatally transient ventricular hypertrophy, most often involving the interventricular septum, which can produce subaortic stenosis. Alternatively, this process can produce a more global hypertrophic cardiomyopathy, yielding abnormal myocardial function. These infants may demonstrate clinical symptoms resulting from diminished cardiac output, left ventricular outflow tract obstruction, and congestive heart failure, which may relate to abnormal systolic or diastolic function.

Considerable speculation remains concerning the pathophysiology of myocardial and septal hypertrophy in the IDM. Early theories centered around an increase

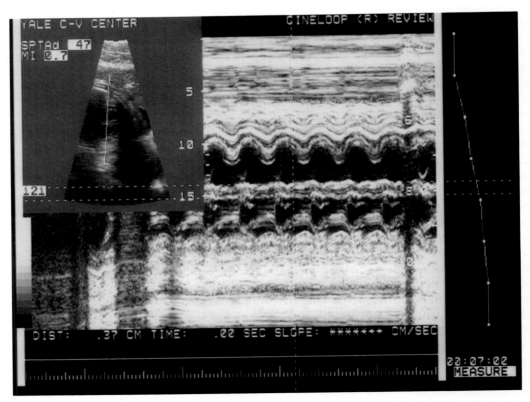

Fig. 14-11. Duplex image incorporating four-chamber view of the heart (inset box, upper left) with M-mode measurement of interventricular septum in a class B diabetic woman at 30 weeks' gestation. Septum is 4 mm thick.

in glycogen deposition in the myocardium. Gutgesell et al[82] described microscopic findings in the myocardium of IDMs similar to those found in adults with idiopathic hypertrophic subaortic stenosis, with disarray of hypertrophic septal myocardial fibers. Insulin has been implicated as the stimulus for the exuberant septal and myocardial growth.[83] Glucose crosses the placenta by facilitated diffusion, a process that is not modified even with maternal hyperglycemia. The fetus will normally respond to an increased carbohydrate load with an increased endogenous insulin production. The subsequent hyperinsulinemic state is a stimulus for myocardial hypertrophy, as first described by Breitweser et al.[83] The neonatal heart is rich in insulin receptors,[84] which may make the myocardium responsive to such changes in carbohydrate metabolism.

Many echocardiographic studies have demonstrated the increased propensity for the IDM to develop hypertrophic cardiomyopathy. The hypertrophic changes almost always involve the interventricular septum but may also involve both ventricular walls. Various terminology has been used to identify this abnormality, including asymmetric septal hypertrophy of the IDM, disproportionately thickened septum, ventricular septal hypertrophy, and hypertrophic cardiomyopathy of the IDM. Whatever the name, the diagnosis of disproportionate septal hypertrophy is made by demonstrating an interventricular septal thickness that is at least 1.3 times the thickness of the posterior wall of the left ventricle[85] or demonstrating ventricular wall thickness greater than 2 SD above the mean for gestational age. Normative data for fetal and newborn myocardium thickness have been determined echocardiographically in offspring of women with and without diabetes.[86,87] Table 14-5 gives normal ventricular wall dimensions during the third trimester.

There has long been speculation about the relationship between the degree of maternal glycemic control and the development of fetal cardiac hypertrophy. With the advent of echocardiography in the late 1970s, Mace et al[88] reported that there was a gross correlation between the degree of maternal diabetic control and infant septal hypertrophy. More recently, Veille et al[89] studied fetuses of 20 to 41 weeks' gestation and found that 75 percent of fetuses of diabetic mothers had evidence of septal hypertrophy, defined as septal thickness greater than 2 SD above the mean of age. In addition, they reported that the ratio of septal thickness to the anteroposterior cardiac dimension was significantly greater in the fetuses of diabetic mothers when compared with normal fetuses and that this relationship was maintained when the anteroposterior dimension was indexed to the fetal weight.[90] Sheehan et al[90]

estimated that approximately 35 percent of IDMs will have some degree of septal hypertrophy and concluded that better maternal diabetic control reduced the incidence of fetal septal hypertrophy. Experience at the Yale Fetal Cardiovascular Center has demonstrated that even with strict maternal glucose control, fetuses of diabetic mothers have measurable cardiac hypertrophy, although not necessarily to a clinically significant degree.[86] Furthermore, in our experience, some fetuses with hypertrophic cardiomyopathy will show a diminution or even resolution of the hypertrophic myocardium before birth, with improved maternal diabetic control.

The reported prevalence of septal hypertrophy among fetuses of diabetic women varies, perhaps as a result of varying study populations, varying definitions of normal limits, laboratory differences, and differences and evolution of echocardiographic technique. However, most echocardiographic studies of the fetus of the diabetic mother suggest the frequent occurrence of hypertrophic cardiomyopathy in these patients as well as the importance of maintaining euglycemia in the pregnant woman.

Hypertrophic cardiomyopathy may have varied physiologic consequences for fetal cardiac hemodynamics. Rasanen and Kirkinen[91] used third-trimester fetal echocardiography to study 18 fetuses of diabetic women and compared them with 51 normal pregnancies, finding that in comparison with normal fetuses, fetuses of diabetic mothers had decreased biventricular myocardial fractional shortening, smaller left ventricular stroke volume, and diminished left ventricular output. In normal fetuses, left ventricular fractional and circumferential shortening is greater than that of the right ventricle; however, this relationship was not found in the fetuses of the diabetic women.[91] Also, this study demonstrated that when AC was doubled with growth in the normal fetus, cardiac output increased 10-fold, whereas in the fetus of the diabetic mother, the increase in cardiac output was only threefold.[91] These findings suggest that the fetus of the diabetic mother has a smaller stroke volume and cardiac output relative to fetal size. This may result from the apposition of the thickened interventricular septum to the mitral valve during systole, which then leads to dynamic left ventricular outflow tract obstruction and diminished cardiac output. In addition, the thickened septum and myocardium lead to abnormal diastolic

Table 14-5. Comparison of Cardiac Wall Thickness in Diabetic and Normal Patients 34 to 40 Weeks' Gestation

	Normal	Diabetic
Interventricular septum	4.9 ± 0.3	6.1 ± 0.7[a]
Right ventricular free wall	3.2 ± 0.3	5.7 ± 0.8[b]
Left ventricular free wall	3.3 ± 0.4	6.4 ± 0.6[b]

[a] P <.05.
[b] P <.01.
(Data from Weber et al[86])

filling properties of the left ventricle, which can decrease right to left flow across the foramen ovale, thus diminishing left ventricular stroke volume. In support of these data, Walther et al,[92] using Doppler echocardiography, noted a strong negative correlation between interventricular septal thickness and cardiac output.

Septal hypertrophy and cardiomegaly in and of themselves do not necessarily impair cardiac function. As a result, some infants born with septal or myocardial hypertrophy may be completely asymptomatic, whereas others may demonstrate a clinical septum of decreased myocardial performance and diminished cardiac output. Hypertrophic cardiomyopathy in the neonate of a woman with diabetes may lead to signs and symptoms of pulmonary congestion, cyanosis, poor cardiac output, and systolic murmur, making it difficult to distinguish this syndrome from other forms of congenital heart disease. Besides echocardiography, two-dimensional real-time, M-mode, pulsed-wave Doppler, and color flow Doppler mapping permit the immediate and accurate diagnosis of hypertrophic cardiomyopathy, as well as the exclusion of congenital structural cardiac anomalies. The natural history of the hypertrophic cardiomyopathy resulting from maternal diabetes is one of complete spontaneous resolution, usually within the first 6 months of life and certainly by the end of the first year. If hypertrophic changes of the myocardium continue beyond this time, one must consider the diagnosis of idiopathic or familial hypertrophic cardiomyopathy.

Fetal Echocardiography in the Diabetic Pregnancy

Because abnormalities of cardiac structure and function resulting from either diabetic embryopathy or diabetic hypertrophic fetopathy can easily be demonstrated, fetal echocardiography is an important part of the prenatal evaluation of the pregnant woman with diabetes. This should be accomplished with both midtrimester scanning as well as third-trimester evaluation. We have developed a protocol for fetal echocardiographic evaluation in the pregnant woman with diabetes at the Yale Fetal Cardiovascular Center that includes a fetal echocardiogram at 18 to 24 weeks' gestation to define the structural integrity of the heart and a follow-up study at 32 to 34 weeks' gestation, both to re-evaluate cardiac structure and to evaluate any devel-

opment of hypertrophic cardiomyopathy. Earlier evaluation by vaginal sonography may be considered, although evidence of possible evolution of fetal cardiac anomalies[93] suggests that attempts at early diagnosis of cardiac anomalies (13 to 15 weeks) should be corroborated by a repeat evaluation between 18 and 22 weeks of gestation.[94,95]

A complete fetal echocardiographic examination should incorporate the following standard views:

The four-chamber view
The left ventricular long-axis view, with visualization of the aortic outflow tract
The short-axis view, with visualization of the pulmonary outflow tract and ductus arteriosus
The longitudinal view of the aortic arch[96–101]

These views will provide details of the intracardiac anatomy and evaluation of the conotruncus and left ventricular outflow tract. The scan should also include an evaluation of the relationship of the great arteries to one another. A normal crossing relationship virtually excludes the possibility of TGA.

The echocardiographic features of the fetus with diabetic hypertrophic cardiomyopathy include restricted ventricular filling, dynamic left or right ventricular outflow tract obstruction, and global myocardial hypertrophy.[82,88] Some of or all these findings may be present in any individual fetus and to varying degrees. It is virtually unheard of to find clinically significant hypertrophic cardiomyopathy in the IDM without concomitant fetal macrosomia. The diagnosis of hypertrophic cardiomyopathy can be made using the fetal echocardiographic views mentioned above. M-mode measurements of the septal and ventricular wall may be helpful in these cases. These measurements should be taken just below the atrioventricular valves from a long-axis view of the left ventricle, taking care to orient the M-mode cursor perpendicular to the interventricular septum.

M-mode and real-time two-dimensional echocardiography can be used to evaluate the ventricular septum, which should measure less than 6 mm during the third trimester.[86] Also, the movement of the mitral valve can be assessed. During systole, the anterior leaflet of the mitral valve may be seen to be closely opposed to the interventricular septum, a phenomenon known as systolic anterior motion. This is believed to occur as a result of the mitral valve being pulled or "sucked" toward the septum by the Venturi effect, which has been created by obstruction distal to the mitral valve in the left ventricular outflow tract. One may also note mid-systolic closure of the aortic valve, which can also be seen with M-mode echocardiography.

Color flow Doppler mapping has been an important addition to the fetal echocardiogram, as it can demonstrate sites of functional stenosis or dynamic obstruction. Color Doppler flow mapping can be applied to the two-dimensional image or, alternatively, to the M-mode image to assess the precise point in the cardiac cycle when turbulence begins. Pulsed-wave Doppler is used to assess ventricular inflow patterns of the fetus with evidence of hypertrophic cardiomyopathy. Quantitative assessment of left ventricular outflow tract obstruction can be made with both pulsed-wave and directed continuous-wave Doppler techniques.

Summary

The metabolic milieu that exists in the pregnant woman can adversely affect normal fetal cardiac growth and development. When diabetes mellitus is present during the first trimester, there can be abnormal cardiovascular organogenesis. The congenital heart disease resulting from this metabolic abnormality appears to be related to abnormal neural crest cell migration and resulting malformations of the conotruncus. Defects such as DORV and truncus arteriosus may result. Because cardiac looping and septation occur between the third and sixth postconceptual weeks, maintaining strict metabolic control both before and after conception is a reasonable strategy to minimize the incidence of structural heart disease in the fetus of the woman with diabetes.

When diabetes mellitus is present in the third trimester, there is a strong association with the development of fetal hypertrophic cardiomyopathy, which may lead to abnormalities such as left ventricular outflow tract obstruction, diminished cardiac output, and congestive heart failure. This hypertrophic cardiomyopathy typically resolves spontaneously within the first 6 months of postnatal life. Although debate continues, this phenomenon most likely results from fetal hyperinsulinemia in response to the transplacental transmission of maternal hyperglycemia. There is reason to be-

lieve that good control of carbohydrate metabolism in the pregnant diabetic woman can decrease the likelihood of structural and functional heart disease in her offspring. Fetal echocardiography has become the cornerstone for accurate prenatal diagnosis of the cardiovascular abnormalities associated with maternal diabetes mellitus.

GASTROINTESTINAL ABNORMALITIES

The most common gastrointestinal disorders associated with diabetes are small bowel atresia, left colon syndrome, and imperforate anus.[102] Imperforate anus is thought by some to be a variation on the caudal regression theme. Small bowel atresia has been reported to occur in 1 to 300 to 1 in 1,500 live births.[103,104] It is often associated with polyhydramnios. Duodenal atresia is a common form of small bowel obstruction that can be associated with Down syndrome.[105,106] Colonic atresia is a rare cause of intestinal obstruction accounting for less than 10 percent of obstructions. Associated anomalies are rare, as colonic atresia is the result of a local intrauterine vascular accident.[107]

Prenatal Diagnosis

Sonographic findings in small bowel atresia are characterized by dilated sonolucent "masses" that occupy the fetal abdominal cavity (Fig. 14-12). The classic "double-bubble" finding (Fig. 14-13) described in duodenal atresia can also be seen in jejunal atresia. Unfortunately, the double-bubble picture is not always present before 24 weeks' gestation, resulting in the possibility of a false-negative diagnoses in the second trimester. Ultrasound during the third trimester is therefore necessary. Determination of disaccharidase activity in the amniotic fluid before the 22nd week of gestation can also be helpful in making the diagnosis.[108]

The sonographic diagnosis of colonic atresia is based on the detection of enlarged echo-free colonic loops in the lower abdomen and active peristalsis. The biometric measurement of the colon is above the 95th percentile. Polyhydramnios is less frequent than with proximal lesions.

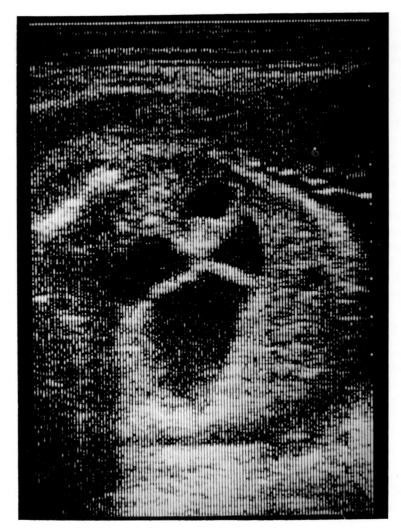

Fig. 14-12. Transverse section of the fetal abdomen demonstrating multiple loops of dilated bowel. This picture can be consistent with either ileal or jejunal atresia and is usually associated with increased amniotic fluid volume.

Management and Outcome

Isolated small bowel obstruction is a treatable condition after birth and is associated with a reasonable outcome. Prognosis depends on the site of the obstruction, the length of the remaining bowel, delayed diagnosis, and associated anomalies. The more distal the obstruction, the better the prognosis. Therefore, in the setting of diabetes, the benefit of second-trimester diagnosis (versus third-trimester identification) of small bowel obstruction would be to alert the physician to the possibility of other life-threatening anomalies. In the case of duodenal atresia, karyotyping is necessary to exclude aneuploidy.

Diagnosis at any time during gestation will allow the physician the opportunity to adjust the timing and place of delivery and to optimize outcome for the infant with bowel obstruction.

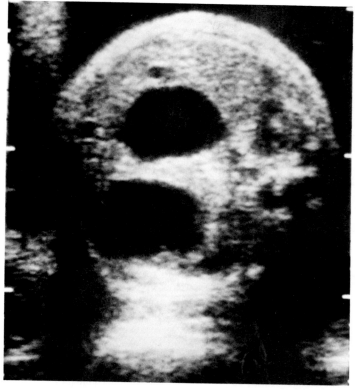

Fig. 14-13. Transverse section of the fetal abdomen depicting the two echolucent areas, the so-called double-bubble sign characteristic of duodenal atresia.

GENITOURINARY ABNORMALITIES

The most common renal anomalies occurring with increased frequency in diabetes are duplication of the collecting system and renal agenesis.[109] Although hydronephrosis has been mentioned as being associated with diabetes, it is unclear whether this is due to a well-defined obstructive lesion.

Prenatal Diagnosis

Ureteral duplication is a treatable abnormality that can be diagnosed by noting a cystic structure adjacent to the kidney. These may or may not be associated with hydronephrosis on the affected side, but oligohydramnios is not a feature of the condition unless another renal abnormality is present. Ultrasound investigation in the first trimester[110] has shown that by using high-resolution and high-frequency transducers, it is possible to visualize kidneys in virtually all embryos by 12 weeks. In 50 percent of cases, one can even visualize a fetal bladder at that time (Fig. 14-14). In renal agenesis, oligohydramnios is the rule from the 16th week of gestation and is associated with absence of kidneys and a fetal bladder (Fig. 14-15). Although we are aware of some diminution in amniotic fluid volume occurring in a case of renal agenesis at 13 weeks of gestation, we are unaware of the condition causing oligohydramnios in the first trimester. The amount of amniotic fluid present in a gestational sac at 12 weeks is not as dependent on fetal urination as in later gestation.

The very finding that alerts the physician to the possibility of renal agenesis impairs one's ability to unerringly diagnose this lethal anomaly. Although kidneys can normally be visualized in the second trimester, the

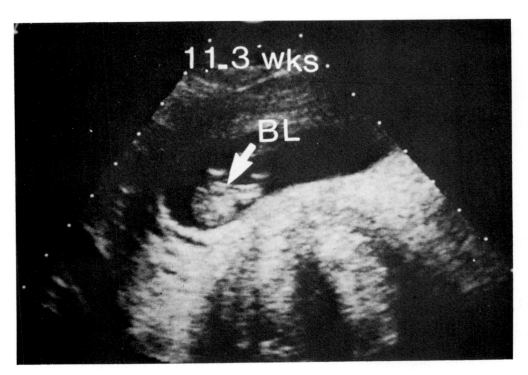

Fig. 14-14. Ultrasound scan of a fetus at approximately 11 weeks in whom the fetal bladder is visualized (BL).

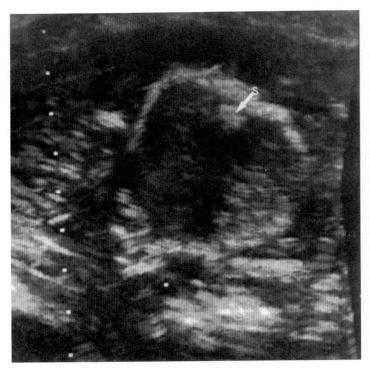

Fig. 14-15. Transverse scan of the abdomen illustrating the absence of kidneys in a patient with renal agenesis. S, spine. (From Reece and Hobbins,[112] with permission.)

absence of the amniotic fluid "window" renders renal visualization very difficult. The problem is compounded by the fact that fetal adrenal may undergo hypertrophy, creating the suspicion that something is present in the area where the kidneys usually reside.

Management and Outcome

Bilateral renal agenesis is a lethal congenital anomaly. Termination may be considered when the diagnosis is made. Aggressive care should not be delivered in view of the dismal prognosis.

OTHER ABNORMALITIES

Caudal Regression Syndrome

Although caudal regression syndrome occurs most frequently in diabetic pregnancies (200 times more common than in normal pregnancies), it is still a relatively rare condition that complicates 1 in 200 to 1 in 500 diabetic pregnancies.[111,112] Because this lesion occasionally occurs in the absence of mechanical diabetes, it cannot be considered absolutely pathognomonic. The abnormality probably results from a defect in the midposterior axis mesoderm of the embryo occurring before the fourth week postconception. This results in the absence of hypoplasia of caudal structures (Fig. 14-16).

Prenatal Diagnosis

The diagnosis can be made by noting a shortened spine and markedly abnormal lower limbs. In most cases, this diagnosis is possible during the early second trimester. However, Baxi and colleagues[113] recently reported the diagnosis of sacral agenesis at 9 weeks' gestation using transvaginal ultrasound.

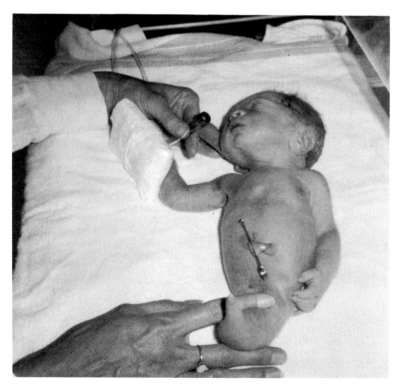

Fig. 14-16. Neonate afflicted with caudal regression syndrome. The spectrum of this abnormality can be quite varied.

Management and Outcome

Termination of pregnancy is an option that may be offered to the parents if the diagnosis is made before the period of viability; otherwise, the patient can be managed expectantly. A loss of motor function is common in infants with sacral agenesis, but sensory function is normally preserved.

Polyhydramnios

Although severe polyhydramnios occurs infrequently in diabetes in the absence of fetal anomalies, slightly excessive amounts of amniotic fluid are often seen in women with diabetes. The proposed mechanisms for hydramnios are the following:

1. Increased amniotic fluid osmolality due to increased glucose
2. Fetal polyuria resulting from fetal hyperglycemia
3. Decreased fetal swallowing

Experimental work has not provided strong support for any of these hypotheses.[114]

Although the most likely reason for the generous fluid volume is increased fetal urine production in women with diabetes,[115] Wladimiroff et al[116] did not demonstrate an increased fetal urine production by sequential estimations of bladder volume over time. Because of problems in methodology, the report does not necessarily rule out increased fetal urine production as a cause for the relative hydramnios in diabetic women. It has been our anecdotal experience that fetal bladder size in many cases of hydramnios in classes A, B, and C women with diabetes appears to be enlarged.

Central nervous system anomalies are the most common fetal malformations associated with hydramnios and constitute about 45 percent of the total. Anencephaly accounts for approximately 80 percent of the central nervous system anomalies, and gastrointestinal abnormalities represent about 30 percent of all anomalies.[117]

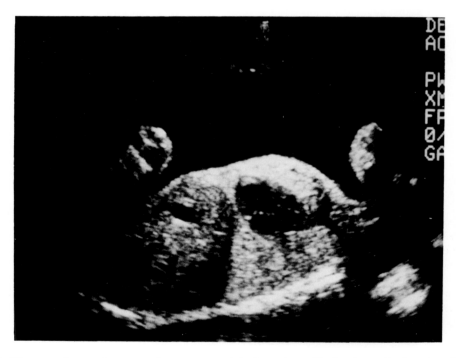

Fig. 14-17. Ultrasound scan demonstrating severe polyhydramnios with the fetus displaced to the posterior uterine area. This fetus was later diagnosed to have a tracheoesophageal fistula.

Prenatal Diagnosis

The sonographic diagnosis is made by measuring a single vertical amniotic fluid pocket of 8 cm or more or an amniotic fluid index greater than 24 cm when using the four-quadrant technique.[117] In addition, the sonographic evaluation of a gestation complicated by hydramnios reveals excessive amniotic fluid with displacement of the fetus toward the posterior aspect of the uterine cavity. Fetal extremities appear to be separated by vast spaces of amniotic fluid (Fig. 14-17).

CONCLUSION

Ultrasound provides much essential information about the fetus of the woman with diabetes and should be used liberally in the management of a pregnant diabetic patient. A first-trimester scan should be used to date the pregnancy and to document fetal viability; a second-trimester scan (about 20 weeks) should allow the perinatologist to rule out most serious fetal anomalies, and a third-trimester examination should be directed to assessing fetal growth. Particular attention should be directed toward ultrasound clues that might suggest fetal macrosomia or IUGR. In general, judicious use of ultrasound should decrease the likelihood of surprises in a condition that is notoriously unpredictable.

REFERENCES

1. Eik-Nes SH, Okland O, Aure JC et al: Ultrasound screening in pregnancy: a randomized controlled trial. Lancet 1:347, 1984
2. Pedersen JF, Molsted-Pederson L: Early growth retardation in diabetic pregnancy. BMJ 1:18, 1979
3. Keys TC, Cousins L, Moore TR: Early fetal growth in insulin dependent diabetics. Proceedings of the 32nd Annual Meeting of the Society for Gynecological Investigation, Phoenix, AZ March 1985
4. Cousins LC, Key TC, Schorzman L, Moore TR: Ultrasonographic assessment of early fetal growth in insulin-treated diabetic pregnancies. Am J Obstet Gynecol 159: 1186, 1988
5. Brown ZA, Mills JL, Metzger BE et al: Early sonographic evaluation for fetal growth delay and congenital malformations in pregnancies complicated by insulin-requiring diabetes. Diabetes Care 15:613, 1992
6. Reece EA, Goldstein I, Pilu G et al: Fetal cerebellar growth unaffected by intrauterine growth retardation: a new parameter for prenatal diagnosis. Am J Obstet Gynecol 157:632, 1987
7. Hill LM, Guzick D, Fries J et al: The transverse cerebellar diameter in estimating gestational age in the large for gestational age fetus. Obstet Gynecol 75:981, 1990
8. Hadlock FP, Harrist RB, Shah YP et al: Estimating fetal age using multiple parameters: a prospective evaluation in a racially mixed population. Am J Obstet Gynecol 156:955, 1987
9. Burrow GN, Ferris TF: Medical Complications during Pregnancy. WB Saunders, Philadelphia, 1982
10. Houchang D, Modanlou HD, Dorchester WL et al: Macrosomia—maternal, fetal and neonatal implications. Obstet Gynecol 55:420, 1980
11. Gabbe SG, Mesman JH, Freeman RK et al: Management and outcome of class A diabetes mellitus. Am J Obstet Gynecol 127:465, 1977
12. Elliott JP, Garite TJ, Freeman RK et al: Ultrasonic prediction of fetal macrosomia in diabetic patients. Obstet Gynecol 60:159, 1982
13. Goldrich JM, Kirkman K: The large fetus: management and outcome. Obstet Gynecol 52:26, 1978
14. Pedersen IM, Tystrup I, Pedersen J: Congenital malformations in newborn infants of diabetic women. Correlation with maternal diabetic vascular complications. Lancet 1:1124, 1964
15. Wladimiroff JW, Bloemsma CA, Wallenburg HCS: Ultrasonic diagnosis for the large-for-date infant. Obstet Gynecol 52:285, 1978
16. Tamura RK, Sabbagha RE, Depp R et al: Diabetic macrosomia: accuracy of third trimester ultrasound. Obstet Gynecol 67:828, 1986
17. Shepard MJ, Richards VA, Berkowitz RL et al: An evaluation of two equations for predicting fetal weight by ultrasound. Am J Obstet Gynecol 152:47, 1982
18. Ogata ES, Sabbagha R, Metzger BE et al: Serial ultrasonography to assess evolving fetal macrosomia. JAMA 243:2405, 1980
19. Elliott JP, Garite TJ, Freeman RK et al: Ultrasonic prediction of fetal macrosomia in diabetic patients. Obstet Gynecol 60:159, 1982
20. Yarkoni S, Reece EA, Wan M et al: Intrapartum fetal weight estimation: a comparison of three formulae. J Ultrasound Med 5:707, 1986
21. Campbell S, Thoms A: Ultrasound measurement of the fetal head to abdomen circumference ratio in the assessment of growth retardation. Br J Obstet Gynaecol 84:165, 197

22. Yarkoni S, Schmidt W, Jeanty P et al: Clavicular measurement: a new parameter for fetal evaluation. J Ultrasound Med 4:467, 1985

23. Langer OD, Levy J, Brustman L et al: Glycemic control in gestational diabetes—how tight is tight enough: small for gestational age versus large for gestational age. Am J Obstet Gynecol 161:646, 1989

24. Jovanovic-Pederson L, Peterson CM, Reed GF et al: Maternal postprandial glucose levels and infant birth weight: the diabetes in early pregnancy study. Am J Obstet Gynecol 164:103, 1991

25. Parafitt VJ, Clark JD, Turner GM, Hartog M: Maternal postprandial glucose levels influence infant birth weight in diabetic pregnancy. Diabetes Res 19:133, 1992

26. Lin CC, River J, River P et al: Good diabetic control early in pregnancy and favorable fetal outcome. Obstet Gynecol 67:51, 1986

27. Persson B, Stangenberg M, Hansson U, Norlander E: Gestational diabetes (GDM): comparative evaluation of two treatment regimens, diet versus insulin and diet. Diabetes, suppl. 2, 34:101, 1985

28. Coustan DR, Imarah J: Prophylactic insulin treatment of gestational diabetes reduces the incidence of macrosomia, operative delivery, and birth trauma. Am J Obstet Gynecol 150:836, 1984

29. Leiken E, Jenkins JH, Graves WL: Prophylactic insulin in gestational diabetes. Obstet Gynecol 70:587, 1987

30. Buchanan TA, Kjos SL, Montoro MN et al: Use of fetal ultrasound to select metabolic therapy for pregnancies complicated by mild gestational diabetes. Diabetes Care 17:275, 1994

31. Vohr BR, Lipsitt LP, Oh W: Somatic growth of children of diabetic mothers with reference to birth size. J Pediatr 97:196, 1980

32. Pettitt DJ, Nelson RG, Saad MF et al: Diabetes and obesity in the offspring of Pima Indian women with diabetes during pregnancy. Diabetes Care, suppl. 1, 16:310, 1993

33. Sabbagha RE: Intrauterine growth retardation. p. 103. In Sabbagha RE (ed): Diagnostic Ultrasound. Harper & Row, Hagerstown, MD, 1980

34. Jeanty P, Romero R, Hobbins JC: Fetal limb volume: a new parameter to assess fetal growth and nutrition. J Ultrasound Med 4:273, 1985

35. Goldstein I, Reece EA, Pilu G et al: Cerebellar measurements with ultrasonography in the evaluation of the fetal head growth and development. Am J Obstet Gynecol 156:1056, 1987

36. Laurin J, Marsal K, Persson PH: Ultrasound measurement of fetal blood flow in predicting fetal outcome. Br J Obstet Gynaecol 94:90, 1987

37. Arduini D, Rizzo G, Romaini C, Mancuso S: Fetal blood flow velocity waveforms as predictors of growth retardation. Obstet Gynecol 70:7, 1987

38. Brook CGD: Consequences of intrauterine growth retardation. BMJ 286:164, 1983

39. Milunsky A (ed): Genetic Disorders and the Fetus: Diagnosis, Prevention, and Treatment. 3rd Ed. Johns Hopkins University Press, Baltimore, 1992

40. Miller E, Hare JW, Cloherty JP et al: Elevated maternal hemoglobin A1c in early pregnancy and major congenital anomalies in infants of diabetic mothers. N Engl J Med 304:1331, 1981

41. Pinter E, Reece EA, Leranth CZ et al: Yolk sac failure in embryopathy due to hyperglycemia: ultrastructural analysis of yolk sac differentiation in rat conceptuses under hyperglycemic culture conditions. Teratology 33:363, 1986

42. Fuhrmann K, Reiher H, Semmler K et al: Prevention of congenital malformations in infants of insulin-dependent diabetic mothers. Diabetes Care 6:219, 1983

43. Kitzmiller JL, Gavin LA, Gin GD et al: Preconception management of diabetes continued through early pregnancy prevents the excess frequency of major congenital anomalies in infants of diabetic mothers. JAMA 265:731, 1991

44. Goldman JA, Dicker D, Feldberg et al: Pregnancy outcome in patients with insulin-dependent diabetes mellitus with preconceptional diabetic control: a comparative study. Am J Obstet Gynecol 155:293, 1986

45. Steel JM, Johnstone FD, Hepburn DA, Smith AF: Can prepregnancy care of diabetic women reduce the risk of abnormal babies? BMJ 301:1070, 1991

46. Soler NG, Walsh CH, Malins JM: Congenital malformations in infants of diabetic mothers. J Med 178:303, 1976

47. Cunningham ME, Walls WJ: Ultrasound in the evaluation of anencephaly. Radiology 118:165, 1976

48. Campbell S: Early prenatal diagnosis of neural tube defects by ultrasound. Clin Obstet Gynecol 20:35, 1977

49. Goldstein RB, Filly RA: Prenatal diagnosis of anencephaly: spectrum of sonographic appearance and distinction from the amniotic band syndrome. AJR 151:547, 1988

50. Milunsky A: Prenatal diagnosis of neural tube defects. The importance of serum alpha-fetoprotein screening in diabetic pregnant women. Am J Obstet Gynecol 142:1030, 1982

51. Wald NJ: Maternal serum alpha-fetoprotein measurement in antenatal screening for anencephaly and spina bifida in early pregnancy. Report of U.K. collaborative study on alpha-fetoprotein in relation to neural tube defects. Lancet 1:1323, 1977

52. Pilu G, Romero R, Goldstein I et al: Subnormal cerebellum size in fetuses with spina bifida. Am J Obstet Gynecol 158:1052, 1994

53. Nicolaides KH, Campbell S, Gabbe SG et al: Ultrasound

screening for spina bifida: cranial and cerebellar signs. Lancet 2:72, 1986

54. Cowchock S, Ainbender E, Prescott G et al: The recurrence risk of neural tube defects in the United States: a collaborative study. Am J Med Genet 5:309, 1980

55. Naeye C: Congenital malformations in offspring of diabetes. Ph.D. thesis. Harvard University, Boston, 1967

56. Chervenak FA, Jeanty P, Cantraine F et al: The diagnosis of fetal microcephaly. Am J Obstet Gynecol 149:512, 1984

57. Ferencz C, Rubin JD, McCarter RJ, Clark EB: Maternal diabetes and cardiovascular malformations: predominance of double outlet right ventricle and truncus arteriosus. Teratology 41:319, 1990

58. Becerra JE, Muin JK, Cordero JF, Erickson JD: Diabetes mellitus during pregnancy and the risks for specific birth defects: a population-based cases-control study. Pediatrics 85:1, 1990

59. Hoffman JIE, Christianson R: Congenital heart disease in a cohort of 19,502 births with long-term follow-up. Am J Cardiol 42:641, 1978

60. Mitchell SC, Korones SB, Behrendes HW: Congenital heart disease in 56,109 births: incidence and natural history. Circulation 43:323, 1971

61. Rowland TW, Hubbell JP, Nadas AS: Congenital heart disease in infants of diabetic mothers. J Pediatr 53:579, 1958

62. Kleinman CS, Santulli TV: Ultrasonic evaluation of the fetal human heart. Semin Perinatol 7:90, 1983

63. Smythe JF, Copel JA, Kleinman CS: Outcome of prenatally detected cardiac malformations. Am J Cardiol 69:1471, 1992

64. Reece EA, Gabrielli S, Abdalla M: The prevention of diabetes-associated birth defects. Semin Perinatol 12:292, 1988

65. Miller E, Hare JW, Cloherty JP et al: Elevated maternal hemoglobin A1c in early pregnancy and major congenital anomalies in infants of diabetic mother. N Engl J Med 304:1331, 1981

66. Key TC, Giuffrida R, Moore TR: Predictive value of early pregnancy glycohemoglobin in the insulin-treated diabetic patient. Am J Obstet Gynecol 156:1096, 1987

67. Ylinen K, Aula P, Stenman U et al: Risk of minor and major fetal malformations in diabetics with high haemoglobin A1c values in early pregnancy. BMJ 289:345, 1984

68. Leslie RDG, Pyke DA, John PN, White JM: Haemoglobin A1 in diabetic pregnancy. Lancet 2:958, 1978

69. Mills JL, Knopp RH, Simpson JL et al: Lack of relation of increased malformation rates in infants of diabetic mothers to glycemic control during organogenesis. N Engl J Med 318:671, 1988

70. Shields LE, Gan EA, Murphy CNM et al: The prognostic value of hemoglobin A1c in predicting fetal heart disease in diabetic pregnancies. Obstet Gynecol 81:954, 1993

71. White P: Diabetes mellitus in pregnancy. Clin Perinatol 1:331, 1974

72. Kirby ML: Cardiac morphogenesis. Recent research advances. Pediatr Res 21:219, 1987

73. Rychter Z: Analysis of relations between aortic arches and aorticopulmonary septation. Birth Defects 14:443, 1978

74. Leatherbury L, Connuck DM, Gauldin HE, Kirby ML: Hemodynamic changes and compensatory mechanisms during early cardiogenesis after neural crest ablation in chick embryos. Pediat Res 30:509, 1991

75. Goldmuntz E, Driscoll D, Budarf ML et al: Microdeletions of chromosomal region 22q11 in patients with congenital conotruncal cardiac defects. J Med Genet 30:807, 1993

76. Wilson TA, Blethen SL, Vallone A et al: DiGeorge anomaly with renal agenesis in infants of mothers with diabetes. Am J Med Genet 47:1078, 1993

77. Soler NG, Walsh CH, Malins JM: Congenital malformations in infants of diabetic mothers. Q J Med 45:303, 1976

78. Miller JD, Wilson HM: Macrosomia, cardiac hypertrophy, erythroblastosis, and hyperplasia of the islands of Langerhans in infants of diabetic mothers. J Pediat 23:251, 1943

79. Driscoll SG, Bernischke K, Curtis GW: Neonatal deaths among infants of diabetic mothers: post-mortem findings in ninety-five infants. Am J Dis Child 100:818, 1960

80. Naeye RL: Infants of diabetic mothers: a quantitative, morphologic study. Pediatrics 35:980, 1965

81. Gutgesell H, Mullins C, Gillette P et al: Transient hypertrophic subaortic stenosis in infants of diabetic mothers. J Pediatr 89:120, 1976

82. Gutgesell H, Speer M, Rosenberger H: Characterization of the cardiomyopathy in infants of diabetic mothers. Circulation 61:441, 1980

83. Breitweser JA, Meyer RA, Sperling MA et al: Cardiac septal hypertrophy in hyperinsulinemic infants. J Pediatr 96:535, 1980

84. Steven J, Whitsett JA: Insulin binding to neonatal human, guinea pig and rat myocardial membranes. Pediatr Res 13:482, 1979

85. Way GL, Wolfe RR, Eshaghpour E et al: The natural history of hypertrophic cardiomyopathy in infants of diabetic mothers. J Pediatr 95:1020, 1979

86. Weber HS, Copel JA, Reece EA et al: Cardiac growth in fetuses of diabetic mothers with good metabolic control. J Pediatr 118:103, 1991

87. Allan LD, Joseph MC, Boyd EGCA et al: M-mode echocardiography in the developing human fetus. Br Heart J 47:573, 1982

88. Mace S, Hirschfeld SS, Riggs T et al: Echocardiographic abnormalities in infants of diabetic mothers. J Pediatr 95:1013, 1979

89. Veille JC, Sivakoff M, Hanson R, Fanaroff AA: Interventricular septal thickness in fetuses of diabetic mothers. Obstet Gynecol 79:51, 1992

90. Sheehan PW, Rowland TW, Shal BL: Maternal diabetic control and hypertrophic cardiomyopathy in infants of diabetic mothers. Clin Pediatr 25:266, 1986

91. Rasanen J, Kirkinen P: Growth and function of human fetal heart in normal, hypertensive and diabetic pregnancy. Acta Obstet Gynecol Scand 66:349, 1987

92. Walther F, Siassi B, King J, Wu P: Cardiac output in infants of insulin dependent diabetic mothers. J Pediatr 107:109, 1985

93. Rice MJ, McDonald RW, Sahn DJ: The evolution of fetal heart disease. p. 219. In Copel JA, Reed KL (eds): Doppler Ultrasound in Obstetrics and Gynecology. Raven, New York, 1995

94. Gembruch U, Knopfle G, Bald R, Hansmann M: Early diagnosis of fetal congenital heart disease by transvaginal echocardiography. Ultrasound Obstet Gynecol 3:310, 1993

95. Copel JA, Kleinman CS: Early screening for fetal cardiac anomalies. Ultrasound Obstet Gynecol 3:308, 1993

96. Benacerraf BR, Pober BR, Sanders SP: Accuracy of fetal echocardiography. Radiology 165:847, 1987

97. Shime J, Bertrand M, Hagen-Ansert S et al: Two-dimensional and M-mode echocardiography in the human fetus. Am J Obstet Gynecol 148:679, 1984

98. Axel L: Real-time sonography of fetal cardiac anatomy. AJR 141:283, 1983

99. DeVore GR, Donnerstein RL, Kleinman CS et al: Normal anatomy as determined by real-time-directed M-mode ultrasound. Am J Obstet Gynecol 144:249, 1982

100. Huhta JC, Hagler DJ, Hill LM: Two-dimensional echocardiographic assessment of normal fetal cardiac anatomy. J Reprod Med 29:162, 1984

101. Nimrod C, Nicholson S, Machin G et al: In utero evaluation of fetal cardiac structure: a preliminary report. Am J Obstet Gynecol 148:516, 1984

102. Kucera J: Rate and type of congenital anomalies among offspring of diabetic women. J Reprod Med 7:61, 1971

103. Phelhan JT: Jejunal atresia and stenosis. Pediatr Surg 46:470, 1959

104. De Lorimier A, Fonkalsrud EW, Hays DM: Congenital atresia of the jejunum and ileum. Surgery 65:819, 1969

105. Miro J, Bard H: Congenital atresia and stenosis of duodenun: the impact of a prenatal diagnosis. Am J Obstet Gynecol 158:555, 1988

106. Young DG, Wilkinson AW: Abnormalities associated with neonatal duodenal obstruction. Surgery 63:832, 1968

107. Freeman NV: Congenital atresia and stenosis of the colon. Br J Surg 53:595, 1966

108. Morin PR, Potier M, Dallaire L et al: Prenatal detection of intestinal obstruction: deficient fluid disaccharidases in affected fetuses. Clin Genet 18:217, 1980

109. Gabbe SG, Cohen AW: Diabetes mellitus in pregnancy. p. 1097. In Bolognese RJ, Schwartz R, Schneider J (eds): Perinatal Medicine: Management of the High Risk Fetus and Neonate. Williams & Wilkins, Baltimore, 1982

110. Alexander ES, Spitz HB, Clark RA: Sonography of polyhydramnios. AJR 138:343, 1982

111. Soler NG, Walsh CH, Malins JM: Congenital malformations in infants of diabetic mothers. Br J Med 178:303, 1976

112. Reece EA, Hobbins JC: Ultrasonography and diabetes mellitus with pregnancy. p. 297. In: Sanders RC, James AE (eds): The Principles and Practice of Ultrasonography in Obstetrics and Gynecology. Appleton & Lange, E. Norwalk, CT, 1985

113. Baxi L, Warren W, Collins MH, Timor-Tritsch IE: Early detection of caudal regression syndrome with transvaginal screening. Obstet Gynecol 75:486, 1990

114. Reece EA, Hobbins JC: Diabetic embryopathy: pathogenesis, prenatal diagnosis and prevention. Obstet Gynecol Surv 41:325, 1986

115. Jacoby HE, Charles D: Clinical conditions associated with hydramnios. Am J Obstet Gynecol 94:910, 1966

116. Wladimiroff JW, Barentsen R, Wallenburg HCS et al: Fetal urine production in a case of diabetes associated with polyhydramnios. Obstet Gynecol 46:100, 1975

117. Carlson DE, Platt LD, Mederais AL et al: Quantifiable polyhydramnios: diagnosis and management. Obstet Gynecol 75:989, 1990

118. Pederson J, Pedersen-Molsted L: Congenital malformations: the possible role of diabetes care outside pregnancy. Ciba Found Symp 265, 1979

119. Fuhrmann K, Reiber H, Semmler K et al: The effect of intensified conventional insulin therapy before and during pregnancy on the malformation rate of offspring of diabetic mothers. Exp Clin Endocrinol 83:173, 1984

120. Kitzmiller J, McCoy D, Grin F et al: A regional perinatal program to present congenital anomalies in infants of diabetic mothers, abstracted. Proc Soc Gynecol Invest 56, 1986

121. Steel JM: Preconception, conception, and contraception. p. 601. In Reece EA, Coustan DR (eds): Diabetes Mellitus in Pregnancy: Principles and Practice. Churchill Livingstone, New York, 1988

122. Tamura RK: Diabetes mellitus and accelerated fetal growth. p. 165. In Sabbagha RE (ed): Diagnostic Ultrasound Applied to Obstetrics and Gynecology. JB Lippincott, Philadelphia, 1994

123. Deter RL, Harrist RB: Detection of growth abnormali-

ties. p. 387. In Chervenak FA, Isaacson GC, Campbell S (eds): Ultrasound in Obstetrics and Gynecology. Little, Brown, Boston, 1993

124. Gramellini D, Folli MC, Raboni S et al: Cerebral-umbilical Doppler ratio as a predictor of adverse perinatal outcome. Obstet Gynecol 79:416, 1992

125. Reece EA, Goldstein I, Hobbins JC (eds): Fundamentals of OB/GYN Ultrasound. Appleton & Lange, E. Norwalk, CT, 1994

126. Reece EA, Hobbins JC, Mahoney MJ, Petrie RH (eds): Medicine of the Fetus and Mother. JB Lippincott, Philadelphia, 1992

15

Fetal Biochemical and Biophysical Assessment

FRANK MANNING

The potential adverse effect of chronic maternal glucose imbalance, the salient pathologic characteristic of diabetes, on fetal health is well documented. In the days before the discovery of insulin therapy, few diabetic women achieved pregnancy, and in those that did, the perinatal loss rate was at least 65 percent.[1] Most of these perinatal deaths occurred as sudden stillbirths. The introduction of insulin therapy and with it the ability to regulate maternal plasma glucose concentration effected a profound change on pregnancy outlook in diabetes; the proportion of women with diabetes able to conceive increased, and of those, the proportion ending in a live birth rose dramatically. This therapeutic advance has continued with a progressive improvement in outcome as the clinical ability to control blood glucose fluctuations advanced, such that even before the introduction of modern highly sophisticated antepartum testing methods, the perinatal mortality rate had declined significantly.[2] Therefore, at the outset of any consideration of the contemporary role of antepartum testing in the management of the diabetic pregnancy, it needs to be stressed that the primary therapeutic aim is to effect tight control of maternal glucose concentration, an end point that now is progressively more attainable with the introduction of the new insulin products, the modern delivery systems, (including for some patients), the use of subcutaneous insulin infusion pumps, and the products for self-glucose monitoring. The role of antepartum evaluation is directed toward the identification and timely intervention of those residual fetuses who continue to exhibit evidence of perinatal compromise even within the milieu of relatively normal glucose homeostasis or when such normal homeostasis has not been accomplished.

PERINATAL DEATH AND COMPROMISE AMONG DIABETIC PREGNANCIES: PATHOPHYSIOLOGIC MECHANISMS

The fetus of the diabetic pregnancy is subject both to the common causes of perinatal compromise and to some unique and highly specific risk factors, and both adverse consequences occur at a disproportionately higher rate among women with diabetes.

Chronic Uteroplacental Insufficiency

Chronic uteroplacental insufficiency, as manifested by growth failure, oligohydramnios, and increased placental vascular resistance, as evidenced by abnormal flow velocities in the umbilical artery, occurs less frequently among diabetic pregnancies in general than in the nondiabetic population. In some specific diabetic subgroups, namely, those exhibiting long-standing disease (White's class C and D) and those with end organ damage (White's class T, F, and H), it occurs at a significantly higher rate (Table 15-1). Thus, for example, in the study population of 5,895 consecutive diabetic pregnancies seen in the Fetal Assessment Unit (1981–1993), the incidence of mild intrauterine growth retardation (IUGR) (<10th to >3rd birthweight percentile for gestational age and sex) was 2.3 percent, and severe IUGR (≤3rd percentile) was 1.1 percent (Manning FA, unpublished data, 1994). By contrast, in the nondiabetic population (73,255 assessed pregnancies), the incidence of mild IUGR was 4.6 per-

251

Table 15-1. Chronic Uteroplacental Insufficiency: Clinical Markers

	Study Population				Nondiabetic
	Pregnant Diabetic Women (N = 5,894)				Nondiabetic
Clinical Marker	Gestational (diet ± insulin) (N = 4,657) (%)	Class B (N = 408) (%)	Class C or Greater (N = 830) (%)	All Insulin-dependent (N = 1,238) (%)	Nondiabetic High-Risk (N = 73,255) (%)
Intrauterine growth retardation (<10th–>3rd)	15 (0.032)	6 (1.7)	22 (2.6)	28 (2.3)	3,368 (4.6)[a]
Intrauterine growth retardation (≤3rd)	5 (0.01)	2 (0.48)	11 (1.3)	13 (1.9)	1,758 (2.4)[a]
Oligohydramnios (≤2 cm largest vertical pocket)	139 (0.3)	6 (1.3)	18 (2.1)	24 (1.9)	735 (1)[a]
Absent diastolic[b] flow umbilical artery	4/1,600 (0.5)	3/201 (1.5)	9/402 (2.5)	12 (1.9)	N/A

[a] $P < .001$ as compared with all insulin-dependent diabetics.
[b] Introduced from 1987 onward—not routine.
(Data from Fetal Assessment Unit Data—University of Manitoba 1980–1994.)

cent and severe IUGR was 2.4 percent. Lagnew et al[3] reported a similar finding, noting an incidence of IUGR (<10th percentile) of 4.2 percent among 614 diabetic pregnancies. Among our patients with gestational diabetes mellitus (GDM) (White's class A_1 A_2), the occurrence of growth failure is so extremely rare (<0.1 percent) as to evoke considerable clinical concern portending an ominous outcome. The interpretation of birthweight percentiles as a manifestation of adequate placental function in the diabetic fetus is subject to some challenge because it is possible that any growth-restraining effect of placental dysfunction could be masked by the somatotropic influence of a glucose-rich milieu. In the fetal lamb, the effect of progressive placental embolic damage on fetal growth can be ameliorated by fetal intravenous hyperalimentation but not by intragastric feeding in utero.[4,5]

The incidence of oligohydramnios in the diabetic fetus with intact membranes and an intact genitourinary tract is significantly less than that observed in the nondiabetic high-risk population (Table 15-1). This difference may reflect a lower incidence of uteroplacental insufficiency among diabetic patients. Again, however, this assumption is open to challenge because daily fetal urine production may be increased in the presence of fetal hyperglycemia, the effect presumably being due to an increased solute load to the fetal kidney.[6]

The incidence of abnormal Doppler umbilical artery flow velocities, a measure of placental resistance, is very low among GDM pregnancies and increases among insulin-dependent diabetic mellitus (IDDM) pregnancies (Table 15-1).

Placental sonography in the detection of evolving abruption is an emerging art. Notwithstanding the lack of fixed ultrasound criteria, in our experience, there is no suggestion that the incidence of chronic abruption is altered among diabetic pregnancies.

Chronic uteroplacental failure in diabetic pregnancies virtually never occurs in the absence of associated hypertension. Hypertension, either chronic or pregnancy-induced, occurs more frequently in women with diabetes than in their nondiabetic counterparts.[7]

Developmental Anomalies

The emergence, differentiation, organization, and functional arrangement of the structural elements of the developing embryo is exceedingly complex and depends on exquisitely sensitive timing, occurring within a normal hormonal and metabolic milieu. In women with poorly controlled diabetes, the critical organogenesis phase, occurring in the first 7 to 10 weeks of pregnancy is subject to a variety of noxious influences. These may include an excess of glucose, which may yield a substrate-driven interruption in the timing sequences[8]; an altered intracellular pH and electrolyte balance; abnormal fluctuations in fetal insulin levels and somatomedins,[9] which may yield abnormal somatotropic signals and local depletion of critical differentiation cofactors (e.g., arachidonic acid depletion),[10] and the occurrence of potential teratogens such as ketones.[11] By whatever mechanism, the incidence of developmental anomalies (8 to 9 percent) is increased by three- to fivefold among diabetic pregnancies as compared with the nondiabetic pregnancies (2 to 3 percent).[12,13] There must, however, be considerable variability among diabetic populations, since in our experience the incidence of major anomalies among 1,258 IDDM mothers was less than 3 percent. Although the fetus of a mother with diabetes is subject to the same wide range of anomalies as in nondiabetic pregnancy, certain system anomalies occur at a disproportionately higher frequency. Cardiac anomalies and, in particular, ventricular septal defects and complex lesions such as transposition of the great vessels occur about five times more frequently,[14] and central nervous system malformation, in particular, neural tube defects and holoprosencephaly, occur about 10 times more frequently.[15] The sacral agenesis/caudal dysplasia complex is reported to occur up to 400 times more commonly among fetuses of mothers with diabetes.[16]

Three critical aspects need be addressed in regard to anomalies among women with diabetes.

First, these malformations make a significant contribution to the overall perinatal mortality rate of offspring of mothers with diabetes. In the days preceding good maternal glucose control, anomalies accounted for only about 10 percent of all perinatal deaths. The progressive betterment of glucose control and decreased perinatal mortality overall have increased the relative contribution of anomalies up to 50 percent.[17] This trend has continued such that in our population, in whom "tight" glucose control is the norm, the proportion of perinatal deaths attributable to anomalies now exceeds 90 percent.

Second, advances in ultrasound imaging have made it possible to identify major structural/functional anomalies with greater precision and at progressively earlier gestational ages. In our experience, the detection of neural tube defects now approaches 100 percent[18] and the detection of major and lethal anomalies in high-risk populations, including pregnancies complicated by diabetes, is now 86 percent. It is of interest to contrast the high anomaly detection rate with the much lower rate recently reported in the "Radius" study.[19] In our experience, anomaly detection and classifica-tion by prognosis has had a powerful impact on management and outcome.

Third, there is now convincing evidence that the rate of anomalies among diabetic fetuses can be reduced. There are at least three studies that indicate that periconceptional "tight" glucose regulation (mean glucose level, <100 mg/dl) effects a significant reduction in anomalies.[20-22] Concurrently, the use of folic acid supplementation in the preconceptional and embryonic period effects a significant decrease in the incidence of neural tube defects.[23,24]

Fatal Respiratory Distress Syndrome

In pregnant women with uncontrolled or poorly controlled diabetes, the incidence of severe and fatal respiratory distress syndrome (RDS) is increased relative to perinates of comparable age in nondiabetic pregnancies,[25] and death from RDS in the term diabetic infant is reported.[26] This concern has had a profound impact on the management of pregnancies complicated by diabetes. Amniocentesis for determination of lecithin/sphingomyelin (L/S) ratio and phospholipid profile became a common technique. The distribution of L/S results is skewed toward immaturity in poorly controlled diabetic women.[27,28] However, in well-controlled diabetic women there is no significant difference from nondiabetic women in either the distribution of L/S results,[28] the predictive accuracy of the L/S alone or in combination with the nonlecithin phospholipids,[28] or the incidence of RDS by age cohort.[29,30] Concurrently, the management of RDS has undergone radical changes (e.g., new respiratory methods, artificial surfactants), and as a consequence, neonatal mortality has declined dramatically. In our current experience, the neonatal mortality rate among infants of diabetic mothers (IDMs) of 34 weeks or greater approaches 0 percent. The now near-universal usage of ultrasound assessment in our pregnant population with diabetes for purposes of pregnancy dating (optimal window, 8 to 18 weeks) has drastically reduced the occurrence of uncertain fetal age. The use of late pregnancy (>28 weeks) serial fetal assessment has eliminated the arbitrary delivery of women with GDM at or before term and extended the planned delivery date in uncomplicated women with IDDM closer to or at term. As a consequence of these management changes, the use of amniocentesis in the pregnancy complicated by diabetes has become very uncommon. By 1987, amniocentesis was performed for lung maturity in only 14 percent of cases[31] and, at present, the procedure is reverted to in less than 5 percent of cases. In our current experience, the occurrence of fatal RDS in the pregnancy complicated by diabetes after 34 weeks' gestation is now exceedingly rare, having not occurred in the past 3 years (>1,400 diabetic pregnancies).

Diabetes-Specific Perinatal Mortality

In uncontrolled or poorly controlled IDDM, sudden and unexpected stillbirth is a frequent complication, estimated to occur in 10 to 30 percent of pregnancies.[32] Both extremes of glucose concentration abnormalities (i.e., hyperglycemia and hypoglycemia) can result in this tragic consequence.

Maternal hyperglycemia is invariably associated with fetal hyperglycemia[33,34] (Fig. 15-1). Fetal hyperglyce-

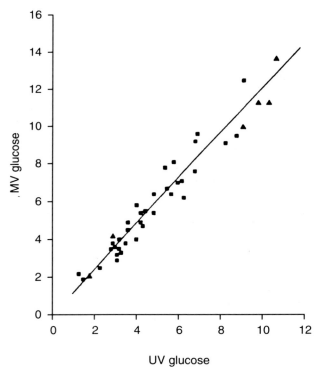

Fig. 15-1. Relationship between maternal venous (MV) and umbilical venous (UV) blood glucose concentration. Data obtained from antepartum cordocentesis in 41 diabetic pregnancies. (From Salverser et al,[33] with permission.)

mia can induce fetal compromise up to lethality by a variety of pathophysiologic processes either independently or in concert. Aerobic glycolysis is substrate-driven and in a glucose-rich environment may yield an increase in oxygen demand and relative tissue hypoxia. Anaerobic glycolysis is also substrate-driven. In the human fetus, hyperglycemia correlates directly with lactic acid concentration and inversely with pH and oxygen partial pressure.[35] In the extreme, lactic acidemia in the fetus may be fatal. The simultaneous occurrence of fetal hypoxemia, the trigger to the anerobic glycolytic pathway, and fetal hyperglycemia is a potentially lethal combination. In her elegant experiments of induced isocapnic hypoxemia in twin fetal lamb chronic preparations, Shelly demonstrated that the rate of development of acidemia was greatly accelerated and the reversibility reduced in the lamb receiving a glucose infusion as compared with the lamb receiving saline. In the primate *(Macacca mulatta),* fetal insulin infusion results in metabolic acidemia, profound bradycardia, and acute fetal deterioration to death.[36] Although speculative, because fetal electrolytes were not measured in these experiments, one explanation for this acute effect is fetal hypokalemia and cardiac dysrhythmia.

The time of day of the sudden stillbirth among the uncontrolled or poorly controlled diabetic patient has not been studied systematically, and in view of the rarity of this catastrophe with modern management, it is now virtually impossible to determine. It was my clinical impression, however, that most of these sudden fetal deaths occurred in the late evening and early morning hours, at a time when the mother was most likely to be recumbent and therefore at risk of supine hypotension, at a time when fetal biophysical activities were peaking and oxygen demand was high,[37,38] and at a time when paradoxical (fasting-induced) hyperglycemia was most likely to occur. It seems reasonable to assume that some of these sudden fetal deaths occurred as a consequence of the hypoxemia/hyperglycemia effect.

In some species (e.g., sheep), fetal hypoglycemia, often profound, may occur either spontaneously or as an effect of maternal fasting[39] and is not associated with adverse fetal consequence. In the primate fetus, including humans, fetal hypoglycemia does not occur spontaneously but rather occurs only in the presence of profound maternal hypoglycemia or fetal hyperinsulinemia, either responsive (to hyperglycemia) or experimental.[39] The primate fetus does not tolerate hypoglycemia and deterioration and death is the rule. In the poorly controlled human with diabetes, wide fluctuations in maternal blood sugar are common, and degrees of hypoglycemia up to severe (insulin shock) may occur. It is likely that, in these cases, hypoglycemia is a cause of sudden fetal death. Indeed, the last "sudden" fetal death that occurred in our practice was associated with severe maternal hypoglycemia: this woman with IDDM was being fasted overnight for cesarean section, developed severe hypoglycemia (<2 mmol/L), and the fetus was dead by morning.

Maternal ketoacidosis is another rare but potentially lethal cause of sudden fetal deterioration.

FETAL ASSESSMENT IN THE DIABETIC PREGNANCY

Biochemical Methods

Before the introduction of dynamic biophysical variable monitoring, objective estimation of fetal risk in diabetes was based on the measurement of a variety of substances in maternal blood, including heat-stable (placental) alkaline phosphatase, leucine aminopeptidase (oxytocinase), human placental lactogen, and most commonly, serum or urinary estriols.[41] These measures bore a passing relationship to perinatal risk but were neither very sensitive nor specific.[40,41] Our clinical group, like others, abandoned these biochemical indices years ago, without any visible detrimental consequence whatsoever.

The key and only essential biochemical marker of perinatal risk in diabetic pregnancies is the *maternal glucose concentration*. It may be argued that most of the dramatic reduction in perinatal morbidity and mortality among diabetic patients is a direct consequence of glucose monitoring and control. Self-monitoring of blood glucose using glucose oxidase-impregnated reagent strips and a reflectance meter coupled with aggressive insulin therapy now permits excellent control in the ambulatory outpatient setting.[42] The goal of "tight" control is to maintain the morning fasting value between 60 and 90 mg/dl, the premeal nadirs between 60 and 100 mg/dl, and the postprandial peaks at 120

mg/dl or less. The overnight fasting values should not drop below 60 mg/dl.[2]

Maternal serum α-fetoprotein (AFP) is of proven value in screening for open neural tube defects and other anomalies and so is of special importance in women with diabetes. The serum AFP values tend to be lower among IDDM women, averaging about 60 to 70 percent of the nondiabetic pregnancy value.[43,44] Therefore, the cut-off value in neural tube screening by maternal serum AFP needs to be adjusted downward by about one-third.

Biophysical Methods

In modern perinatal medicine, all methods of fetal assessment are ultrasound-based. The palate of methods is broad and can be categorized by gestational age and indication. Dynamic ultrasound imaging is used for determination of fetal morphometrics, primarily for dating purposes and serial assessment of growth and for determination of fetal morphology. Sequenced ultrasound evaluation is strongly recommended for all pregnancies complicated by diabetes. The initial scan yields maximal information when performed between 16 and 18 weeks' gestation ("dating scan"). Fetal morphometrics at this age are highly predictive of true fetal age (±7 days), and morphometric screening for central nervous system and major gastrointestinal anomalies is quite reliable. Cardiac and renal anomalies may not be as easily diagnosed at this gestation. A second scan is recommended at 24 to 28 weeks' gestation to confirm normal fetal growth velocity and to further assess fetal morphology. In addition to the general anatomic survey, there should be a focused cardiac, facial, and limb scan at this time.

The ultrasound-based methods for evaluation of fetal well-being can be subdivided into three groupings: antepartum fetal heart rate testing (nonstress test [NST], contraction stress test [CST], computer-assisted heart rate analysis, acoustic stimulation), umbilical artery and other fetal vessel Doppler flow velocity waveform analysis, and the composite fetal biophysical profile score. The choice of testing method(s) varies from center to center and by individual preference. By whatever method selected, the focus ought to be detection of the fetus in jeopardy early enough to effect therapeutic intervention.

The most commonly used testing method is the NST,

performed twice weekly from 28 to 32 weeks on-wards.[45] This testing method alone may not be optimal because the incidence of false-positive tests is high, ranging from 8 to 15 percent,[46,47] and is increased in the immature fetus (≤32 weeks) and because the false-negative rate (death within 1 week of a normal test) is relatively high in general (>2 per 1,000)[48] and even higher in pregnancies complicated by diabetes (14 per 1,000).[49] Most groups that use the NST as the primary test rely on the CST or the biophysical profile score as a means of evaluating the nonreactive NST and base subsequent management on these added data. Our group does not use the NST as a primary testing method in women with diabetes.

The CST remains a valuable test in the evaluation of the diabetic fetus.[50] Some groups, most notably that of Freeman and associates at Long Beach Memorial Hospital in California, use the CST as the primary test-ing method in women with IDDM, beginning testing at about 32 weeks and then weekly thereafter with mid-week NST testing.[3] The fetal biophysical profile score is used as a backup test, particularly in very preterm gestation. The incidence of positive CST results in women with diabetes is about 11 to 12 percent.[50] Un-fortunately, the incidence of false-positive CST is high, on average about 30 percent.[51] By contrast, the false-negative rate for the CST (death within 1 week of a normal test) is remarkably low (0.6 per 1,000).[52,53]

Fetal Doppler Velicometry

Although there are clinical proponents of umbilical artery velicometry in the assessment of the diabetic pregnancy,[54] the method has not been proved to con-vey any advantage.

Fetal Biophysical Profile Scoring

Fetal biophysical profile scoring (BPS) is a dynamic ultrasound-based assessment of a composite of acute (fetal breathing, movement, tone, heart rate reactivity) and chronic (amniotic fluid volume) indices of fetal health.[55,56] The effect of fetal hypoxemia and acidemia (asphyxia) on these variables is described in detail elsewhere.[57] The fetal BPS is a powerful predictor of fetal acidemia in the high-risk population (r = .517;

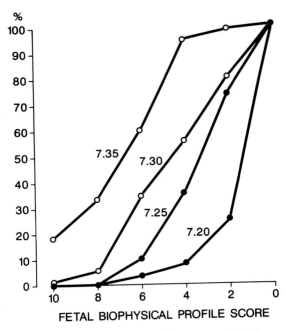

Fig. 15-2. Fetal biophysical profile score and fetal venous pH. Numbers next to graph lines indicate percentage of ob-servation for each biophysical profile score that fell below an arbitrary umbilical venous pH.

$P < .001)^{57}$ (Fig. 15-2). In diabetic pregnancies, a signif-icant correlation between the fetal BPS and umbilical venous pH is reported (r = .46; $P < .01$). The some-what-lower correlation between BPS and diabetes is most likely a reflection of the higher incidence of mild and clinically innocuous acidemia among fetuses of mothers with diabetes.

Fetal BPS has proved to be a reliable method of fetal assessment in the pregnancy complicated by diabetes. In the initial study of the method, Johnson et al re-ported on 238 well-controlled diabetic pregnancies (50 IDDM) tested twice weekly from as early as 28 weeks' gestation.[31] In this small series, the incidence of abnormal BPS results was 3.3 percent and there were no stillbirths and no neonatal deaths unrelated to anomaly (corrected perinatal mortality rate, 0 per 1,000). Dicker et al[58] reported their experience in 98 IDDM pregnancies managed by twice-weekly fetal BPS from 28 weeks onward: 2.9 percent of 978 BPS results were abnormal, prompting intervention, and there were no perinatal deaths. Our group reported an initial

Table 15-2. Interpretation of Fetal Biophysical Profile Score Results and Recommended Clinical Management Based on These Results

Test Score Result	Interpretation	PNM Within 1 Week Without Intervention	Management
10/10 8/10 (normal fluid) 8/8 (NST not done)	Risk of fetal asphyxia extremely rare	<1/1,000	Intervention only for obstetric and maternal factors; no indication for intervention for fetal disease
8/10 (abnormal fluid)	Probable chronic fetal compromise	89/1,000	Determination that there is functioning renal tissue and intact membranes— if so, deliver for fetal indications
6/10 (normal fluid)	Equivocal test, possible fetal asphyxia	Variable	If the fetus is mature—deliver; in the immature fetus, repeat test within 24 hours—if <6/10, deliver
6/10 (abnormal fluid)	Probable fetal asphyxia High probability of fetal asphyxia	89/1,000 91/1,000	Deliver for fetal indications Deliver for fetal indications
4/10	Fetal asphyxia almost certain	125/1,000	Deliver for fetal indications
2/10 0/10	Fetal asphyxia certain	600/1,000	Deliver for fetal indications

Abbreviations: PNM, perinatal mortality; NST, nonstress test.

experience in 1,161 diabetic pregnancies managed by twice-weekly fetal BPS from 28 weeks onward[59] (Table 15-2). The incidence of abnormal BPS results was less than 2 percent. Three perinatal deaths (all stillbirths) occurred among the 1,161 diabetic women studied (corrected perinatal mortality rate, 2.58 per 1,000). In the past 3 years (1990–1993 inclusive), we have used the BPS method in 2,116 diabetic pregnancies: the intervention rate for an abnormal score remains below 2 percent, and the corrected perinatal mortality rate was 2.1 per 1,000 (Table 15-3). Two aspects of the fetal BPS in fetuses of diabetic mothers warrant further comment. The incidence of fetal breathing movement is

Table 15-3. Biophysical Profile Scoring in Diabetic Pregnancies

Study	No. of Patients	Incidence of Abnormal BPS (%)	Corrected PNM[a]
Johnson et al[31]	238	3.3	0
Manning et al[59]	1,161	<2	2.58 (3 deaths)
Dicker et al[58]	98	2.9	0
Manning[b]	2,116	<2	2.1 (5 deaths)

Abbreviations: BPS, biophysical profile scoring; PNM, perinatal mortality.
[a] Lethal anomalies excluded.
[b] Unpublished data 1990–1993 inclusive.

related to maternal glucose, rising about 30 minutes after the maternal peak.[60] This effect appears to be related to relative hypoglycemia because glucose infusion in normoglycemic lambs does not alter the incidence of breathing movements.[61] In human pregnancies complicated by diabetes, the incidence and intensity of fetal breathing movements often appear enhanced. There is no experimental nor clinical evidence, however, to suggest that a rise in fetal glucose can override the suppressor effect of hypoxemia on the fetal central respiratory center. Accordingly, the absence of fetal breathing movements is a predictor of hypoxemia in the diabetic fetus, as in the nondiabetic. Extreme maternal hyperglycemia can evoke an ominous fetal breathing pattern typified by tachypnea (respiratory rate, ≥100 beats per minute) that persists unabated for prolonged observation periods (>1 hour). This rare pattern of fetal breathing movements is not reassuring and may be associated with fetal compromise and death.[62]

Amniotic fluid volume is often increased in diabetes, particularly when maternal glucose has been poorly controlled. Asphyxia-related oligohydramnios occurs as a result of reflex redistribution of cardiac output, yielding relative renal hypoperfusion. There is neither experimental nor clinical evidence to suggest that this reflex and its renal consequence are altered in any way in the fetus of the diabetic mother. Accordingly, the observation of oligohydramnios in these fetuses is as predictive of chronic asphyxia as in nondiabetic fetuses. However, given that there must be a measurable period between the onset of the reflex and the development of oligohydramnios (mean interval, 17 days), it would follow that this latent period would be longer in fetuses with increased amniotic fluid volume. Accordingly, the observation of normal amniotic fluid volume in the diabetic pregnancy, although reassuring, ought to be less so than in the nondiabetic. To date, we are unable to prove that this theoretical limitation exists and therefore continue to rely on normal amniotic fluid as an indicator of well-being in the fetus of the diabetic pregnancy.

SUMMARY

The advances in care of the pregnant woman with diabetes have yielded among the most spectacular gains in perinatal medicine. The perinatal mortality rate has plummeted from the 60 to 70 percent level of the pre-insulin days to the lower level of 1 percent today. The stillbirth rate has fallen by more than 600-fold in the past six decades. It is becoming evident that "tight" control of maternal glucose coupled with antepartum fetal surveillance can reduce corrected perinatal mortality to about 2 per 1,000 and perhaps even lower. The advances in periconceptional prevention therapies for anomalies hold promise of further reducing the perinatal loss rate with this common condition. The pregnancy complicated by diabetes can now be categorized as a manageable "at-risk" condition, with a high expectation of a healthy mother and child. It remains our duty to continue to practice and improve on the clinical methods that have yielded these gains.

REFERENCES

1. Gabbe SG: Management of diabetes in pregnancy: six decades of experience. p. 456. In Pitkin RM, Zlatnick F (eds): The Yearbook of Obstetrics and Gynecology. Yearbook Medical Publishers, Chicago 1977
2. Landon MB, Gabbe SG: Diabetes mellitus and pregnancy. Obstet Gynecol Clin North Am 19:633, 1992
3. Lagnew DC, Pircon RA, Towers CV et al: Antepartum fetal surveillance in patients with diabetes: when to start? Am J Obstet Gynecol 168:1820, 1993
4. Charlton V, Johengen M: Fetal intravenous nutritional supplementation ameliorates the development of embolization induced growth retardation in sheep. Pediatr Res 22:55, 1987
5. Charlton V, Johengen M: Effect of intrauterine nutritional supplementation on fetal growth retardation. Biol Neonate 48:125, 1985
6. Kurjack A, Kirkinen P, Latin V et al: Ultrasound assessment of fetal kidney function in normal and complicated pregnancies. Am J Obstet Gynecol 141:266, 1981
7. Hanson U, Persson B: Outcome of pregnancies complicated by type 1 insulin dependent diabetes in Sweden: acute pregnancy complications, neonatal mortality and morbidity. Am J Perinatol 10:330, 1993
8. Freinkel N, Lewis NJ, Akazama S et al: The honeybee syndrome: implications of the teratogenicity of mannose in rat-embryo culture. N Engl J Med 310:225, 1984
9. Sadler TW, Phillips LS, Balkan W et al: Somatomedin inhibitors from diabetic rat serum alter growth and development of mouse embryos in culture. Diabetes 35:861, 1986
10. Goldman AS, Baker L, Piddington R et al: Hyperglycemic-induced teratogenesis is mediated by a functional deficiency of arachodonic acid. Proc Natl Acad Sci USA 82: 8227, 1985
11. Sadler TW, Horton WE Jr: Mechanism of diabetes induced congenital malformation as studied in mammalian embryo culture. p. 51. In Jovanovic L, Peterson CM, Fuhrman K (eds): Diabetes in Pregnancy: Teratology, Toxicity and Treatment. Praeger Ltd., New York, 1986
12. Simpson JL, Elias S, Martin AO et al: Diabetes in pregnancy. I. Prospective study of anomalies in offspring of mothers with diabetes mellitus. Am J Obstet Gynecol 146:263, 1983
13. Mills JL, Kropp RH, Simpson JP et al: Lack of relations of increased malformation rates in infants of diabetic mothers to glycemia control during organogenesis. N Engl J Med 318:671, 1988
14. Landon MB: Diabetes mellitus and other endocrine diseases. p. 1097. In Gabbe SG, Niebyl JR, Simpson JL (eds): Obstetrics: Normal and Problem Pregnancies. Churchill Livingstone, New York, 1991
15. Reece EA, Hobbins JC: Diabetic embryopathy: pathogenesis, prenatal diagnosis and prevention. Obstet Gynecol Surv 41:325, 1986
16. Kucera J: Rate and type of congenital anomalies among offspring of diabetic women. J Reprod Med 7:61, 1971
17. Simpson JL, Elias S, Martin AO et al: Diabetes in pregnancy—North Western University Series (1977–1981). I. Prospective study of anomalies in offspring of mothers

with diabetes mellitus. Am J Obstet Gynecol 146:263, 1983

18. Kyle PM, Harman CR, Evans JA et al: Life without amniocentesis: elevated maternal serum alpha-fetoprotein (MSAFP) in the Manitoba Program 1986–1991. J Ultrasound Obstet Gynecol (in press)

19. Ewigman BG, Crane JP, Frigoletto FD et al: Effect of perinatal ultrasound screening on perinatal outcome. N Engl J Med 329:821, 1993

20. Furhamm K, Reiher H, Semmler K et al: Prevention of congenital malformation in infants of insulin-dependent diabetic mother. Diabetes Care 6:219, 1983

21. Mills JL, Baker L, Goldman A: Malformation in the infants of diabetic mothers occur before the seventh gestational week: implication for treatment. Diabetes 28:292, 1979

22. Kitzmiller JL, Gavin LA, Gin GD et al: Preconception management of diabetes continued through early pregnancy prevents the excess frequency of major congenital anomalies in infants of diabetic mothers. JAMA 265:731, 1991

23. Smithells RW, Sheppard S, Scorah CJ et al: Apparent prevention of neural tube defects by periconceptual vitamin supplementation. Arch Dis Child 56:911, 1981

24. Medical Research Council Vitamin Study 1991: Prevention of neural tube defects. Lance 2:131, 1991

25. Kulovich MV, Gluck L: The lung profile. II. Complicated pregnancies. Am J Obstet Gynecol 135:64, 1979

26. Ylinen K: High levels of hemoglobin A_{1c} associated with delayed fetal lung maturation in insulin-dependent diabetic pregnancies. Acta Obstet Gynecol Scand 66:263, 1987

27. Ojomo EO, Coustan DR: Absence of evidence of pulmonary maturity at amniocentesis in term infants of diabetic mothers. Am J Obstet Gynecol 163:954, 1990

28. Piper JM, Langer O: Does maternal diabetes delay fetal pulmonary maturity. Am J Obstet Gynecol 168:783, 1993

29. Mimouri F, Miodovnik M, Whitsett JA et al: Respiratory distress syndrome in infants of diabetic mothers in the 1980's: no direct adverse effect of maternal diabetes with modern management. Obstet Gynecol 69:191, 1987

30. Kjos SL, Walther FJ, Montoro M et al: Prevalence and etiology of respiratory distress in infants of diabetic mothers: predictive value of fetal lung maturation tests. Am J Obstet Gynecol 163:898, 1990

31. Johnson JM, Lange IR, Harman CR et al: Biophysical profile scoring in the management of the diabetic pregnancy. Obstet Gynecol 72:841, 1988

32. Beard RW, Turner RC, Oakley N: Fetal response to glucose loading. Postgrad Med J 47:68, 1971

33. Salverser DR, Freeman J, Brudenell JM et al: Prediction of fetal acidemia in pregnancies complicated by maternal diabetes mellitus by biophysical profile scoring and fetal heart rate monitoring. Br J Obstet Gynaecol 100:227, 1993

34. Shelly JH, Bassett JM, Milner RDG: Control of carbohydrate metabolism in the fetus and newborn. Br Med Bull 31:37, 1975

35. Carson BS, Phillips AF, Simmons MA et al: Effects of a sustained insulin infusion upon glucose uptake and oxygenation in the ovine fetus. Pediatr Res 14:147, 1980

36. Patrick JE, Natale R, Richardson B: Patterns of human fetal breathing activity at 34–35 weeks gestational age. Am J Obstet Gynecol 132:507, 1978

37. Patrick JE, Campbell K, Carmichael L et al: Patterns of gross body movements over 24 hour observation intervals during the last 10 weeks of pregnancy measured with a realtime scanner. Am J Obstet Gynecol 142:363, 1982

38. Boddy K, Dawes GS: Fetal breathing. Br Med Bull 32:1, 1975

39. Druzin M, Socol M, Murata Y, Manning FA: Fetal bradycardia and death following profound experimental hypoglycemia in the primate fetus, abstracted. Proc SGI 1980

40. Spellacy WN, Buhi WC, Birk SA: The effectiveness of human placental lactogen measurement as an adjunct in decreasing perinatal death. Am J Obstet Gynecol 121:835, 1975

41. Ray DA, Yeast JD, Freeman RK: The current role of daily serum estriol monitoring in the insulin dependent diabetic woman. Am J Obstet Gynecol 154:1257, 1986

42. Landon MB, Gabbe SG: Glucose monitoring and insulin administration in the pregnant diabetic patient. Clin Obstet Gynecol 28:496, 1985

43. Wald NJ, Cuckle HS, Boreham J et al: Maternal serum alpha-fetoprotein and diabetes mellitus. Br J Obstet Gynaecol 86:101, 1979

44. Wald NJ, Cuckle HS: Biochemical detection of neural tube defects and Down's syndrome. p. 269. In Turnbull AC, Chamberlain G (eds): Obstetrics. Churchill Livingstone, Edinburgh, 1989

45. Landon MB, Gabbe SG, Sachs L: Management of diabetes mellitus and pregnancy: a survey of obstetricians and maternal-fetal medicine specialists. Obstet Gynecol 75:635, 1990

46. Lavery JP: Non-stress fetal heart rate testing. Clin Obstet Gynecol 25:689, 1982

47. Landon MB, Larger O, Gabbe SG et al: Fetal surveillance in pregnancies complicated by insulin-dependent diabetes mellitus. Am J Obstet Gynecol 167:617, 1992

48. Devoe LD: The non-stress test. p. 378. In Eden RD, Boehm FH (eds): Assessment and Care of the Fetus. Physiological, Clinical and Medicolegal Principles. Appleton-Lange, E. Norwalk, CT, 1990

49. Barrett J, Salyer S, Boehm F: The non-stress test: an evaluation of 1000 patients. Am J Obstet Gynecol 141:153, 1981

50. Gabbe SG, Mestman JH, Freeman RK et al: Management

and outcome of diabetes mellitus classes B-R. Am J Obstet Gynecol 129:723, 1977

51. Collea J, Holls W: The contraction stress test. Clin Obstet Gynecol 25:707, 1982

52. Freeman RK, Anderson G, Dorchester WA: A prospective multi-institutional study of antepartum fetal heart rate testing. I. Risk of perinatal mortality and morbidity according to antepartum fetal heart rate test results. Am J Obstet Gynecol 143:771, 1982

53. Brudenell JM: Fetal monitoring in the diabetic pregnancy. p. 118. In Spencer JD (ed): Fetal Monitoring: Physiological and Technique of Antenatal and Intrapartum Assessment. Castle House Publication Ltd., Kent, England, 1989

54. Landon MB, Gabbe SG, Bruner JP et al: Doppler umbilical artery velocimetry in pregnancy complicated by insulin-dependent diabetes. Obstet Gynecol 73:961, 1989

55. Manning FA, Platt LD, Sipos L: Antepartum fetal evaluation: development of a fetal biophysical profile. Am J Obstet Gynecol 136:787, 1980

56. Manning FA: The fetal biophysical profile score. In: Aspects of Fetal Life. Appleton-Lange, E. Norwalk, CT, 1994

57. Manning FA, Snijders R, Harman CR et al: Fetal biophysical profile score. VI. Correlation with antepartum umbilical venous fetal pH. Am J Obstet Gynecol 169:755, 1993

58. Dicker D, Feldberg D, Yeshaya A et al: Fetal surveillance in insulin dependent diabetic pregnancy: predictive value of the biophysical profile. Am J Obstet Gynecol 159:800, 1988

59. Manning FA, Morrison I, Lange IR et al: Fetal assessment based on fetal biophysical profile scoring: experience in 12620 referred high risk pregnancies. I. Perinatal morbidity by frequency and etiology. Am J Obstet Gynecol 151:343, 1985

60. Patrick J, Natale R, Richardson B et al: Patterns of human fetal breathing activity at 34–35 weeks gestational age. Am J Obstet Gynecol 132:507, 1978

61. Richardson B, Hohimer AR, Mueggler P et al: Effects of glucose concentration on fetal breathing movements and electrocortical activity in fetal lambs. Am J Obstet Gynecol 142:678, 1982

62. Manning FA, Heaman M, Boyce D et al: Intrauterine fetal tachypnea. Obstet Gynecol 58:398, 1981

16

Testing for Gestational Diabetes

MARSHALL W. CARPENTER

The association between type II, non-insulin-dependent diabetes mellitus and the prior obstetric history of large babies, stillbirths, and neonatal deaths has been observed for several decades.[1] The inference that this association is the result of subclinical maternal diabetes has been confirmed by studies that relate glucose intolerance during pregnancy and subsequent perinatal mortality or morbidity rates. The concept of gestational diabetes mellitus (GDM, pregnancy-related glucose intolerance that remits after delivery) was initially articulated in 1965.[2] Initial studies showed an association between the degree of glucose intolerance and perinatal mortality rates in selected patient series[3] and population-based studies.[4,5] Subsequent observations have associated the presence of GDM with fetal macrosomia[6,7]; neonatal morbidities, such as hypoglycemia, polycythemia, and hyperbilirubinemia[8]; and an increased risk of later maternal glucose intolerance in the nonpregnant state.[9] Similarly, well-defined treatment protocols have been shown to reduce perinatal morbidity and operative delivery rates and decrease perinatal mortality rates to population norms,[7,10–13] resulting in the view that GDM is a treatable disorder.[14–16]

This chapter discusses diagnostic criteria for the oral glucose tolerance test and for the intravenous glucose tolerance test (IVGTT). In addition, proposed screening tests are examined, including historical factors, glycosylated hemoglobin and other blood protein levels, and other oral challenge tests. The diagnostic use of amniotic fluid glucose, insulin, and C-peptide, as well as postpartum evaluation of women with suspected diabetic fetopathy are also examined.

REQUIREMENTS FOR DIAGNOSTIC AND SCREENING TESTS

Standards for a medical diagnostic test derive from an understanding or consensus about the natural history of the disorder to be diagnosed and its pathogenesis of morbidity. Clinical and laboratory signs are used to define the disorder and form the standard against which various diagnostic tests are judged.

The studies that established the association of GDM with perinatal morbidity defined GDM based on threshold blood glucose concentrations after an oral glucose load. In this case, the diagnostic test does not identify morbidity directly but rather the pregnancy at risk. In gravid women with GDM, additional tests may help document the presence of macrosomia, fetal asphyxia, or the risk of neonatal morbidity. In the following discussion, the glucose tolerance test (oral or intravenous) is viewed as the diagnostic test, whereas the various means of identifying gravid women in whom the tolerance test should be performed are viewed as screening tests.

The diagnostic (or confirmatory) test should meet several functional requirements.[17] The test procedure should be clearly defined and easily performed in various clinical situations and laboratories. The interpretation of the test should be simple, even if the derivation of the limits of normality are complex and controversial (such as with the oral glucose tolerance test). The test should be evaluated for reproducibility of test function among individual subjects and among testing centers. Diagnostic (or confirmatory) tests should have a high sensitivity and specificity based on studies of

Table 16-1. Parameters of Diagnostic Tests

		Condition	
	Test result	Present	Absent
Sensitivity: a ÷	Abnormal	a	b
(a + c)			
Specificity: d ÷	Normal	c	d
(b + d)			

Positive predictive
 accuracy: a ÷
 (a + b)

Negative predictive
accuracy:
d ÷ (c + d)

Note that sensitivity and specificity are independent of the prevalence of a condition [(a + c) ÷ (a + b + c + d)], whereas positive and negative predictive accuracy are a function of the condition's prevalence.

subjects with known diagnoses and appropriate unaffected controls. The positive and negative predictive accuracies of the diagnostic test are evaluated by applying the test to varying populations, thereby establishing the test's clinical utility and cost (Table 16-1).

The screening test, the means by which patients are selected for definitive testing, should be well defined, easily administered, inexpensive, and reproducible. The screening test should have a high sensitivity, identifying most individuals who have the disorder, but it need not have the high specificity demanded of the diagnostic test. The following discussion illustrates many of the above criteria for screening and diagnostic tests.

ORAL GLUCOSE TOLERANCE TEST

The oral glucose tolerance test has commonly been used in clinical investigation and practice because it models the physiologic events after a meal and is easily administered. Several earlier studies (Table 16-2) have addressed the methodologic issues of establishing norms for the oral glucose tolerance test.

Most studies lack information relating glucose tolerance test thresholds to subsequent rates of perinatal morbidity.[3,5,18–21] High tolerance test criteria may define an obvious high-risk group of gravid women[5] but may not identify the larger number of pregnant women whose fetuses remain at risk from maternal glucose

intolerance. Low tolerance test thresholds may inappropriately label normal-risk gravid women as having GDM. Some studies were limited by not justifying the choice of diagnostic threshold,[3,21] not defining the population tested,[3,18,21] having an inadequate sample size, or choosing nonspecific outcomes such as perinatal mortality that may follow other maternal morbidities independent of GDM.[3] Gillmer et al[20] correlated the depression in neonatal blood glucose with the total increase in blood glucose concentrations above baseline values in a 3-hour oral glucose tolerance test performed in late pregnancy, although diagnostic threshold values were not chosen. Glucose tolerance test criteria were not examined in the study.

O'Sullivan and Mahan's[22] study of the prevalence of late diabetes after gestational glucose intolerance from an unselected group of pregnancies has formed the basis for the glucose tolerance test criteria in pregnancy that are most commonly used in North America. With glucose tolerance test data from 752 subjects, upper limits for normal were selected statistically and defined as two standard deviations (SD) above the mean for each of four glucose values in the 3-hour test. Glucose intolerance was identified when at least two test values met or exceeded these limits (Table 16-3). This yielded the prevalence of GDM of approximately 2 percent sought by the authors. O'Sullivan et al[4] documented a fourfold increased perinatal mortality rate among 187 pregnant women who were identified as having GDM in this manner. These mathematically derived criteria were also validated by finding a 60 percent prevalence of abnormal glucose tolerance 16 years later in women previously identified as having GDM.[9] By this means, criteria for glucose tolerance during pregnancy were developed that identified pregnancies at risk of perinatal mishap in a small proportion of the general population.

In O'Sullivan's studies, whole blood was tested using the Somogyi-Nelson method for measuring reducing substances. Several later studies have attempted to transliterate his findings to present methods of glucose oxidase or hexokinase assays of plasma. Plasma glucose values have been shown to be 14 percent higher than those in whole blood obtained from the same samples using the same assay method.[23] Amankwah et al[24] added 13 percent to O'Sullivan's Somogyi-Nelson values and rounded these numbers to the nearest 5 mg/dl. The National Diabetes Data Group (NDDG)[14]

Table 16-2. Proposed Criteria for Oral Glucose Tolerance Test During Pregnancy

| Author[a] | Oral Glucose Load (g) | Sample Time and Glucose Values (mg/dl) | | | | | | | Medium | Method | Criteria for Abnormal Test |
		Fasting	30 Min	60 Min	90 Min	120 Min	150 Min	180 Min			
Carrington et al.[3] 1957	100					170			Whole blood	Folin-Wu	120-min value met or exceeded
O'Sullivan and Mahan[22] (1964)	100	90		165		143		127	Whole blood	Somogyi-Nelson	Two values met or exceeded
Chen et al.[18] (1972)	100	110		185		130		118	Plasma	Glucose oxidase	Three values met or exceeded
Macafee et al.[5] (1974)	50	180		180		140		180	Plasma	Glucose oxidase	120-min and any other value met or exceeded
Gillmer et al.[20] (1975)	50	+[b]	+	+	+	+	+	+	Plasma	Glucose oxidase	≥42 area units above baseline
Amankwah et al.[24] (1977)	100	100		180		160		140	Plasma	Glucose hexokinase	Two values met or exceeded
NDDG[14] (1979)	100	105		190		165		145	Plasma	Glucose oxidase	Two values met or exceeded
Merkatz et al.[19] (1980)	75	105		185		140		125	Plasma	Glucose oxidase	Two values met or exceeded
Mestman[21] (1980)	100	110		200		150		130	Plasma	Glucose oxidase	Two values met or exceeded
Carpenter and Coustan[28] (1982)	100	95		180		155		140	Plasma	Glucose oxidase	Two values met or exceeded

[a] Numbers in parentheses represent year of study publication.
[b] + = time of sampling.

Table 16-3. Criteria for 100-G Oral Glucose Tolerance Test in Pregnancy (mg/dl glucose)

Time	O'Sullivan and Mahan[22a]	NDDG[14] Adaption	Carpenter and Coustan[26] Adaptation
Preglucose	90	105	95
1 hr	165	190	180
2 h	145	165	155
3 h	125	145	140

[a] O'Sullivan and Mahan rounded chi-square + 2 SD values to nearest 5 mg/dl.

reinterpreted O'Sullivan's data for glucose oxidase methods on plasma by increasing O'Sullivan's criteria by 15 percent; these criteria were reaffirmed by the American Diabetes Association in 1985.[25] However, neither attempt to transliterate O'Sullivan's data took into consideration the change in method in addition to the change in the medium tested. The Somogyi-Nelson method has been shown to identify other saccharides in addition to glucose. The glucose oxidase or hexokinase methods are specific for glucose and generally result in a 5-mg/dl decrease in measured values in the range of glucose concentrations documented in these tests.[26,27] Criteria for the 100-g glucose tolerance test proposed by Carpenter and Coustan[28] take both issues into consideration when interpreting O'Sullivan's criteria. Sacks et al[29] performed simultaneous Somogyi-Nelson assays in whole blood and glucose oxidase assays in plasma in 994 unselected pregnant women undergoing 3-hour glucose tolerance tests, confirming that the Somogyi-Nelson assay resulted in glucose values 2 to 6 percent higher than the glucose oxidase assay. Patients whose glucose tolerance test results fall between the Carpenter and Coustan and NDDG criteria have the same probability of insulin treatment (26 percent) as those meeting the NDDG criteria (30 percent)[30] and the same probability of fetal macrosomia.[31]

Because O'Sullivan's original criteria were developed from a statistical model, it remains uncertain whether even the most "accurate" transliteration of them to modern testing methods is relevant. For example, even when only one value of the 3-hour glucose tolerance test is abnormal, surveillance of such pregnancies demonstrates the frequent need for insulin treatment, and application of such treatment in a randomized trial has been shown to reduce the macrosomia rate significantly to nondiabetic values compared with that in nontreated controls.[32] Still unexamined is the correlation of a glucose tolerance test with perinatal morbidity in the context of modern obstetric practice by means of blinding physicians to the results of the tolerance test. Such a study of appropriate size would address the utility of the test for diagnosis and intervention in pregnancy.

In contrast to common practice in North America, much of the rest of the world uses a 75-g oral glucose tolerance test during pregnancy, according to criteria adopted by the World Health Organization.[15] A multicenter study of the effect of pregnancy on the 75-g, 2-hour test enlisted 1,009 mostly unselected pregnant women.[33] Based on the 95th percentile, fasting, 1-hour, and 2-hour values in subjects whose pregnancies were beyond 16 weeks' gestation, diagnostic values of 7, 11, and 9 mM, respectively, were suggested. The authors suggested that impaired glucose tolerance during pregnancy be diagnosed if the test produced an abnormal 2-hour glucose value and if either the fasting or the 1-hour limit were met. These criteria resulted in 10 women diagnosed as having impaired glucose tolerance and 2 with World Health Organization criteria for diabetes mellitus for an incidence of 1.2 percent in a sample group with a mean maternal age of 27 years.

However, the utility of these criteria for the identification of perinatal morbidity still requires examination.

INTRAVENOUS GLUCOSE TOLERANCE TEST

The IVGTT was adapted for use in pregnancy by Silverstone et al.[34] The unit of measurement of the test, the k value, is a measure of the percent decrease of glucose over time, according to the equation, $\log_e y = \log_e A - kt$, where y is the blood glucose concentration in milligrams per deciliter, A is the y intercept, and t is the elapsed time in minutes. The value k then becomes the index of tolerance. The disappearance curve for glucose after rapid intravenous injection is, therefore, a logarithmic function and can be plotted on semilogarithmic paper as a straight line. The slope, k, can be computed by dividing the difference between the natural logs of any two glucose values, A and B, by the intervening time interval in minutes multiplied by 100, according to the following equation.

$$k = \frac{\log_e A - \log_e B}{\text{time B} - \text{time A (in minutes)}} \times 100$$

Posner's et al[35] table provides the means of transposing the quotient of a 10-minute level and a 60-minute glucose level to a k value (Table 16-4). Silverstone et al[34,36] described mean and lower 95 percent confidence limit k values during the three trimesters of pregnancy, derived from a visually fitted slope derived from six data points at 10-minute intervals during the 1-hour test. Subjects used for these studies were known to have normal fasting blood sugar levels and be free of glycosuria. The subjects also had no family history of diabetes and no history of macrosomia, liver disease, thyroid disease, cardiac disease, or hypertension. The patients were also not taking drugs that might affect their glucose tolerance. The lower limit of normal for k in the first trimester (-2 SD) was 1.37; in the second trimester, 1.18; and in the third trimester, 1.13. Values below this level were regarded as abnormal.

O'Sullivan et al[37] reported on 232 randomly selected pregnancies tested in the third trimester and 11 weeks' postpartum with an IVGTT. They found a mean k of 2.02 in late pregnancy and 2.53 postpartum. They

Table 16-4. Posner et al's[35] Intravenous Glucose Tolerance Test k Values Derived From Quotients[3]

Q	k	Q	k	Q	k
1.284	0.50	1.568	0.90	1.916	1.30
1.290	0.51	1.576	0.91	1.925	1.31
1.297	0.52	1.584	0.92	1.935	1.32
1.303	0.53	1.592	0.93	1.944	1.33
1.310	0.54	1.600	0.94	1.954	1.34
1.316	0.55	1.608	0.95	1.964	1.35
1.323	0.56	1.616	0.96	1.974	1.36
1.330	0.57	1.624	0.97	1.984	1.37
1.336	0.58	1.632	0.98	1.994	1.38
1.343	0.59	1.640	0.99	2.004	1.39
1.350	0.60	1.649	1.00	2.014	1.40
1.357	0.61	1.657	1.01	2.024	1.41
1.364	0.62	1.665	1.02	2.034	1.42
1.370	0.63	1.674	1.03	2.044	1.43
1.377	0.64	1.682	1.04	2.054	1.44
1.384	0.65	1.690	1.05	2.065	1.45
1.391	0.66	1.699	1.06	2.075	1.46
1.398	0.67	1.707	1.07	2.086	1.47
1.405	0.68	1.716	1.08	2.096	1.48
1.412	0.69	1.725	1.09	2.110	1.49
1.419	0.70	1.733	1.10	2.117	1.50
1.426	0.71	1.742	1.11	2.128	1.51
1.433	0.72	1.751	1.12	2.138	1.52
1.441	0.73	1.759	1.13	2.149	1.53
1.448	0.74	1.768	1.14	2.160	1.54
1.455	0.75	1.777	1.15	2.171	1.55
1.462	0.76	1.786	1.16	2.182	1.56
1.470	0.77	1.795	1.17	2.193	1.57
1.477	0.78	1.804	1.18	2.204	1.58
1.484	0.79	1.813	1.19	2.214	1.59
1.492	0.80	1.822	1.20	2.226	1.60
1.499	0.81	1.831	1.21	2.237	1.61
1.507	0.82	1.844	1.22	2.247	1.62
1.514	0.83	1.850	1.23	2.259	1.63
1.522	0.84	1.859	1.24	2.271	1.64
1.530	0.85	1.863	1.25	2.282	1.65
1.537	0.86	1.878	1.26	2.294	1.66
1.545	0.87	1.887	1.27	2.307	1.67
1.553	0.88	1.896	1.28	2.316	1.68
1.561	0.89	1.906	1.29	2.329	1.69

[a] Q = 10-min glucose/60-min glucose.
(From Posner et al,[35] with permission.)

found 11 percent of patients had third trimester values less than or equal to 1.34. Hadden et al[38] found 16 percent of selected patients had k values less than or equal to 1.40, but neither series observed an excessive perinatal mortality rate in pregnancies with low k values.

Several studies have compared the IVGTT with an oral glucose tolerance test using varying criteria for each test in subjects with low[39] and high[36,40,41] a priori risks for GDM. These studies show a poor correlation between the two tests, although none have performed tests in a large, unselected group of pregnant women and none have related test results to perinatal morbidity.

The IVGTT offers some theoretic advantages over the oral glucose tolerance test. The k value allows easier analysis of glucose tolerance data and is, in most circumstances, independent of the method of glucose measurement. Finally, it is unaffected by variation in gastric emptying and other phenomena that may vary from patient to patient. On the other hand, the IVGTT is more expensive and is nonphysiologic in that glucose is infused in a bolus, peripherally, and is not subject to the usual influence of gastrointestinal physiology.

SCREENING TESTS

Historical and Clinical Risk Factors

Historical and clinical risk factors have been advocated as indications for an oral glucose tolerance test in pregnancy, thus functioning, as a group, as a screening test.[42] Reproductive history (e.g., prior offspring weighing 9 lb or more, fetal death, neonatal death, congenital anomaly, and prematurity), family history of diabetes, and clinical findings (e.g., obesity, excessive weight gain during pregnancy, glycosuria, proteinuria, and hypertension) have been advocated as factors that mandate an oral glucose tolerance test. Apart from obesity and glycosuria, O'Sullivan et al[43] found the presence of these risk factors in 37 percent of an unselected indigent population. In this study, historical risk factors had a sensitivity of 0.63 in contrast to the 50-g challenge test, which had a sensitivity of 0.79 at a cutoff level of 130 mg/dl using Somogyi-Nelson methods in whole blood (approximately 143 mg/dl by the glucose oxidase method in plasma). Others have found that historical and clinical risk factors identify only 50 percent of cases of GDM.[44–46] Historical and clinical risk factors, therefore, have a high prevalence and function with a low test sensitivity, both of which are undesirable for a screening test.

Maternal age has also been advocated as a criterion for subsequent testing. The largest study of unselected population-based screening found an incidence of GDM of 3.8 percent in women 30 to 34 years of age but only 0.7 percent in those younger than age 21.[46] However, the presently advocated GDM screening protocol of providing an oral glucose challenge only in women 30 years of age or older and in younger women with risk factors, results in a sensitivity of only 65 percent at a cutoff of 140 mg/dl.[42] Because most pregnancies occur in younger women, a screening sensitivity of 90 percent is reached at this threshold only if all pregnant women are screened with an oral glucose challenge. Consequently, screening for GDM in all gravid women, with some sort of glucose challenge test, is desirable.

Glucose Challenge Test

Several studies have proposed oral glucose challenge test criteria for further testing with an oral glucose tolerance test. These studies vary in patient selection, the documentation of test conditions and results, and the rationale for the choice of a screening test threshold. Most studies are a sequential series of patients or appear to be a random sampling of patients, although two studies appear to be selected patient samples.[18,24] Three studies did not provide explicit documentation of either testing method or whether whole blood, plasma, or serum was used for testing.[18,19,47] In several investigations, a uniform screening protocol was not used.[19,20,44,48] Three studies documented test parameters, so as to provide the basis for comparison with other later studies.[19,28,43] In only one study, was there universal confirmatory testing of the screening test result.[43] Because of O'Sullivan's universal confirmation of the 50-g oral glucose challenge screening test and because of its high sensitivity for detecting GDM, this type of screening test is most commonly used in North America. However, there is no agreement about what threshold of this screening test should be used to require the confirmatory 3-hour, 100-g oral glucose tolerance test. In a population-based study, universal screening for GDM was performed in more than 6,000

subjects with a 50-g challenge and glucose oxidase method in plasma with follow-up 3-hour glucose tolerance testing in all with screening test values 130 mg/dl or higher.[46] Ten percent of all subjects with GDM had screening test values between 130 and 139 mg/dl. However, the increased sensitivity for GDM achieved by performing confirmatory testing of screening values in this range would result in an increase in confirmatory testing from 14 to 23 percent with its attendant costs.

Glucose Polymer Challenge Tests

Glucose polymer is an inexpensive, commercially available glucose saccharide mixture containing 3 percent glucose, 7 percent maltose, 55 percent maltotrios, and 85 percent polysaccharides. Its osmotic load is one-fifth that of glucose and has been reported to be associated with less gastrointestinal symptoms. The potential improvement in patient comfort in using this preparation and its correlation with tests performed with glucose solution have, consequently, been investigated[49–52] (Table 16-5. Reece et al[51] observed a high degree of correspondence between the two solutions employed in the 1-hour challenge test (κ = 0.62; P <0.0001). Women expressed a preference for the Polycose drink, and had less gastrointestinal symptoms. A moderate level of agreement between the results of 3-hour glucose tolerance tests using the two solutions (κ = 0.45; P <0.001) has also been demonstrated.[52] These result suggest that the glucose polymer is an effective alternative to glucose.

Testing State

There is a gradual impairment of glucose tolerance during the second trimester of pregnancy, which results in elevated blood glucose concentrations and increased insulin/glucose ratios after meals in the normal gravid woman. Conversely, there is a decrease in fasting blood glucose in mid-to-late pregnancy. These normal changes persist until delivery. As a result, testing protocols suggest that, in asymptomatic patients without signs of diabetes, screening and definitive testing for GDM be delayed until the second half of pregnancy, usually 24 to 28 weeks after the last menstrual period.

Studies that examined glucose screening test criteria have not documented patient feeding before the glu-

Table 16-5. Tests for Gestational Diabetes Using Glucose Versus Polymer Saccharide Solutions

Author	Methods	Results
Court et al[49] (1984)	Single-blind trial, women at risk for GDM 50-g polymer vs. 50-g glucose tests Outcomes Symptoms, incremental area under 2-hour curve	Polymer ingestion followed by less symptoms and associated with comparable curve area
Court et al[50] (1985)	Open label trial of duplicate oral tolerance tests, unselected pregnancies 100-g polymer vs. 100-g glucose Outcomes Mean plasma glucose, incremental area	Mean plasma glucose and incremental area under 2-hour curve were comparable in polymer vs. glucose tests; correlation between 1st and 2nd test was better using polymer solution
Reece et al[51] (1987)	Open label observational trial of polymer test followed by glucose test 50-g, 1-hour challenge test Outcome Proprotion with abnormal tests	Polymer test abnormal in 5 of 7 glucose-abnormal tests; glucose test abnormal in 5 of 8 polymer-abnormal tests
Reece et al[52] (1989)	Open label observational trial of polymer test followed by glucose test 100-g, 3-hour tolerance test Outcome Proprotion with abnormal tests	Polymer test abnormal in 2 of 4 glucose-abnormal tests; glucose test abnormal in 2 of 4 polymer-abnormal tests

Abbreviation: GDM, gestational diabetes mellitus.

cose screening test. In a recent study, a 50-g oral glucose screening test was administered in the fasting state and 1 hour after a standard 600-calorie breakfast in a randomized crossover trial.[53] There were 46 confirmed normal subjects and 24 patients with GDM studied. There were no differences in test results under the two conditions among normal individuals. The test result was significantly higher among patients with GDM if they were fasting (173.9 ± 28.8 mg/dl) than if the test followed a standard breakfast (154.8 ± 24.1 mg/dl). These findings contrast with those of Lewis et al[54] who found that, among those with GDM, glucose levels 1 hour after 50-g glucose ingestion were similar in the fasting state as in the 1-hour postmeal but lower in the 2-hour postmeal state. Nondiabetic subjects had higher glucose levels 1 hour after the 50-g glucose ingestion if this was performed in the fasting state. A cross-sectional study of the effect of postmeal interval on the 50-g 1-hour challenge test demonstrated an increased insulin response but no change in glycemic response when the test was performed within 3 hours of a preceding meal.[55] Overall, these data suggest that, if a patient has eaten, a 130-mg/dl test threshold is appropriate to maximize test sensitivity. If it can be documented, however, that the patient is in a fasting state, then a different screening test threshold, perhaps 140

to 145 mg/dl, can yield similar test sensitivity of about 90 percent and potentially improve the specificity relative to the glucose tolerance test. Nevertheless, the utility of being able to perform the screening test in the context of the antepartum office visit, without regard to the timing and content of the last meal is so great that using the test threshold of 130 mg/dl would be preferred so as to maximize test sensitivity at the cost of a slightly reduced test specificity in those patients who may be in a fasted state at the time of the screening test.

Fasting, Random, and Postmeal Glucose Studies as Screening Tests

Glucose values obtained without a glucose challenge have been investigated as screening tests. Such tests, if workable, would have the advantage of avoiding the administration of a glucose solution.

The fasting plasma glucose concentration is less likely to be elevated than postprandial values in GDM.[56–58] O'Sullivan et al[4] found that only 2 percent of unselected patients had fasting whole blood levels greater than or equal to 90 mg/dl. In another study of 1,697 gravid women, no GDM was identified among those having fasting plasma glocuses less than 90 mg/

dl.[59] However, glucose tolerance testing was performed only on women with historical risk factors and in a small sample of those without.

Stangenberg et al[60] examined 6,969 random blood glucose levels from 1,500 pregnant women without any "signs or symptoms of diabetes." They found a mean of 83 mg/dl and a 95th percentile of 114 mg/dl. With a threshold of 116 mg/dl, 11.6 percent of the 1,500 subjects had an abnormal value; of those, 10 (5.8 percent) had an abnormal glucose tolerance test result. However, with the exception of 30 patients who had fasting glycosuria, no confirmatory testing was performed in the rest of the 1,500 patients. The overall prevalence of GDM identified in this group (0.9 percent) was substantially less than that in O'Sullivan's study performed with universal confirmatory testing. This suggests that a protocol that uses random blood glucose levels may have a substantial false-negative rate.

Lind and Anderson[61] performed plasma glucose measurements on 2,043 patients between 28 and 32 weeks' gestation. Subjects who ate within 2 hours and those who ate more than 2 hours earlier had 99th percentile values of 109 and 100 mg/dl, respectively. In the 32 (1.4 percent) subjects whose levels exceeded this cutoff, 2 had unequivocal diabetes, and 4 had impaired glucose tolerance, according to World Health Organization criteria.[15] This low prevalence of GDM (0.26 percent) was partly the result of the higher glucose tolerance test criteria used in the study. That only 1.7 percent of the unselected screened population was actually tested with a glucose tolerance test suggests that a substantial proportion of patients with GDM in this population may have been undetected.

Coustan et al[62] found that a standardized 600-calorie meal could be used to identify gravid women with known GDM, but only at a 1-hour postmeal glucose threshold of 100 mg/dl could a 90 percent test sensitivity be achieved. This threshold (mean plus 0.85 SD in a group of 46 nondiabetic subjects) would require confirmatory testing in more than 20 percent of screened subjects.

Glycated Blood Proteins in the Diagnosis of Gestational Diabetes

Glycated hemoglobins and other proteins have been investigated as screening tests for GDM (Table 16-6). Glycation is the slow and almost irreversible binding of glucose or a phosphorylated sugar to hemoglobin or other blood proteins. Because it is dependent on the concentration of the reactants and because the red blood cell concentration of glucose approximates that in extracellular fluid, glycated hemoglobin has been investigated as a diagnostic test for nongestationally related diabetes. Using ion exchange chromatography, nonfractionated glycohemoglobin was measured in 167 patients undergoing a glucose tolerance test and in 105 known diabetic patients.[63] A significant difference in mean glycohemoglobin values could be demonstrated in the group with a normal glucose tolerance test result compared with those with an abnormal one, even if the patients appeared to maintain fasting and postprandial euglycemia apart from the tolerance test. Hall et al[64] used affinity chromatography on fresh and postincubation aliquots of hemoglobin to measure total and stable glycohemoglobin levels on 53 patients referred for glucose testing. Those who had impaired glucose tolerance and diabetes mellitus, according to World Health Organization criteria, had significantly greater total and stable glycohemoglobin levels than those with normal glucose tolerance test results. In this small number of patients, there was no overlap in values of stable glycosylated hemoglobin when normal subjects were compared with those with impaired glucose tolerance or diabetes mellitus.

GDM, however, may not present with the same constant elevations of blood sugar levels as in nonpregnant states. Gravid women with GDM have fasting blood sugar concentrations that are low by comparison with those in nonpregnant individuals. In addition, normal nondiabetic gravid women have significantly elevated postabsorptive glucose values compared with those in the nonpregnant woman. Because of increased erythropoiesis, red blood cells are younger in pregnancy, and hemoglobin is less glycated. Finally, disturbances in glucose tolerance may have only occurred for a brief period, as a result of the hormonal milieu changing rapidly from relative insulin sensitivity to that of insulin resistance as the pregnancy progresses. For all these reasons, a measure of chronic hyperglycemia, such as glycated hemoglobin, may not be effective in distinguishing normal from gestational diabetic gravid women. Hemoglobin A_{1c} (HbA_{1c}) values in nondiabetic women have been shown to fall during pregnancy from the first through the third trimester and then to rise postpartum.[65] In another study, however,

Table 16-6. Tests for Gestational Diabetes Using Fructosamine or Glycated Hemoglobin Assays versus Oral Glucose Challenge Tests

Author	Methods	Results
Roberts et al[74] (1983)	Observed pregnancies tested with GTT and fructosamine within 4 weeks; normal fructosamine was <95th percentile for normal pregnancy; 79 gravidae tested by 3-hour 100-g GTT	17 of 20 (85%) with abnormal GTT had elevated fructosamine Specificity = 95%
Roberts et al[75] (1990)	Observed 507 unselected pregnancies tested with 28 and 36 week 100-g GTT; fructosamine at 36 weeks	Compared to 36-week GTT, sensitivity of 28-week GTT was 81% and for 36-week fructosamine was 50%
Nasrat et al[76] (1990)	Observed unselected pregnancies; tested 2nd and 3rd trimester with fructosamine and GTT; fructosamine abnormal at 90th percentile	Fructosamine had 50% sensitivity for abnormal GTT
Comtois et al[77] (1989)	Compared fructosamine and fructosamine/protein; 100-g GTT in 100 pregnancies with risk of GDM	Similar fructosamine levels; fructosamine/protein elevated in only 3/13 GDM
Fadel et al[17] (1979)	HbA$_1$ (microcolumn technique) in 53 normal and 22 GDM tested for clinical risk	5.8 ± 1.0% vs. 7.0 ± 1.3% (ns); only 5/23 GDM had HbA$_1$ values ≥2 SD
Shah et al[68] (1982)	HbA$_1$ (ion-exchange chromatography, abnormal >8.8%); 50-g, 1-hour (≥140 mg/dl), 100-g GTT; 90 subjects at clinical risk	Similar HbA$_1$ in those with and without GDM HbA$_1$: sensitivity 22%, specificity 90% 50-g challenge: sensitivity 83%, specificity 56%
Artal et al[69] (1984)	HbA$_1$ (ion-exchange chromatography, abnormal >7.0%); 100-g GTT (higher than ADA criteria); 82 random patients	Similar HbA$_1$ in those with and without GDM HbA$_1$: sensitivity 73%, specificity 34%
McFarland et al[70] (1984)	HbA$_1$ (thiobarbituric acid technique) in 17 normal and 22 GDM identified by glucose screening	0.49 ± 0.07 vs. 0.54 ± 0.06 nM hydorxymethylfurfural/mg protein (P < .05); high degree of overlap between those with and without GDM
Cousins et al[71] (1984)	HbA$_1$ (fast hemoglobin test, abnormal >6.8%); 50-g, 1-hour (≥150 mg/dl), 100-g GTT; 806 unselected subjects	Similar HbA$_1$ in those with and without GDM HbA$_1$: sensitivity 80%, specificity 57% 50-g challenge: sensitivity about 80%, specificity 92%

Abbreviations: GTT, 3-hour glucose tolerance test; GDM, gestational diabetes mellitus; HbA$_1$, hemoglobin A$_1$.

the HbA$_{1c}$ concentration was reported to be elevated in normal pregnancy.[66]

Fadel et al,[67] using a microcolumn chromatographic method to identify HbA$_1$ and O'Sullivan's criteria for GDM, compared HbA$_1$ values among 23 nondiabetic nonpregnant women, 53 normal pregnant women, and 22 patients with GDM. The latter had significant elevations in HbA$_1$, although there was considerable overlap in the distribution of values among groups.

Shah et al[68] measured HbA$_1$ using ion-exchange chromatography and applied the NDDG criteria for GDM in a group of patients with risk factors for it. Glucose tolerance tests were performed in those patients who had a 50-g oral glucose challenge test result of 140 mg/dl or more or who later presented with other clinical data suggestive of this disorder. Of the 18 patients identified with GDM, 15 had an abnormal oral challenge test result, and only 4 had an abnormal glycated hemoglobin value. This indicates a test sensitivity of 27 percent for glycated hemoglobin in the identification of GDM in this at-risk group. A high proportion of the elevated glycated hemoglobin values (five of nine) were found in gravid women without GDM.

Artal et al[69] measured HbA$_1$ with ion-exchange chromatography and more restrictive criteria for an oral glucose tolerance test to define GDM in an at-risk group of gravid women. A low HbA$_{1c}$ cutoff of 7 percent was used as a screening test for GDM. This low HbA$_{1c}$ value gave a test sensitivity of 73 percent but was very nonspecific (34 percent). McFarland et al[70] found no difference in glycated hemoglobin levels between 41 women with normal glucose tolerance and 12 women with GDM by the NDDG criteria.

Cousins et al[71] performed 1-hour, 50-g glucose challenge tests and glycated hemoglobin levels on 806 consecutive unselected prenatal patients. This group used the NDDG criteria for GDM. The effect of the test threshold of the glucose challenge test and the HbA$_1$ test on sensitivity and specificity were compared. The authors performed glucose tolerance testing on all subjects with a challenge test result of 150 mg/dl or more. Assuming that this scheme would identify 80 percent of patients with GDM, the authors calculated the specificity of the glucose challenge test to be 92 percent at 150 mg/dl. An HbA_1 threshold of 6.8 achieved a sensitivity of 80 percent but had a specificity of only 57 percent at this cutoff. If the HbA_1 threshold is increased (9.2 percent), so that a specificity of 92 percent is reached, the sensitivity falls to about 36 percent. These data, obtained from an unselected pregnancy sample, do not support the use of glycated hemoglobin as a screening test for GDM.

It is unknown whether fractions of glycosylated hemoglobin, which have been tested in the nonpregnant population and found to be effective, would perform equally well in the identification of women with GDM. Studies in the use of the stable fraction of HbA_{1c} may show this to be a more effective screening tool. Other glycosylated plasma proteins have a potential as markers for GDM. Glycosylated albumin has a shorter half-life than that of glycosylated hemoglobin and may be more effective in identifying women with an acute rise in mean daily blood glucoses. Jones et al[72] showed a more rapid decline in glycated albumin than glycated hemoglobin among nonpregnant patients with types I and II diabetes undergoing initial insulin treatment.

Leiper et al,[73] using affinity chromatography, examined glycated albumin, glycated plasma proteins, and glycated hemoglobin in 14 insulin-dependent diabetic gravid women. A decrease of more than 50 percent in the former markers was noted after 4 weeks of improved metabolic control. Not until 12 weeks, however, did glycated hemoglobin levels decrease significantly.

Another marker for abnormalities of glucose hemostasis is fructosamine, an indicator of the glycation of plasma proteins. Roberts et al[74] showed a significant difference in fructosamine levels among women with GDM versus those without GDM. Using the 95th percentile cutoff for nondiabetic gravid women, the authors found a test sensitivity of 0.85 and specificity of 0.95 for fructosamine. However, the same authors[75] found that, in an unspecified sample of 507 pregnant women, a 100-g glucose load at 28 weeks had a sensitivity for GDM diagnosed at 36 weeks of 81 percent compared with a sensitivity of 50 percent for fructosamine tests performed at 4-week intervals during pregnancy.

Nasrat et al[76] found no association in unselected pregnant women between fructosamine and second or third trimester fasting glucose levels or birth weight and found a fructosamine sensitivity of only 50 percent for GDM using the 90th percentile value. The low sensitivity of fructosamine for GDM has also been noted by other investigators.[77]

AMNIOTIC FLUID STUDIES

In both normal and diabetic pregnancies, amniotic fluid glucose levels have been noted to correlate with simultaneous maternal plasma glucose concentrations and to rise acutely in response to a maternal glucose load. Insulin content or concentration in amniotic fluid is associated with increased amniotic fluid glucose and may provide a more stable marker for diabetic fetopathy. Using a solid-phase system for radioimmunologic insulin determination, Weiss et al[78] measured total insulin concentration in amniotic fluid in 487 samples of fluid, noting a slight upward trend between 28 and 42 weeks' gestation. In a subsequent study, 75 women with a family history of diabetes underwent an oral glucose tolerance test that consisted of a glucose load of 1 g/kg and capillary blood glucose samples obtained in the fasting state and 2 hours after glucose ingestion.[79] This test was performed between 20 and 28 weeks' gestation. At various times after 28 weeks, amniotic fluid total insulin concentrations were determined. Of the 25 patients with postprandial plasma glucose values in excess of 200 mg/dl, 9 showed evidence of diabetic fetopathy in the infant at birth. Another five infants with diabetic fetopathy were found among subjects with lower postprandial glucose tolerance test values. All 14 infants showing evidence of diabetic fetopathy had elevated amniotic fluid total insulin concentrations.

In addition, the proinsulin connecting peptide, C-peptide, has been measured in amniotic fluid as a marker for fetal insulin production. Assays for C-peptide offer advantages over those for insulin because C-peptide is not bound by anti-insulin antibodies and is minimally extracted by the liver, and assays are not affected by the presence of proinsulin. Levels of amniotic fluid C-peptide correlate well with standardized infant birth weight and the degree of diabetic control.[80] One study found an association of total amniotic fluid content of C-peptide with the presence of neonatal morbidity but not C-peptide concentration.[81]

Amniotic fluid biochemical markers for diabetic fetopathy should be distinguished from tests designed to identify gravid women with abnormal glucose tolerance. The former test is best applied to pregnant women already known to have glucose intolerance who are, thus, at risk of diabetic fetopathy. Amniotic fluid studies, therefore, serve as confirmatory tests and are, therefore, required to have high test specificity and sensitivity. Conversely, glucose challenge tests are designed to identify gravid women with disturbances in glucose homeostasis, only some of whom will have evidence of diabetic fetopathy. Challenge tests, therefore, serve as screening tests, identifying a small group of gravid women at high risk. The circumstances justifying measurements of amniotic fluid glucose, insulin, proinsulin, or C-peptide level in diabetes-complicated pregnancies are, as yet, undefined.

POSTPARTUM IDENTIFICATION OF PRE-EXISTING GESTATIONAL DIABETES

Most women having large babies do not have glucose intolerance identifiable during the pregnancy. In circumstances in which universal screening is not performed during pregnancy, when a woman has a large offspring, postpartum testing may identify antecedent GDM. This information would allow counseling about the risk of glucose intolerance in subsequent pregnancies and later in life.

Glucose homeostasis and insulin sensitivity appear to change within the first few days after delivery. This may be due to altered diet, increased nocturnal activity, and possibly increased glucose utilization induced by lactation, as well as the abrupt cessation of placental influence. MacDonald et al[82] performed a 50-g glucose challenge in the early puerperium on 357 women who had been tested for glucose tolerance during their preceding pregnancy. They were able to document a slight drop in fasting and 2.5-hour postchallenge glucose values in the puerperium. In 12 nondiabetic women, Lind et al[83] showed a significant drop in fasting plasma insulin levels by the second postpartum day. They performed a glucose tolerance test in the early puerperium and again 6 weeks after delivery. Using the incremental area under the glucose tolerance curve, these authors were able to show a continued improvement in glucose hemostasis between that noted in the early puerperium and several weeks postpartum. Carpenter et al[84] performed a 100-g, 3-hour oral glucose tolerance test within 48 hours postpartum in 37 subjects with GDM and 28 with screening test results of less than 130 mg/dl during pregnancy. The sum of the 1- and 2-hour incremental (the postprandial minus the fasting glucose value) glucose values were used to distinguish normal from subjects with GDM. A threshold value of 110 mg/dl yielded a sensitivity of 80 percent and a specificity of 90 percent for antecedent GDM. This test has not been validated patients with macrosomic fetuses.

O'Sullivan and Mahan[22] examined the prevalence of glucose intolerance in the immediate postpartum period among women diagnosed for the first time during pregnancy as having GDM. They identified glucose intolerance by a 100-g glucose challenge, used the same criteria for glucose intolerance as used during the pregnancy, and found a prevalence of 1.8 percent. This study is notable because these patients were sampled sequentially from a presumably normal population of indigent women. Coustan and Lewis[85] identified 72 gravid women with GDM using universal screening. Follow-up in these patients included a fasting and 2-hour postbreakfast test 5 weeks postpartum using fasting value of 105 mg/dl or a 2-hour postmeal value of 120 mg/dl as upper limits. The authors found an 18 percent prevalence of abnormal glucose tolerance by these criteria among their subjects.

Based on these studies, follow-up testing for the purpose of identifying women with continuing impaired glucose tolerance or diabetes should not be done until 5 to 6 weeks postpartum. The NDDG[14] recognizes a 75-g oral glucose challenge test as diagnostic for impaired glucose tolerance in the nonpregnant state if plasma glucose values of 115 mg/dl at fasting, 200 mg/dl at 1 hour, or 140 mg/dl at 2 hours are met or exceeded. The appropriate timing and utility of any glucose challenge testing for the diagnosis of preceding GDM is unknown, however.

C-peptide is secreted in equal molar proportions with insulin. Umbilical cord levels of C-peptide can be measured by assays that eliminate interference by transplacental passage of maternal insulin antibodies and are unaffected by fetal proinsulin. Sosenko et al[86] measured C-peptide levels in 79 infants of diabetic mothers and 62 infants of nondiabetic mothers. They found significantly elevated cord levels in the offspring of diabetic mothers. The degree of elevation correlated well with the presence of hypoglycemia and macrosomia. The earliest assay performed was at 34 weeks.

Weiss et al[87] measured cord blood insulin concentrations by solid-phase radioimmunoassay in 180 mature newborns to obtain a normal range of values and in 221 babies who weighed more than 4,000 g at birth. The umbilical cord insulin level in these cases correlated with increased 1- and 2-hour postprandial glucose tolerance test plasma glucose values, which suggests antecedent GDM. This suggests that either cord C-peptide or insulin levels, with appropriate documentation, may be shown to identify antecedent GDM. Hoegsberg et al[88] found a similar association between fetal macrosomia at birth and cord blood insulin concentrations. However, in contrast to Weiss et al, they could not demonstrate higher antenatal glucose challenge test glucose values in mothers of macrosomic infants.

GLUCOSE TOLERANCE IN TWIN PREGNANCY

The insulin resistance that characterizes the latter half of pregnancy is due, in part, to increased placental secretion of human chorionic somatomammotropin and to increased consumption of insulin by the placenta. A further degeneration of glucose homeostasis might thus be expected in twin pregnancy. Dwyer et al[89] examined the function of a 50-g 3-hour glucose tolerance test in 288 patients with twins and compared the results with those of patients with singleton pregnancies at 32 to 34 weeks' gestation. Women with twin pregnancies had significantly lower fasting plasma glucose levels, but there were not differences in 1-, 2-, and 3-hour glucose levels after glucose ingestion. The incidence of GDM, however, was significantly higher (5.6 percent) than in singleton pregnancies (2.5 percent).

Naidoo et al[90] examined IVGTT results using a glucose load of 0.5 g/kg in 20 twin and 20 singleton pregnancies matched for age, parity, weight, height, and gestational age. Mean glucose disappearance rates did not differ between twin pregnancies and singleton pregnancies. Fasting insulin levels were slightly but not significantly higher in twin pregnancies than in singleton ones. However, all postinfusion insulin levels were significantly higher in twin pregnancies. These data suggest that the 50-g oral glucose challenge test may function appropriately as a screening test in women with twin pregnancies. However, because of the increased requirements for insulin secretion during a twin pregnancy, the likelihood of GDM is probably increased in pregnancies with twin fetuses.

REFERENCES

1. Paton DM: Pregnancy in the prediabetic patient. Am J Obstet Gynecol 56:558, 1948
2. Jackson WPV: Studies in prediabetes. BMJ 2:690, 1965
3. Carrington ER, Shuman CR, Reardon HS: Evaluation of the prediabetic state during pregnancy. Obstet Gynecol 9:664, 1957
4. O'Sullivan JB, Charles D, Mahan CM, Dandrow RV: Gestational diabetes and perinatal mortality rate. Am J Obstet Gynecol 116:901, 1973
5. Macafee CAJ, Beischer NA: The relative value of the standard indications for performing a glucose tolerance test in pregnancy. Med J Aust 1:911, 1974
6. Dandrow RV, O'Sullivan JB: Obstetric hazards of gestational diabetes. Am J Obstet Gynecol 96:1144, 1966
7. Coustan DR, Imarah J: Prophylactic insulin treatment of gestational diabetes reduces the incidence of macrosomia, operative delivery, and birth trauma. Am J Obstet Gynecol 150:836, 1984
8. Warner RA, Cornblath M: Infants of gestational diabetic mothers. Am J Dis Child 117:65, 1975
9. O'Sullivan JB: Long term follow-up of gestational diabetes. In Camerini-Davalos RA, Cole HS (eds): Early Diabetes in Early Life, Third International Symposium. Academic Press, San Diego, 1975
10. Haworth JC, Dilling LAL: Effect of abnormal glucose tolerance in pregnancy on infant mortality rate and morbidity. Am J Obstet Gynecol 122:555, 1975
11. Gabbe SG, Mestman JH, Freeman RK et al: Management and outcome of class A diabetes mellitus. Am J Obstet Gynecol 127:465, 1977
12. O'Sullivan JB, Gellis SS, Dandrow RV, Tenney BO: The potential diabetic and her treatment in pregnancy. Obstet Gynecol 17:683, 1966

13. Coustan DR, Lewis SB: Insulin therapy for gestational diabetes. Obstet Gynecol 51:306, 1978
14. Anonymous: National Diabetes Data Group. Classification and diagnosis of diabetes mellitus and other categories of glucose intolerance. Diabetes 28:1039, 1979
15. WHO Expert Committee on Diabetes Mellitus: World Health Organization Technical Report Series 646. World Health Organization, Geneva, 1980
16. Frienkel N, Hadden D: Summary and recommendations of the Second International Workshop-Conference on Gestational Diabetes Mellitus. Diabetes 34:123, 1985
17. Sackett DL, Haynes RB, Tugwell P: The selection of diagnostic tests. In Clinical Epidemiology. Little, Brown, Boston, 1985
18. Chen W, Palav A, Tricon V: Screening for diabetes in a prenatal clinic. Obstet Gynecol 40:567, 1972
19. Merkatz JR, Duchon MA, Yamashita TS, Housen HB: A pilot community based screening program for gestational diabetes. Diabetes Care 3:453, 1980
20. Gillmer MDG, Beard RW, Brooke FM, Oakley MW: Relation between maternal glucose tolerance and glucose metabolism in the newborn. BMJ 3:402, 1975
21. Mestman JH: Outcome of diabetes screening in pregnancy and perinatal morbidity in infants of mothers with mild impairment in glucose tolerance. Diabetes Care 3:447, 1980
22. O'Sullivan JB, Mahan CM: Criteria for the oral glucose tolerance test in pregnancy. Diabetes 13:278, 1964
23. Mager M, Farest G: What is "true" blood glucose? A comparison of three procedures. Am J Clin Pathol 44:104, 1965
24. Amankwah KS, Prentice RL, Flleury FJ: The incidence of gestational diabetes. Obstet Gynecol 49:497, 1977
25. Anonymous: Proceedings of the Second International Workshop-Conference on Gestational Diabetes Mellitus: Diabetes 34:123, 1985
26. Henry EJ: Clinical Chemistry: Principles and Technics. 1st Ed. Hoeber Medical, New York, 1965
27. Niejadlik DC, Dube AH, Adamko SM: Glucose measurements and clinical correlations. JAMA 224:1743, 1973
28. Carpenter MW, Coustan DR: Criteria for screening tests for gestational diabetes. Am J Obstet Gynecol 144:768, 1982
29. Sacks DA, Abu-Fadil S, Greenspoon JS, Fotheringham N. Do the current standards for glucose tolerance testing in pregnancy represent a valid conversion of O'Sullivan's original criteria? Am J Obstet Gynecol 161:638, 1989
30. Neiger R, Coustan DR: Are the current ACOG glucose tolerance test criteria sensitive enough? Obstet Gynecol 78:1117, 1991
31. Magee MS, Walden CE, Benedette TJ et al: Influence of diagnostic criteria on the incidence of gestational diabetes and perinatal morbidity. JAMA 269:609, 1993
32. Langer O, Anyaegbunam A, Rustman L et al: Management of women with one abnormal glucose tolerance test value reduces adverse outcome in pregnancy. Am J Obstet Gynecol 161:642, 1989
33. Lind T, Phillips PR, the Diabetic Study Group of the European Association for the Study of Diabetes: Influence of pregnancy on the 75-g OGTT: a prospective multicenter study. Diabetes 40:8, 1991
34. Silverstone FA, Solomons E, Rubricius J: The rapid intravenous glucose tolerance test in pregnancy. J Clin Invest 40:2180, 1961
35. Posner NA, Silverstone FA, Brewer J, Heller M: Simplifying the intravenous glucose tolerance test. J Reprod Med 27:633, 1982
36. Silverstone FA, Posner NA, Pomerance W et al: Application of the intravenous and oral glucose tolerance tests in pregnancy. Diabetes 20:476, 1971
37. O'Sullivan JB, Snyder PJ, Sporer AC et al: Intravenous glucose tolerance test and its modification by pregnancy. J Clin Endocrinol Metab 31:33, 1970
38. Hadden DR, Harley JMG, Kajtar TJ, Montgomery DAD: A prospective study of three tests of glucose tolerance in pregnant women selected for potential diabetes with reference to the fetal outcome. Diabetologia 7:87, 1971
39. Ocampo PT, Coseriu VG, Quilligan EF: Comparison of standard oral glucose tolerance test and rapid intravenous glucose tolerance test in normal pregnancy. Obstet Gynecol 24:508, 1964
40. Singh MM, Arshat H: Comparison of oral and intravenous glucose tolerance tests in the diagnosis of diabetes in pregnancy. Br J Obstet Gynaecol 85:536, 1978
41. Cooper A, Granat M, Sharf M: Glucose intolerance during pregnancy II. A comparative study of diagnostic screening methods. Obstet Gynecol 53:495, 1979
42. Management of Diabetes Mellitus in Pregnancy, ACOG Technical Bulletin 92. American College of Obstetricians and Gynecologists, Washington, DC, May 1986
43. O'Sullivan JB, Mahan CM, Charles D, Dandrow RV: Screening criteria for high-risk gestational diabetic patients. Am J Obstet Gynecol 116:895, 1973
44. Lavin JP, Barden TP, Miodovnik M: Clinical experience with a screening program for gestational diabetes. Am J Obstet Gynecol 141:491, 1981
45. Marquette GP, Klein VR, Niebyl JR: Efficacy of screening for gestational diabetes. Am J Perinatol 2:7, 1985
46. Coustan DR, Nelson C, Carpenter MW et al: Maternal age and screening for gestational diabetes: a population-based study. Obstet Gynecol 73:557, 1989
47. Lind T, McDougall AN: Antenatal screening for diabetes mellitus by random blood glucose sampling. Br J Obstet Gynaecol 88:346, 1981
48. Beard RW, Gillmer MDG, Oakley NW, Gunn PJ: Screening for gestational diabetes. Diabetes Care 3:468, 1980

49. Court JD, Stone RP, Killip M: Comparison of glucose and glucose polymer for testing oral carbohydrate tolerance in pregnancy. Obstet Gynecol 64:251, 1984

50. Court JD, Mann SL, Stone PR et al: Comparison of glucose polymer and glucose for screening and tolerance tests in pregnancy. Obstet Gynecol 66:491, 1985

51. Reece EA, Holford T, Tuck S et al: Screening for gestational diabetes: one-hour carbohydrate tolerance test performed by a virtually tasteless polymer of glucose. Am J Obstet Gynecol 156:132, 1989

52. Reece EA, Gabrielli S, Abdalla M et al: Diagnosis of gestational diabetes by the use of a glucose polymer. Am J Obstet Gynecol 160:383, 1989

53. Coustan DR, Widness JA, Carpenter MW et al: Should the 50 gram one hour screening test for gestational diabetes be administered in the fasting or fed state? Am J Obstet Gynecol 154:1031, 1986

54. Lewis GF, McNally C, Blackman JD et al: Prior feeding alters the response to the 50-g glucose challenge test in pregnancy. Diabetes Care 16:1551, 1993

55. Berkus MD, Stern MP, Mitchell BD et al: Does fasting interval affect the glucose challenge test? Am J Obstet Gynecol 163:1282, 1990

56. Gillmer MDG, Beard RW, Brooke FM, Oakley NW: Carbohydrate metabolism in pregnancy. BMJ 3:399, 1975

57. Muck BR, Hommel G: Plasma insulin response following intravenous glucose in gestational diabetes. Arch Gynakol 223:259, 1977

58. Turner RC, Harris E, Bloom SR, Uren C: Relation of fasting plasma glucose concentration to plasma insulin and glucagon concentrations. Diabetes 26:166, 1977

59. Guttorn E: Practical screening for diabetes mellitus in pregnant women. Acta Endocrinol (Copenh), suppl. 182:11, 1974/1975

60. Stangenberg M, Persson B, Nordlanden E: Random capillary blood glucose and conventional selection criteria for glucose tolerance testing during pregnancy. Diabetes Res 2:29, 1985

61. Lind T, Anderson J: Does random blood glucose sampling outdate testing for glycosuria in the detection of diabetes during pregnancy? BMJ 4:289, 1984

62. Coustan DR, Carpenter MW, Widness JA et al: The "breakfast tolerance test": screening for gestational diabetes with a standardized mixed nutrient meal. Am J Obstet Gynecol 157:1113, 1987

63. Lev-Ran A, VanderLaan WP: Glycohemoglobins and glucose tolerance. JAMA 241:912, 1979

64. Hall PM, Cook JGH, Sheldon J et al: Glycosylated hemoglobins and glycosylated plasma proteins in the diagnosis of diabetes mellitus and impaired glucose tolerance. Diabetes Care 7:147, 1984

65. Widness JA, Schwartz HC, Kahn CB et al: Glycohemoglobin in diabetic pregnancy: a sequential study. Am J Obstet Gynecol 136:1024, 1979

66. Schwartz HC, King KC, Schwartz AL: Effects of pregnancy on hemoglobin A₁c in normal, gestational diabetic, and diabetic women. Diabetes 25:1118, 1976

67. Fadel HE, Hammond SD, Huff TA, Harp RJ: Glycosylated hemoglobins in normal pregnancy and gestational diabetes mellitus. Obstet Gynecol 54:322, 1979

68. Shah BD, Cohen AW, May C, Gabbe SG: Comparison of glycohemoglobin determination and the one-hour oral glucose screen in the identification of gestational diabetes. Am J Obstet Gynecol 144:774, 1982

69. Artal R, Mosley GM, Dorey FJ: Glycohemoglobin as a screening test for gestational diabetes. Am J Obstet Gynecol 148:412, 1984

70. McFarland KF, Murtiashaw M, Baynes JW: Clinical value of glycosylated serum protein and glycosylated hemoglobin levels in the diagnosis of gestational diabetes mellitus. Obstet Gynecol 64:516, 1984

71. Cousins L, Dattel BJ, Hollingsworth DR, Zettner A: Glycosylated hemoglobin as a screening test for carbohydrate tolerance in pregnancy. Am J Obstet Gynecol 150:455, 1984

72. Jones IR, Owens DR, Williams S et al: Glycosylated serum albumin: an intermediate index of diabetic control. Diabetes Care 6:501, 1983

73. Leiper JM, Talwar D, Robb DA et al: Glycosylated albumin and glycosylated proteins: rapidly changing indices of glycaemia in diabetic pregnancy. Q J Med 218:225, 1985

74. Roberts AB, Court DJ, Henley P et al: Fructosamine in diabetic pregnancy. Lancet 2:998, 1983

75. Roberts AB, Baker JR, Metcalf P, Mullard C: Fructosamine compared with a glucose load as a screening test for gestational diabetes. Obstet Gynecol 76:773, 1990

76. Nasrat HA, Ajabnoor MA, Ardawi MSM: Fructosamine as a screening test for gestational diabetes mellitus: a reappraisal. Int J Gynecol Obstet 34:27, 1990

77. Comtois R, Desjarlais F, Nguyen M, Beauregard H: Clinical usefulness of estimation of serum fructosamine concentration as screening test for gestational diabetes. Am J Obstet Gynecol 160:651, 1989

78. Weiss PAM, Lichtenegger W, Winter R, Purstner P: Insulin levels in amniotic fluid—management of pregnancy in diabetes. Obstet Gynecol 51:393, 1978

79. Weiss PAM, Hofman H, Winter R et al: Gestational diabetes and screening during pregnancy. Obstet Gynecol 63:776, 1984

80. Lin CC, River P, Moawad AH et al: Prenatal assessment of fetal outcome by amniotic fluid C-peptide levels in pregnant diabetic women. Am J Obstet Gynecol 141:671, 1981

81. Stangenberg M, Persson B, Vaclavinkova V: Amniotic fluid

volumes and concentrations of C-peptide in diabetic pregnancies. Br J Obstet Gynaecol 89:536, 1982

82. MacDonald HN, Good W, Schwarz K, Stone J: Serial observations of glucose tolerance in pregnancy and the early puerperium. Br J Obstet Gynaecol 78:489, 1971

83. Lind T, Harris VG: Changes in the oral glucose tolerance test during the puerperium. Br J Obstet Gynaecol 83:460, 1976

84. Carpenter MW, Coustan DR, Widness JA et al: Postpartum testing for antecedent gestational diabetes. Am J Obstet Gynecol 159:1128, 1988

85. Coustan DR, Lewis SB: Insulin therapy for gestational diabetes. Obstet Gynecol 51:306, 1978

86. Sosenko IR, Kitzmiller JL, Loo SW et al: The infant of the diabetic mother: correlation of increased cord C-peptide levels with macrosomia and hypoglycemia. N Engl J Med 301:859, 1979

87. Weiss PAM, Hofmann H, Purstner P et al: Fetal insulin balance: gestation diabetes and postpartal screening. Obstet Gynecol 64:65, 1984

88. Hoegsberg B, Gruppuso PA, Coustan DR: Hyperinsulinemia in macrosomic infants of nondiabetic mothers. Diabetes Care 16:32, 1993

89. Dwyer PL, Oats JN, Walstab JE, Beischer NA: Glucose tolerance in twin pregnancy. Aust NZ J Obstet Gynaecol 22:131, 1982

90. Naidoo L, Jailal I, Moodley J, Desai R: Intravenous glucose tolerance tests in women with twin pregnancy. Obstet Gynecol 66:500, 1985

17

Management of Gestational Diabetes

DONALD R. COUSTAN

The most important step in the management of gestational diabetes mellitus (GDM) is its diagnosis. Once this has been achieved, almost every type of management protocol has been associated with a reduction in the perinatal mortality rate. This is probably a reflection of the increased maternal and fetal surveillance prompted by this diagnosis along with general improvements in perinatal care. Currently, the perinatal mortality rate is no longer the only yardstick by which successful care is measured. The management of high-risk situations is also directed toward lowering perinatal morbidity rates. This chapter outlines a plan of management that includes the above considerations.

GOALS OF MANAGEMENT

As discussed in an earlier chapter, the perinatal mortality rate is increased in diabetic pregnancies when hyperglycemia is allowed to persist unchallenged. There is evidence that mean whole blood glucose levels above 100 mg/dl in diabetic mothers are associated with a significant increase in the perinatal mortality risk,[1] and most large centers currently strive to maintain average plasma glucose concentrations below 120 mg/dl; even more stringent goals are reported by a number of investigators. We assume that the fetus whose mother experiences hyperglycemia only during pregnancy is equally sensitive to mild elevations of circulating glucose levels as is the fetus of the long-standing diabetic woman. For this reason, to prevent perinatal loss, it is reasonable to utilize the same strict standards for metabolic control in the patient with

GDM as in women with overt diabetes. Similarly, although perinatal deaths are reported to occur at nearly the background level in properly diagnosed and managed GDM-associated pregnancies, surveillance of the fetus for signs of compromise may be reasonable. This point remains controversial and is primarily a cost versus benefit issue.

In most large series of GDM pregnancies, even though reasonable standards for glucose control have reportedly been met, a residual increase in perinatal morbidity has remained. The morbidities reported include fetal macrosomia, operative delivery, birth trauma, and neonatal complications such as hypoglycemia, hyperbilirubinemia, plethora, and hypocalcemia. The prevention of such problems is the primary challenge remaining for those who manage pregnancies complicated by GDM.

ATTAINING THE GOALS

Dietary Therapy

The cornerstone of management in pregnancies with overt diabetes or GDM is diet. Specific recommendations for dietary therapy in diabetic pregnancy are given in Chapter 12 and are not repeated here. It is worthwhile, however, to re-emphasize that, no matter how nutritionally sound a diet prescription might be, it is useless if it is not followed by the patient. Therefore, it is particularly important to be aware of cultural and individual preferences when nutritional counseling is provided.

Glucose Monitoring

Although standard in earlier protocols, urine testing for glucose has now been abandoned in the management of overt diabetes and GDM. Although urinary thresholds for glucose excretion are lowered in response to the increased renal plasma flow in pregnancy, causing postprandial glycosuria in many women, the absence of glycosuria does not ensure euglycemia.

The standard of care for monitoring glucose metabolism in pregnant women with overt diabetes is self-monitoring of blood glucose levels (SMBG) four to six times daily. A case could be made for similar standards in GDM. However, in most series, approximately 3 percent of pregnancies are complicated by this condition (as opposed to 0.5 percent with overt diabetes), and the cost of such frequent SMBG in all women with GDM would be significant. Furthermore, there is a learning curve for SMBG such that data from the first week or two are not as reliable as those obtained after the patient has accumulated experience in the use of this technology. Given the relatively low perinatal mortality rate in prospectively identified GDM, intensive monitoring of glucose levels may not be justified in all such individuals. Nevertheless, more than 20 percent of women with GDM will manifest hyperglycemia (individual plasma glucose levels of >120 mg/dl 2 hours after or >130 mg/dl 1 hour after a meal), despite the prescription of a diet appropriate for diabetic pregnancy.[2-4] Presumably, these pregnancies are at increased risk of perinatal mortality, and more intensive treatment should be undertaken. The Third International Workshop-Conference on Gestational Diabetes Mellitus[5] concluded

> It was noted that the utility of SMBG in the patient with mild GDM, not requiring insulin, although reasonable and logical, has not been formally proven and its costs and benefits require study.

To identify the higher-risk GDM women, some authors have advocated weekly testing of fasting plasma glucose to recategorize those women whose fasting values exceed a threshold, such as 100 or 105 mg/dl, as facing perinatal risks similar to those seen in overt diabetes.[6] Although it has been demonstrated that fasting hyperglycemia connotes a different, and more significant, mechanism of disorder in maternal carbohydrate metabolism compared with isolated postprandial hyperglycemia, the fetal consequences of hyperglycemia have not been linked specifically to the time of day. Indeed, the fetus may respond with increased pancreatic insulin formation and release no matter what time hyperglycemia occurs. Freinkel[7] reported higher birthweights, and higher corrected birthweights, among 58 infants of GDM mothers with normal fasting plasma glucose levels than among 106 infants of normal mothers. At least three other studies of diabetic pregnancies have now demonstrated that postprandial glucose determinations are more predictive of fetal macrosomia than are fasting values.[8-10] Thus, although fasting hyperglycemia may be a relatively specific marker for general maternal hyperglycemia, its absence does not preclude abnormal maternal fuel metabolism with resultant fetal hyperinsulinemia, leading to macrosomia and other morbidities.

Many investigators suggest using both fasting and postprandial circulating glucose measurements to evaluate maternal glycemia in gestational diabetes. The Third International Workshop-Conference on Gestational Diabetes Mellitus[5] noted that

> The use of insulin is now widely recommended when standard dietary management does not consistently maintain normal fasting plasma glucose <5.8 mM [105 mg/dl] and/or the 2-h postprandial plasma glucose <6.7 mM [120 mg/dl]. Data from many sources indicate that the upper limit for normal values for fasting plasma glucose may be lower than 5.8 mM when specific assay methods and gestational age are taken into account.

In our center, women with GDM have at least one "set" of circulating glucose measurements done weekly. Each "set" consists of a fasting, a 2-hour post-breakfast, and a late afternoon level. All can be performed on a single day, or they may be split into different days for patient convenience. We assume that the day on which blood is being tested is probably the "best" day for an individual (i.e., the day on which she is most likely to adhere to her dietary regimen). Thus, if a single value is above our goal (fasting level >100 mg/dl or either of the two postprandial values >120 mg/dl), the treatment is intensified. This intensification may consist of more frequent monitoring or institution of insulin therapy. If the value is only mildly elevated and more frequent monitoring is elected, a second high value dictates immediate insulin therapy to minimize fetal jeopardy.

The use of glycosylated hemoglobin measurements as the sole means to ascertain the adequacy of diabetic control is impractical because there is a delay of up to 1 month between changes in glycemia and their reflection in glycosylated hemoglobin values. Furthermore, these measurements are not nearly sensitive enough to detect the mild degree of maternal hyperglycemia that should prompt a therapeutic response in GDM.

Oral Hypoglycemic Agents

Currently, oral hypoglycemic agents are not recommended for use during pregnancy. Although there are some series in which such drugs were used successfully,[11,12] these agents are contraindicated on theoretical grounds. Most of the oral agents work by stimulating pancreatic β-cells to produce and release insulin. The sulfonylureas are known to cross the placenta and would be expected to stimulate fetal pancreatic insulin release. Because the adverse fetal consequences of maternal GDM are believed to be related to fetal hyperinsulinemia, any agent that increases fetal insulin production would be expected to worsen the outcome in such pregnancies. There is a least one report of perinatal death among 6 of 18 diabetic pregnancies treated with sulfonylureas during the third trimester, although no contemporaneous nontreated control group was available for comparison.[13] Adverse neonatal consequences were predicted for these drugs used during pregnancy[14] and have been reported.[15,16] Data are lacking regarding the use of some of the newer agents that may work more by changing insulin receptor dynamics than by stimulating insulin release. Using an in vitro isolated perfused placental cotyledon model, Elliott et al[17] demonstrated that glyburide, one of the second-generation oral agents, crosses the human placenta minimally.

Insulin Therapy

When permissible glucose levels have been exceeded, insulin should be instituted to reduce perinatal mortality risks, as outlined above. The topic of insulin therapy has been extensively covered in Chapter 11, so only those specific issues relevant to GDM are discussed here.

Because of the theoretical advantage of a decreased antibody response, human (rather than pork or beef) insulin should be prescribed for women with GDM. These individuals generally require insulin only temporarily but are at increased risk of developing diabetes later in life. Because the cost of human insulin is now similar to that of highly purified pork or beef insulin, there is no reason to prescribe nonhuman varieties.

Pregnancy is a time of intensified central and peripheral insulin resistance. For this reason, women with GDM generally require, and tolerate, considerably higher starting doses of insulin than do nonpregnant diabetic individuals. For the woman with GDM who requires insulin because of hyperglycemia despite dietary treatment, we initiate insulin therapy at a dose of 30 U/d. This is given as 20 U of NPH and 10 U of regular insulin, mixed in the same syringe, and injected 15 to 30 minutes before breakfast each morning. Because insulin resistance seems to reach its maximum in the third trimester, we usually start with one-half of the above dose if treatment is required before 28 weeks of gestation, particularly if the patient is lean. The mixture of intermediate- and short-acting insulins, given in the proportion of 2:1, is based on the pattern of insulin release in normal nondiabetic women in the third trimester of pregnancy[18] (Fig. 17-1).

If hyperglycemia persists despite the above starting dose of insulin, adjustments are made in specific components. For example, if glucose levels are high 2 hours after breakfast, the regular insulin dose is increased. If the afternoon glucose level is high, the NPH insulin dose is increased. Despite normal circulating glucose levels in the afternoon (when NPH insulin is at its peak of absorption), if evening or fasting glucose levels are elevated, a second insulin injection is administered just before the evening meal. Further modifications of the insulin regimen are similar to those recommended for the overt diabetic patient and are covered in Chapter 11.

Symptomatic hypoglycemia is exceedingly rare, in our experience, among GDM individuals treated with this insulin regimen. Nevertheless, all patients are instructed in recognizing a hypoglycemic episode, in treating it, and in reporting this occurrence to us.

When insulin therapy is required because of maternal hyperglycemia, most patients are asked to begin SMBG at an initial frequency of four times each day:

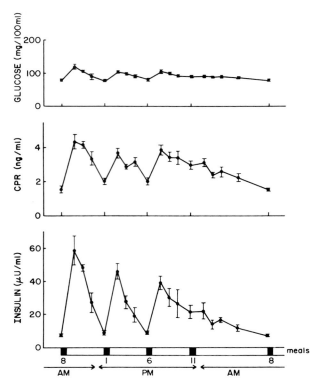

Fig. 17-1. Serum glucose, insulin, and C-peptide (CPR) levels in six normal women in the third trimester of pregnancy (mean ± standard error of the mean). (From Lewis et al,[18] with permission.)

fasting and 2 hours after each meal. These results are used to guide further refinements in insulin dosage.

Insulin to Prevent Morbidity (Prophylactic Insulin)

The above discussion of *therapeutic* insulin presupposes that insulin treatment is being instituted because of maternal hyperglycemia and is necessary because of the increased perinatal mortality risk demonstrated in hyperglycemic overt diabetic women. However, most women with GDM are in apparently good control with dietary therapy, never exceeding the abovementioned thresholds of glycemia that would trigger the prescription of the therapeutic insulin.

According to the classic Pedersen[19] hypothesis, maternal hyperglycemia is responsible for fetal hypergly-

cemia that, in turn, causes fetal hyperinsulinemia. It is this fetal hyperinsulinemia that is responsible for fetal macrosomia and the other fetal and neonatal morbidities associated with diabetic pregnancies. Theoretically, then, maternal glycemic control should eliminate these types of morbidity. Furthermore, those women with GDM who maintain good metabolic control while receiving dietary therapy should not give birth to macrosomic or otherwise morbid infants. In many series, however, an excess rate of macrosomia and other morbidity has been reported despite relatively good metabolic control.[20-23] At least three possible explanations for this phenomenon come to mind:

1. The standard thresholds for "euglycemia" are not low enough to prevent fetal islet cell stimulation
2. Glucose is not being measured often enough to document true euglycemia
3. The fetal pancreas is stimulated to produce and release insulin by substances other than glucose that are elevated in GDM but are not routinely measured

Any or all of these phenomena may be operative in GDM, and there is evidence to support all three.

In 1980, Roversi et al[24] reported on an uncontrolled series of 235 pregnancies with GDM (by standard diagnostic criteria) in which the maximal tolerated dose of insulin was administered, using hypoglycemic symptoms as the end point of therapy. The incidence of macrosomia (>4,000 g) was only 2.6 percent, and the operative delivery rate (i.e., primary cesarean section, vacuum extraction, or forceps) was 14.5 percent. The mean plasma glucose levels were approximately 90 mg/dl before the initiation of treatment and 70 mg/dl during therapy. Although no untreated control group was available for comparison, the incidence of macrosomia reported was extremely low, and this suggests that such aggressive attempts to lower maternal glucose levels may be rewarded with further improvements in outcome. Langer et al[25] reported on a series of 334 women with GDM and 334 normal controls. Those whose average blood glucose level was greater than 104 mg/dl manifested a fourfold higher prevalence of infants above the 90th percentile of birthweight for gestational age than did those whose blood glucose concentrations averaged 87 to 104 mg/dl. There was no difference in infants who were small for dates. Once the average blood glucose level was less than 87 mg/dl, small-for-gestational-age infants were 2.5 times more likely, and large-for-gestational-age infants were 2.6 times less likely. Thus the customary goal of postprandial glucose values of less than 120 mg/dl may not be low enough.

Goldberg et al[4] reported on a series of 58 gravid women with GDM who performed SMBG four times daily and were compared with a historical control group followed more conventionally. Insulin therapy, used in 50 percent of the SMBG patients and 21 percent of the control patients, was prescribed if the fasting whole blood glucose level exceeded 95 mg/dl or the 1-hour postprandial values exceeded 120 mg/dl. The incidence of macrosomia (≥4,000 g) was reduced from 24 percent in the control group to 9 percent in the SMBG group. Similarly, the incidence of large-for-gestational-age (≥90th percentile) infants was 41 percent in the control group and 12 percent in the SMBG group. Thus, more frequent measurement of circulating glucose levels may allow for more complete detection of maternal hyperglycemia, even when conventional thresholds are used. This, in turn, may allow for more effective prevention of morbidity.

The third possibility, that maternal hyperglycemia is only one of several possible stimuli for fetal hyperinsulinemia, is more theoretical. Nonglucose secretogogues for the fetal islet cell, such as certain amino acids,[26] are known to exist, but evidence linking maternal hyperaminoacidemia with perinatal morbidity in GDM is sparse. Horska et al[27] reported higher amniotic fluid levels of nine amino acids among diabetic pregnancies compared with controls. Persson et al[28] described a significant relationship between maternal plasma branched chain amino acid levels and amniotic fluid C-peptide levels in diabetic pregnancies. Similarly, Freinkel and Metzger[29] found, in GDM pregnancies, correlations between birthweight and maternal levels of alanine, serine, and leucine.

Weiss et al[30,31] used amniotic fluid and cord blood insulin levels as a bioassay for fetal islet cell hyperactivity in diabetic pregnancies. Amniotic fluid insulin levels above the 97th percentile for gestational age were highly predictive of "diabetic fetopathy," even in some women with normal oral glucose tolerance test results.[30] Similarly, in one-fourth of 335 neonates weighing more than 4,000 g, cord blood insulin levels exceeded the 97th percentile even though the mothers had not been antepartally identified as GDM individu-

als. Thus, fetal insulin production or release (or both) may be a sensitive marker for the derangement in metabolism that results in morbidity in these infants. The authors suggest serial measurement of amniotic fluid insulin levels in GDM pregnancies and using the results to guide therapeutic decision making as to insulin administration. Although no randomized trial of amniocentesis in this context has been reported, the findings of Weiss et al lend credence to the hypothesis that maternal glycemia is not the only issue of importance in determining the effects of GDM on the fetus.

Prophylactic Insulin

In an attempt to reduce the adverse perinatal outcomes, O'Sullivan et al,[32] in 1966, randomized women into two groups: 305 were treated with prophylactic insulin (10 U/d NPH), and 306 constituted an untreated control group. A third cohort of 328 nondiabetic pregnant women served as normal controls (Table 17-1). O'Sullivan et al found that 13 percent of the untreated women with GDM gave birth to babies weighing more than 9 lb (4.1 kg) compared with 4 percent of normal gravid women. Although no influence of prophylactic insulin treatment on the perinatal mortality rate was evident, a subsequent reanalysis of the data showed that insulin treatment was associated with a significant reduction in perinatal mortality rate for the subset of women with GDM who were aged 25 years or older and treated with insulin before the 32nd week of pregnancy.[33] Unfortunately, data from these studies do not address such issues as operative delivery and birth trauma.

In a second randomized trial of prophylactic insulin,

Table 17-1. Randomized Trial of Prophylactic Insulin

	Treatment Group		
	Gestational Diabetic Patient		
	Insulin[a]	No Treatment	Normal Control
No.	305	306	324
Babies >9 lb	13	40	12
(%)	(4.3)	(13.1)[b]	(3.7)

[a] 10 U NPH insulin every morning.
[b] P <.01.
(Modified from O'Sullivan et al,[32] with permission.)

50 percent of untreated GDM women, but only 36 percent of diet-treated and 7 percent of insulin-treated (20 U NPH and 10 U regular insulin each morning) women delivered babies weighing more than 8.5 lb (3.85 kg).[34] When birthweights were corrected for fetal gender, birth order, maternal height and midpregnancy weight, and gestational age, significant differences persisted. The series was too small to demonstrate differences in operative delivery rates or birth trauma. A third study also found prophylactic insulin effective in preventing fetal macrosomia.[35]

Persson et al[36] reported on a randomized clinical trial of prophylactic insulin (8 to 12 U/d) in which the difference in macrosomia between the treated and untreated groups was not clinically or significantly different, with macrosomia being exceedingly rare in both groups. Approximately 20 percent of the subjects in each group were entered into the study after 36 weeks of gestation, when it is unlikely that treatment would have had any effect on macrosomia. Thus, three of the four published randomized clinical trials of prophylactic insulin reported a significant lowering of the incidence of fetal macrosomia with this intervention.

A number of other series that were not randomized noted a lowering of the macrosomia rate with insulin treatment of GDM.[37,38] We reviewed 445 consecutive pregnancies complicated by GDM[39] (Table 17-2) and categorized the patients according to the type of treatment initially prescribed. There were 146 who received no particular treatment, 184 who received a therapeutic diet, and 115 who were treated with prophylactic insulin (20 U NPH and 10 U regular insulin each morning, as a starting dose) and diet. Babies larger than 4,000 g were born to 18 percent of both the untreated and diet-treated mothers but to only 7 percent of those given prophylactic insulin. In addition, operative deliveries (i.e., primary cesarean sections, midforceps, and midcavity vacuum extraction) were necessary in 28 percent of the untreated, 30 percent of the diet-treated, and only 16 percent of the prophylactic insulin-treated patients. Similarly, birth trauma occurred in 14 percent of the untreated, 13 percent of the diet-treated, and only 5 percent of insulin-treated pregnancies. These differences could not be explained by confounding variables. Women treated with prophylactic insulin had, if anything, more severe GDM (as evidenced by the degree of glucose tolerance test abnormality). Neither could such variables as maternal obesity and weight gain, duration of treatment, and gestational age at diagnosis or delivery account for the effect seen. This study thus provides a link between the previously reported prophylactic insulin effect of lowering the incidence of macrosomia and the predicted secondary effect of lowering the incidence of operative delivery and birth trauma.

Although it is highly likely that prophylactic insulin is effective in preventing macrosomia in the infants of GDM mothers, it is also clear that its use involves treating all such patients in order for there to be the potential of benefit for less than one-half of their babies (i.e. those who would otherwise be macrosomic). If the avoidance of macrosomia is desirable to the patient and health care provider, ideally, it should be possible to single out those pregnancies at greatest risk and prescribe treatment. Daily SMBG with therapeutic insulin when fairly conservative thresholds are exceeded has been described previously. Buchanan et al[40] applied ultrasound at 29 to 33 weeks' gestation to women with GDM and normal fasting glucose levels who were treated by diet alone. If the abdominal circumference exceeded the 75th percentile for dates, subjects were randomized to either continued diet therapy or to insulin treatment. The use of insulin was associated with a reduction in large-for-gestational age babies from 45 to 13 percent ($P < .04$), a rate similar to that of 14

Table 17-2. Retrospective Study of Prophylactic Insulin

	Treatment Group		
	Prophylactic Insulin	Diet	Untreated
No.	115	184	146
Birthweight >4,000 g (%)	8 (7)[a]	34 (18.5)	26 (17.8)
Birthweight >90th percentile (%)	9 (7.8)[b]	33 (17.9)	32 (21.9)
Operative delivery[c] (%)	17/104 (16)[a]	52/171 (30)	39/137 (28)
Birth trauma (%)	5 (4.8)[a]	23 (13.4)	20 (13.7)

[a] $P < .05$.
[b] $P < .01$.
(Modified from Coustan and Imarah,[39] with permission.)

percent, which occurred when the abdominal circumference was below the 75th percentile. If replicated, this approach seems reasonable.

The benefits of any form of treatment must be weighed against the risks of that treatment. In the case of prophylactic or therapeutic insulin for GDM, the risks to be considered include the immediate risk of hypoglycemia and the possible long-term risk of temporary exposure to insulin. As discussed above in the section, *Insulin Therapy,* symptomatic hypoglycemia in women with GDM who are treated with insulin during the third trimester is exceedingly rare unless a meal is omitted.

The potential long-term risks have received more consideration. It has been hypothesized that brief exposure to exogenous insulin sensitizes an individual, which might then result in an anamnestic response if exposure to exogenous insulin occurs at a later date. It has even been suggested that such brief exposure to insulin might make the later appearance of diabetes more likely. When O'Sullivan and Mahan[41] followed the patients participating in their randomized trial of prophylactic insulin, they found that the incidence of diabetes among the insulin-treated and control groups was similar 16 years after the index pregnancies. In fact, women treated with prophylactic insulin during their pregnancies appeared to be less likely to have severe diabetes than did those in the untreated control group. Thus, there is no evidence to suggest that insulin treatment increases the long-term risks of women with GDM. The current availability of human insulin should lower even further any concerns about theoretical risks.

FETAL EVALUATION

Because the perinatal mortality risk of GDM has diminished markedly with more thorough screening programs and intense surveillance of glycemia, antepartum monitoring in such patients has become the subject of debate, particularly as to whether the potential benefit outweighs the cost. In 1977, Gabbe et al[42] reported on a series of 261 women with GDM and recommended that women with uncomplicated pregnancies, GDM, and fasting euglycemia, be allowed to go to 40 weeks before antepartum surveillance is instituted. Landon and Gabbe[43] reported on a second series

of 97 women with GDM. Insulin was instituted if the fasting plasma glucose level exceeded 105 mg/dl on one occasion or the 2-hour postprandial plasma glucose concentration exceeded 120 mg/dl on repeated occasions; these parameters were measured weekly. Twenty-eight women (29 percent) required insulin. Beginning at 28 weeks' gestation, all patients recorded fetal activity daily. Antepartum surveillance with nonstress tests was begun in all patients by 40 weeks of gestation. However, those requiring insulin (29 percent) and those not insulin treated who had chronic hypertension (5 percent), pregnancy-induced hypertension (8 percent), or a previous stillbirth (1 percent) were followed with weekly nonstress tests and twice-weekly urinary estriol measurements from 34 weeks. Thus, 43 percent required antepartum surveillance before 40 weeks. No perinatal deaths occurred, and only six patients (6 percent) required intervention for suspected fetal jeopardy. These authors recommend that antepartum fetal surveillance with nonstress tests be used before term only in insulin-requiring GDM pregnancies and in those not treated with insulin who manifest hypertension, prolonged pregnancy, and other risk factors. Some centers, including our own, have been hesitant to attempt to discriminate among individuals with GDM and have continued to recommend universal antepartum assessment. We use weekly testing, beginning at 36 weeks' gestation in uncomplicated GDM. The particular test used should be that which is most commonly performed in a given center and may consist of nonstress tests, contraction stress tests, biophysical profiles, or combinations of these.

DELIVERY

The timing and mode of delivery in diabetic pregnancies are discussed in Chapter 22. The principles enumerated for the overt diabetic patient are equally applicable to those for patients with GDM. Macrosomia is every bit as much a problem here as in the offspring of "true" diabetic women. Consequently, a careful evaluation of fetal size is necessary before choosing the mode of delivery; primary cesarean section, without a trial of labor, for the obviously large baby is reasonable in many cases. Fetal weight estimations based on abdominal palpation are notoriously inaccurate, particularly with large babies. Even ultrasound estimates of fetal weight, using traditional formulas, have less than optimal ability to discriminate macrosomic from more normal-sized fetuses.[44,45] Other formulas have been derived to assess macrosomia, and other fetal structures have been assessed in an attempt to predict shoulder dystocia.[46,47] Attempts have been made to measure shoulder soft tissue width with ultrasound[48] and by computed tomography[49] and to measure fetal fat thickness with magnetic resonance imaging,[50] although none of these approaches enjoys widespread support at present. Because of the difficulties encountered in predicting fetal weight and shoulder dystocia, guidelines for the mode of delivery must be inexact and subject to refinement as new data emerge. Currently, we opt for cesarean section in most, if not all, cases of GDM where the estimated fetal weight is 4.5 kg or more. When the estimated weight is between 4 and 4.5 kg, clinical judgment as to the size of the pelvis and the patient's previous obstetric history play a major role in decision making. There is also a down-side risk to "overly" diagnosing macrosomia by ultrasound. Levine et al[51] found that the false-positive diagnosis of a large-for-gestational-age fetus was associated with a greater likelihood of the diagnosis of abnormal labor and of elective cesarean section compared with that in pregnancies with similar sized babies who were not diagnosed ultrasonically to be large-for-gestational age.

If the gravid woman with GDM has been euglycemic and has developed no complications (such as hypertensive disorders), there is little indication for preterm delivery. However, if the fetus is growing rapidly near term, induction of labor before macrosomia makes vaginal delivery problematic might be considered. In a retrospective review of mostly nondiabetic mothers, whose fetuses were estimated to weigh above the 90th percentile at term, Combs et al[52] found a higher cesarean section rate with elective induction for macrosomia. Kjos et al[53] found no difference in cesarean section rates when insulin-requiring GDM women at 38 weeks' gestation were randomized to elective induction or expectant management.

RECOMMENDATIONS

It is clear that the most important step in the management of GDM is the recognition of this disorder. All such women should be given dietary counseling and should be monitored at least weekly for fasting and postprandial hyperglycemia. Should hyperglycemia occur, insulin should be administered to restore glucose homeostasis and reduce perinatal mortality risks. Intervention to reduce perinatal morbidity is less clear. We feel comfortable in providing our patients with appropriate information about macrosomia and its consequences and offering them various options, including prophylactic insulin or SMBG performed four times each day to identify those patients with GDM and even mild sporadic derangements of carbohydrate metabolism and begin them on insulin therapy. If and when confirmatory data from appropriately controlled studies become available, it may become practical in the future to identify those women with GDM who require insulin therapy by performing ultrasound in the early third trimester or by sampling amniotic fluid at regular intervals and to treat only those fetuses manifest apparent macrosomia or hyperinsulinemia.

It is most important to acknowledge that the lack of perinatal mortality risk is no longer an appropriate end point for success in the management of GDM and to adopt a thoughtful and coherent approach to the prevention of other types of morbidity.

REFERENCES

1. Karlson K, Kjellmer I: The outcome of diabetic pregnancies in relation to the mother's blood sugar level. Am J Obstet Gynecol 112:213, 1972
2. Neiger R, Coustan DR: Are the current ACOG glucose tolerance test criteria sensitive enough? Obstet Gynecol 78:1117, 1991
3. Drexel H, Bichler A, Sailer et al: Prevention of perinatal morbidity by tight metabolic control in gestational diabetes. Diabetes Care 11:761, 1988
4. Goldberg JD, Franklin B, Lasser D et al: Gestational diabetes: impact of home glucose monitoring on neonatal birth weight. Am J Obstet Gynecol 154:546, 1986
5. Metzger BE, the Organizing Committee: Summary and recommendations of the Third International Workshop-Conference on Gestational Diabetes Mellitus. Diabetes, suppl. 2, 40:197, 1991.
6. Freinkel N, Metzger BE: Gestational diabetes: problems in classification and implications for long-range prognosis. Adv Exp Med Biol 189:47, 1985
7. Freinkel N: Of pregnancy and progeny. Diabetes 29:1023, 1980

8. Jovanovic-Peterson L, Peterson CM, Reed GF et al: Maternal postprandial glucose levels and infant birth weight: the Diabetes in Early Pregnancy Study. Am J Obstet Gynecol 164:103, 1991

9. Parfitt VJ, Clark JDA, Turner GM, Hartog M: Maternal postprandial blood glucose levels influence infant birth weight in diabetic pregnancy. Diabetes Res 19:133, 1992

10. Combs CA, Gavin LA, Gunderson E et al: Relationship of fetal macrosomia to maternal postprandial glucose control during pregnancy. Diabetes Care 15:1251, 1992

11. Coetzee EJ, Jackson WPU: Metformin in management of pregnant insulin-dependent diabetics. Diabetologia 16:241, 1979

12. Sutherland HW, Stowers JM, Cormack JD, Bewsher PD: Evaluation of chlorpropamide in chemical diabetes diagnosed during pregnancy. BMJ 3:9, 1973

13. Malins JM, Cooke AM, Pyke DA, Fitzgerald MG: Sulphonylurea drugs in pregnancy. BMJ 3:187, 1964

14. Adam PAJ, Schwartz R: Diagnosis and treatment: should oral hypoglycemic agents be used in pediatric and pregnant patients? Pediatrics 42:819, 1968

15. Kemball ML, McIver C, Milner RDG et al: Neonatal hypoglycaemia in infants of diabetic mothers given sulphonylurea drugs in pregnancy. Arch Dis Child 45:696, 1970

16. Piacquadio K, Hollingsworth DR, Murphy H: Effects of in-utero exposure to oral hypoglycaemic drugs. Lancet 338:866, 1991

17. Elliott BD, Langer O, Schenker S, Johnson RF: Insignificant transfer of glyburide occurs across the human placenta. Am J Obstet Gynecol 165:807, 1991

18. Lewis SB, Wallin JD, Kuzuya H et al: Circadian variation of serum glucose, C-peptide immunoreactivity and free insulin in normal and insulin-treated diabetic pregnant subjects. Diabetologia 12:343, 1976

19. Pedersen J: The Pregnant Diabetic and Her Newborn. 2nd Ed. Williams & Wilkins, Baltimore, 1977

20. Fadel HE, Hammond SD: Diabetes mellitus and pregnancy: management and results. J Reprod Med 27:56, 1982

21. Miller JM: A reappraisal of "tight control" in diabetic pregnancies. Am J Obstet Gynecol 147:158, 1983

22. Widness JA, Cowett RM, Coustan DR et al: Neonatal morbidities in infants of mothers with glucose intolerance in pregnancy. Diabetes, suppl. 2, 34:61, 1985

23. Berk MA, Mimouni F, Miodovnik M et al: Macrosomia in infants of insulin-dependent diabetic mothers. Pediatrics 83:1029, 1989

24. Roversi GD, Gargiuolo M, Nicolini E et al: Maximal tolerated insulin therapy in gestational diabetes. Diabetes Care 3:489, 1980

25. Langer O, Brustman L, Anyaegbunam A et al: Glycemic control in gestational diabetes mellitus—how tight is tight enough: small for gestational age versus large for gestational age? Am J Obstet Gynecol 161:646, 1989

26. Phillips AF, Dubin JW, Raye JR: Alanine-stimulated insulin secretion in the fetal and neonatal lamb. Am J Obstet Gynecol 136:597, 1980

27. Horska S, Rasov M, Vondracek J: Amino acids in the amniotic fluid of diabetic mothers. Biol Neonate 37:204, 1980

28. Persson B, Pschera H, Lunell NO et al: Amino acid concentrations in maternal plasma and amniotic fluid in relation to fetal insulin secretion during the last trimester of pregnancy in gestational and type I diabetic women and women with small-for-gestational-age infants. Am J Perinatol 3:98, 1986

29. Freinkel N, Metzger BE: Pregnancy as a tissue culture experience: the critical implications of maternal metabolism for fetal development. p. 3. In Elliot K, O'Connor M (eds): Pregnancy Metabolism: Diabetes and the Fetus. Ciba Foundations Symposium no. 63. Excerpta Medica, Amsterdam, 1979

30. Weiss PAM, Hofmann H, Winter R et al: Gestational diabetes and postpartal screening. Obstet Gynecol 64:65, 1985

31. Weiss PAM, Hofmann H, Purstner P et al: Fetal insulin balance: gestational diabetes and postpartal screening. Obstet Gynecol 64:65, 1985

32. O'Sullivan JB, Gellis SS, Dandrow RV, Tenney BO: The potential diabetic and her treatment during pregnancy. Obstet Gynecol 27:683, 1966

33. O'Sullivan JB, Mahan CM, Charles D, Dandrow RV: Medical treatment of the gestational diabetic. Obstet Gynecol 43:817, 1974

34. Coustan DR, Lewis SB: Insulin therapy for gestational diabetes. Obstet Gynecol 51:306, 1978

35. Thompson DJ, Porter KB, Gunnells DJ et al: Prophylactic insulin in the management of gestational diabetes. Obstet Gynecol 75:960, 1990

36. Persson B, Stangenberg M, Hansson U, Nordlander E: Gestational diabetes mellitus (GDM): comparative evaluation of two treatment regimens, diet versus insulin and diet. Diabetes. suppl. 2, 34:101, 1985

37. Zoupas C, Mastrantonakis E, Diakakis I et al: The importance of insulin administration in gestational diabetics: Acta Endocrinol (Copenh), suppl., 265:26, 1984

38. Berne C, Wibell L, Lindmark G: Ten-year experience of insulin treatment in gestational diabetes. Acta Paediatr Scand Suppl 320:85, 1985

39. Coustan DR, Imarah J: Prophylactic insulin treatment of gestational diabetes reduces the incidence of macrosomia, operative delivery, and birth trauma. Am J Obstet Gynecol 150:836, 1984

40. Buchanan TA, Gonzalel M, Kjos SL et al: Use of fetal ultrasound to select metabolic therapy for pregnancies complicated by mild gestational diabetes. Diabetes Care 17:275, 1994

41. O'Sullivan JB, Mahan CM: Insulin treatment and high risk groups. Diabetes Care 3:482, 1980

42. Gabbe SG, Mestmann JH, Freeman RK et al: Management and outcome of class A diabetes mellitus. Am J Obstet Gynecol 127:465, 1977

43. Landon MB, Gabbe SG: Antepartum fetal surveillance in gestational diabetes mellitus. Diabetes, suppl. 2, 34:50, 1985

44. Tamura RK, Sabbagha RE, Dooley SL et al: Real-time ultrasound estimations of weight in fetuses of diabetic gravid women. Am J Obstet Gynecol 153:57, 1985

45. Tamura RK, Dooley SL: The role of ultrasonography in the management of diabetic pregnancy. Clin Obstet Gynecol 34:526, 1991

46. Bracero LA, Baxi LV, Rey HR, Yeh M-N: Use of ultrasound in antenatal diagnosis of large-for-gestational-age infants in diabetic patients. Am J Obstet Gynecol 152:43, 1985

47. Elliott JP, Garite TJ, Freeman RK et al: Ultrasonic prediction of fetal macrosomia in diabetic patients. Obstet Gynecol 60:159, 1982

48. Mintz MC, Landon MB, Gabbe SG et al: Shoulder soft tissue width as a predictor of macrosomia in diabetic pregnancies. Am J Perinatol 6:240, 1989

49. Kitzmiller JL, Mall JC, Gin GD et al: Measurement of fetal shoulder width with computed tomography in diabetic women. Obstet Gynecol 70:941, 1987

50. Jovanovic-Peterson L, Crues J, Durak E, Peterson CM: Magnetic resonance imaging in pregnancies complicated by gestational diabetes predicts infant birthweight ratio and neonatal obesity. Am J Perinatol 10:432, 1993

51. Levine AB, Lockwood CJ, Brown B et al: Sonographic diagnosis of the large for gestational age fetus at term: does it make a difference? Obstet Gynecol 79:55, 1992

52. Combs CA, Singh NB, Khoury JC: Elective induction versus spontaneous labor after sonographic diagnosis of fetal macrosomia. Obstet Gynecol 81:492, 1993

53. Kjos SL, Henry OA, Montoro M et al: Insulin-requiring diabetes in pregnancy: a randomized trial of active induction of labor and expectant management. Am J Obstet Gynecol 169:611, 1993

18
Obstetric Complications

LARRY COUSINS

As the year 2000 approaches, it is assumed that the increased experience in the prevention, diagnosis, and treatment of diabetes has lessened the frequency and severity of complications of diabetes. At the federal level, the U.S. Department of Health and Human Services has proposed specific health goals for the year 2000 for pregnancy regarding diabetes-related complications.[1] Within the obstetric area, increased attention to pregnancy complicated by diabetes is indicated by (1) an increasing body of published literature regarding all aspects of diabetic pregnancies; (2) the development and expansion of local and statewide programs directed at the diagnosis and management of diabetic pregnancies;[2] and (3) the development of specialty and society councils or special interest groups (e.g., American Diabetes Association, Society of Perinatal Obstetricians).

To better define the published experience with maternal morbidity among diabetic pregnancies, A Medline literature search was used to review the English language literature from 1986 to 1993. The Med-line search was identical in design to that used in an earlier review (1965–1985) of obstetric complications.[3] The reports reviewed during both intervals were obtained from computer searches instructed to look for

1. obstetric/maternal risks, complications, or morbidity in diabetic pregnancies
2. antepartum, intrapartum, or postpartum complications in diabetic pregnancies
3. specific complications in diabetic pregnancies (e.g., toxemia, pre-eclampsia, ketoacidosis, hydramnios, and so forth)

The results of the computer searches were processed identically to identify reports with usable data.

Specifically, the computer search reports were reviewed to identify papers with information relevant to the issue of obstetric complications among diabetic pregnancies. To be considered for inclusion in the compiled data, it was necessary for the report to meet the following criteria:

1. The paper was published in English during the earlier (1965–1985) or later (1986–1993) intervals.
2. The diabetic patients were identified according to White's classification or categorized into gestational diabetes mellitus (GDM) and overt (prepregnant) diabetes.
3. The reports cited a specific rate for one or more of the maternal complications of interest.

The questions asked of both reviews were

1. What is the incidence of specific maternal complications among diabetic gravidas?
2. Is there an increased incidence of these complications among diabetic compared with nondiabetic women?
3. If question 2 is answered affirmatively
   A. How good (e.g., prospective, controlled) are the data supporting the conclusion?
   B. Is there a difference in incidence rates between classes of diabetes?
   C. Why are specific complications increased?
4. Are there documented ways to decrease the incidence of specific maternal complications?
5. Does improved medical or obstetric care decrease long-term maternal morbidity?

An additional purpose of the more recent review (1986–1993) was to compare the literature experience during these two intervals to determine whether there are differences in the incidence of individual complications between intervals among specific diabetic classes or categories.

Comparison of the literature searches during the two intervals reveals some interesting similarities and differences. The two computer searches, over significantly different time intervals, 21 years and 8 years, had approximately the same number of reports with potentially usable data (Table 18-1). Detailed review of those reports demonstrated usable data for 24 and 25 complications, respectively. Table 18-1 reflects that not only were there more publications per year regarding obstetric complications in the 1986 to 1993 interval but that the later reports presented more nondiabetic comparison data and dealt with a greater number of specific complications. The increased availability of nondiabetic comparison data in the later interval allows us to address more confidently the second question noted above. Surprisingly, in the later interval the overt diabetic subjects were *less* often categorized into specific White's classes even though a greater total number of diabetic pregnancies (6,070) were reported than in the earlier interval (5,288).[3] This less-frequent classification into White's classes precludes between-class comparisons in the 1986 to 1993 series (Table 18-2). The reason for this difference in classification between the two intervals is not clear.

Despite the limitations of the reviewed literature, the individual reports and the cumulative experience of the two series provide an overview of obstetric morbidity in diabetes-complicated pregnancy. The complications reported in both series include pre-eclampsia, pregnancy-induced hypertension, chronic hypertension, hypertension (total), diabetic ketoacidosis (DKA), hydramnios, preterm labor, primary cesarean section, repeat cesarean section, pyelonephritis, and maternal mortality. In the 1986 to 1993 series, spontaneous preterm delivery, total preterm delivery, predelivery hospitalization days, and postcesarean infectious rates were also compared between diabetic categories (Table 18-2). Complications not included in the data compilation because of limited or nonexistent information that met inclusion criteria were spontaneous abortion and chronic hypertension with superimposed pre-eclampsia. Medical complications of diabetes such as retinopathy, nephropathy, and neuropathy are not considered in this report.

Chi-square analysis of the compiled data was used to test the hypothesis that the presence of an individual complication and the diabetic categories are independent. If the P value of the analysis was less than .05, the hypothesis that the complication and the diabetic categories are independent was rejected. The results of the chi-square analysis for the diabetic category and each complication are listed in Table 18-2. The incidence or prevalence rates noted were calculated by dividing the number of pregnancies affected with the particular complication by the total number of pregnancies described. The diabetic categories were gestational, classes B and C combined, and classes D, F, and R combined. These categories were selected on the basis of sample size and pathophysiologic considerations (i.e., gestational versus prepregnant diabetes and vascular disease absent versus present). Table 18-2 summarizes the reviewed data from the 1965 to 1985[3] and 1986 to 1993 series and provides compiled incidence rates for specific complications in the various diabetic categories. Table 18-3 summarizes the studies that report specific complications among various diabetic classes and the rates seen in nondiabetic control subjects. The results of diabetic versus control comparisons within an individual report are indicated by the P values.

Table 18-1. Comparisons of 1965 to 1985[a] and 1986 to 1993 Literature Reviews of Obstetric Complications Among Diabetic Pregnancies

Years Searched	1965–1985[a]	1986–1993
No. of "relevant" references	52	56
No. of references with usable data[b]	24	25
No. of reports with nondiabetic comparison data	8	13
No. of complications with diabetic and nondiabetic comparison rates	6	14
No. of diabetic-nondiabetic comparisons of individual complications	16	33
Total no. of diabetic pregnancies	5,288	6,070
No. of cases of GDM/overt diabetes	1,781/3,375	2,401/3,677
No. of cases of White's class B	1,191	562
No. of cases of White's class C	935	493
No. of cases of White's class D,F,R, etc.	960	711

[a] Data from Cousins,[3]
[b] See text for specific computer search instructions and inclusion criteria.

Table 18-2. Number of Diabetic Pregnancies Reported and Incidence of Specific Complications According to Years of Review and Diabetic Categories

Complication	Years[a]	GDM No.	GDM %	Classes B and C No.	Classes B and C %	Classes ≥D No.	Classes ≥D %	P^b
PET/PIH	1965–1985	791	10.0	729	8.0	350	15.7	<.005
	1986–1993	1,530	13.7	488	14.1	304	27.0	<.005
Hypertension								
Chronic	1965–1985	142	9.9	411	8.0	118	16.9	<.02
	1986–1993	81	2.5	—	—	—	—	—
Total	1965–1985	128	14.6	612	14.5	353	30.9	<.005
	1986–1993	334	3.3	224	21.0	196	40.0	<.001
DKA	1965–1985	169	0	400	8.3	282	7.1	<.005
	1986–1993	277	0.7	—	—	—	—	—
Hydramnios	1965–1985	133	5.3	199	17.6	167	18.6	<.005
	1986–1993	656	2.0	—	—	—	—	—
Pyelonephritis	1965–1985	124	4.0	356	2.2	264	4.9	NSD
	1986–1993	247	1.2	—	—	—	—	—
PTL	1965–1985	58	0	183	7.7	86	4.7	<.005
	1986–1993	247	8.1	—	—	—	—	—
PTD								
Spontaneous	1965–1985	—	—	—	—	—	—	—
	1986–1993	166	14.6	118	28.0	113	24.0	<.025
Total	1965–1985	—	—	—	—	—	—	—
	1986–1993	717	7.3	224	19.0	205	37.6	<.001
Cesarean section								
Primary	1965–1985	532	12.4	359	44.0	97	56.7	<.005
	1986–1993	255	15.1	—	—	—	—	—
Repeat	1965–1985	532	9.8	359	13.4	97	19.6	<.02
	1986–1993	97	16.5	—	—	—	—	—
Total	1965–1985	800	20.4	554	41.9	175	58.3	<.005
	1986–1993	1,155	23.1	—	—	—	—	—
Maternal mortality	1965–1985	All diabetic women 3/2,614 = 0.11%						—
	1986–1993	All diabetic women 9/6,070 = 0.14%						—

Abbreviations: PET/PIH, pre-eclampsia/pregnancy-induced hypertension; DKA, diabetic ketoacidosis; PTL, preterm labor, PTD, preterm delivery; NSD, no significant difference; GDM, gestational diabetes mellitus.
[a] Data for 1965–1985 review from Cousins.[3]
[b] Chi-square analysis for independence of complication and diabetic category.

PRE-ECLAMPSIA AND PREGNANCY-INDUCED HYPERTENSION

The incidence of pre-eclampsia and pregnancy-induced hypertension among the more than 2,300 classified diabetic patients in the 1986 to 1993 review ranged from 13.7 percent among GDM patients to 14.1 percent in classes B and C and 27 percent among class D or greater subjects (Table 18-2). As was seen in the 1965 to 1985 review,[3] chi-square analysis of the presence of pre-eclampsia and pregnancy-induced hypertension and the diabetic categories is highly significant (Table 18-2), indicating that pre-eclampsia and pregnancy-induced hypertension and the diabetic categories were not independent.

Although originally it was planned to compare complication rates between review periods, it became apparent that in the case of pre-eclampsia and pregnancy-induced hypertension this would not be appropriate. The reservations regarding such comparisons are based on variations in the two series and precision of the diagnosis from one interval to the other. Specifically, in the earlier review most reports failed to differentiate between pregnancy-induced hypertension and pre-eclampsia,[3] whereas in the later series, authors

Table 18-3. Within-Study Comparisons of Specific Complications Rates in Diabetic and Nondiabetic (Control) Pregnancies

| Complications | Diabetes | | Control | | |
	Class	%	%	P	References
PET/PIH					
PIH	G	3.8	3.7	NSD	Jacobson & Cousins[7]
PIH	B–T	13.1	5.6	<.05	Siddiqi et al[11]
PIH	B–F	16.0	7.7	<.001	Rosenn et al[8]
PET	G–F	9.9	4.3	<.05	Garner et al[6]
PET & PIH	G	14.0	7.0	<.01	Nordlander et al[9]
PET & PIH	G	19.8	6.1	<.001	Suhonen & Terano[12]
PET & PIH	B–F	21.0	5.0	<.001	Hanson & Persson[5]
Hypertension					
Chronic	G	2.5	0.3	<.05	Suhonen & Terano[12]
Total	G	3.3	13.0	<.05	Langer et al[25]
Hydramnios	G	2.0	0.7	NSD	Goldman et al[30]
	G	2.1	0.5	<.01	Jacobson & Cousins[7]
	B–F	26.4	0.6	<.001	Rosenn et al[8]
Pyelonephritis	G	1.3	0.7	NSD	Goldman et al[30]
	G	1.0	0.3	NSD	Jacobson & Cousins[7]
	B–F	3.6	1.4	NSD	Rosenn et al[8]
Preterm labor	G	6.2	7.1	NSD	Jacobson & Cousins[7]
	G	9.3	7.2	NSD	Goldman et al[30]
	B–F	31.0	20.0	<.01	Mimouni et al[36]
Preterm delivery					
Spontaneous	B–F	16.1	12.0	NSD	Rosenn et al[8]
Total	G	9.4	6.9	NSD	Goldman et al[30]
	B–F	24.6	6.0	<.001	Hanson & Persson[5]
	B–F	30.0	12.0	<.001	Rosenn et al[8]
	B–F	26.2	9.7	<.01	Greene et al[24]
Cesarean section					
Primary	G	13.4	12.9	NSD	Jacobson & Cousins[7]
Repeat	G	16.5	6.0	<.001	Jacobson & Cousins[7]
Total	G	19.0	11.0	<.05	Nordlander et al[9]
	G	29.9	18.8	<.01	Jacobson & Cousins[7]
	G	31.0	16.0	<.01	Suhonen & Terano[12]
	G	35.0	22.0	<.005	Goldman et al[30]
	B–F	45.2	12.0	<.001	Hanson & Persson[5]
	B–F	53.0	11.6	<.01	Gregory et al[41]
Post-cesarean section infection	G	12.4	5.9	<.05	Jacobson & Cousins[7]
	B–F	13.4	3.2	<.05	Diamond et al[47]

Abbreviations: PET, pre-eclampsia; PIH, pregnancy-induced hypertension.

usually did so. Also, among the overt diabetic categories, the reader cannot be confident that the proportion of a specific White's class within a diabetic category (e.g., classes B and C or class D or greater) is comparable in the two review periods. It is not clear, for example, that the proportion of classes B and C subjects is comparable in the 1965 to 1985 period as in the 1986 to 1993 interval. This lack of classification details is unfortunate because it prevents determining whether there is a change over time in the incidence of pre-eclampsia and pregnancy-induced hypertension. This question is relevant given the previous data[3] that suggested a significant decrease in pre-eclampsia and pregnancy-induced hypertension from a 1963 review[4] to the overall rate of 11.7 percent reported from the 1965 to 1985 review.[3] Finally, comparisons between the 1965 to 1985 and 1986 to 1993 reviews are not appropriate because there is overlapping of calendar years during which reported patients were actually cared for even though the years of the two literature reviews do not overlap.[5–9]

The significance of pregnancy-induced hypertension and pre-eclampsia complicating diabetic pregnancies is emphasized by several observations. These include (1) the incidence of the conditions in the diabetic categories in the earlier[3] and more recent reviews (Table 18-2); (2) the significantly increased incidence of the complication with advancing diabetic class (Table 18-2); (3) the finding in most studies in which nondiabetic comparative data are available that the complication is significantly more frequent among diabetic than control subjects (Table 18-3); and (4) the observation that pre-eclampsia and pregnancy-induced hypertension were the second most common cause for nonspontaneous (i.e., medically indicated or iatrogenic) preterm delivery.[8]

Table 18-3 lists reports with comparisons of rates of pre-eclampsia and pregnancy-induced hypertension in diabetic and nondiabetic pregnancies. These reports suggest the following:

1. The rate of pregnancy-induced hypertension among GDM subjects is not significantly different from controls.[7] This finding is consistent with the earlier report of Gabbe et al.[10]

2. In a composite group of overt diabetic subjects, the incidence of pregnancy-induced hypertension was more than two times more frequent than in control pregnancies.[8,11]

3. When cases complicated by pre-eclampsia and pregnancy-induced hypertension were combined, the incidence was significantly more common among GDM pregnancies than controls.[9,12]

4. In a large Scandinavian report, Hanson and Persson[5] found the combined incidence of pre-eclampsia and pregnancy-induced hypertension among a composite group of overt diabetic patients to be four times higher than the rate in control patients (based on national statistics). These data,[5] along with a smaller report by Garner et al,[6] demonstrated an increased incidence of pre-eclampsia among class D or greater diabetes than the classes B and C category. Among the diabetic categories, there was an interesting concordance in rates of pre-eclampsia and pregnancy-induced hypertension between the large Scandinavian report[5] and the recent review: classes B and C, 16 percent and 14 percent, respectively, and class D or greater, 27 percent and 27 percent, respectively.

Given the high rate of pre-eclampsia and pregnancy-induced hypertension among the more advanced diabetic classes, the morbidity implications of pre-eclampsia and reports indicating a preventative effect of low-dose aspirin therapy on the development of pre-eclampsia,[13–19] it is tempting to consider the use of low-dose aspirin in diabetic gravidas of class D or greater. This question should be examined with prospective, randomized, placebo-controlled trials.

Finally, the reader is directed to the papers of Combs et al[20] and Rosenn et al,[8] reporting a significant association between poor glycemic control and pre-eclampsia or pregnancy-induced hypertension. Combs and associates reported that among overt diabetic patients whose 12- to 16-week glycosylated hemoglobin value was greater than 9 percent, the adjusted odds ratio for the later development of pre-eclampsia was 1.4 compared with those diabetic patients with a glycohemoglobin level of 9 percent or less ($P < .05$). Rosenn and co-workers[8] found significantly higher glycosylated hemoglobin levels in all trimesters among insulin-dependent diabetic women with pregnancy-induced hypertension as compared with normotensive diabetic women. These findings suggest that improved glycemic control in diabetes-complicated pregnancies may reduce the risk of acute hypertensive complications.[8,20]

CHRONIC HYPERTENSION

In the 1986 to 1993 review, only six papers presented usable data regarding chronic hypertension.[6,11,12,20–22] Of these, one identified two chronic hypertensive patients among 81 GDM patients.[12] The 2.5 percent incidence of chronic hypertension among these GDM patients was significantly higher than the rate (0.3 percent) seen in a nondiabetic control group. The control subjects were significantly younger and leaner than the GDM group, and the control incidence of 0.3 percent is less than the commonly reported incidence of chronic hypertension among a general prenatal population of 2 percent.[23] Among overt diabetic women, the reported incidence of chronic hypertension ranged from 11 percent in a group of classes B to R subjects[21] to 44 percent in a small group of class T diabetic subjects.[22] In reports with usable data regarding chronic hypertension among overt diabetic women, 92 patients of the group of 685 (13.4 percent) manifested chronic hypertension.[11,20,21] Because of the limitations in diabetes classification in the later review, it is not possible to make meaningful comparisons between the 1965 to 1985[3] and 1986 to 1993 reviews (Table 18-2). As noted above, Suhonen and Teramo[12] reported a higher incidence of chronic hypertension among GDM subjects than in their control group. The current review did not find reports that demonstrated whether this difference between GDM and control subjects would persist if the subjects were matched for weight, age, smoking, and other variables known to influence the incidence of chronic hypertension.

TOTAL HYPERTENSIVE COMPLICATIONS

The cumulative incidence of total hypertensive complications was 3.3 percent in 334 GDM subjects, 21 percent among 224 classes B and C subjects, and 40 percent among 196 class D or greater diabetic subjects.[24,25] Analysis of the relationship of diabetic categories in the presence of any hypertensive complication indicated that the two variables were not independent (Table 18-2). Langer et al[25] reported on 334 GDM women, with an identical number of controls matched for obesity, race, and parity. There was a significant difference between total hypertensive complications in the GDM patients (3.3 percent) and control subjects (13 percent). This lower incidence of total hypertensive complications among GDM patients is surprising given the significantly younger age of the control subjects. This finding of a lower incidence of total hypertensive complications among GDM patients than controls is discordant with the experience regarding pre-eclampsia, pregnancy-induced hypertension, and chronic hypertension summarized above as well the data in the 1965 to 1985 review.[3]

The report of Greene et al[24] of a large experience of insulin-requiring overt diabetic women from the Joslin Clinic is instructive in several ways. It demonstrates a significantly higher incidence of hypertensive complications among overt diabetic women with vascular disease compared with those without vascular disease. Their data also showed that preterm delivery was significantly more common among hypertensive (relative risk = 2.0) than nonhypertensive diabetic

subjects. Finally, the data indicate that pre-eclampsia was the single most important cause of premature delivery in this diabetic group.

The incidence of total hypertensive complications among overt diabetic categories in the 1986 to 1993 review was numerically greater than the incidence noted in the 1965 to 1985 review (Table 18-2). Given that the rates in the reviews resulted from presumably varying contributions from pregnancy-induced hypertension, pre-eclampsia, and chronic hypertension patients, it is unclear whether this numerical difference represents a true change in the incidence of total hypertensive problems among overt diabetic patients.

In conclusion, total hypertensive complications are increased among overt diabetic women as compared with controls. Furthermore, the incidence of these complications is greater in overt diabetic women with vascular disease than among those without vascular disease. Most information available suggests that total hypertensive complications are greater in GDM than control subjects. The availability of reports with control and GDM data are limited to that of Langer et al,[25] and these data suggest that control, not GDM, subjects had a higher incidence of total hypertensive complications.

DIABETIC KETOACIDOSIS

Three reports[26–28] in the 1986 to 1993 review provided usable series data regarding DKA. From GDM series of 127 and 150 GDM pregnancies, Kilvert et al[27] and Nagy[28] each reported one case of DKA, for an overall incidence of 0.7 percent (Table 18-2). Kilvert et al[27] reported 10 cases of DKA among 508 overt diabetic women. This report summarizing their experience with DKA between 1971 and 1990 noted that there was no obvious change in the incidence of DKA from the earlier to the later portion of this interval. As summarized earlier, β-agonist therapy continues to be associated with ketoacidosis.[3] Consequently, β-agonist therapy of diabetic subjects not only has maternal morbidity consequences but significant perinatal risks as well. Among seven cases of DKA secondary to β-agonist therapy, one resulted in a perinatal loss for a perinatal mortality of 14 percent.[27] Montoro et al[26] reported the experience with 20 pregnant DKA patients cared for at Los Angeles County/University of Southern California Medical Center between 1972 and 1987. These DKA patients were categorized into perinatal mortality versus survival cases. Of the 20 DKA pregnancies, 7 experienced perinatal losses (35 percent). These infants died at a mean gestational age of 31 weeks. This group with perinatal losses had higher serum glucose, blood urea nitrogen, and osmolality levels, as well as greater insulin requirements and duration of ketoacidosis than the survivor group. In this series of 20 subjects, there were no maternal mortalities or fetal mortalities after the start of treatment.

Despite improvement in the prevention and medical management of ketoacidosis, several clinical variables have been associated with the onset of DKA among pregnant subjects. Rodgers and Rodgers[29] reviewed the experience at the State University of New York at Buffalo between 1980 and 1990 as well as the medical literature between 1970 and 1990 to define variables associated with the onset of DKA during pregnancy. In a combined experience of 37 admissions, they found that, in descending order of frequency, the following conditions were identified as the primary contributors to the development of DKA: β-agonist use (30 percent), emesis (27 percent), poor physician management (13 percent), patient noncompliance (11 percent), undiagnosed diabetes (8 percent), infection (5 percent), and undiagnosed pregnancy and insulin pump failure (3 percent each). In a known pregnancy with a compliant patient receiving care, DKA is preventable. In most instances, prevention can be accomplished without hospitalization. Prevention of DKA among known diabetic gravida women requires optimal glycemic control in the well subject, patient compliance with medical recommendations (especially those regarding sick-day rules), increased attention to self-blood glucose monitoring and insulin dosage arrangement when illness occurs, and early and increased frequency of communication between caregiver and patient during times of illness. If, despite these steps, glycemic control significantly deteriorates, prompt hospitalization and aggressive inpatient management is indicated.

HYDRAMNIOS

Among the reports in the 1986 to 1993 review presenting usable data regarding hydramnios, three presented data from GDM subjects[7,30,31] and one reported their experience with overt diabetic women.[8] Three of the reports provided nondiabetic control data.[7,8,30] In previous reports, the diagnosis of hydramnios was based most often on a clinical assessment.[3] Among the more recent reports, ultrasound assessment was used.[8,30] Nevertheless, only one of the papers specified the ultrasound criterion used, deepest vertical pocket greater than 8 cm.[30] Among GDM subjects, the incidence of hydramnios ranged from 2.0 to 2.1 percent.[3,7,31] Among control subjects,[7,30] the incidence of hydramnios was 0.5 to 0.7 percent. In the population-based study of Jacobson and Cousins,[7] there was a statistically significant difference in rates between GDM and control subjects. In the single report among overt diabetics, the incidence of hydramnios was 26.4 percent, more than 40 times the rate seen among controls (0.6 percent).[8]

The etiology of hydramnios among diabetic pregnancies is not established. The concentration of glucose and other solutes in amniotic fluid is not related to amniotic fluid volume.[32] Increasing amniotic fluid volume has been associated with increased output of fetal urine measured sonographically.[33] Although infants of overt diabetic women are at increased risk for congenital anomalies and such anomalies may be associated with an increased incidence of hydramnios, most infants of hydramniotic diabetic pregnancy are structurally normal. Historically, there has been a concern that hydramnios would be associated with an increased incidence of premature rupture of membranes or preterm labor. The experience regarding hydramnios and preterm delivery was conflicting in the 1965 to 1985 review.[3] Mimouni et al,[34] in a detailed analysis of premature labor rates among overt diabetic patients, failed to find any significant correlation between hydramnios and preterm labor. Rosenn et al[8] found no significant association between preterm labor and hydramnios. These authors did find that the presence of hydramnios was significantly associated with elevated mean glucose levels. Glycosylated hemoglobin levels were significantly higher in all trimesters among subjects with hydramnios as compared with the group without hydramnios.

Whether the incidence of hydramnios as a complication of diabetic pregnancies is decreasing over time remains to be answered. Ballard et al[35] found a significant reduction from the 1956 to 1969 period to the 1970 to 1978 period. Diamond et al[36] reported a nonsignificant decrease from the 1977 to 1979 period to the 1980 to 1982 period. The cumulative incidence rates of hydramnios among GDM subjects (shown in Table 18-2) are consistent with a decrease over time. However, caution in assessing such temporal changes is warranted given the varying criteria used to define hydramnios. The existing data support the conclusion that hydramnios is significantly more common among overt diabetic women than control subjects (Table 18-3).

PYELONEPHRITIS

Pyelonephritis was reported in 1.2 percent of 247 GDM women (Table 18-2) and 10 of 254 (3.6 percent) type 1 diabetic women.[8] The 1965 to 1985 review cumulative data indicated that the presence of pyelonephritis and diabetic categories were independent[3] (Table 18-2). In the more recent review, the two studies reporting pyelonephritis among GDM cohorts[7,30] found no difference in the GDM pyelonephritis rates of 1.3 percent[30] and 1.0 percent[7] and the rates in the control groups, 0.7 percent and 0.3 percent, respectively. The pyelonephritis rates in the diabetic subgroups in the recent review are not remarkably different from those reported in 1965 to 1985 review (Table 18-2). The pyelonephritis data summarized in Table 18-3 represent the only reports in the English literature between 1965 and 1993 with comparative nondiabetic control data, and they found no significant differences between diabetic and control rates. The authors of these reports did not comment on whether the presence of pyelonephritis was associated with increased perinatal mortality, as previously suggested by Pedersen and Molsted-Pedersen.[37]

PRETERM LABOR

Preterm labor complicated 8.1 percent of the 247 GDM pregnancies reported with usable data.[7,30] Among overt diabetic pregnancies, the cumulative incidence of preterm labor was 30 percent (136 of 453) and ranged in three reports from 23 to 31 percent.[8,26,34] The reports with nondiabetic control data indicate no significant difference in the preterm labor rate between GDM and control subjects, but a significantly increased rate in overt diabetic women[7,8,30,34] (Table 18-3). Mimouni and associates[34] found the relative risk of preterm labor among 181 overt diabetic women to be 1.64 times the rate seen in their nondiabetic control population ($P < .01$). They reported a significantly higher 28-week glycosylated hemoglobin level among diabetic subjects with preterm labor as compared with diabetic women who did not have preterm labor. The mechanism linking preterm labor and diabetes is uncertain, but Mimouni et al[34] reported a significant correlation between preterm labor and urogenital infections (candida and trichomoniasis). Molsted-Pedersen[38] speculated that hormonal relationship differences between diabetic and nondiabetic women may explain the increased frequency of preterm labor in diabetic pregnant women.

Treatment of preterm labor is multifaceted. Parenteral tocolytic options include β-agonist (e.g., ritodrine, terbutaline) and magnesium sulfate. Oral tocolytics include β-agonists, calcium channel blockers (e.g., nifedipine), and indomethacin. Indomethacin can also be given by rectal suppository. Because of the potent metabolic effects of β-agonists and the absence of data demonstrating significant differences in efficacy between β-agonist and magnesium sulfate tocolysis, many centers would opt to use magnesium sulfate as the tocolytic of first choice in the treatment of preterm labor in diabetic pregnancies. As noted previously, the treatment of preterm labor with β-agonist, with or without glucocorticoids, can produce DKA.[3] Use of glucocorticoids to accelerate pulmonary function has also been associated with significant elevation of blood glucose levels. In the event that β-agonist tocolysis or glucocorticoids are used, more intensive blood glucose monitoring and insulin therapy must be available. An insulin infusion titrated according to frequent fingerstick blood glucose determinations is effective.[39] The glycemic goal of such therapy is to achieve and maintain normal capillary blood glucose levels (70 to 100 mg/dl).

SPONTANEOUS PRETERM DELIVERY

Only a portion of women who experience preterm labor deliver prematurely (i.e., spontaneously). This difference occurs because some diagnoses of preterm labor are falsely positive, other patients stop contracting and deliver at term, and in other instances, the diagnosis of preterm labor is correct but the patient is successfully treated, delivery is delayed, and the patient delivers at term. Preterm delivery is one of the most important contributors to perinatal mortality in diabetic gestations.[38] Molsted-Pedersen[38] reported a Scandinavian experience of 397 diabetic pregnancies from 1974 to 1977. Among GDM subjects, the incidence of spontaneous preterm labor with delivery was 14.6 percent; among classes B and C diabetic women, 28 percent; and among class D or greater diabetic women, 24 percent (Table 18-2). In reports that did not classify overt diabetic patients into the various White's classes, the incidence of spontaneous preterm labor and delivery ranged from 16 to 23 percent.[8,34] Combining the Molsted-Pedersen overt diabetic classes, the incidence of spontaneous labor and delivery was 26 percent.[38] Rosenn et al[8] reported the incidence of spontaneous labor and delivery to be 16.1 percent and was not significantly different than the rate of 12 percent among 508 control subjects. As other centers report their experience with spontaneous preterm labor and delivery, it will allow us to judge whether the findings of these initial controlled reports are confirmed. In the interim given the significantly higher incidence of preterm labor among overt diabetic pregnancies and the morbidity associated with preterm delivery, the clinician must make every effort to treat preterm labor, thereby, attempting to avoid preterm delivery.

TOTAL INCIDENCE OF PRETERM DELIVERY

In a more recent review, authors more clearly differentiated between subjects manifesting preterm labor, preterm delivery after preterm labor and total preterm delivery rates than in the earlier review.[3] The more specific diagnostic categories allow more refined assessments, as suggested in the data summarized in Table 18-2. Among 717 GDM subjects, the total preterm delivery rate was 7.3 percent. Among classes B and C and class D or greater groups, the total preterm delivery rates were 19.0 percent and 37.6 percent, respectively. Analysis of these data indicated that the total preterm delivery rate was not independent of the diabetic categories. Among studies reporting the total preterm delivery rates,[5,8,20,22,24,30,31,40] four papers presented nondiabetic control rates[5,8,24,30] (Table 18-3). Goldman et al[30] reported no significant difference in the preterm delivery rate between GDM and control subjects matched for age, parity, and ethnicity. By contrast, studies with control data reporting total preterm delivery rates among overt diabetic pregnancies all reported a significantly higher rate among diabetic than nondiabetic women[5,8,24] (Table 18-3). Furthermore, consistent with the nonindependence of diabetic categories and total preterm delivery rates is the large Joslin Clinic report of Greene and associates.[24] The authors found an approximately twofold higher total preterm delivery rate among class D or greater than among classes B and C diabetic women. Undoubtedly, several factors contribute to the increased total preterm delivery rate among overt diabetic pregnancies as compared with GDM and nondiabetic subjects. Such factors include (1) increased hypertensive complications in overt diabetes[5,24]; (2) an increased incidence of chronic hypertension[20–22]; (3) an increased rate of preterm labor[26,34]; and (4) a yet-to-be quantitated discomfort on the part of the caregiver with continuing a diabetic pregnancy to term because of concerns regarding intrauterine fetal demise, accelerated fetal growth, increased risk of cephalopelvic disproportion, shoulder dystocia, and so forth.

Greene and associates[24] most clearly quantitated the contribution of various conditions to preterm delivery rates among insulin-dependent overt diabetic women. These data emphasize the dramatic impact of hypertensive complications on preterm delivery rates. In this experience, overall diabetic women had a 3.22 relative risk of prematurity compared with control subjects. However, this risk was significantly affected by the mother's blood pressure status. The relative risk of prematurity for normotensive diabetic women was 2.08, whereas among hypertensive diabetic women the risk rose to 5.19.

CESAREAN SECTION

Twelve of the twenty-five references in the 1986 to 1993 review had usable data regarding cesarean section. Ten of these papers reported total cesarean section data,[5,9,12,22,26,28,30,31,41,42] two reported primary cesarean section rates,[7,40] and one reported repeat cesarean rates.[7] Five of the twelve presented nondiabetic control data for comparison (Table 18-3). Among GDM women, the incidence of primary cesarean section ranged from 13.4 to 18.4 percent.[7,40] The 13.4 percent primary cesarean rate among 97 GDM subjects was comparable with the 12.9 percent rate in the simultaneously followed control group.[7] From the same report, the repeat cesarean rate among GDM women was 16.5 percent, significantly greater than the 6.0 percent rate among control subjects.

Only four of the reports dealt with cesarean section among overt diabetic women,[5,22,26,41] and two of these reports were small series of specific diabetic patient types (9 class T diabetic women,[22] 20 DKA patients[26]). In the paper by Gregory et al,[41] the primary cesarean section rate among overt diabetic women was 24.7 percent and the repeat cesarean section rate was 27 percent, for a total cesarean rate of 52 percent. Hanson and Persson[5] reported a total cesarean rate of 45.2 percent among a large group of overt diabetic women. Among GDM women, the total cesarean section rate ranged from 21 to 35 percent. Of the four studies with nondiabetic control rates among GDM women, all reported a significantly higher total cesarean section rate in diabetic than in control groups (Table 18-3). As would be expected among overt diabetic women, the total cesarean section rate was significantly higher than the rate seen in the nondiabetic controls[5,41] (Table 18-3).

Given the greater likelihood of other obstetric and medical complications, the total cesarean rate differences between overt diabetic pregnancies and control women are understandable. The significant difference in total cesarean rates between GDM and control subjects is noteworthy (Table 18-3). Regarding GDM to control subject comparisons, the reports of Goldman et al[30] and Suhonen and Teramo[12] are especially provocative. These authors point out that the cesarean section rate among GDM women was higher than control women despite the absence of differences between groups in the macrosomia rate, incidence of large-for-gestational age infants, or labor abnormalities.

Goldman et al[30] suggested that this finding may be "related to patterns of physician decision making." Suhonen and Teramo[12] also reported a significantly higher total cesarean section rate among GDM than control subjects. This difference in total cesarean section rate occurred even though there was no significant difference between groups in mean birth weight, neonatal relative weights, or macrosomia (defined as

>4,500 g). Given the insensitivity of currently available methods for diagnosing large-for-gestational age or macrosomic infants, and risk assessing for shoulder dystocia in combination with the common experience of an increased incidence of large-for-gestational age infants, macrosomia, and shoulder dystocia among infants of GDM women, physicians may more quickly opt for cesarean section at the first sign of a problem or question rather than continuing with a trial of labor. It is suggested that in the absence of other complications (Table 18-4), GDM pregnancies should be followed expectantly. The elements of such management include (1) meticulous glucose control (mean fasting capillary whole blood glucose level of ≤90 mg/dl and mean 1-hour postprandial capillary whole blood glucose level of ≤120 mg/dl; (2) daily fetal movement counts from 26 to 28 weeks' gestation; (3) a late pregnancy ultrasound for estimated fetal weight, amniotic fluid index, and anthropometric assessment; and (4) antenatal testing if the patient is undelivered at 40 weeks' gestation. This approach is a modification of that recommended by Fadel and Hammond,[43] which was associated with a 7 percent primary cesarean section rate. This approach is also consistent with recommendations of the California Diabetes and Pregnancy Program.[44]

In the absence of superimposed complications (Table 18-4), this expectant management approach is also advocated for overt diabetic women. Routine preterm delivery, as widely practiced in the past, is not appropriate. The philosophy of avoiding early delivery, coupled with meticulous attention to maternal and fetus status, allows the fetus and the labor mechanism to mature and the inducibility of the cervix to improve.

Table 18-4. Factors Influencing the Timing of Delivery of Diabetic Pregnancies

Suboptimal glycemic control
Maternal hypertension
Macrosomia
Decreased fetal activity
Suspicious fetal biophysical test
Poor maternal compliance
Maternal vascular disease
Hydramnios
Poor obstetric history
Prior intrauterine demise

The presence of one or more risk factors listed in Table 18-4 may demand preterm delivery. In the absence of such risk factors, the major concerns regarding an expectant management approach include intrauterine fetal demise and macrosomia with consequent shoulder dystocia. The former is minimized by establishment of euglycemia, monitoring the pregnancy for other maternal or fetal complications, and antenatal biophysical testing (e.g., fetal movement counts, nonstress test). The risk of shoulder dystocia is minimized by careful evaluation of the fetus and mother. A later pregnancy ultrasound at 37 to 38 weeks allows for estimation of fetal weight and head-body proportions. This ultrasound information, maternal physical examination, possibly radiologic assessment by pelvimetry, and maternal past obstetric history provides the information that guides the judicious obstetrician's intrapartum management. In labors in which there is a suspicion of macrosomia (>4000 g) or fetal head-trunk disproportion, it is important to avoid injudicious use of forceps or vacuum extraction.

PREDELIVERY HOSPITALIZATION DAYS

Outpatient evaluation and management of pregnancies complicated by diabetes is currently the standard[44] and is associated with excellent perinatal outcomes.[7,45,46] In most instances, hospitalization is unnecessary as long as the patient is involved in a comprehensive patient evaluation and care program, motivated and compliant, and does not develop superimposed maternal or fetal complications. Despite the current philosophy of outpatient management of diabetic pregnancies, these women are more likely to be hospitalized than nondiabetic gravid women because of a "carry-over" philosophy from earlier years of late pregnancy hospitalization for more intensive maternal-fetal monitoring in anticipation of a preterm delivery or because of hospitalization for superimposed complications. In the 1965 to 1985 review of the English literature,[3] there were no data quantitating the experience with predelivery hospitalization of diabetic women. In more recent review, two papers reported such data. Gregory and associates,[41] reporting from University Hospital Nottingham, dichotomized their experience into two intervals (1977 to 1983 and 1984 to 1990). The 81 overt diabetic subjects in the later interval entered care at 8 weeks' gestation, delivered at 37.5 weeks, and spent significantly fewer predelivery days in the hospital (mean, 5.3 days) than the 58 women (mean, 15 days) in the earlier interval who entered care at 12 weeks and delivered at 37 weeks. Nagy,[31] in reporting the experience with 409 GDM pregnant women in Deprescen, Hungary, cared for between 1985 and 1991, noted that the mean number of predelivery hospitalization days for diet-controlled GDM women was 6.0 days and for diet- and insulin-treated GDM patients, the value was 7.6 days. The authors of these reports did not specify what the indications for hospitalization were in their centers.[31,41] Gregory et al[41] explained the reduction in antenatal hospital days by the increased experience in outpatient management by the diabetes team and the introduction of an obstetric day care unit for fetal monitoring.

POSTOPERATIVE INFECTIONS

Jacobson and Cousins[7] reported a significantly higher rate of infectious complications among 97 GDM subjects (12.4 percent) than found in the population-based control group (5.9 percent) ($P < .05$). The difference in infectious complication rates between the two groups were related to the difference in the repeat cesarean section rate (diabetic women greater than control women). When the difference in repeat cesarean sections was controlled for, there was no significant difference in infectious complication rates between the groups. Diamond and associates[47] compared overt diabetic subjects undergoing cesarean section to a case control group of nondiabetic women. Overall, the incidence of post-cesarean section endometritis or wound infections was significantly greater among the diabetic women (14.1 percent) compared with control subjects (3.2 percent). The significant difference between diabetic and nondiabetic subjects persisted when the patients were categorized into either high-risk (those with ruptured membranes or labor before cesarean) or low-risk (absence of rupture of membrane or labor preceding cesarean) categories. The incidence of post-cesarean section endometritis or wound infection in the low-risk diabetic and nondiabetic subjects was 9.1 percent and 1.8 percent, respectively ($P < .05$). Corresponding rates among the high-risk diabetic and nondiabetic subjects was 25.0 percent and 6.3 percent, respectively ($P < .05$). These authors reported that post-cesarean section and infectious morbidity were independent of White's classification but *not* of glycemic control. High-risk diabetic women in poor control had a higher rate of postoperative infections than high-risk diabetic women in good control ($P < .05$).

Why should there be a difference in conclusions between these two controlled studies dealing with GDM and overt diabetic pregnancies?[7,47] What is the relationship between infection rates and diabetes mellitus? What is the relationship between deterioration in glycemic control and infection rates and infection-related processes? There is a growing body of data supporting a link between hyperglycemia and infection. These data suggest a vicious circle among hyperglycemia, impairment in various cellular and humoral processes involved in host resistance to infection, increased infection rates, and infection-induced metabolic alterations that predispose to or perpetuate hyperglycemia, thereby completing the circle.[48] The role or contribution, if any, of the normal immunologic changes of pregnancy to differences in infection rates between diabetic and nondiabetic gravida women is uncertain. The pregnancy literature regarding this vicious circle is unrevealing.[3,7,8] A variety of in vivo and in vitro human studies in nonpregnant subjects, as well as experimental animal studies, suggests that hyperglycemia is associated with a compromise in processes involved with host defenses. These processes include decreased leukocyte glycolysis[49] with the potential for reduction in metabolic energy necessary for internalization of infectious particles,[50] impaired chemotaxis,[51–54] decreased in vitro phagocytosis,[55,56] a reduction in intracellular bactericidal activity against various pathogens,[57,58] impaired cell-mediated immune response (indicated by a reduction in phytohemagglutinin-induced lymphocyte transformation,[59] decreased peripheral blood lymphocyte response to staph phage lysate,[60] and a compromise in various tissue factors (e.g., impaired blood flow secondary to vascular insufficiency or a reduction in tissue oxygen levels predisposing to the risk of anaerobe growth or oxygen-dependent leukocyte bactericidal activity). Reports with nondiabetic control data are consistent with the hypothesis that hyperglycemia is significantly correlated to the risk of infection.[51–54,56,57,59,60]

The presence of infection has the potential to exaggerate or perpetuate hyperglycemia as a consequence of infection-induced changes. These changes include an increase in adrenal glucocorticoids,[61] enhanced hepatic conversion of L-alanine to glucose,[62] increased peripheral tissue glycolysis,[63–65] increased fasting growth hormone levels,[66] and increased plasma catecholamines.[67] These infection-induced metabolic-endocrinologic alterations result directly or indirectly (e.g., via increased insulin resistance) in hyperglycemia.

The overt diabetic pregnancy data of Diamond and associates[47] are consistent with the nonpregnancy studies. The failure to demonstrate an increased rate of infectious complications associated with GDM may be due to the generally good glycemic control present among GDM subjects.[7]

Obviously, it would be advantageous for other centers to report their experience with both perioperative and nonoperative infectious morbidity to see whether they would corroborate the findings of Diamond and associates.[47] The information among nonpregnant overt diabetic subjects indicating that hyperglycemia increases the risk of infections provides another argument for careful attention to metabolic control in diabetic pregnancies.

MATERNAL MORTALITY

Nine maternal mortalities were reported among the 6,070 diabetic pregnancies in the 1986 to 1993 review (0.14 percent). This rate is comparable with the incidence reported in the 1965 to 1985 review[3] (Table 18-2). The nine mortalities in the more recent review were derived from two reports.[22,68] The multicenter series of nine renal transplant patients by Ogburn et al[22] reported one mortality in a 28-year-old subject who had diabetes for 15 years and whose pregnancy occurred 2 years after renal transplant. She was normotensive with an early pregnancy creatinine clearance of 45 ml/min and had a history of vasculopathy with ulcers on both feet that had required amputations of several toes. She had been noncompliant with medical recommendations before her pregnancy and had a first trimester glycosylated hemoglobin level of 15 percent (normal, 6.0 to 8.8 percent). Her hemoglobin level was 8.5 g/dl, and an electrocardiogram demonstrated nonspecific ST changes without evidence of ischemia or infarction. At 21 weeks' gestation, she was found unconscious, and her glucose level on arrival at the hospital was 140 mg/dl. Resuscitative efforts were unsuccessful. An autopsy revealed pulmonary edema without pulmonary embolus or myocardial infarction. Reece et al,[68] in reviewing 1 class H case of their own and 12 in the literature between 1953 and 1986, compiled eight maternal mortalities. The series of 13 patients ranged from 23 to 38 years of age. Of the 13 patients, 12 presented with myocardial infarction and 1 with severe angina and positive coronary arteriogram. The coronary disease diagnosis was established before pregnancy in 3, during pregnancy in 8, and postpartum in 2 subjects. Of the five maternal survivors, three had their cardiac diagnosis established before pregnancy and two in the first trimester. Although the numbers were small, of the three class H patients diagnosed before pregnancy, all mothers and infants survived. By contrast, among those class H subjects in which the diagnosis was not made until pregnancy, the maternal mortality was 8 of 10 and fetal mortality was 5 of 9.

The composite maternal mortality rate of 0.14 percent in the 1986 to 1993 review was greater than 10 times the maternal mortality rate reported in the United States between 1974 and 1978.[69] The experience of both the 1965 to 1985 review[3] and the more recent review are consistent with the thesis that the maternal mortality risk is greater in overt diabetic women than among GDM women. Nevertheless, even among GDM women, the potential for maternal mortality as a complication of hypertension, infection, or ketoacidosis (e.g., secondary to β-agonist) must not be overlooked. To minimize this risk, not only must antenatal medical and obstetric care be state of the art but comprehensive preconception medical evaluation and patient education are imperative. This latter point especially relates to the overt diabetic women with the potential for or with documented vascular disease. Not only does optimal preconception evaluation and care optimize perinatal outcome, it has the potential to allow improved patient counseling (regarding risks, long-term prognosis, antepartum care elements, and so forth) and a current assessment for the presence or absence of end organ complications (e.g., retinopathy, nephropathy, coronary artery disease, neuropathy).

CONCLUSIONS

The following conclusions are based on two sequential reviews of the English literature regarding obstetric complications in diabetic pregnancies. The initial re-

view covering the years 1965 to 1985 has been previously published.[3] The conclusions from that review have been supplemented by a review of the years 1986 to 1993. The reviewed literature supports the following conclusions:

1. All hypertensive complications (pregnancy-induced hypertension, pre-eclampsia, chronic hypertension) for which there is a reasonable database are significantly more common in class D or greater diabetic pregnant women than nondiabetic pregnant women. Comparing GDM to control subjects (Table 18-3) when pre-eclampsia and pregnancy-induced hypertension cases are combined, the incidence is greater in GDM than control subjects. Two controlled reports have failed to find a significant difference between GDM and control subjects in the incidence of pregnancy-induced hypertension.[7,10] Chronic hypertension was significantly more common among GDM than control subjects.

2. Hydramnios is more common in overt diabetic than GDM and control subjects.[3] In the more recent literature reviewed, two controlled reports found similar rates of hydramnios in GDM and control subjects[7,30] (Table 18-3). In one, the difference was statistically significant,[7] whereas in the other, using a more objective assessment of amniotic fluid volume, the difference was not statistically significant.[30]

3. DKA is more common among overt diabetic women than GDM subjects but remains a possibility even among GDM women[3] (Table 18-2).

4. There is no demonstrable difference in the incidence of pyelonephritis between the diabetic subgroups or in comparing diabetic categories to control subjects (Table 18-3).

5. The reports with control data suggest there was no significant difference in the preterm labor rates between GDM and control subjects, whereas the rate among overt diabetic pregnancies is greater than in control subjects (Table 18-3). Preterm delivery after spontaneous labor was not independent of the diabetic categories (Table 18-2). In view of this, it is interesting that the only report with control data that met inclusion criteria did not find a significant difference in the incidence of preterm delivery after spontaneous labor when comparing overt diabetic with control subjects.[8] In all papers with control data reporting total preterm delivery rates, overt di-

abetic pregnancies were found to be significantly more likely to deliver prematurely.[5,8,24]

6. Primary, repeat, and total cesarean section rates were not independent of diabetic categories.[3] Among GDM women, although the rate of primary cesarean section did not differ from controls, the repeat cesarean section rate was significantly higher.[7] Total cesarean section rates were significantly greater in GDM and overt diabetic groups (Table 18-3). Post-cesarean section infectious morbidity was found to be more common among GDM and overt diabetic groups than control subjects (Table 18-3). The increased rate among GDM women appeared to be explainable on the basis of the increased rate of repeat cesarean sections among GDM women as compared with control subjects.[7]

7. The maternal mortality rate among diabetic gravida women appears to be greater than 10 times the rate in nondiabetic women.

8. More recent reports indicate that improved glycemic control is associated with a significant reduction in various obstetric complications among overt diabetic women. These complications include preeclampsia and pregnancy-induced hypertension,[8,20] hydramnios,[8] preterm labor,[34] and postoperative endomyometritis.[47]

ACKNOWLEDGMENT

I gratefully acknowledge the excellent assistance of Ms. Sue Halvin in the preparation of this manuscript.

REFERENCES

1. Department of Health and Human Services, Public Health Service: Healthy People 2000. DHHS Publication (PHS) 91-50213, 1990

2. Cousins L, Kitzmiller J, Schneider J et al: The California Diabetes and Pregnancy Program: Implementation of a multi-center experience with diabetic pregnancies. J Perinatol 12:173, 1992

3. Cousins LM: Pregnancy complications among diabetic women: review 1965–1985. Obstet Gynecol Surv 42:140, 1987

4. Kyle G: Diabetes in pregnancy. Intern Med, suppl. 3, 59: 1, 1963

5. Hanson U, Persson B: Outcome of pregnancies complicated by type 1 insulin-dependent diabetes in Sweden: acute pregnancy complications, neonatal mortality and morbidity. Am J Perinatol 10:330, 1993

6. Garner PR, D'Alton ME, Dudley DK et al: Preeclampsia in diabetic pregnancies. Am J Obstet Gynecol 163:505, 1990

7. Jacobson JD, Cousins L: A population-based study of maternal and perinatal outcome in patients with gestational diabetes. Am J Obstet Gynecol 161:981, 1989

8. Rosenn B, Miodovnik M, Combs CA et al: Poor glycemic control and antepartum obstetric complications in women with insulin-dependent diabetes. Int J Gynaecol Obstet 43:21, 1993

9. Nordlander E, Hanson U, Persson B: Factors influencing neonatal morbidity in gestational diabetic pregnancy. Br J Obstet Gynaecol 96:671, 1989

10. Gabbe S, Mestman J, Freeman R et al: Management and outcome of class A diabetes mellitus. Am J Obstet Gynecol 127:465, 1977

11. Siddiqi T, Rosenn B, Mimouni F et al: Hypertension during pregnancy in insulin-dependent diabetic women. Obstet Gynecol 17:514, 1991

12. Suhonen L, Teramo K: Hypertension in preeclampsia in women with gestational glucose intolerance. Acta Obstet Gynecol Scand 72:269, 1993

13. Beaufils M, Uzan S, Donsimoni R, Colau JC: Prevention of preeclampsia by early anti-platelet therapy. Lancet 1: 840, 1985

14. Wallenburg HC, Dekker GA, Makovitz JW, Rotmans P: Low dose aspirin prevents pregnancy induced hypertension and preeclampsia in angiotensin-sensitive primigravidae. Lancet 1:1, 1986

15. Schiff P, Peleg E, Goldenberg M et al: The use of aspirin to prevent pregnancy-induced hypertension and lower the ratio of thromboxane 2 to prostacyclin in relatively high risk pregnancies. N Engl J Med 312:351, 1989

16. Collins R, Wallenburg HC: Pharmacological prevention and treatment of hypertensive disorders in pregnancy. p. 512. In Chalmers I, Enkin M, Kirse MJ (eds): Effective Care in Pregnancy and Childbirth. Vol. 1. Pregnancy. Oxford University Press, Oxford, 1989

17. McParland P, Pearce JM, Chamberlain GPT: Doppler ultrasound and aspirin in recognition and prevention of pregnancy-induced hypertension. Lancet 335:1552, 1990

18. Uzan S, Beaufils M, Beart G et al: Prevention of fetal growth retardation with low dose aspirin: findings of the EPREDA trial. Lancet 337:1427, 1991

19. Imperiale TF, Petrulif AS: A meta-analysis of low-dose aspirin for the prevention and pregnancy induced hypertensive disease. JAMA 226:260, 1991

20. Combs CA, Rosenn B, Kitzmiller JL et al: Early pregnancy

proteineuria in diabetes related to preeclampsia. Obstet Gynecol 82:801, 1993

21. Diamond MP, Shah DM, Hester RA et al: Complication of insulin-dependent diabetic pregnancy by preeclampsia and/or chronic hypertension: analysis of outcome. Am J Perinatol 2:263, 1985

22. Ogburn PL, Kitzmiller JL, Hare JW et al: Pregnancy following renal transplantation in class T diabetes mellitus. JAMA 255:911, 1986

23. Pritchard JA, MacDonald PC, Grant NF (eds): Williams Obstetrics. 17th Ed. Appleton & Lange, E. Norwalk, CT, 1985

24. Greene MF, Hare JW, Krache M et al: Prematurity among insulin-requiring diabetic gravid women. Am J Obstet Gynecol 161:106, 1989

25. Langer O, Levy J, Brustman L et al: Glycemic control in gestational diabetic mellitus—how tight is tight enough: small for gestational age vs. large for gestational age? Am J Obstet Gynecol 161:646, 1989

26. Montoro MN, Myers VP, Mestman JH et al: Outcome of pregnancy in diabetic ketoacidosis. Am J Perinatol 10:17, 1993

27. Kilvert JA, Nicholson HO, Wright AD: Ketoacidosis in diabetic pregnancy. Diabetic Med 10:278, 1993

28. Nagy G: Late complications of gestational diabetes—maternal effects. Zentralbl Gynakol 115:450, 1993

29. Rodgers BD, Rodgers DE: Clinical variables associated with diabetic ketoacidosis during pregnancy. J Reprod Med 36:797, 1991

30. Goldman M, Kitzmiller JL, Abrams B et al: Obstetrics complications with GDM. Effects of maternal weight. Diabetes, suppl. 2, 40:79, 1991

31. Nagy G: Management of gestational diabetes. Zentralbl Gynakol 115:147, 1993

32. Cassady G: Amniocentesis. Clin Perinatol 1:87, 1974

33. VanOtterlo L, Wladimiroff J, Wallenberg H: Relationship between fetal urine production and amniotic fluid volume in normal pregnancy and pregnancy complicated by diabetes. Br J Obstet Gynaecol 84:205, 1977

34. Mimouni F, Miodovnik M, Siddiqi TA et al: High spontaneous premature labor rated in insulin-dependent diabetic pregnant women: an association with poor glycemic control and urogenital infection. Obstet Gynecol 1972:175, 1988

35. Ballard J, Holroyde J, Tsang R et al: High malformation rates in decreased mortality in infants of diabetic mothers managed after the first trimester of pregnancy (1956–1978). Am J Obstet Gynecol 148:1111, 1984

36. Diamond M, Vaughn W, Salyer S: Efficacy of outpatient management of insulin-dependent diabetic pregnancies. J Perinatol 5:2, 1985

37. Pedersen J, Molsted-Pedersen L: Prognosis of the outcome of pregnancy in diabetes. Acta Endocrinol 50:70, 1965

38. Molsted-Pedersen L: Premature labor and perinatal mortality in diabetic pregnancy—obstetric consideration. p. 392. In Carbohydrate Metabolism in Pregnancy in the Newborn. In Sutherland HW, Stowers JM (eds). New York, Springer-Verlag, 1979

39. Cousins LM. Obstetrical management in fetal surveillance in the pregnant diabetic. p. 345. In Brody S, Ueland K (eds): Endocrine Disorders in Pregnancy. Appleton-Century-Crofts, E. Norwalk, CT, 1989

40. Philipson EH, Kalhan SC, Edelberg SC, Williams TG: Maternal obesity as a risk factor in gestational diabetes. Am J Perinatol 2:268, 1985

41. Gregory R, Scott AR, Mohajer M, Tattersall RB: Diabetic pregnancy 1977–1990: have we reached a plateau? J Coll Physicians Lond 26:162, 1992

42. Kjos SL, Henry OA, Montoro M et al: Insulin-requiring diabetes in pregnancy: randomized trial of active induction of labor and expected management. Am J Obstet Gynecol 169:611, 1993

43. Fadel H, Hammond S: Diabetes mellitus in pregnancy. J Reprod Med 27:56, 1982

44. Guidelines for Care. Sweet Success, California Diabetes and Pregnancy Program. Department of Health Services, Maternal and Child Health Branch. State of California, 1992

45. Gabbe SG: Management of diabetes mellitus in pregnancy. Am J Obstet Gynecol 153:824, 1985

46. Freinkel N, Dooley SL, Metzger BE: Care of the pregnant woman within insulin-dependent diabetes mellitus. N Engl J Med 313:96, 1985

47. Diamond MP, Enteman SS, Salyer SL et al: Increased risk of endometritis in wound infection after casearean section in insulin-dependent diabetic women. Am J Obstet Gynecol 155:297, 1986

48. Rayfield EJ, Ault MJ, Keusch GT et al: Infection and diabetes: the case for glucose control. Am J Med 72:439, 1982

49. Esmann V: The diabetic leukocyte. Enzyme 13:32, 1972

50. Sbarra AJ, Karnovisky ML: The biochemical basis of phagocytosis. 1. Metabolic changes during the injection of particles by polymorphonuclear leukocytes. J Biol Chem 234:1355, 1959

51. Perillie PE, Knowlan JP, Fench SC: Studies of the resistance to infection in diabetic mellitus: local exudative cellular response. J Lab Clin Med 59:1008, 1962

52. Brayton RG, Stokes PE, Schwartz MS, Louria DB: Effective alcohol in various diseases on leukocyte mobilization, phagocytosis in the intracellular bacterial killing. N Engl J Med 282:123, 1970

53. Mowat AG, Baum J: Chemotaxis of polymorphonuclear leukocytes from patients with diabetes mellitus. N Engl J Med 284:621, 1971

54. Molenaar DM, Palumbo PJ, Wilson WR, Ritts RE: Leukocyte chemotaxis in diabetic patients and their nondiabetic first degree relatives. Diabetes 25:880, 1976

55. Bybee JD, Rogers DE: The phagocytic activity of polymorphonuclear leukocytes obtained from patient with diabetes mellitus. J Lab Clin Med 64:1, 1964

56. Bagdade JD, Root RK, Bulger RJ: Impired leukocyte function in patients with poorly controlled diabetes. Diabetes 23:9, 1974

57. Knowlan CN, Beaty HN, Bagdade JD: Further characterization of the impaired bacterialcidal function of granulocytes in patients with poorly controlled diabetes. Diabetes 27:889, 1978

58. Rayfield EJ, Keusch GT, Gilbert HS et al: Does diabetic control affect susceptibility to infection? Clin Res 26:425a, 1978

59. MacCuish AC, Urbaniak SJ, Campbell CJ: Phytohemagglutinin transformation and circulating lymphocyte subpopulation in insulin-dependent diabetic patients. Diabetes 23:708, 1974

60. Casey JI, Heeter BJ, Klyschevich KA: Impaired response of lymphocytes of diabetic subject to antigen of *Staphylococcus aureus*. J Infect Dis 136:495, 1977

61. Beisel WR, Rapoport MI: Interrelations between adrenocortical functions and infectious illness. N Engl J Med 280:541,596, 1969

62. Long CL, Kinney JM, Geiger JW: Nonsuppressability of gluconeogenesis of glucose in septic patients. Metabolism 25:193, 1976

63. Yeung CY, Lee VWY, Yeung MB: Glucose disappearance rate in neonatal infection. J Pediatr 82:486, 1973

64. Guckian JC: Role of metabolism in pathogenesis of bacteremia due to *Diplococcus penumoniae* in rabbits. J Infect Dis 127:1, 1973

65. Felig P, Brown WV, Levine RA, Clatchskin G: Glucose homeostasis in viral hepatitis. N Engl J Med 283:1436, 1970

66. Rayfield EJ, Curnow RT, George DT, Beisel WR: Impaired carbohydrate metabolism during mild viral illnesses. N Engl J Med 289:618, 1973

67. Griffiths J, Groves AC, Leung FY: Hypertriglyceridemia and hypoglycemia in gram-negative sepsis in the dawn. Surg Gynecol Obstet 136:897, 1973

68. Reece EA, Egan JF, Coustan DR et al: Coronary artery disease in diabetic pregnancies. Am J Obstet Gynecol 154:150, 1986

69. Beuhler J, Kaunitz A, Hogue C et al: Maternal mortality in women age 35 years or older: United States. JAMA 255:53, 1986

19
Diabetic Retinopathy

LOIS JOVANOVIC-PETERSON
CHARLES M. PETERSON

Before 1922, few infants of diabetic mothers survived.[1] With the advent of insulin, the infant survival rate improved, but it was not until the 1980s that the mortality rate dropped to a rate near that of the general population.[2] Although infant survival seems to be directly related to the degree of maternal glucose control,[3,4] there is still controversy regarding the impact of pregnancy per se on the maternal health status.[5–9] This chapter specifically covers the literature on pregnancies complicated by diabetic retinopathy and attempts to tease out the variables that influence the natural history of retinopathy during pregnancy.

NATURAL HISTORY IN NONPREGNANT INDIVIDUALS

Diabetic retinopathy is the result of retinal arteriolar and capillary endothelial cell damage, basement membrane thickening, and pericyte damage.[10] Diabetic retinopathy is a progressive disorder that has two distinct clinical stages: background (preproliferative) and proliferative.[11] For research purposes, these stages are subdivided into several grades based on a specific set of defined criteria and objective findings,[12] as summarized in Table 19-1.

The nonproliferative type is also known as background retinopathy (Fig. 19-1). An intermediate category, known as preproliferative retinopathy, is used, as are more subtle gradings of the severity of the changes in retinopathy (Fig. 19-2). Proliferative retinopathy requires the growth of new capillaries on the retina (Fig. 19-3). These may extend into the vitreous and rupture, causing vitreous hemorrhage, which is usually only a minor visual threat. The hemorrhage typically resolves over a period of several weeks after it has appeared as a sudden unilateral clouding or loss of vision. If the blood in the vitreous organizes and does not clear, vision may be impaired. It is for this reason that the surgical procedure of vitrectomy was developed. The real threat to vision is that, subsequent to the hemorrhage, there will be scarring and traction

Table 19-1. Grading System for Diabetic Retinopathy: Modified Airlie House Diabetic Retinopathy Classification Based on the Seven Standard Fundus Photographs

Clinical Grouping	Description of Retina
Normal	No retinopathy
Minimal background	Microaneurysms or blot hemorrhages only
Mild background	Hemorrhages easily visible with an ophthalmoscope and questionable presence of hard exudates, soft exudates, and intraretinal microvascular abnormalities, and/or venous beading
Moderate background	Numerous hemorrhages and definite presence of both hard and soft exudates with obvious intraretinal microvascular abnormalities and venous beading; lesions localized to less than two fields of the seven standard fields of the fundus photographs
Severe background	Same lesions as moderate, but presence of these lesions in greater than or equal to two fields of the fundus photographs
Proliferative retinopathy	Presence of neovascularization

(From Early Treatment Diabetic Retinopathy Study Research Group,[12] with permission.)

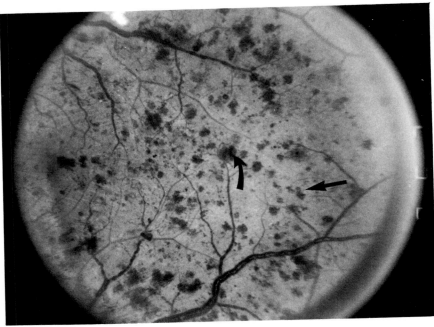

Fig. 19-1. Microaneurysms and dot and blot hemorrhages in the retina. Hemorrhages are large and have irregular margins. Smaller hemorrhages cannot be distinguished from microaneurysms.

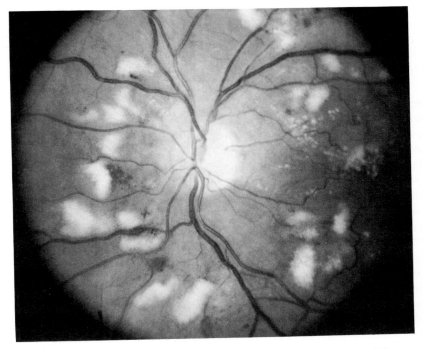

Fig. 19-2. Multiple cotton-wool spots surround the optic disc in a pregnant diabetic woman.

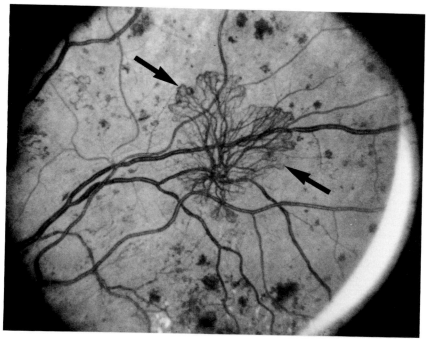

Fig. 19-3. A neovascular frond (arrows) of proliferative diabetic retinopathy that is made up of irregular, small vessels.

detachment of the retina, resulting in permanent visual loss.

By and large, background retinopathy does not threaten vision. It is characterized by the appearance of exudates, microaneurysms, and small red dot hemorrhages in the retina. Unless these occur in the perimacular area, visual symptoms do not occur. Background retinopathy is extremely common in diabetes and is practically universal if carefully sought after the patient has had the disease for 20 years. Background retinopathy is usually not clinically apparent in casual examinations with the ophthalmoscope in patients who have had diabetes for less than 10 years.

Preproliferative retinopathy is a transitional stage toward proliferative retinopathy. Fortunately, not all background retinopathy progresses to proliferative retinopathy. When this transitional stage occurs, there is increasing evidence that early and vigorous photocoagulation may prevent subsequent proliferation and visual loss. The characteristic lesions in preproliferative retinopathy are intraretinal microvascular abnormalities and soft, or cotton-wool, exudates.

The mechanisms that cause retinal damage appear similar to the more general effect of diabetes on the systemic microvascular system. Putative mechanisms include circulatory damage and ischemia, endothelial deposits, platelet plugs, cholesterol plaques, myofibril hypertrophy, and hyperglycemia-induced hypercoagulation.[13] The evidence that retinopathy is a consequence of excessive elevation of blood glucose levels and the sequelae of these elevations is consistent with a demonstrated inhibition of retinopathy by strict glycemic control in diabetic dogs.[14] Unfortunately, retinopathy in humans is not as easily studied. It is clear that the duration of diabetes is a strong risk factor for diabetic retinopathy. The Wisconsin Epidemiologic Study of Diabetic Retinopathy (WESDOR) found that the prevalence of retinopathy in patients with an onset of diabetes before age 30 was 17 percent after five years and up to 97.5 percent at greater than 15 years' duration.[15,16] The severity of retinopathy was related to the duration of diabetes, level of glycosylated hemoglobin, age at examination, presence of proteinuria, and higher diastolic blood pressure. Similar prevalence data have been reported in several other studies.[17-21] Although the WESDOR did not address pregnancy per se, they did find that the number of previous pregnancies did not affect retinopathy prevalence rates.

ROLE OF HYPERGLYCEMIA AS A CAUSE

Evidence directly indicating the importance of metabolic control has become available as a result of prospective studies of diabetes in human subjects.

Two randomized, prospective trials have recently been reported. The first was a study from Sweden in which 102 patients with insulin-dependent diabetes mellitus (IDDM), nonproliferative retinopathy, normal serum creatinine concentrations, and unsatisfactory blood glucose control were randomly assigned to intensified insulin treatment or standard insulin treatment.[22] They were then evaluated at 1.5, 3, 5, and 7.5 years. The two groups maintained a separation in their glycosylated hemoglobin levels of 1.4 percent (P = .001). Over the study period, the two groups had a significant difference in the prevalence of proliferative retinopathy requiring photocoagulation (27 percent versus 52 percent, P = .01). The second study confirmed the first study but had a sample size 10 times larger. The latter study, The Diabetes Control and Complications Trial was a National Institutes of Health-funded multicenter study that finally provided the definitive answer as to the relationship of retinopathy and glucose levels in nonpregnant people.[23] This trial recruited 1,441 type I, IDDM patients and randomized them into two groups of glycemic control. Those patients in the standard care group maintained a mean glycosylated hemoglobin of 9.0 percent, and those patients in the intensive care group maintained a mean glycosylated hemoglobin of 7.2 percent. The intensive care group had a 50 percent lower prevalence rate of new-onset retinopathy or progression of retinopathy compared with that in the standard case group.

RAPID NORMALIZATION OF GLUCOSE

Several studies have also shown dramatic reversal of diabetic retinopathy after only 2 to 3 months of insulin infusion pump therapy.[24-26] Although these studies are promising, other studies have implicated rapid normalization of blood glucose level as a causal factor in accelerating diabetic retinopathy.[23,27] This progression of retinopathy has been characterized mainly by the appearance of nerve fiber layer infarctions and intraretinal vascular lesions, which appear to be secondary to decreased blood flow.[28]

The effects of normalization of blood glucose levels on various stages of pre-existing diabetic retinopathy are unknown. The risk of returning an abnormal retinal circulation that has adapted to an elevated blood glucose level to an environment of normal blood glucose level is undetermined. The current methods of achieving tight control of glucose levels also result in episodes of hypoglycemia, the effects of which on pre-existing diabetic retinopathy are unknown. Hypoglycemia has been implicated as a causative factor in the development of vitreous hemorrhage in proliferative diabetic retinopathy,[29,30] but these cases are anecdotal.

Preliminary reports and our own experience suggest that retinopathy may continue to progress after the achievement of tight control of glucose levels. These reports are unable to determine whether the natural progression of the disease was unaffected or normalization of blood glucose levels actually adversely affected diabetic retinopathy. In our cases (presented later), the onset of visual symptoms appeared to be related to the achievement of good control of blood glucose levels.

Drash et al[31] reported on four children with Mauriac syndrome (marked hyperglycemia and growth retardation) who initially presented with minimal diabetic retinopathy. When the diabetes was controlled, the degree of retinopathy progressed rapidly in all four children, with the development of microaneurysms, hemorrhages, exudates, and macular edema. The three older children went on to develop proliferative retinopathy, and one patient became blind in one eye. This report, although distressing, may be related to the association of the onset of diabetic complications with the onset of puberty. All these patients were prepubertal when first seen and progressed through puberty during the period of diabetic control.

Tamborlane et al[32] reported equally disturbing vitreous hemorrhages in 2 of 10 patients, 1 within 3 months after the start of tight control of glucose levels. The ages of these 2 patients were not stated, and both started with proliferative retinopathy. Nevertheless, these two case studies have led at least one advocate of tight control of glucose levels to recommend that such control not be attempted in patients with a history of underinsulinization and severe retinopathy.[33]

In our own experience, two patients with well-documented control of blood glucose levels reported changes in vision shortly after the normalization of these levels.[34] However, our third patient with background retinopathy had macular edema that developed 2 weeks after acute normalization of her twice-normal glucose levels and resolved completely after 9 months of maintenance of normoglycemia with an insulin infusion pump.

These observations suggest that, as a prevention measure against retinopathy, normoglycemia may be the treatment goal for diabetic nonpregnant patients. In patients with predisposed retinae, acute normalization of blood glucose levels should be avoided. Instead, the process should proceed with caution. Once normoglycemia is achieved, however, its maintenance may be accompanied by improvement in the diseased retina.

The lessons to be learned from the studies of nonpregnant diabetic patients are as follows:

1. The duration of diabetes is closely associated with the presence of retinopathy[35]
2. Hyperglycemia, as documented by an elevated hemoglobin A_{1c} level, is associated with an increased risk of retinopathy[22,23]
3. The severity of retinopathy at the beginning of an observation period is thought to be significant in predicting subsequent changes in retinopathy[36]
4. Current age or age at the time of the examination has been found to be related to the severity of retinopathy[35]
5. Hormonal influence may potentiate retinopathy[37]
6. Hypertension potentiates retinopathy[38]
7. Rapid normalization of blood glucose may accelerate retinopathy[31,32]
8. Smoking accelerates retinopathy

We now turn to the diabetic pregnant woman and look for evidence of a "pregnancy risk factor" for diabetic retinopathy over and above those observations in nonpregnant populations.

DOES PREGNANCY CHANGE THE NATURAL HISTORY?

Peptide and steroid hormones have been implicated as accomplices in diabetic retinopathy for decades.[37,39] Regression of proliferative retinopathy in patients with pituitary infarctions has been reported.[38,39] This observation resulted in the use of hypophysectomy as a treatment for patients with proliferative retinopathy. Although the retinopathy did regress, the life span of these patients was shortened, perhaps secondary to the steroid doses needed to sustain viability. The hypothesis that growth hormone might be the primary villain was strengthened when Merimee et al[40] observed that ateliotic dwarfs, who are totally deficient in growth hormone, do not develop retinopathy, even with more than 15 years of documented hyperglycemia.

Pregnancy is associated with a marked elevation in placental lactogen, which has many growth hormone-like effects.[41] Because of this and elevations in other hormones that cause vascular changes, such as estrogen, progesterone, and cortisol, pregnancy may in fact accelerate retinopathy.

Hypertension has also been linked to the severity of retinopathy.[15,16,42–45] Studies in which antihypertensive agents have been used to slow the progression of diabetic nephropathy have also suggested that such therapy may retard the progression of retinopathy.[45,46] In our own study, in which we used a nonmydriatic camera to screen for diabetic retinopathy in the diabetic population in Santa Barbara County, we noted that those patients with evidence of retinopathy had significantly higher blood pressure than did those patients who had no evidence of retinopathy.[47] The relationship of hypertension to retinopathy may be particularly important during pregnancy because, in up to 20 percent of IDDM women, pregnancy-induced hypertension develops.[48] Rosenn et al[49] reported progression of retinopathy in 51 of 154 pregnancies among IDDM women. They found that hypertension, be it pregnancy-induced or pre-existing chronic hypertension, was the most important risk factor associated with progression of retinopathy in pregnancy. Using logistic regression analysis, these authors showed that the association of hypertension with the progression of retinopathy persisted after controlling for the effects of poor glycemic control and of rapid changes in glycemic control.

Investigators have reported differing findings regarding the effects of pregnancy per se on diabetic retinopathy. Many reports show that, for women with minimal or no retinopathy at the onset of pregnancy, although there may be minor progression, vision-threatening retinopathy generally does not occur. Of 234 pregnancies followed at the Rikshospitalet in Oslo, Norway, from 1970 to 1977, new incidence or progression of retinopathy during pregnancy was reported in 68 pregnancies.[50] Rodman et al[51] reported that 85 percent of patients with background retinopathy experienced progression during pregnancy. Soubrane et al[52] followed the course of diabetic retinopathy by repeated fluorescein angiography during pregnancy in 22 diabetic women. The mean number of microaneurysms increased consistently throughout pregnancy and decreased after pregnancy but not to the number encountered before pregnancy. Other observers have also reported that progression seemed to be accelerated during pregnancy.[53,54] By contrast, Stephens et al[55] found that, of 114 pregnancies in 78 diabetic women, retinopathy developed during only 2 pregnancies.

When a woman starts her pregnancy with more severe retinopathy, the likelihood that retinopathy will progress increases. Thus, the duration of diabetes is an independent risk factor for the progression of retinopathy in pregnancy. Dibble et al[18] reported that, in 3 of 19 patients with only background retinopathy, proliferative changes developed during pregnancy. Horvat et al[56] conducted a 12-year prospective study during which they surveyed 107 women with latent diabetes and 160 with clinical diabetes. In the latter group, background retinopathy was present or occurred during gestation in 40 women. Vision remained stable in all except 4 patients (10 percent) who progressed to pro-

liferative retinopathy. Only 1 woman had new vessels develop in one eye during pregnancy, whereas the other 3 had proliferative changes noted after completing their pregnancies. Eleven women had proliferative retinopathy with one case appearing de novo during pregnancy. These individuals had an average duration of diabetes of 21 years in contrast to 13.5 years for women with background retinopathy. In this study, retinopathy was noted to fluctuate during the index and subsequent pregnancies. Not infrequently, changes occurred in both directions at one time, with one part of the eye getting better while another part worsened. The authors concluded that pregnancy was not associated with an increased risk to the mother of retinal changes and visual loss.

Moloney and Drury[53] followed 53 pregnant patients with IDDM by retinal photography every 6 weeks and for 6 months postpartum. Thirty-three (62 percent) had retinopathy at first examination, and in eight others (15 percent), it developed as pregnancy advanced. They reported progressive changes as gestation progressed with a moderate increase in microaneurysms, hemorrhages in 30 (56.6 percent), and soft exudates in 15 (28.3 percent). Four women had neovascularization for the first time with further deterioration with advancing pregnancy. By 6 months after delivery, background changes had regressed to control levels, and neovascularization showed some regression. Again, development and progression of retinopathy were related to the duration of diabetes, and every pregnant patient who had diabetes for 10 years or longer had retinopathy. Increased doses of insulin and polyhydramnios were risk factors for retinal hemorrhage. Of interest, low fasting blood glucose levels (better control) late in pregnancy were associated significantly with soft exudates. Pregnancy had no visible effect in

Table 19-2. Progression of Diabetic Retinopathy in Pregnancy Stratified by Initial Retinal Findings

Author (Year)	No. of Pregnancies	No. (%) with Progression Given the Initial Findings		
		None	Background	Proliferative
Horvat et al[56] 1980	160	13/118 (11)	11/35 (31)	1/7 (14)
Moloney and Drury[53] 1982	53	8/20 (40)	15/30 (50)	1/3 (33)
Dibble et al[18] 1982	55	0/23 (0)	3/19 (16)	7/13 (54)
Ohrt[57] 1984	100	4/50 (8)	15/48 (31)	1/2 (50)
Rosenn et al[49] 1992	154	18/78 (23)	28/68 (41)	5/8 (63)

the retinae of patients who had diabetes for less than 2 years, but thereafter, it did accelerate the development of retinopathy. Also in conjunction with a strict metabolic control management protocol during pregnancy, the course of retinopathy changed with an increase in hemorrhages and soft exudates. These changes were of short duration and usually resolved within 6 weeks.[54]

Table 19-2 summarizes the above reports in which diabetic retinopathy was assessed before and after pregnancy and presents findings of progression based on the initial examination.[18,49,53,56,57] These studies clearly show that the severity of retinopathy at the onset of pregnancy is an independent risk factor for progression. When a woman had no retinopathy early in pregnancy, the risk of progression varied from 0 to 40 percent. When a woman had background retinopathy at the start of her pregnancy, her risk of progression increased to 16 to 50 percent; however, when a woman had proliferative retinopathy at the start of her pregnancy, her risk was as high as 63 percent.

PROSPECTIVE TRIALS IN PREGNANCY

Differences in the conclusions reported from some of these studies may have resulted from lack of objective recording and assessment of the retinal lesions and inappropriate comparison groups or none at all. Klein et al[58] reported on a prospective study to determine the effect of pregnancy on diabetic retinopathy. The control group for the IDDM (type I diabetes) pregnant women was composed of nonpregnant IDDM women. After adjusting for glycosylated hemoglobin, current pregnancy was significantly associated with progression ($P < .005$). Diastolic blood pressure had a lesser effect on the probability of progression. This group also reported that, when the duration of diabetes is controlled for in the analysis, parity is not a risk factor for retinopathy.

Price et al[59] found that the course of pregnancy is closely related to the severity of the eye disease at the start of the pregnancy. Those patients without retinopathy do not develop significant retinopathy and have relatively uncomplicated pregnancies. Those patients with retinopathy tended also to have progressive eye disease and obstetric complications. Of note, the infant outcome was satisfactory despite the high-risk pregnancies.

Larinkari et al[60] followed 40 consecutive pregnant IDDM women randomized at the end of the first trimester to receive conventional insulin treatment or constant subcutaneous insulin infusion (CSII). Nine women randomized to CSII declined the treatment. Two of eighteen women who were receiving conventional treatment had some deterioration of retinopathy compared with 5 of 13 in the CSII group and 3 of 9 who declined pump treatment. In most women, retinal deterioration was mild, but two patients who received CSII developed acute ischemic retinopathy, which progressed to a proliferative stage despite laser treatment. The decrease in hemoglobin A_{1c} level in these two patients was among the greatest and fastest in the study. These findings are analogous to those mentioned earlier in this chapter in poorly controlled nonpregnant patients after the institution of tight glucose control.

Serup[61] described the influence of pregnancy on diabetic retinopathy in a prospective study in Copenhagen initiated in 1979. In this protocol, three ophthalmologic examinations were performed during pregnancy and three in the year after delivery. Of the 145 women enrolled in the study, about one-half of the patients with retinopathy had deterioration during pregnancy. All improved to some extent after delivery. In a few women with background retinopathy at the onset of pregnancy, proliferative retinopathy developed, which commonly disappeared during the early postpartum period. No severe changes with respect to vitreous hemorrhages or severe proliferative changes occurred. In only one case was postpartum photocoagulation necessary to arrest retinal proliferative changes at the optic disc. Thus, Serup[61] agrees with Moloney and Drury[53] that pregnancy may interfere with the spontaneous course of diabetic retinopathy, resulting in a deterioration during pregnancy followed by some regression after delivery. Complete remission of retinopathy was noted in women who did not have it at conception but in whom it developed during gestation. These findings led to the conclusion that treatment with photocoagulation during pregnancy and in the 8 to 12 months after delivery should be restricted. This is in contrast to the approach of others who advise treatment before, during, and after pregnancy for proliferative retinopathy.[62]

Phelps et al[63] noted that, in pregnancies managed

by intensive therapy to normalize the blood glucose level, 55 percent of retinal abnormalities worsened. Deterioration of background retinopathy correlated significantly with the levels of plasma glucose at entry and with the improvement in glycemia achieved. They concluded that the abrupt institution of improved diabetic control during pregnancy may be one factor in the deterioration of background retinopathy of pregnancy.

In a preliminary report of the Diabetes in Early Pregnancy Study Group, the eyes of 18 pregnant type I diabetic women were photographed in the first and third trimesters of pregnancy to evaluate the effect of normoglycemia on retinopathy.[64] The mean duration of diabetes was 18 years. All women achieved normoglycemia within 1 month of conception and maintained normoglycemia to term. Retinopathy was photo-graphically documented monthly with seven standard stereoscopic fields. In 21 of 36 eyes (58.3 percent), the level of retinopathy increased. Of 12 patients who had hemoglobin A_1 levels lower than 7.0 percent (normal <7.0 percent), 8 increased at least one level in one or both eyes (66.7 percent). Renal disease (50 percent depression of the creatinine clearance rate and proteinuria greater than 150 mg/24 h) appeared to be associated with progression to more severe levels of retinopathy. Eight of nine patients who had cystoid macular edema had proteinuria greater than 1.0 g/24 h. Photocoagulation therapy prevented loss of ambulatory vision. A report of the entire study population of diabetic women in the Diabetes in Early Pregnancy Study Group[65] showed that patients with mild or more severe retinopathy at conception were at high risk of progression of retinopathy during pregnancy. The

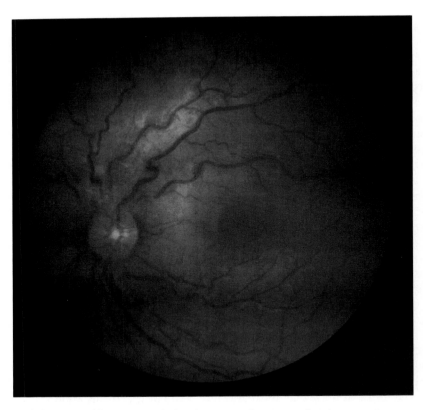

Fig. 19-4. Retina of a 35-year-old woman with the diagnosis of gestational diabetes mellitus. Note the corkscrew development of the smaller retinal vessels. Tortuosity of the retinal vessels does not necessarily infer any form of retinopathy. It may actually be a genetic marker for glucose intolerance in some persons.

rates of progression from nonproliferative retinopathy to proliferative retinopathy were 6.76 percent and 30 percent in patients whose baseline retinopathy levels were mild and moderate, respectively. Elevated glycosylated hemoglobin levels at entry above six standard deviations above the mean of a normal pregnant population were associated with a statistically significant increased risk of progression. Among women with the highest initial glycosylated hemoglobin concentrations, those who improved the most in metabolic control during early pregnancy were the most likely to progress ($P = .03$).[65] In the Diabetes in Early Pregnancy study, as in the study by Phelps, et al[63] rapid normalization of blood glucose may have been a major independent variable in the progression of retinopathy.

Although gestational diabetic women do not have a risk of diabetic retinopathy during the index preg-

nancy because of the recent onset of their hyperglycemia, 50 percent of these women have marked tortuosity of their retinal vessels[66] (Fig. 19-4). This tortuosity is not a result of the pregnancy because it did not regress up to 1 year postpartum. It is hypothesized that retinal vessel tortuosity may be a marker for those women in whom type II (non-insulin-dependent) diabetes will develop because 50 percent of women with gestational diabetes go on to have frank diabetes as they age.[67–69] Further reports are necessary to confirm this hypothesis.

WHEN TO TREAT PREGNANT WOMEN

A retina that has been treated with photocoagulation therapy for proliferative diabetic retinopathy is shown in Figure 19-5. There are no randomized trials of preg-

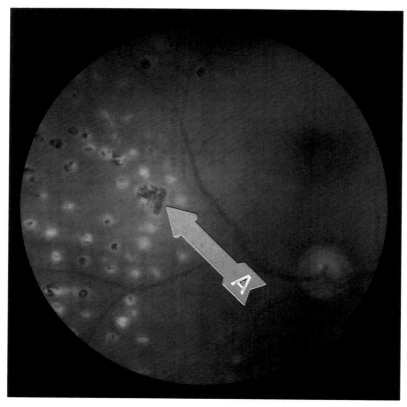

Fig. 19-5. This woman received photocoagulation or laser therapy for neovascularization of her retinal vessels. Laser treatment appears on the photograph as dark and light spots (arrow A on the retina).

nant women with retinopathy in which photocoagulation therapy has been the study variable. We can only learn from the trials reported in nonpregnant patients.[70] The Diabetic Retinopathy Study recommended photocoagulation therapy for significant neovascularization of the optic nerve head and in those patients with any neovascularization in the presence of vitreous hemorrhage. The controversy about photocoagulation therapy during pregnancy concerns the known observations that retinopathy regresses postpartum and thus photocoagulation therapy may not be necessary.[62] Most centers treat significant neovascularization rather than risk a retinal hemorrhage. The definitive study remains to be presented.

SUMMARY

This review of retinopathy in pregnant and nonpregnant patients provides the rationale for identifying the following risk factors that accelerate the natural progression of retinopathy during pregnancy.

1. Pregnancy per se is an independent risk factor that accelerates retinopathy
2. Hypertension potentiates this acceleration
3. Hyperglycemia at the start of pregnancy also potentiates this acceleration
4. Rapid normalization of blood glucose markedly accelerates the progression of retinopathy
5. The duration of diabetes and state of the retina at the beginning of the pregnancy influence the rate of acceleration

Prudent therapy suggests that treatment in pregnancy should be planned to allow normalization of blood glucose slowly, bringing the glycosylated hemoglobin to less than six standard deviations above the mean of a normal population over a period of at least 6 to 9 months before conception.[71] In addition, while awaiting clinical trials, photocoagulation treatment for proliferative retinopathy that presents during pregnancy would appear prudent, according to the recommendations of the Diabetic Retinopathy Study Group,[70] despite the possibility that retinopathy may regress spontaneously postpartum.

REFERENCES

1. Jovanovic L, Peterson CM: Optimal insulin delivery for the pregnant diabetic patient. Diabetes Care, suppl. 1, 5: 24, 1982
2. Coustan DR: Management of the pregnant diabetic. p. 311. In Olefsky JM, Sherwin RS (eds): Diabetes Mellitus: Management and Complications. Churchill Livingstone, New York, 1985
3. Karlsson K, Kjellmer I: The outcome of diabetic pregnancies in relation to the mother's blood sugar level. Am J Obstet Gynecol 112:213, 1972
4. Jovanovic L, Druzin M, Peterson CM: Effect of euglycemia on the outcome of pregnancy in insulin-dependent diabetic women as compared with normal control subjects. Am J Med 71:921, 1981
5. White P: Pregnancy and diabetes, medical aspects. Med Clin North Am 49:1015, 1965
6. Cassar J, Kohner EM, Hamilton AM et al: Diabetic retinopathy and pregnancy. Diabetologia 15:105, 1978
7. Hare JW, White P: Pregnancy in diabetes complicated by vascular disease. Diabetes 26:953, 1977
8. Sharma WK, Archer DB, Hadden DR et al: Morbidity and mortality in patients with diabetic retinopathy. Trans Ophthalmol Soc UK 100:83, 1980
9. Carstensen LL, Frost-Larsen K, Fuglebjerg S, Nerup J: Does pregnancy influence the prognosis of uncomplicated insulin-dependent juvenile-onset diabetes mellitus? Diabetes Care 5:1, 1982
10. Palmberg P, Smith M, Waltman S et al: The natural history of retinopathy in insulin-dependent juvenile-onset diabetes. Ophthalmology 88:613, 1981
11. Early Treatment Diabetic Retinopathy Study Research Group: Manual of Operations, Early Treatment Diabetic Retinopathy Study, 5-1–5-10. Maryland Medical Research Institute, Baltimore, 1985
12. Early Treatment Diabetic Retinopathy Study Resarch Group: Grading diabetic retinopathy from stereoscopic color fundus photographs: an extension of the modified Airlie House classification. ETDRS report number 10. Ophthalmology 98:786, 1991
13. Bresnick GH, Davis MD, Myers FL, deVenecia G: Clinicopathologic correlations in diabetic retinopathy. II. Clinical and histologic appearance of retinal capillary microaneurysms. Arch Ophthalmol 95:1215, 1977
14. Engerman RL: Animal models of diabetic retinopathy. Trans Am Acad Ophthalmol Otolaryngol 81:710, 1976
15. Klein R, Klein BEK, Moss S et al: The Wisconsin Epidemiologic Study of Diabetic Retinopathy. III. Prevalence and risk of diabetic retinopathy when the age at diagnosis is less than thirty years. Arch Ophthalmol 102:520, 1984

16. Klein R, Klein BEK, Moss S et al: The Wisconsin Epidemiologic Study of Diabetic Retinopathy. III. Prevalence and risk of diabetic retinopathy when the age at diagnosis is greater than thirty years. Arch Ophthalmol 102:527, 1984

17. Job D, Eschwege E, Guyot-Argenton C et al: Effect of multiple daily insulin injections on the course of diabetic retinopathy. Diabetes 25:463, 1976

18. Dibble CM, Kochenour NK, Worley RJ et al: Effect of pregnancy on diabetic retinopathy. Obstet Gynecol 59:699, 1982

19. Pirart J: Diabète et complications dégénératives. Présentation d'une étude prospective portant sur 4400 cas observés entre 1947 et 1973. Diabete Metab 3:97, 1977

20. Cunha-Vaz JG, Fonseca JR, Faria De Abreu JR, Ruas MA: Detection of early retinal changes in diabetes by vitreous fluorophotometry. Diabetes 28:16, 1979

21. Waltman SR, Oestrick C, Krupin T et al: Quantitative vitreous fluorophotometry: a sensitive technique for measuring early breakdown of the blood retinal barrier in young diabetic patients. Diabetes 27:85, 1978

22. Reichard P, Nilsson B-Y, Rosenqvist U: The effect of long-term intensified treatment on the development of microvascular complications of diabetes mellitus. N Engl J Med 329:304, 1993

23. The Diabetes Control and Complications Trial Research Group (DCCT): The effect of intensive treatment of diabetes on the development and progression of long-term complications in insulin-dependent diabetes mellitus. N Engl J Med 29:977, 1993

24. Lawson PM, Champion MC, Canny C et al: Continuous subcutaneous insulin infusion (CSII) does not prevent progression of proliferative and preproliferative retinopathy. Br J Ophthalmol 66:762, 1982

25. Irsigler K, Kritz H, Najemnik C: Reversal of florid diabetic retinopathy. Lancet 2:1068, 1979

26. Kohner EM: The effect of diabetes on retino-vascular function. Acta Diabetol, suppl. 1, 8:135, 1971

27. Van Ballegooie E, Hooymans JMM, Timmerman Z et al: Rapid deterioration of diabetic retinopathy during treatments with continuous subcutaneous insulin infusion. Diabetes Care 7:236, 1984

28. Brinchmann-Hansen O, Dahl-Jorgensen K, Hanssen KF et al: Effects of intensified insulin treatment on various lesions of diabetic retinopathy. Am J Ophthalmol 100:644, 1985

29. Murata M, Yoshimoto H: Morphological study of the pathogenesis of retinal cottonwool spot. Jpn J Ophthalmol 27:362, 1983

30. Tasman W: Diabetic vitreous hemorrhage and its relationship to hypoglycemia. Mod Probl Ophthalmol 20:413, 1979

31. Drash AL, Daneman D, Travis L: Progressive retinopathy with improved metabolic control in diabetic dwarfism (Mauriac's syndrome). Diabetes, suppl. 2, 29:1A, 1980

32. Tamborlane WV, Puklin JE, Bergman M et al: Long-term improvement of metabolic control with the insulin pump does not reverse diabetic microangiopathy. Diabetes Care, suppl. 1, 5:58, 1982

33. Engerman RL: Perspectives in diabetes: pathogenesis of diabetic retinopathy. Diabetes 38:1203, 1989

34. Jovanovic-Peterson L, Peterson CM. Diabetic retinopathy. Clin Obstet Gynecol 34:516, 1991

35. Klein R, Klein BEK, Moss SE et al: Retinopathy in young-onset diabetic patients. Diabetes Care 8:311, 1985

36. Groop LC, Teir S, Koskimies PH et al: Risk factors and markers associated with proliferative retinopathy in patients with insulin-dependent diabetes. Diabetes 35:1397, 1986

37. Barnes AJ, Kohner EM, Johnston DG, Alberti KGMM: Severe retinopathy and mild carbohydrate intolerance: possible role of insulin deficiency and elevated circulating growth hormone. Lancet 1:1465, 1985

38. Rand LI, Krolewski AS, Aiello LM et al: Multiple factors in the prediction of risk of diabetic retinopathy. N Engl J Med 313:1433, 1985

39. Larinkari J, Laatikainen L, Ranta T: Metabolic control and serum hormone levels in relationship to retinopathy in diabetic pregnancy. Diabetologia 22:327, 1982

40. Merimee TJ, Zapf J, Froesch ER: Insulin-like growth factors: studies in diabetics with and without retinopathy. N Engl J Med 309:527, 1983

41. Peterson LP, Kundu N: Endocrine assessment of high-risk pregnancies. Obstet Gynecol Ann 9:169, 1980

42. Kostraba JN, Klein R, Dorman JS et al: The epidemiology of Diabetes Complications Study IV. Correlates of diabetic background and proliferative retinopathy. Am J Epidemiol 133:381, 1991

43. Janka HU, Warram JH, Rand LJ, Krowlewski AS: Risk factors for progression of background retinopathy in long-standing IDDM. Diabetes 38:460, 1989

44. Chase HP, Garg SK, Jackson WE et al: Blood pressure and retinopathy in type I diabetes. Ophthalmology 97:155, 1990

45. Norgaard K, Feldt-Rasmussen B, Deckert T: Is hypertension a major independent risk factor for retinopathy in type I diabetes? Diabetic Med 8:334, 1991

46. Jackson WE, Holmes DL, Garg SK et al: Angiotensin-converting enzyme inhibitor therapy and diabetic retinopathy. Ann Ophthalmol 24:99, 1992

47. Lewis JM, Jovanovic-Peterson L, Ahmadizadeh I et al: The Santa Barbara County Diabetic Screening Feasibility Study: significance of diabetes duration and systolic blood pressure. J Diabet Complications 8:51, 1994

48. Cousins L: Pregnancy complications among diabetic women: review 1965–1985. Obstet Gynecol Surv 42:140, 1987

49. Rosenn B, Miodovnik M, Kranias et al: Progression of diabetic retinopathy in pregnancy: association with hypertension in pregnancy. Am J Obstet Gynecol 166:1214, 1992

50. Jervell J, Moe N, Skjaeraasen J et al: Diabetes mellitus and pregnancy: management and results at Rikshospitalet, Oslo, 1970–1977. Diabetologia 16:151, 1979

51. Rodman HM, Singerman LJ, Aiello LM: Diabetic retinopathy: effects of pregnancy and laser therapy, abstracted. Diabetes 29:1A, 1980

52. Soubrane G, Canivet J, Coscas G: Influence of pregnancy on the evolution of background retinopathy. Int Ophthalmol Clin 8:249, 1985

53. Moloney JBM, Drury IM: The effect of pregnancy on the natural course of diabetic retinopathy. Am J Ophthalmol 93:745, 1982

54. Rodman HM, Singerman LJ, Aiello LM, Merkatz IR: Diabetic retinopathy and its relationship to pregnancy. p. 321. In Merkatz ER, Adams PAJ (eds): The Diabetic Pregnancy: A Perinatal Perspective. Grune & Stratton, Orlando, FL, 1979

55. Stephens JW, Page OC, Hare RL: Diabetes and pregnancy: a report of experiences in 119 pregnancies over a period of ten years. Diabetes 12:213, 1963

56. Horvat M, Maclean H, Goldberg L, Crock GW: Diabetic retinopathy in pregnancy: a 12-year prospective survey. Br J Ophthalmol 64:398, 1980

57. Ohrt V: The influence of pregnancy on diabetic retinopathy. Acta Endocrinol (Copenh), suppl. 277, 112:122, 1986

58. Klein BEK, Moss SE, Klein R: Effect of pregnancy on progression of diabetic retinopathy. Diabetes Care 13:34, 1990

59. Price JH, Hadden DR, Archer DB, Harley DG: Diabetic retinopathy in pregnancy. Br J Obstet Gynaecol 91:11, 1984

60. Larinkari J, Laatikainen L, Ranta T et al: Metabolic control and serum hormone levels in relationship to retinopathy in diabetic pregnancy. Diabetologia 22:327, 1982

61. Serup L: Influence of pregnancy on diabetic retinopathy. Acta Endocrinol (Copenh), suppl. 277, 112:122, 1986

62. Klein BEK: Diabetic Retinopathy During Pregnancy, p. 77. In Jovanovic L (ed): Controversies in the Field of Pregnancy and Diabetes. Springer-Verlag, New York, 1988

63. Phelps RL, Sakol P, Metzger BE et al: Changes in diabetic retinopathy during pregnancy: correlations with regulation of hyperglycemia. Arch Ophthalmol 104:1806, 1986

64. Chang S, Fuhrmann M, Jovanovic L: The Diabetes in Early Pregnancy Study Group (DIEP): pregnancy, retinopathy, normoglycemia: a preliminary analysis. Diabetes, suppl., 35:3A, 1986

65. The Diabetes in Early Pregnancy Study Group: Metabolic control and progression of retinopathy, abstracted. Presented at the National American Diabetes Association Meeting, New Orleans, LA, June 11, 1994.

66. Boone MI, Farber ME, Jovanovic-Peterson L, Peterson CM. Increased retinal vascular tortuosity in gestational diabetes mellitus. Ophthalmology 96:251, 1989

67. Mestman JH: Follow-up studies in women with gestational diabetes mellitus. p. 191. In Weiss PAM, Coustan DR (eds): Gestational Diabetes. Springer-Verlag, New York, 1988

68. O'Sullivan JB: Subsequent morbidity among gestational diabetic women. p. 174. In Sutherland HW, Stowers JM (eds): Carbohydrate Metabolism in Pregnancy and the Newborn: Incorporating the Proceedings of the International Colloquium at Aberdeen, Scotland. Churchill Livingstone, Edinburgh, 1984

69. Stowers JM, Sutherland HW, Kerridge DF: Long-range implications for the mother: the Aberdeen experience. Diabetes, suppl. 2, 34:106, 1985

70. The Diabetic Retinopathy Study Research Group: Photocoagulation treatment of proliferative diabetic retinopathy: the second report of Diabetic Retinopathy Study findings. Ophthalmology 85:82, 1978

71. Laatikainen L, Teromo K, Hieta-Heikurainen et al: A controlled study of the influence of continuous subcutaneous insulin infusion treatment on diabetic retinopathy during pregnancy. J Intern Med 221:367, 1987

20
Diabetic Nephropathy

JOHN L. KITZMILLER
C. ANDREW COMBS

Diabetic nephropathy, with its link to cardiovascular disease, is the major cause of deaths related to diabetes mellitus and is also the most important complication of diabetes that affects the outcome of pregnancy. Perinatal problems associated with diabetic nephropathy include congenital malformations, fetal growth retardation, stillbirth, and preterm delivery with associated neonatal disorders. Maternal hazards consist of possible renal failure during or after pregnancy, superimposed pre-eclampsia, the frequent association of nephropathy with proliferative retinopathy and macular edema, and the risk of eventual morbidity or death from macrovascular disease. Despite the possible complications, such women and their mates frequently desire to have a child. Optimal outcomes for mothers and babies are produced when a multidisciplinary approach is used at a perinatal center with perinatologists, nephrologists, diabetologists, and neonatologists interacting effectively. Patient care must be supported by diabetes educators, dietitians, medical social workers, and obstetric nurses who specialize in high-risk pregnancy. With such an approach, perinatal outcome has improved dramatically for women with diabetic nephropathy, but concerns persist about preservation of maternal health.

There are many unanswered questions regarding diabetic nephropathy and pregnancy. To consider them, we must have an understanding of the background of the natural history and pathogenesis of this disorder. There has been an acceleration of information and hypotheses about diabetic nephropathy in the 1980s and 1990s. There are new data on structure-function relationships in the kidneys,[1-3] on the possible damaging role of hyperfiltration early in the course of diabetes,[4] on the identification of incipient nephropathy as microalbuminuria,[5,6] and on interacting biochemical pathways that link hyperglycemia to changes in the kidneys.[7]

Obstetric physicians who care for women with diabetic nephropathy often view the pregnancy as such an important time that the perspective of the natural or remedied course of diabetic nephropathy may be lost. Optimal long-term maternal and child health occurs when health care providers consider the full continuum of the stages of living with diabetes proceeding through the childbearing years. The effectiveness of medical therapy in the years before pregnancy strongly influences the degree of complications noted during gestation. By contrast, the rationale and goals of treatment during pregnancy must include effects on long-term maternal health as well as short-term perinatal outcome.

DEFINITION AND EPIDEMIOLOGY

Overt clinical diabetic nephropathy in insulin-dependent diabetes mellitus, type I diabetes (IDDM) is characterized by persistent proteinuria (>0.5 g/24 h *total protein* excretion, or >200 µg/min or >300 mg/24 h urinary *albumin* excretion [UAE]), hypertension, declining glomerular filtration rate (approximately 12 ml/min/y), and eventual end-stage renal failure with uremia.[8,9] Diabetic nephropathy is the leading cause of end-stage renal disease (ESRD) in Western nations.[10] Renal failure is a leading cause of death for diabetic adults of all ages, but proteinuria also predicts at least

315

a 10-fold increased mortality rate from macrovascular disease, especially myocardial infarction and congestive heart failure, in both IDDM and non-insulin-dependent mellitus, type II diabetes (NIDDM).[11–15] Because of the high morbidity and mortality rates, research has focused on early changes in renal function and structure that could predict advanced diabetic nephropathy and identify subjects for treatment to prevent it.[9] The concept of *incipient* diabetic nephropathy is defined by repetitive subclinical increases in urinary excretion of albumin, known as microalbuminuria (two of three samples of 20 to 200 μg/min or 30 to 300 mg/24 h),[5,8] although a subset of patients with IDDM and NIDDM may show a decline in renal function without significant increases in the excretion of albumin.[16]

The prevalence of microalbuminuria in IDDM of more than 10 years' duration has been reported to be 15 to 30 percent[6] and is highest with (1) poor glycemic control marked by even modestly elevated glycohemoglobin,[17,18] (2) hypertension,[19–21] (3) elevated low-density lipoprotein-cholesterol,[21] and (4) smoking.[22] Of new cases of IDDM, 7 to 10 percent develop microalbuminuria within 5 years.[19,21,23] Studies conducted before widespread use of glycohemoglobin and self-monitoring of blood glucose indicated that the disease in 85 percent of women with microalbuminuria progressed to diabetic nephropathy.[24–27] However, in a clinical setting devoted to strict metabolic control in 1985 to 1991, only 31 percent of 79 patients with persistent microalbuminuria had diabetic nephropathy after 5 years of follow-up, compared with 2 percent of normoalbuminuric patients.[23] Progression was associated with higher glycohemoglobin and blood pressure levels. The authors concluded that calculation of the annual increase in UAE (microalbuminuria progression rate of >5%/y) was a more specific method of identifying patients in whom diabetic nephropathy will develop.[23]

Ongoing changes in diabetes management seem to be yielding a declining incidence of nephropathy in IDDM. Until recently, macroproteinuria developed gradually over 20 to 30 years of diabetes in 30 to 50 percent of women, and approximately 60 percent of cases progressed to renal failure by 10 years of clinical proteinuria.[9,28] The annual incidence of new cases of diabetic nephropathy was 3 percent according to Andersen et al.[29] More recent data show an incidence of 0.5 percent at 12 years' duration of IDDM, rising to 2.0 percent at 16 years.[30] The incidence peaks at 15 to 18 years of diabetes and is highest in women with diabetes diagnosed before age 20[30] or in the age interval of 25 to 35 years,[31] demonstrating the relevance to childbearing. For cases of IDDM diagnosed in the 1960s in Scandinavia, and thus exposed to modern diabetes management, the cumulative incidence of diabetic nephropathy was 9 to 16 percent at a 20-year duration of diabetes.[30,32]

For women with NIDDM, the prevalence of microalbuminuria is approximately 26 to 30 percent after 10 years of diabetes,[33] and in 6 to 15 percent, diabetic nephropathy develops after 10 to 20 years.[33,34] For this group, the cumulative incidence of renal failure is approximately 11 percent,[35] lower than in IDDM, but in NIDDM, the prevalence of coronary artery disease is 20 percent with microalbuminuria and 40 to 50 percent with macroproteinuria (duration diabetes 5 to 8 years).[33]

Because 50 to 70 percent of cases of IDDM never develop diabetic nephropathy in spite of decades of diabetes, research has focused on factors that influence the susceptibility to nephropathy. Substantially more diabetic nephropathy is found in diabetic siblings of patients with this disorder than in diabetic controls,[36] and this could indicate genetic predisposition, such as differences in the angiotensin-converting enzyme (ACE) gene,[37] or familial clustering of other influences, such as poor glycemic control, hyperlipidemia, or hypertension.[36] The concept that a parental history of hypertension[38,39] or increased sodium-lithium countertransport in erythrocytes[39,40] predisposes to diabetic nephropathy remains controversial.[41–43] Hypertension may be concurrent with[20] or follow the onset of microalbuminuria.[19] Sodium-lithium countertransport activity can be associated with an elevated lipid profile.[21] The Steno hypothesis states that diabetic nephropathy reflects widespread vascular damage and thus represents genetic susceptibility to the deleterious effects of hyperglycemia.[44] Deckert et al.[6] expanded the concept to include possible common genetic susceptibility factors for both diabetic nephropathy and macrovascular disease (premature atherosclerosis) and explored the complex possible common pathogenesis of albuminuria and atherosclerosis.

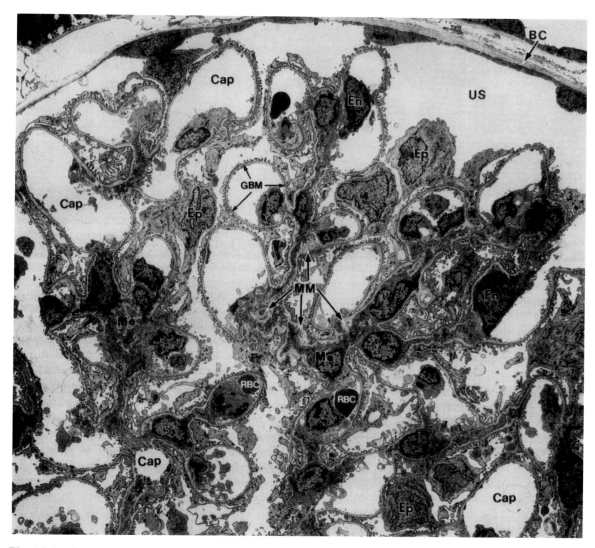

Fig. 20-1. Electron micrograph of the glomerulus, consisting of three cell types (visceral epithelial [Ep], endothelial [En], and mesangial [Me]), and glomerular extracellular matrices (glomerular basement membrane [GBM] and mesangial matrix [MM]). The parietal epithelium lines Bowman's capsule (BC). US, urinary space; RBC, red blood cell. (Original magnification × 2,500.) (From Kanwar et al,[45] with permission.)

RENAL STRUCTURE/FUNCTION RELATIONSHIPS

This discussion of the microanatomy of the glomerulus is taken mainly from the excellent review by Kanwar et al.[45] The main glomerular tuft is a network of capillaries made up of three cell types: epithelial podocytes, endothelium, and mesangium (Fig. 20-1). The visceral epithelium lies in the urinary or Bowman's space that covers the outer aspect of the glomerular basement membrane (GBM), and the podocyte foot processes are anchored on to the GBM. Podocytes and foot processes are covered by a thick glycocalyx made up of negatively charged sialoglycoproteins and heparan sulfate proteoglycans (HS-PG) and other sugar residues and proteins. Slit diaphragms intervene between the

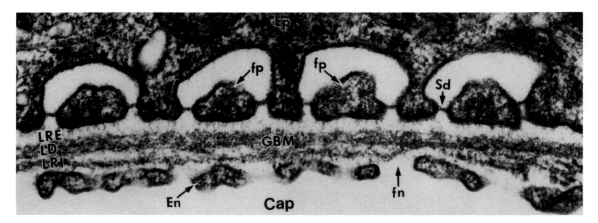

Fig. 20-2. Electron micrograph of the ultrafiltration unit. Note epithelial foot processes [fp] of epithelial cell [Ep] with intervening slit diaphragms [Sd], GBM, and fenestrated [fn] endothelium [En]. The GBM consists of lamina densa [LD] and lamina rarae interna [LRI] and externa [LRE]. (Original magnification × 50,000.) (From Kanwar et al,[45] with permission.)

foot processes (Fig. 20-2). The attenuated and fenestrated cytoplasm of the endothelial cells invests the GBM from the inside. The coat of the endothelium is thin and contains neuraminic acid residues and other glycoproteins, including negatively charged proteoglycans. The sialoglycoproteins and HS-PG impart electronegativity to the capillary surface, preventing adsorption of plasma proteins and blood cells. Mesangial cells are in the stalk of the glomerular tuft (intercapillary regions) (Fig. 20-1) and produce extracellular mesangial matrix. Mesangial cells phagocytose particulate matter in the glomerular circulation and have contractile properties in response to angiotensin II, which may help regulate intraglomerular hemodynamics. Various antigens and bioactive receptors are demonstrated in the mesangial cells.

A complex network of two types of extracellular matrix (ECM) supports the glomerular cells, GBM, and mesangial matrix (Figs. 20-1 and 20-2). The GBM lies between the epithelial and endothelial cells of the peripheral capillary loops, whereas the central mesangial matrix forms the stalk region of the glomerulus in which mesangial cells are embedded. The GBM is an amorphous scaffold with a central dense region made up mostly of type IV collagen, with loosely interwoven fibrils of collagen and HS-PG on either side.[45] The sulfate radicals hold water in between the polysaccharide chains of the proteoglycans and maintain the GBM as

a hydrated gel matrix, which contributes to a constant solute flow across the gel membrane. Both extracellular matrices are made up of many glycoproteins synthesized by glomerular cells; laminin, collagen IV, and HS-PG are of special importance in diabetes. The mesangial matrix has a higher turnover rate compared with the GBM, which may benefit the clearance of large numbers of adsorbed macromolecules. The turnover rates of various glycoproteins also differ, with HS-PG far exceeding that of type IV collagen, which probably contributes to ultrafiltration because circulating cations bind to anionic sulfate radicals. The matrix glycoproteins self-aggregate and interact with one another by specific binding domains, forming a complex normal or pathologic macromolecular structure (Fig. 20-3).

The kidneys receive approximately 20 percent of the cardiac output and approximately 20 percent of the plasma is ultrafiltered into Bowman's space, with most of the filtrate reabsorbed by the tubules. The glomerular filtration rate (GFR) depends on (1) the huge glomerular capillary filtering surface, (2) the relatively high hydrostatic pressure gradient across glomerular capillary walls related to relaxed preglomerular arterioles and constricted postglomerular arterioles, and (3) the greater permeability of the glomerular capillary wall than other capillaries in the body.[46] As Kanwar et al[45] noted, the formation of the ultrafiltrate "is heavily

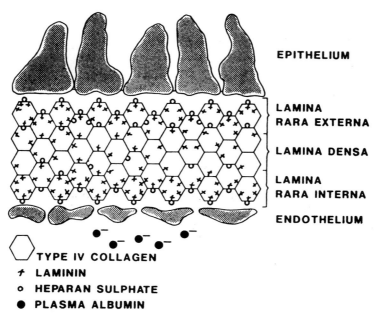

EPITHELIUM

LAMINA RARA EXTERNA

LAMINA DENSA

LAMINA RARA INTERNA

ENDOTHELIUM

⬡ TYPE IV COLLAGEN
⨏ LAMININ
○ HEPARAN SULPHATE
● PLASMA ALBUMIN

Fig. 20-3. Extracellular matrix glycoproteins and the structure of the glomerular basement membrane. Heparan sulfate-proteoglycan (HSPG) and plasma albumin are negatively charged. (From Deckert et al,[6] with permission.)

influenced by the integral interplay between the various cell types of the glomerulus and its extracellular matrices, which are responsive in turn to hormonal and hemodynamic fluctuations. . . . The structural integrity of the cellular and extracellular components and the delicate interplay between them are essential" in maintaining normal glomerular function.

A variety of renal lesions have been described in patients with diabetes. Diffuse glomerulosclerosis is the most common, present in about 75 percent of patients with diabetic nephropathy.[47] In this lesion, there is periodic acid-Schiff-positive material in the capillary walls and mesangium. The capillary basement membrane is usually thickened, mesangial cells and substance are increased, and mesangial cells may eventually be replaced by matrix.[48] Formation of nodules in the matrix, the nodular glomerulosclerosis described by Kimmelstiel and Wilson,[49] is found in about one-half of diabetic patients with macroproteinuria.[47] The nodules usually are found at the periphery of the glomerulus and are made up of hyaline material deposited on the inner aspects of the capillary loops. As the glomerulosclerotic lesions progress, capillary lumina are obliterated, and there is a balance between oc-cluded, hyalinized glomeruli and open glomeruli with marked mesangial expansion.[50] The lesions of diabetic nephropathy include hyalinization of arterioles and interstitial fibrosis.[47] Various exudative lesions have also been described in diabetic nephropathy, but their functional meanings are obscure.

CLINICAL COURSE

Investigators of diabetic renal disease have tried to correlate the structural changes with parameters of renal function in assessing the course of diabetic nephropathy.[1–3,50] These studies of renal function and structure carried out in subjects with diabetes of short to longer duration now allow us to differentiate early and advanced stages of the development of diabetic nephropathy. The five stages originally described by Mogensen are well accepted[9,51,52]: (1) early hypertrophy-hyperfunction; (2) early glomerular lesions without albuminuria; (3) incipient nephropathy characterized by microalbuminuria; (4) overt clinical nephropathy characterized by macroproteinuria, declining glomerular filtration, and hypertension; and (5) end-stage diabetic renal disease with uremia[9] (Table 20-1). Mogensen's diagram of the progression of changes in renal function in IDDM is reproduced in Figure 20-4.

Stage 1

At the time of the diagnosis of diabetes, there is increased kidney size and glomerular volume and generalized hyperfiltration marked by GFR greater than 150 ml/min.[4,53] This is accompanied by glomerular hypertrophy with an enlarged capillary surface area and presumed increased intraglomerular pressure.[9,54,55] At this early stage of diabetes, there is no abnormal proteinuria in the resting state, but exercise produces a fivefold increase in the rate of urinary excretion of albumin.[56,57] In this first stage, the GBM and mesangial thicknesses are not greater than those in controls.[58] Improved glycemic control with insulin treatment reverses the elevation in GFR and the exercise-induced proteinuria.[56,57]

Stage 2

Over the next 3 to 7 years of diabetes,[52] at least in patients with imperfect control of hyperglycemia, there is a persistent 20 to 30 percent increase in GFR, greater than the expansion in extracellular fluid volume, so that there is a real renal hyperfunction.[59] Renal plasma

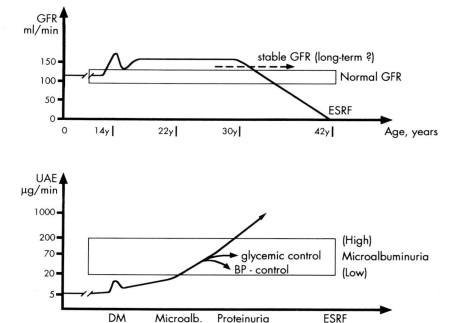

Diabetic nephropathy
Intervention in microalbuminuria

Fig. 20-4. Urinary albumin excretion rate (UAE), and glomerular filtration rate (GFR), in the course of diabetes. Usually, blood pressure starts to increase in insulin-dependent diabetes mellitus (IDDM) after an increase in UAE, indicating incipient diabetic nephropathy (microalbuminuria). When UAE reaches 70 µg/min (101 mg/24 h), GFR starts to decline. Overt diabetic nephropathy is characterized by proteinuria and often by large increases in blood pressure (BP) and further linear decline in GFR. The figure also shows that microalbuminuria and GFR can be stabilized by antihypertensive treatment (AHT) and excellent metabolic control (and possibly by a low protein diet). ESRF, end-stage renal failure. (Modified from Mogensen,[51] with permission.)

Table 20-1. Stages in Renal Involvement in Insulin-Dependent Diabetes Mellitus

Stage and Time Sequence	Designation	Main Characteristics	Main Structural Changes	GFR (ml/min)	Albumin Excretion (mg/24 h)	Blood Pressure	Suggested Main Pathophysiologic Change
Stage I At clinical diagnosis	Hyperfunction and hypertrophy stage	Large kidneys and glomerular hyperfiltration	Glomerular hypertrophy; normal BM and mesangium	150	May be increased but readily reversible	Normal	Glomerular volume expansion and increased intraglomerular pressure
Stage II In short-term diabetes (1–15 y)	"Silent" stage with normal UAE, but structural lesions present	Normal UAE	Increased BM thickness and mesangial expansion	With or without hyperfiltration[a,b]	Normal (often increased in stress situations)	Normal	Changes as indicated above but variable (dependent on metabolic control), in addition, increased accumulation of BM and BM-like material
In long-term diabetes (>15 y)			No or few studies	With or without hyperfiltration[a,b]	Normal (often increased in stress situations)	Normal or slightly elevated	
Stage III Early Late	Incipient DN (microalbuminuria)	Persistently elevated UAE	Severity probably in between II and IV	160 130	30–105 105–300 (considerable range)	Often elevated compared with healthy subjects; also elevated during exercise	Glomerular closure probably starts in this stage; in some patients, high intraglomerular pressure
Stage IV Early	Overt DN	Clinical proteinuria	Further increase in BM thickening and mesangial expansion	130–70	>300	Often frank hypertension	High rate of glomerular closure and advancing mesangial expansion
Intermediate			Increasing rate of glomerular closure	70–30	Increasing clinical proteinuria	Hypertension in almost all patients	Hyperfiltration in remaining glomeruli (deleterious?)
Advanced			Hypertrophy of remaining glomeruli	30–10		Hypertension in almost all patients	
Stage V	Uremia	End-stage renal failure	Generalized glomerular closure	0–10	Decreasing (due to nephron closure)	High but often controlled by dialysis treatment	Advanced lesions and glomerular closure

Abbreviations: DN, diabetic nephropathy; GFR, glomerular filtration rate; UAE, urinary albumin excretion; BM, basement membrane.
[a] Changes probably present in all stages when glycemic control imperfect.
[b] Possible marker of future nephropathy (if GFR >150 ml/min).
(Modified from Mogensen and Schmitz,[9] with permission.)

Table 20-2. Possible Factors That May Influence Progression to Incipient or Clinical Diabetic Nephropathy[a]

Glomerular hyperfiltration in single nephrons	High dietary protein intake
High vascular permeability in general	Low level of heparan sulfate
Genetic disposition to hypertension	Angiotensin II excess

Hypersecretion of growth hormone, other growth factors?

Degree of hyperglycemia, or genetically determined susceptibility to hyperglycemia
  Advanced glycation end products alter extracellular matrix and cellular proteins
  Increased secretion of mesangial matrix with disruption of collagen architecture
  High level of aldose reductase activity (accumulation of polyols, depletion of myoinositol)
  Auto-oxidation of glucose, formation of reactive oxygen species
  De novo synthesis of diacylglycerol, activation of protein kinase C
    Increased endothelial permeability
    Mesangial cell contraction
    Synthesis of prostaglandins
    Extracellular matrix proteins
    Quenched responses to nitric oxide

[a] Multiple interactions are probable.
(Data from Mogensen and Schmitz,[9] Deckert et al,[6] Hirsch,[52] Brownlee,[94] and Derubertis and Craven.[111])

flow is not always increased at this stage and actually may be decreased relative to the mass of renal tissue. Therefore, the increased GFR is not simply due to increased blood flow.[56] Most investigators relate the increase in GFR to an increased capillary filtration surface area.[60,61] There is progression in exercise-induced proteinuria with increased albumin excretion related to increases in systolic blood pressure.[56,57] In these early years of diabetes, there is a gradual increase in the thickness of the GBM, often followed by mesangial expansion.[50,62–64] Despite the glomerular hyperfiltration and increased GBM thickness in virtually all diabetic persons after 5 years of disease, in 20 to 40 percent of subjects, clinical nephropathy develops, but in the others, it does not. Table 20-2 lists factors that may determine in which patients the disorder will progress.[9,52]

Stage 3

Incipient diabetic nephropathy is characterized by microalbuminuria, with repeatable baseline urinary excretion rates for albumin of 30 to 300 mg/24 h (20 to 200 μg/min).[8] At this stage, GFR is well preserved and may remain above normal, with increased capillary surface area seen in structural studies.[56] The degree of microalbuminuria slowly increases over several years.[57] The annual increase in albumin excretion ranges from 0 to 112 mg/24 h, and the degree is related to glycemic control[65] and to differences in diastolic blood pressure in the range of 75 to 105 mm Hg.[19,56] Although GFR remains high at approximately 140 ml/min, renal plasma flow declines in relation to increasing diastolic pressures. These changes suggest to Mogensen et al[56] that there may be impaired renal vascular autoregulation in this phase of the disorder. It remains controversial whether an initial rise in blood pressure triggers increased UAE. In a prospective study of the development of microalbuminuria in normotensive patients with IDDM, Mathiesen et al[19] found no significant rise in diastolic blood pressure until 3 years of UAE at rates greater than 30 mg/24 h (Fig. 20-5). Chavers et al[64] studied glomerular lesions in 26 patients with IDDM with normoalbuminuria and 22 with microalbuminuria (Table 20-3). Mesangial volume per glomerulus varied in both groups but was significantly increased in patients with the higher levels of UAE, who also had modest increases in blood pressure or slight decreases in creatinine clearance. The authors concluded that microalbuminuric patients are not uniform with regard to glomerular pathologic findings and that increased UAE best predicts diabetic nephropathy when "other features of nephropathy are already present" (mesangial expansion, slight decrease in GFR, and modest hypertension).

Stage 4

Overt clinical DN is characterized by macroproteinuria (UAE >300 mg/24 h, total urinary protein >500 mg/24 h), which can increase rapidly year to year by 1 to 3 g/24 h,[56] and by progressive decline in GFR by 1.0 to 1.2 ml/min/mo.[56,57] Hypertension is common in this stage, and the rate of decline in GFR is related to the diastolic blood pressure level.[56] The glomerular structural correlates of the functional changes of overt clinical diabetic nephropathy include a further increase in GBM thickness and arteriolar hyalinosis, the degree of which is related to both proteinuria and the other result of diabetic microvascular disease, retinopathy.[66] Perhaps the most important marker for overt diabetic

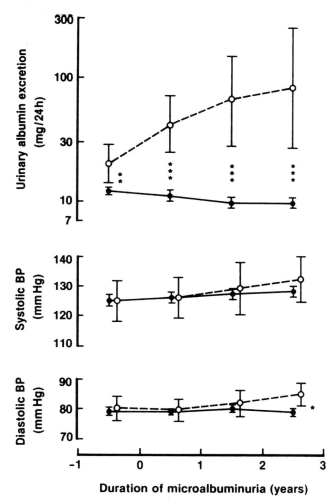

nephropathy is a continuing increase in the total mesangium (cells and matrix) with the mesangial volume fraction enlarging from 33 to 57 percent of the glomerular tuft.[1,3,50,63] Mesangial expansion increases the interface between endothelial capillaries and mesangium and decreases the peripheral capillary filtration surface[1,3,50] (Fig. 20-6). The extent of mesangial expansion correlates better with the decline in creatinine clearance than does the thickness of the GBM or the percentage of glomeruli that have become sclerotic. A compensatory enlargement of open glomeruli may parallel mesangial expansion, thus temporarily preserving the filtration surface.[3,50,67,68] As this process becomes limited, however, and there is an increase in hyalinized, obliterated glomeruli,[50,63] glomerular filtration declines markedly.[3]

Stage 5

End-stage renal failure is characterized by generalized glomerular closure, marked decreases of GFR (creatinine clearance <10 ml/min), rising plasma creatinine and blood urea nitrogen, and increased tubular excretion of β_2-microglobulin.[57] Albumin excretion may decrease as a result of nephron closure.[9] The degree of azotemia is related to the percentage of sclerotic glomeruli that are occluded; it is also possible to observe capillary closure within nonsclerotic glomeruli.[63,67] Worsening hypertension accompanies the renal failure.

Proteinuria

Proteins in the urine of diabetic patients consist mainly of negatively charged, spherically configured albumin with a radius of 36 Å, and neutral IgG with a larger radius of 55 Å.[69] The mechanisms for proteinuria in diabetic nephropathy are not completely understood, and it is probable that no single factor is responsible.[45] Studies have focused on the structural nature of the barrier to permeability, on glomerular hemodynamic function, and on the nature of the proteins filtered.

Tracer studies of normal glomerular filtration led to

Fig. 20-5. Course of urinary albumin excretion (UAE) and blood pressure in IDDM. Fifteen patients developing persistent microalbuminuria (open circles) are compared with 190 patients who continued with normoalbuminuria (closed circles). Duration of diabetes 10 to 30 years. No medication except insulin at enrollment. Antihypertensive therapy added if blood pressure (BP) exceeded 160/95 mm Hg on three consecutive occasions. Persistent microalbuminuria defined as UAE >30 mg/24 h in at least two of three consecutive samples in 2 subsequent years. Patients in whom microalbuminuria developed had significantly higher hemoglobin A_{1c} at enrollment and throughout the course of the study. By multiple regression analysis, initial UAE and hemoglobin A_{1c} had a significant influence on the UAE 5 years later, whereas age, duration of diabetes, systolic and diastolic blood pressure, inverse serum creatinine corrected for weight, and degree of retinopathy were without significant influence. Mean and 95% confidence interval are given. *P <.05, **P <.01, ***P <.001. (Modified from Mathiesen et al,[19] with permission.)

Table 20-3. Glomerular Lesions and Clinical Characteristics of IDDM With or Without Microalbuminuria[a]

	Group 1 (Normal blood pressure and creatinine clearance)	Group 2	Group 3
		(Microalbuminuria)	
No.	26	10	12
Duration of diabetes (yr)	18 ± 8	17 ± 7	21 ± 7
Glycohemoglobin (%)	10 ± 2	11 ± 2	11 ± 2
Blood pressure (mm Hg)	115/73 ± 10/8	113/74 ± 9/8	128/82 ± 17/6
Creatinine clearance (ml/min/1.73²)	114 ± 12	120 ± 24	90 ± 24
Urinary albumin excreted (mg/24 h)	10 ± 4	39 ± 24	93 ± 59
Urinary IgG excreted	3 ± 2	8 ± 7	10 ± 5
Mean glomerular volume ($\times 10^6$ μm³)	1.3 ± 0.3	1.5 ± 1.0	1.4 ± 0.3
Mesangial volume per glomerulus ($\times 10^6$ μm³)	0.26 ± 0.13	0.34 ± 0.35	0.41 ± 0.13[b]
Total peripheral capillary filtration surface per glomerular ($\times 10^6$ μm³)	0.13 ± 0.04	0.15 ± 0.10	0.11 ± 0.03
Thickness of the glomerular basement membrane (mm)	508 ± 109	550 ± 128	625 ± 101[c]

[a] Values are means ± 50. Normal range for glycohemoglobin 5.5–8.5%.
[b] Vs. group 2, two-tailed $P < 0.007$ by Mann-Whitney U test.
[c] Vs. group 1, two-tailed $P < 0.003$ by Mann-Whitney U test.
(Modified from Chavers et al,[64] with permission.)

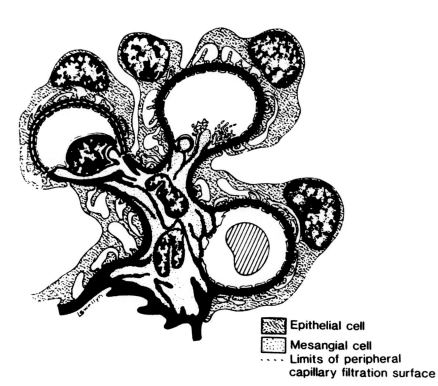

Epithelial cell
Mesangial cell
· · · · Limits of peripheral capillary filtration surface

Fig. 20-6. Schematic representation of the glomerular tuft illustrating the limits of the peripheral capillary filtration surface related to mesangial expansion. (From Mauer et al,[1] with permission.)

the hypothesis of two barriers to the permeability of macromolecules, with the GBM as the primary barrier and subepithelial slit diaphragms as secondary.[45] Viberti et al[70] described the glomerular capillary wall as "a membrane perforated by pores of similar size and uniformly coated by negative electrical charges. The passage of macromolecules across this barrier depends on the size, [configuration], and charge of the circulating molecule, but also on the transglomerular pressure gradient, the driving force in the glomerular filtration of particles." Regarding intraglomerular pressure, it is of interest that infusion of angiotensin II results in the contraction of mesangial cells in culture,[71] reduction of renal plasma flow, an elevation in the transcapillary hydraulic pressure difference, and increased urinary excretion of proteins.[72] These findings suggest to Kanwar et al[45] that "disturbances in the intraglomerular hemodynamics can induce proteinuria even though no detectable structural abnormalities are observed in the filtration unit."

There is also tubular reabsorption of proteins, a process that may be easily saturated, but under conditions of nonsaturation, the tubular reabsorption of proteins is proportional to the filtered load.

At the stage of microalbuminuria in diabetic nephropathy, there is increased fractional excretion of both albumin and IgG at UAE rates of less than 60 μg/min (90 mg/24 h).[70] Studies of the fractional renal clearance of neutral dextrans in the 30- to 60-Å interval in early diabetic nephropathy showed normal glomerular pore size.[69,73] Viberti et al[70] concluded that the microproteinuria was due to increased intraglomerular pressure, which increases the filtration of both albumin and IgG, and is associated with increased capillary filtration surface area. Thus, at this stage, there is a nonselective microproteinuria. Later in the course of incipient nephropathy, when albumin excretion exceeds 60 μg/ml (90 mg/24 h), there is a charge selectivity defect because the polyanion albumin is selectively filtered in greater proportion than the larger size IgG.[74] Histochemical studies demonstrate a loss of the fixed negative electrical charge of the GBM, which allows the more polyanionic albumin to pass.[70,75]

Altered glomerular handling of glycated albumin may also be involved in microproteinuria.[76] Experimental use of a monoclonal antibody against glycated albumin in mice reduced albumin excretion and prevented mesangial matrix accumulation with overexpression of type IV collagen.[77]

With the macroproteinuria of stage 4 clinical diabetic nephropathy, albumin contributes 42 percent of the filtered protein at this stage compared with 7 percent in normal controls.[70] There is also an increase in the fractional clearance of IgG as a result of a continued loss of selectivity for charge and size in the glomerular membrane, increased pore size within the GBM,[69] and a loss of secondary barrier size selectivity in the epithelial layers with more advanced diabetic nephropathy.[70,75,78] Thus, at this stage of heavy proteinuria and low GFR, loss of glomerular pore size selectivity in addition to the depletion of membrane polyanions determines the character of the proteinuria. The cause of the loss of the pore size selectivity is not determined.

PATHOGENESIS

Glomerular Effects of Hyperglycemia

Hyperglycemia induced compositional changes in the GBM and mesangial extracellular matrix that are related to the loss of permselectivity for albumin and the later decrease in GFR. In studies of the biosynthesis of extracellular components in tissue cultures of endothelial cells, excess glucose led to increased expression of collagen IV, laminin, and fibronectin, but not HS-PG, so that the ratio of HS-PG to collagen IV was significantly reduced.[79] In cultured rat glomerular mesangial cells, high concentrations of glucose also enhanced ECM accumulation of collagen IV,[80] fibronectin, and laminin.[81] These in vitro findings may explain the thickened GBM found in diabetic subjects and the relative loss of anionic HS-PG in the ECM,[82] and they fit with observations of increased expression of collagen type IV in the GBM early in the course of diabetic nephropathy[83] and decreased synthesis of HS-PG in GBM of diabetic patients[84,85] and experimental animals.[86,87] The decreased density of HS-PG could also facilitate mesangial expansion because heparan sulfate inhibits mesangial cell growth in the rat.[88]

In addition to decreased expression of anionic proteoglycans, another mechanism that reduces the negative charge of ECM in diabetes is by undersulfation of heparan sulfate[89] as a result of diminished activity of glomerular N-deacetylase, the key enzyme in the sulfation of HS-PG.[90] In poorly controlled diabetic rats, markedly decreased N-deacetylase activity[91] correlates with mean blood glucose levels and albuminuria.[90]

Hyperglycemia also results in increased nonenzymatic glycosylation of collagen IV, fibronectin, and laminin, which decreases their affinity to binding HS-PG,[92] and decreases turnover of glycosylated collagen IV.[93] Both mechanisms could lead to reduced density of anionic HS-PG in the glomerular ECM.[6] The early glycation products formed by a nonenzymatic process adducting glucose to proteins can undergo a complex series of rearrangements to form advanced glycation end products (AGEs), which accumulate over time.[94,95] Macrophages and endothelial, vascular smooth muscle, and mesangial cells contain AGE-specific receptors.[95,96] In vitro, AGE protein stimulates mesangial cell production of fibronectin, laminin, and collagen IV.[97,98] In vivo, deposition of AGEs within the glomerulus can lead to thickening of the GBM, mesangial matrix expansion,[96] and increased endothelial permeability.[99] The effects can be blocked by the AGE-inhibitor aminoguanidine.[100,101]

Glucose autoxidation is another possible cause of glomerular and vascular damage in diabetes.[102] This process is catalyzed by metal ions that yield *reactive oxygen species:* free radicals, hydrogen peroxide, and hydroxyl radicals.[103] The reactive oxygen species, if not neutralized by antioxidants such as vitamin E and C, glutathione, or lipoic acid, can cause peroxidation of membrane lipids and induce oxidation of LDL, both of which are cytotoxic to endothelium.[104] Both processes of peroxidation can increase vascular permeability. In diabetic rats, impaired degradation of hydrogen peroxide was found in isolated glomeruli.[105] In other models, the rate of free radical production is markedly enhanced by early glycation products[106]; furthermore, reactive oxygen species also mediate the reaction of aldehydes with membrane proteins to form AGEs. Thus, "oxidative stress" may amplify the toxic effects of AGEs on endothelium.[104]

Biochemical Processes by Which Hyperglycemia Can Cause Glomerular Injury

Concurrent studies of (1) human tissues, (2) experimental models of diabetes, and (3) cultured endothelial and mesangial cells have provided insights into the metabolic pathways by which hyperglycemia may lead to injury.[6,7,107] One of the first to be studied was activation of the polyol pathway, in which excess glucose is catalyzed by aldose reductase in tissues of diabetic subjects to form sorbitol, with increased formation of fructose leading to nonenzymatic fructosylation, decreased myoinositol uptake, and utilization of reduced nicotinamide adenine dinucleotide (NADH)[6,7,106] (Fig. 20-7). Although there is better evidence for the involvement of polyol pathway activation in the pathology of diabetes in nerve and lens than in diabetic nephropathy, some, but not all, studies show that aldose reductase inhibitors reduce hyperfiltration and subsequent albuminuria in experimental models of diabetes.[108–110] Polyol pathway activation or aldose reductase inhibition may have crossover effects on other

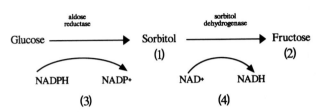

Fig. 20-7. The aldose reductase pathway with demonstrated or postulated biochemical consequences of potential relevance to the pathogenesis of diabetic nephropathy. (1) Increased sorbitol leads to decreased myoinositol and decreased phosphoinoside signaling, which can result in poor CA^{2+} mobilization and mesangial cell contraction; (2) increased fructose leads to increased fructosylation and protein cross-linking associated with increased collagen IV and decreased HS-PG in the glomerular extracellular matrix; (3) decreased NADPH causes decreased GSH:GSSG, facilitating oxidative damage, and increased lipoperoxides; decreased GSH:GSSG also causes increased cyclo-oxygenase activity, resulting in increased free radicals; decreased NADPH also causes increases in the pentose phosphate pathway, contributing to increased triose phosphates in the de novo DAG pathway, resulting in increased protein kinase C activity, increased prostaglandin production, and hyperfiltration; (4) increased NADH causes increased dihydroxyacetone and increases in the de novo DAG pathway, also resulting in increased PKC, increased prostaglandin production, and hyperfiltration. NADPH, reduced form of nicotinamide-adenine dinucleotide phosphate; NADP+, oxidized form of NADP; NADH, reduced form of nicotinamide-adenine dinucleotide; NAD+, oxidized form of NAD; HS-PG, heparan sulfate proteoglycan; GSH, reduced glutathione; GSSG, oxidized glutathione; DAG, diacylglycerol; PKC, protein kinase C. (Modified from Larkins and Dunlop,[7] with permission.)

cellular processes such as impaired regeneration of the reduced forms of natural protective antioxidants, which scavenge radicals by limiting available nicotinamide adenine dinucleotide phosphate (NADPH), and increased nonenzymatic fructosylation of glomerular tissues.[7]

Another cellular action of excess glucose studied in isolated glomeruli and in cultured endothelial and mesangial cells depends on the family of protein kinase C (PKC) isozymes, which are involved in the transduction of extracellular signals by growth factors, hormones, paracrines, and autocoids.[111] Increased PKC activity is detected in glomeruli from diabetic rats[112] and in mesangial cell cultures exposed to high glucose concentrations.[113] The major endogenous cellular mediator of PKC activation is diacylglycerol (DAG), which binds to the regulatory subunit of the enzyme.[111] DAG is formed by de novo synthesis from high intracellular concentrations of glucose.[113,114] Hyperglycemia also leads to increased glomerular eicosanoid generation (prostaglandins E_2 and I_2 and thromboxane A_2)[114] and the process activates PKC in isolated glomeruli[111] and mesangial cells.[115,116]

What are the effects of PKC activation on glomerular endothelial and mesangial cells? PKC activation leads to the development of intercellular gaps in endothelial cell monolayers[117] and to increased permeability to albumin.[118] In mesangial cells, PKC activation modulates contractile responses to angiotensin II[111] and is linked to increased synthesis of eicosanoids.[111,119,120] Inhibitors of PKC block the actions of high concentrations of glucose or thromboxane/prostaglandin endoperoxide analogues, which stimulate matrix protein synthesis in mesangial cells (fibronectin, laminin, and collagen type IV).[120] Activation of PKC is also implicated in the suppression of nitric oxide-mediated increases in glomerular cyclic guanosine monophosphate (cGMP).[111] Since cGMP inhibits mesangial contraction, proliferation, and matrix protein synthesis, this effect of PKC activation may amplify the glomerulotoxic effects of hyperglycemia.[111]

Hyperfiltration

The observation of increased kidney size and glomerular filtration in early diabetes led to the hypothesis that renal hypertrophy and hyperfiltration were responsible for the development of clinical nephropathy.[121–123]

Mogensen and Christensen[26] found that proteinuria was more likely to develop when GFR had been elevated, and Wiseman and Viberti[124] observed a correlation between elevated GFR and increased renal volume in type I diabetes. In this study, hyperfiltration was unlikely in diabetic patients with normal kidney size. However, recent studies correlating renal volume with histopathologic findings or with changes in GFR have not entirely supported the necessity for renal hypertrophy in the pathogenesis of nephropathy. Renal size did not indicate the severity of diabetic renal lesions on biopsy,[125] and renal volume did not decrease with GFR was lowered in response to intensive insulin therapy.[126] Ellis et al[125] and Wiseman et al[126] conclude that renal growth is not a sufficient explanation for the hyperfiltration seen in early diabetes.

The hyperfiltration hypothesis received support from experimental studies in which renal ablation resulted in single-nephron hyperfiltration in the remaining kidney, hypertension, glomerular lesions similar to those of diabetes (increased mesangial area and decreased peripheral capillary surface), and ultimately, glomerulosclerosis.[127,128] In the renal ablation experiments of Hostetter et al[127] and Steffes et al,[128] hyperfiltration was due to elevated flow and increases in the glomerular transcapillary-hydraulic pressure difference. This model of experimental hyperfiltration showed that increased GFR was associated with a fourfold increase in protein excretion as a result of impaired charge and size-selective permeability.[127] A model of streptozotocin-induced diabetes in rats also produced hyperfiltration; a 40-percent increase in GFR was secondary to (1) increased renal plasma flow caused by vasodilation and (2) increased transcapillary pressure difference.[127]

What is the role of hyperglycemia in inducing hyperfiltration? Intravenous glucose infusions raise GFR somewhat in normal controls and produce larger increases in GFR and renal plasma flow in diabetic subjects.[129] In diabetic children[130] and streptozotocin-induced diabetic rats,[131] increased plasma and glomerular ultrafiltrate glucose stimulate sodium-coupled glucose tubular reabsorption and the associated solute-linked water reabsorption. Ditzel et al[130] believe that this could contribute to the increased GFR. Complex hormonal responses occur secondary to hyperglycemia. It is difficult to determine just what factor is responsible for the altered renal hemodynamics and filtration,[132–135] but Hostetter[123] doubts that changes in insulin, glucagon, growth hormone, or catecholamines are responsible for the hyperfiltration. To avoid the systemic hormonal changes that accompany hyperglycemia, Kasiske and colleagues[134] studied the isolated perfused rat kidney from control and diabetic animals. Increased glucose in the perfusate caused vasodilation and increased GFR (increased inulin clearance). Mannitol was used as a control for the osmotic effects of glucose, and it produced a different response (i.e., vasoconstriction). The hyperfiltration produced by glucose was blocked when prostaglandin synthetase inhibitors were administered. Glucose also inhibited the tubular-glomerular feedback mechanism, in which there is usually vasoconstriction in response to an increase in filtered sodium load. Kasiske et al[134] proposed that this inhibition of the feedback mechanism may have a permissive role in the glucose-induced vasodilation seen in their studies. The authors reviewed other evidence that prostaglandin metabolism is altered in the glomerulus in diabetes and that hyperglycemia increases vascular production of prostaglandins.

Finally, hypertension is an important factor in the development of clinical nephropathy, and Parving et al[24] and Hostetter[123] link hypertension to hemodynamic changes that could be associated with increased glomerular filtration of macromolecules and structural endothelial-mesangial abnormalities. Therefore, there is abundant evidence that hemodynamic and hyperglycemic changes lead to hyperfiltration in the glomeruli and this predisposes to the development of the lesions of clinical diabetic nephropathy. However, as noted above, not all diabetic subjects with early hyperfiltration go on to develop diabetic nephropathy; so hyperfiltration may be a predisposing process but is not a sufficient explanation of the pathogenesis of diabetic nephropathy.

Linking the Pathogenesis of Glomerular and Macrovascular Disease in Diabetes

Proteinuria is a risk factor for cardiovascular morbidity in people with diabetes, independent of or associated with the risk factors for the development of atherosclerosis (hypercholesterolemia, decreased high-density lipoproteins, smoking, and hypertension).[11–13] Therefore, many investigators are searching for common pathogenic mechanisms that may link thickening of the basement membrane, endothelial dysfunction, and accumulation of ECM in the glomerulus and large vessels.[6,44,106–108,136] Deckert and colleagues[6] point out the similarities of glomerular mesangial and arterial myomedial cells: mesenchymal origin, with contractile and phagocytic properties; both synthesize collagen IV, fibronectin, laminin, and HS-PG. In susceptible diabetic subjects with albuminuria, both mesangial and myomedial proliferation occur, and the composition of the expanded ECM is similar, with decreased density of HS-PG, which can result in increased postendothelial macromolecular permeability[137] and decreased endothelial binding of lipoprotein lipase and antithrombin III.[44] These processes could contribute to atherogenesis[138] and thrombogenesis.[139,140]

Another hypothesis proposes that circulating or subendothelial AGEs specifically interact with endothelium to alter vascular function.[94,95,107] As noted, AGE receptors on monocytes/macrophages; fibroblasts; and mesangial, endothelial, and smooth muscle cells may mediate cellular proliferation and matrix accumulation.[95] Brownlee[94] and Vlassara et al[95] reviewed the evidence for the role of AGEs in the "atherosclerosis of diabetes" and for prevention of the effects by the AGE inhibitor guanethidine.

INTERVENTIONS
Antihypertensive Agents

Hypertension frequently accompanies chronic renal insufficiency of any cause, including diabetic nephropathy. Several longitudinal studies show that hypertension usually appears after there is already evidence of incipient diabetic nephropathy, suggesting that hypertension is a consequence of the renal disease rather than the cause of it.[19,141,142] Nonetheless, there is widespread agreement that uncontrolled hypertension accelerates the progression from incipient to overt nephropathy and from overt nephropathy to ESRD. Even modest blood pressure elevations that would usually be considered "high-normal" are believed to cause a worsening of diabetic nephropathy.[143] It is therefore natural to hypothesize that strict control of arterial pressure might slow the progression of nephropathy.

Antihypertensive therapy has been extensively investigated in this context. Kasiske et al[144] recently presented a metaregression analysis of 100 studies of various antihypertensive agents for diabetic nephropathy. Regardless of the agent used, the analysis indicated that reduction of arterial pressure resulted in both a decrease in urinary protein excretion and a sparing of GFR ($P < .001$ for both effects). ACE inhibitors appeared to be especially beneficial in this analysis because these agents were associated with an additional decrease in proteinuria and increase in GFR that is independent of their blood pressure-lowering effect ($P < .0001$ and $P < .05$, respectively). The authors noted that "the salutary effect of ACE inhibitors on proteinuria was seen whether or not the patient had hypertension, whether or not the patient had microalbuminuria or clinically apparent proteinuria, and whether the patient had type I or type II diabetes." It seems likely that in addition to their systemic action, ACE inhibitors have a favorable local effect on intrarenal hemodynamics, at least when low sodium intake is used by treated subjects.[145,146]

That ACE inhibitors have a special value in slowing the progression from incipient to overt diabetic nephropathy was confirmed in a subsequent double-blind multicenter trial by the European Microalbuminuria Captopril Study Group.[147] Normotensive patients with incipient nephropathy were randomized to receive either placebo or captopril, 50 mg twice daily, for 2 years. Progression to overt nephropathy was observed in 26 percent of the placebo group versus only 9 percent of the captopril group ($P = .03$).

That ACE inhibitors can slow the progression from overt nephropathy to ESRD was confirmed in a double-blind American collaborative study.[148] Patients with overt nephropathy were randomized to receive either placebo or captopril 25 mg three times daily for a median of 3 years. Other antihypertensive agents were used as needed in both groups with the aim to keep blood pressure below 140/90 mm Hg. In the placebo group, creatinine clearance declined by a mean of 17 ml/min/y versus 11 ml/min/y in the captopril group ($P = .03$). As a result, the captopril group had a 50 percent reduction in the risk of reaching one of the severe end points of the study: dialysis, renal transplantation, or death.[148]

We conclude from these studies that nonpregnant patients with incipient or overt nephropathy should receive an ACE inhibitor even if they are normotensive. However, ACE inhibitors are *contraindicated in pregnancy* because of their serious adverse effects on fetal and neonatal renal function.[149]

Additional antihypertensive therapy is indicated if blood pressure is even modestly elevated. A 1989 consensus statement recommended that such therapy should be started if systolic pressure rises by 20 mm Hg or more or if diastolic pressure rises by 10 mm Hg or more over 2 years.[150] Mogensen et al[151] recommended initiating therapy if the mean arterial pressure exceeds 90 to 95 mm Hg (roughly 120/80 mm Hg). A 1993 consensus statement recommends that the goal of therapy is to keep systolic pressure below 130 mm Hg and diastolic pressure below 85 mm Hg, and lower if tolerated.[152] The latter statement also recommends treatment of isolated systolic hypertension, defined as a systolic pressure of 140 mm Hg or more.

There is a wide choice of agents to use in addition to ACE inhibitors. The 1993 consensus statement concludes that α_1-receptor blockers, calcium antagonists, and low-dose thiazide diuretics may be especially useful.[152] The statement also classifies several agents that should be used "with caution" because of adverse effects on glycemic control and lipid balance, interference potential with hypoglycemia awareness, or other potential complications. These include β-adrenergic blockers, combined α- and β-adrenergic blockers, centrally acting α_2-agonists, potassium-sparing agents, and sympatholytics.[152] Drugs we find to be useful and relatively safe during pregnancy include diltiazem, clonidine, prazosin, and methyldopa. Methyldopa is little used outside of pregnancy because of the poor compliance associated with drowsiness and the rise in blood pressure after 6 to 9 months of use, associated with increased plasma volume.[153] However, methyldopa has been wisely used during pregnancy and has not been found to affect the development of offspring.[154]

Studies of Bakris and colleagues[155,156] indicate that certain calcium antagonists (diltiazem) and ACE inhibitors (isinopril) "attenuate the rise in glomerular capillary pressure, glomerular hypertrophy, and mesangial matrix expansion in diabetic animal models."[146] In a randomized, prospective, parallel group study, these agents resulted in a slower rate of decline in GFR, lower UAE, and a better overall metabolic profile in hypertensive patients with NIDDM and overt nephropathy compared with the combination of a loop diuretic (furosemide) and β-adrenoreceptor antagonist (atenolol), even given a similar level of arterial pressure control in all treatment groups.[146] Diltiazem seems to have a greater effect on lowering proteinuria in diabetic subjects than other calcium antagonists, such as nifedipine.[155–157]

Metabolic Control

Large epidemiologic studies have consistently demonstrated that diabetic nephropathy is related to poor glycemic control in both IDDM and NIDDM. These studies show that higher levels of glycosylated hemoglobin are associated with both incipient and overt nephropathy, and these associations persist in multivariate analyses that control for other factors such as age, duration of diabetes, blood pressure control, and dietary protein intake.[158–162] It has long been hypothesized, therefore, that strict glycemic control would result in improved renal function and would slow the progression of nephropathy to ESRD.

Short-term trials of intensive insulin therapy to achieve normoglycemia for a few weeks to 1 year generally show that such therapy results in improvements in several of the indirect markers of the severity of nephropathy, including microproteinuria, kidney volume, and the amino acid-stimulated rise in GFR.[163–165] Three recent long-term trials of strict metabolic control also show that intensified insulin therapy can indeed prevent or delay the progression from incipient to overt nephropathy and suggest that such therapy might slow the progression to ESRD.

In studies from the Steno Hospital, Denmark, 70 IDDM patients without clinical diabetic nephropathy from 1980 to 1983 were randomized to receive conventional subcutaneous insulin therapy or intensive therapy with insulin pumps and frequent adjustment of insulin dosage based on self-monitoring of blood glucose.[166] Although the design of the trial was to continue therapy for only 2 years, most patients continued over the subsequent 3 to 5 years with the therapy to which they were randomized. Long-term follow-up measures of glycemic control and albuminuria were reported in 1991. Intensive therapy resulted in a large reduction in the number of patients whose disease progressed from incipient nephropathy to overt nephropathy (2 of 9 in the intensive group [22 percent] versus 10 of 10 in the conventional group [$P < .01$]). Of the patients without incipient nephropathy at the time of randomization, none developed nephropathy during the follow-up period.

Similar results were obtained in the Stockholm Diabetes Intervention Study.[167] In 1982, 54 IDDM patients were randomized to receive standard treatment consisting of physician visits every 4 months and (usually) to insulin injections a day. Forty-eight patients were randomized to receive intensified treatment consisting of intensive education, biweekly physician visits, frequent telephone contacts, and (usually) three insulin injections a day with dosages adjusted according to self-monitored blood glucose levels. Follow-up after 7.5 years of therapy was reported in 1993.[168] Nephropathy developed more commonly in those with standard treatment (9 of 54, 17 percent) than in those with intensified treatment (1 of 48, 2 percent, $P = .01$).

The American Diabetes Control and Complications Trial (DCCT) found that intensive treatment reduced the appearance of both incipient and overt nephropathy.[65] In this study, 1,441 IDDM patients from 29 centers were recruited from 1983 to 1989 and randomized to receive either conventional therapy with one or two insulin injections per day or intensive therapy involving frequent physician visits, extensive education and training, and three or more insulin injections per day or insulin pump therapy with dosages adjusted according to self-monitored blood glucose levels. In 1993, the results were reported after an average of 6.5 years of follow-up. Those who received intensive therapy were much less likely than those who received conventional therapy to to develop either incipient nephropathy (albuminuria >40 mg/d; risk reduction = 34 percent) or overt nephropathy (albuminuria >300 mg/d; risk reduction = 54 percent).

Thus, all three trials were consistent in showing that strict metabolic control can often prevent the progression from incipient nephropathy to overt nephropathy. Furthermore, the DCCT showed that such control can also prevent or delay the onset of incipient nephropathy. Unfortunately, these studies did not address the question as to whether strict control can prevent the progression from overt nephropathy to ESRD. In the three trials combined, only six patients had overt nephropathy at the time of randomization, and very few patients had progression to frank renal insufficiency during the course of any of the trials. Thus, there is inadequate statistical power in these studies to answer this question. Older studies suggested that glycemic control alone is inadequate to prevent progression once overt nephropathy is established.[169–171] This does not imply, however, that strict control is not of value for patients with overt diabetic nephropathy. The Steno study, Stockholm study, and DCCT all showed that good glycemic control also prevented the progression of diabetic retinopathy and neuropathy. Thus, intensive therapy with the aim that all diabetic patients should maintain near-normoglycemia is now considered the standard of appropriate care.

Low Protein Diet

In many experimental renal diseases, diets high in protein cause an acceleration of disease progression.[172] In diabetic rats, high protein intake was found to dilate the glomerular afferent arterioles, increase glomerular pressure and blood flow, increase proteinuria, and accelerate glomerular scarring.[173] These observations led to speculation that dietary protein restriction in diabetic nephropathy might be beneficial.

Five studies have reported that a low protein diet (0.6 to 0.8 g/kg body weight) maintained over 1.5 to 3 years indeed resulted in decreased proteinuria and a slowing of the fall of GFR. In the first four of these, the patients served as their own controls during two sequential observation periods.[174–177] Although the results of these studies suggested benefit, the best evidence comes from the more recent randomized trial by Zeller et al.[178] In this study, 35 IDDM patients were randomized to a diet containing 0.6 g/kg/d protein, 0.5 to 1 g/d phosphorus, and 2 g/d sodium versus the patient's usual diet, containing at least 1 g/kg protein and 1 g of phosphorus. After a mean follow-up of 3 years, GFR had declined by 37 ml/min in the control group and only 9.5 ml/min in the low-protein diet group ($P < .05$).[171]

It has been suggested that protein restriction in the 0.6-mg/kg range can result in protein undernutrition.[179] However, other studies have not confirmed this.[180,181] Based on all these studies, we conclude that dietary protein should be restricted to 0.6 to 0.8 mg/kg/d in patients with overt nephropathy. Further investigation is needed to determine whether similar restriction is beneficial for patients with incipient diabetic nephropathy.

Other Interventions

Cigarette smoking was associated with more rapid progression of nephropathy in a recent prospective study.[182] Over a period of 1 year, nephropathy progressed in 53 percent of smokers, in 33 percent of patients who quit smoking, and in only 11 percent of nonsmokers. In this study, blood pressure was well controlled in all patients, and the association of smoking with disease progression was shown by multivariate analysis to be independent of glycemic control. These data add to the many other health reasons to encourage diabetic women to quit smoking.

Several other therapies have been proposed to slow the progression of diabetic nephropathy. These include aldose-reductase inhibitors, glycosylation inhibitors, somatostatin analogs, and prostaglandin synthesis inhibitors. The reader is referred to a review by Tuttle et al[165] for an explanation of the theoretical rationale behind these agents. At this time, there are insufficient clinical data to recommend their use.

PRECONCEPTION EVALUATION AND CARE

With the recognition that excess congenital malformations and spontaneous abortions can be prevented by instituting a program of strict glycemic control before pregnancy is attempted,[183–185] special preconception programs for diabetes management are now in place in many areas of the world.[186,187] Factors associated with preconception glycemic control also reduce congenital anomalies in babies of women with diabetic vascular disease.[185,187]

Evaluation of renal function and staging of nephropathy should be a part of the routine preconception management of every diabetic woman. Probably because of changes in glomerular hemodynamics during pregnancy, proteinuria increases; so it may become difficult or impossible to determine whether incipient or overt diabetic nephropathy is present if the initial renal evaluation is done during gestation. A 24-hour urine specimen should be collected for determination of albumin excretion and creatinine clearance. The albumin assay should be performed by a reference laboratory because numerous technical problems can cause invalid results in laboratories that do not run such assays routinely. A 24-hour collection is preferred to a shorter timed collection because protein excretion follows a diurnal rhythm. Use of a protein/creatinine ratio in a single voided spot urine can lead to large errors.[188]

Modification or initiation of antihypertensive therapy is another important goal of preconception care. Many women with incipient or overt diabetic nephropathy are receiving ACE inhibitors, which are contraindicated during pregnancy.[149] These women should be changed to other agents before conception. There is a wide choice of agents to use, although none is ideal for both mother and fetus. The α_1-receptor blockers and calcium antagonists may be preferred in late pregnancy because of their potential beneficial effect on the long-term course of nephropathy, but there are inadequate data at this time about potential teratogenicity; so alternative agents are preferred in the first trimester. Methyldopa and β-blockers appear to be safe from a fetal viewpoint, but the 1993 Consensus Statement[152] classifies the latter among several agents that should be used "with caution" because of potential adverse effects on glycemic control, potential to interfere with hypoglycemia awareness, or other potential complications. Other agents that must be used "with caution" include combined α- and β-adrenergic blockers, centrally acting α_2-agonists, potassium-sparing agents, and sympatholytics. Balancing these risks, we prefer methyldopa as a first-line agent and use prazosin or clonidine if additional therapy is needed at the beginning of pregnancy. Diltiazem can be added at the end of the first trimester if needed or preferred.

Evaluation for ischemic heart disease should be carried out before conception in patients with overt diabetic nephropathy because these patients have a high risk of significant coronary disease. A careful history and physical examination should be supplemented with an electrocardiogram. Manske et al[189] found that there was virtually no significant coronary disease among diabetic patients with ESRD as long as their age was less than 45, the duration of diabetes was less than 25 years, and there were no ST-T wave changes on the electrocardiogram. If any of these risk factors is present, evaluation by a cardiologist is indicated.

Ophthalmologic evaluation is critical in preparing for pregnancy because almost all women with diabetic nephropathy have some degree of retinopathy. Proliferative retinopathy should be in spontaneous remission or treated by laser photocoagulation before pregnancy because this lowers the chances of recurrence during pregnancy.

Counseling regarding potential pregnancy complications is important once the presence and stage of nephropathy are determined and other evaluations are completed.

PREGNANCY

Maternal Complications

Normal pregnancy is accompanied by a 50 percent increase in renal blood flow and GFR. As a result, there is a doubling of the urinary excretion of albumin and other proteins. With nephropathy, these physiologic changes are superimposed on progressive glomerular disease. The pathophysiologic consequences depend on the stage of nephropathy and probably also on such factors as blood pressure control, glycemic control, and dietary protein intake.

The normal pregnancy-induced rise in GFR is seen in only about one-third of patients with overt diabetic nephropathy[190,191] (Table 20-4). In another third, GFR remains roughly constant, and in the final third, it actually decreases. The decrease may reflect the underlying natural history of the progression of nephropathy, which averages about 10 ml/min/y in nonpregnant IDDM subjects. Jovanovic and Jovanovic[192] reported that the decrease could be prevented in a small group of women with diabetic nephropathy by strictly controlling blood pressure and blood glucose level during pregnancy.

Table 20-4. Changes in Creatinine Clearance during Pregnancy in Women with Diabetic Nephropathy

	Change by Third Trimester		
First Trimester	No. Increased >25% (%)	No. Stable (%)	No. Decreased >15% (%)
>90 ml/min	3 (21)	5 (36)	6 (43)
60–89 ml/min	9 (45)	6 (30)	5 (25)
<60 ml/min	2 (20)	6 (60)	2 (20)
Total	14 (32)	17 (39)	13 (29)

(Data from Kitzmiller et al,[190] Jovanovic and Jovanovic,[192] and Reece et al.[191])

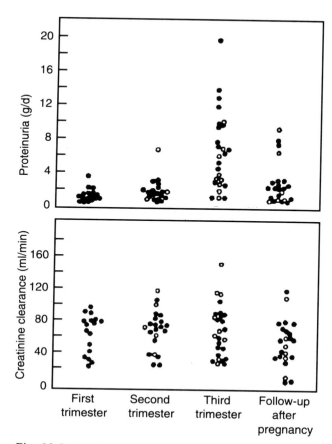

Fig. 20-8. Distribution of levels of proteinuria and creatinine clearance in women with diabetic nephropathy in each trimester of pregnancy and at a follow-up visit 9 to 35 months after delivery. Closed circles, women studied in each trimester; open circles, women not seen in the first trimester. (From Kitzmiller et al,[190] with permission.)

Proteinuria typically increases with pregnancy in nephropathic patients, often reaching levels of 10 g/d or more[190,191] (Fig. 20-8). Although some of this increase may be due to the underlying progression of nephropathy, most is likely caused by the physiologic hyperfiltration of pregnancy because proteinuria generally subsides after delivery. Excessive proteinuria often leads to hypoalbuminemia and then generalized edema, owing to decreased plasma oncotic pressure. Optimal treatment is problematic. Dietary protein supplementation or albumin infusions may be temporarily helpful but can also further increase renal blood flow and protein excretion in a "vicious circle." Diuretics may be helpful, but they must be used judiciously during pregnancy because excessive lowering of plasma volume can adversely affect uteroplacental perfusion.

Blood pressure control often worsens during pregnancy in patients with diabetic nephropathy. The reasons for this are not entirely known but probably involve adjustments in intrarenal and systemic hemodynamics, changes in antihypertensive drug levels attributable to the physiologic hemodilution of pregnancy, and changes in levels of binding proteins. It is not unusual for a patient with diabetic nephropathy to require frequent increases in the dosage of antihypertensive agents as pregnancy progresses. Many patients require multiple-agent therapy, (discussed in the section, *Preconception Evaluation and Care*). In keeping with the 1993 Consensus Statement,[150] we believe that an appropriate goal of therapy is to keep systolic pressure at 130 mm Hg and diastolic pressure at 85 mm Hg. Lower pressures may adversely affect uteroplacental perfusion and fetal oxygenation and growth.

Pre-eclampsia is the most frequent serious maternal complication of diabetic nephropathy. Table 20-5, which shows the results from six series of patients with diabetic nephropathy from 1981 to 1994, indicates that pre-eclampsia complicated more than one-third of the pregnancies.[190–195] Two recent studies suggested that

Table 20-5. Complications of Pregnancy with Overt Diabetic Nephropathy, 1981–94

Complication	No.	%	Reference No.
Pre-eclampsia	69/191	36.0	190–195
Anemia[a]	24/57	42.0	190,191
Perinatal death			
Major malformations	3/130	2.3	190–193,195
IUGR, preterm delivery	3/130	2.3	190–193,195
Total deaths	6/130	4.6	190–193,195
IUGR	24/114	21.0	190,191,193,195
Fetal distress	15/78	19.0	190,191,193,195
Cesarean delivery	75/100	75.0	191,192,193,195
Preterm delivery			
<37 weeks	107/191	56.0	190–195
<34 weeks	47/191	24.0	190–195

Abbreviations: IUGR, intrauterine growth retardation.
[a] Anemia = hematocrit <28% or hemoglobin <10 g/dl.
(Data from Kitzmiller et al,[190] Reece et al,[191] Jovanovic and Jovanovic,[192] Grenfell et al,[193] Combs et al,[194] and Kimmerle et al.[195])

pre-eclampsia may be just as common with incipient nephropathy as it is with overt nephropathy. Winocour et al[196] reported on four women with incipient nephropathy antedating pregnancy, and three developed pre-eclampsia. Combs et al[194] found that the rate of pre-eclampsia in diabetic women depended on the level of proteinuria in early pregnancy (Fig. 20-9). Pre-eclampsia occurred in 10 percent of those with early-pregnancy proteinuria of less than 190 mg/d (no nephropathy, $N = 204$), 40 percent of those with proteinuria of 190 to 499 mg/d (incipient nephropathy, $N = 45$); and 47 percent of those with proteinuria greater than 500 mg/d (overt nephropathy, $N = 62$). The relationship of proteinuria to pre-eclampsia persisted in multiple regression analysis that controlled for the effects of parity, chronic hypertension, retinopathy, and glycemic control. Regarding diabetic women with renal transplants (White's class T), a multicenter survey showed that six of nine developed pre-eclampsia (67 percent) during pregnancy.[197]

It is often difficult to distinguish between "true" pre-eclampsia and a "simple" worsening of chronic hypertension and chronic proteinuria. Indeed, some authors

refer only to a "pre-eclampsia-like syndrome." The distinction is of great practical importance because true pre-eclampsia is usually best treated by delivery, whereas simple exacerbation of hypertension and proteinuria can be managed with hospital bed rest and vigorous antihypertensive therapy. Uric acid levels can be elevated in true pre-eclampsia and in diabetic nephropathy.[190] Occasionally, findings such as hemolysis, thrombocytopenia, or elevated transaminase levels point to pre-eclampsia. However, there is often no finding that allows the diagnosis to be made definitively. In practice, the decision to manage expectantly or to deliver the infant must balance the risks of preterm delivery, indicators of fetal well-being, and the short- and long-term risks of uncontrolled hypertension in the mother.[198]

Low-dose aspirin in the second and third trimester may reduce the rate of pre-eclampsia and resultant preterm delivery in high-risk patients, although there are no data addressing whether this therapy is effective in women with diabetic nephropathy. An ongoing clinical trial by the National Institutes of Health Maternal-Fetal Medicine Units may help to answer this question.

Anemia is another common complication of pregnancy with diabetic nephropathy, resulting from the combination of decreased erythropoietin production in the kidney and the physiologic hemodilution of pregnancy. The degree of anemia is related to the degree of renal dysfunction, as reflected by lower creatinine clearance, and this anemia is not generally associated with abnormal serum iron level studies.[190] In severe cases, synthetic erythropoietin can be used.[199] To avoid hypertensive reactions or hyperviscosity syndromes, the dosage should be kept low with a goal to correct the anemia over several weeks.

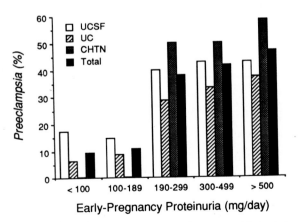

Fig. 20-9. Increased rate of pre-eclampsia with incipient diabetic nephropathy (total proteinuria, 190 to 499 mg/d) and overt nephropathy (>500 mg/d) compared with women without nephropathy (<189 mg/d). Normotensive patients from University of California San Francisco (UCSF), University of Cincinnati (UC), and chronic hypertensive patients from both centers (CHTN). (From Combs et al,[194] with permission.)

Perinatal Outcome

In the 1950s and 1960s, perinatal mortality rates averaged about 30 percent in women with diabetic nephropathy, with losses divided roughly equally among those caused by major malformations, premature delivery brought about because of pre-eclampsia, and severe growth delay with asphyxia as a result of maternal vascular disease.[200] This outlook has improved substantially in the past two decades. Table 20-5 shows that perinatal mortality rates now average less than 5 percent.[190–193] This dramatic improvement has been brought about on several fronts. Improved periconceptional glycemic control has decreased the incidence of major malformations. Advances in perinatal care such as fetal surveillance, sonographic recognition of growth delay, and better control of hypertension have reduced the rate of preterm delivery and have improved the metabolic status of those infants who still require preterm delivery. Advances in neonatal care continue to reduce the mortality and morbidity rates of premature neonates. Despite the improved neonatal survival, pregnancy in women with diabetic nephropathy still carries a high rate of complications that place the fetus and newborn at risk of serious complications.

Intrauterine growth retardation (IUGR) still occurs at roughly twice the rate as in the general population (Table 20-5). The incidence of IUGR is related to the severity of nephropathy and hypertension (Fig. 20-10). It is presumed that strict control of hypertension will reduce the incidence. We generally advise all women with nephropathy to rest in bed in the lateral decubitus position for several hours each day and to avoid vigorous exercise because we believe this will help prevent excess proteinuria and accelerated hypertension. If IUGR is suspected, we advise complete bed rest. We restrict dietary protein intake to 80 g/d in patients with diabetic nephropathy. Lower values may be beneficial

for the long-term course of nephropathy, but we believe that this amount is probably the minimum acceptable for adequate fetal growth.

To prevent excess morbidity from IUGR, hypoxia, and asphyxia, the diagnosis must be made, and fetal surveillance must be undertaken. There are no controlled trials regarding the optimal method of fetal surveillance in diabetic women. We instruct all pregnant women in fetal movement counting. In women with diabetic nephropathy, we use serial sonographic assessments of fetal growth in the late second and third trimester. If there is evidence of growth delay, we begin nonstress testing immediately. Because these tests may have false nonreactivity before 32 weeks of gestation, we rely on the contraction stress test and sonographic biophysical profile as backup tests. If there is mild-to-moderate oligohydramnios remote from term, we start with the contraction stress test and proceed to twice-weekly amniotic fluid volume assessments. Even in the absence of IUGR, we start weekly nonstress testing on all women with diabetic nephropathy by 28 weeks of gestation and increase to twice weekly by 36 weeks of gestation. Umbilical artery Doppler velocimetry has been studied in a few women with diabetic nephropathy. Fetuses with IUGR tend to have abnormal Doppler S/D ratios.[201] However, it is not clear at this time to what extent the Doppler studies

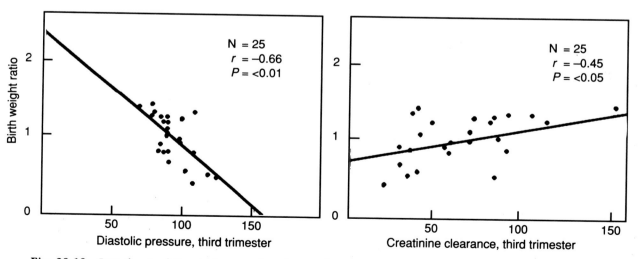

Fig. 20-10. Growth retardation in fetuses of mothers with nephropathy is related to lower creatinine clearance and hypertension. Birthweight ratio is the birthweight divided by median normal birthweight for gestational age. (Modified from Kitzmiller et al,[190] with permission.)

should be used to guide management. We doubt, for example, that delivery is indicated if Doppler study findings are abnormal, but other, more traditional indicators of fetal well-being such as fetal heart rate studies and amniotic fluid volume are normal. Furthermore, Salvesen et al[202] found that fetal acidemia in diabetic pregnancies was not accompanied by abnormal Doppler study results. Evidence of fetal distress is common in fetuses with IUGR and cesarean delivery is frequently required (Table 20-5). The timing of delivery depends on gestational age, evidence of fetal lung maturity, and severity of fetal condition. Vaginal delivery can generally be attempted at any gestational age as long as the intrapartum fetal heart rate tracing is reassuring and there are no obstetric indications for cesarean delivery.

Preterm delivery remains a significant problem (Table 20-5). About one-half of preterm births in women with nephropathy are attributable to pre-eclampsia or accelerated hypertension (Fig. 20-11). Many of the remainder occur because of fetal distress, with or without IUGR.[198] Because preterm delivery is so likely, we believe that these patients should receive care at a tertiary center with an intensive care nursery. Although neonatal mortality rates from prematurity

continue to fall, preterm delivery still carries considerable short-term morbidity from respiratory distress, hyperbilirubinemia, apnea/bradycardia, and a host of other complications. Care of these problems is exceedingly expensive, with neonatal intensive care costs currently averaging more than $2,000/d in the United States.

Long-term neurologic complications can be severe. Using standardized psychomotor assessments, Kimmerle et al[195] found evidence of psychomotor retardation in 8 of 34 infants born to mothers with nephropathy (21 percent). In one case, this was attributed to a major malformation. All but one of the other cases were associated with preterm delivery or IUGR, or both. In five of the cases, the retardation was classified as "severe." Although these outcomes were worse than those reported in earlier series,[190,191] they underscore the importance of preventing IUGR and prematurity.

Maternal Outcome

Historically, there has been a concern that the worsening of hypertension and proteinuria during pregnancy might accelerate the progression of nephropathy to ESRD. Indeed, studies that have reported on long-term follow-up after delivery show that many women do indeed progress to ESRD within a few years. Kitzmiller et al[190] reported that 3 of 23 women progressed to ESRD within 2 years of delivery (13 percent), and Reece et al[191] found that 6 of 27 progressed to ESRD within 3 years (22 percent). Kimmerle et al[195] found progression to ESRD in 8 of 29 women (28 percent) within 1 to 9 years. Biesenbach et al[203] reported ESRD in 5 of 5 women at an average of 29 months postpartum (range, 13 to 42 months). However, it must be borne in mind that nephropathy frequently progresses to ESRD even in the absence of pregnancy; thus these observations do not establish that pregnancy accelerates the process.

Three studies have examined the fall in creatinine clearance during the years immediately after pregnancy in women with diabetic nephropathy.[190,191,195,204] All three found that creatinine clearance fell at an average rate of 8 to 10 ml/min/y of follow-up. This rate is no different from that reported for patients with diabetic nephropathy in general.[9] Thus, pregnancy does not appear to accelerate the process of nephropathy.

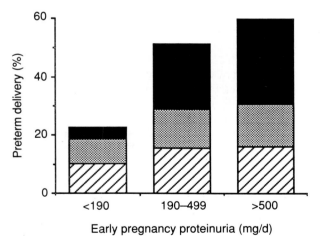

Fig. 20-11. High rate of preterm delivery with incipient nephropathy and overt nephropathy is mainly attributable to increased rate of pre-eclampsia. Solid bars, pre-eclampsia; dotted bars, other indication; hatched bars, spontaneous. (From Combs et al,[194] with permission.)

Diabetic nephropathy is a progressive disease, with or without pregnancy. Until recently, the progression from overt nephropathy to ESRD occurred in an average of about 10 years. It remains to be seen what impact there will be from interventions such as antihypertensive therapy, strict glycemic control, and low-protein diets. Once ESRD occurs, the median survival time is only 3 years, and the 7-year survival rate is only 20 percent. It has been argued that "the poor maternal prognosis is an important reason for discouraging pregnancies [in women with nephropathy] despite the good short-term results."[193] We do not agree with this negative viewpoint.

There are some women for whom the risk of complications is so high that pregnancy is relatively contraindicated. There is a high maternal mortality rate among those who have had myocardial infarctions,[205] so we discourage pregnancy in these women. Women bordering on ESRD (creatinine clearance <30 ml/min, serum creatinine >3 mg/dl) should be considered for renal transplantation or dialysis before pregnancy. Patients in whom hypertension cannot be controlled should be advised that there is a low probability of a successful pregnancy. Women with proliferative retinopathy should be in remission or have laser photocoagulation before becoming pregnant because exacerbations are less frequent under these conditions.

Except for these contraindications, the decision to become pregnant or to continue a pregnancy should largely be one of informed consent. A woman with diabetic nephropathy must be counseled about the progressive nature of the disease. It is important to discuss the implications of a chronic disease on her ability to raise a child and to explore the possibility that she may not survive the child's adolescence. The likely financial burden of pregnancy and neonatal care should be disclosed. After adequate counseling, it is up to the patient and her partner to decide whether to proceed with pregnancy. If this is their wish, with meticulous attention to glycemic control, blood pressure control, diet, bed rest, and fetal surveillance, and excellent outcome can often be obtained.

REFERENCES

1. Mauer SM, Steffes MW, Ellis EN et al: Structural-functional relationship in diabetic nephropathy. J Clin Invest 74:1143, 1984

2. Osterby R, Parving H-H, Nyberg G et al: Morphology of diabetic glomerulopathy and relationship to hypertension. Diabete Metab 15:278, 1989

3. Osterby R, Parving HH, Hommel E et al: Glomerular structure and function in diabetic nephropathy. Early to advanced stages. Diabetes 39:1057, 1990

4. Mogensen CE: Early glomerular hyperfiltration in insulin-dependent diabetes and late nephropathy. Scand J Clin Lab Invest 46:201, 1986

5. Mogensen CE: Microalbuminuria as a predictor of clinical diabetic nephropathy. Kidney Int 31:673, 1987

6. Deckert T, Kofoed-Enevoldsen A, Norgaard K et al: Microalbuminuria: implications for micro- and macrovascular disease. Diabetes Care 15:1181, 1992

7. Larkins RG, Dunlop ME: The link between hyperglycaemia and diabetic nephropathy. Diabetologia 35:499, 1992

8. Mogensen CE, Chachati A, Christensen CK et al: Microalbuminuria: an early marker of renal involvement in diabetes. Uremia Invest 9:85, 1985

9. Mogensen CE, Schmitz O: The diabetic kidney: from hyperfiltration and microalbuminuria to end-stage renal failure. Med Clin North Am 72:1465, 1988

10. Centers for Disease Control: End-stage renal disease associated with diabetes. United States, 1988. MMWR 38:546, 1989

11. Borch-Johnsen K, Andersen PK, Deckert T: The effect of proteinuria on relative mortality in type 1 (insulin-dependent) diabetes mellitus. Diabetologia 28:590, 1985

12. Borch-Johnsen K, Kreiner S: Proteinuria: value as predictor of cardiovascular mortality in insulin-dependent diabetes mellitus. BMJ 294:1651, 1987

13. Jensen T, Borch-Johnsen K, Kofoed-Enevoldsen A, Deckert T: Coronary heart disease in young type 1 (insulin dependent) diabetic patients with and without diabetic nephropathy: incidence and risk factors. Diabetologia 30:144, 1987

14. Pugh JA, Medina R, Ramirez R: Comparison of the course to end-stage renal disease of type 1 (insulin-dependent) diabetic nephropathy. Diabetologia 36:1094, 1993

15. Neil A, Hawkins M, Potok M et al: A prospective population-based study of microalbuminuria as a predictor of mortality in NIDDM. Diabetes Care 16:996, 1993

16. Tsalamandris C, Allen TJ, Gilbert RE et al: Progressive decline in renal function in diabetic patients with and without albuminuria. Diabetes 43:649, 1994

17. D'Antonio JA, Ellis D, Doft BH et al: Diabetes complications and glycemic control: the Pittsburgh Prospective Insulin-Dependent Diabetes Cohort Study status report after 5 yr of IDDM. Diabetes Care 12:694, 1989

18. EURODIAB IDDM Complications Study Group: Microvascular and acute complications in IDDM patients: the EURODIAB IDDM Complications Study. Diabetologia 37:278, 1994

19. Mathiesen ER, Ronn B, Jensen T et al: Relationship between blood pressure and urinary albumin excretion in development of microalbuminuria. Diabetes 39:245, 1990

20. Raal FJ, Kalk WJ, Taylor DR et al: The relationship between the development and progression of microalbuminuria and arterial blood pressure in type 1 (insulin-dependent) diabetes mellitus. Diabetes Res Clin Pract 16:221, 1992

21. Coonrod BA, Ellis D, Becker DJ et al: Predictors of microalbuminuria in individuals with IDDM. Diabetes Care 16:1376, 1993

22. Chase HP, Garg SK, Marshall G et al: Cigarette smoking increases the risk of albuminuria among subjects with type 1 diabetes. JAMA 254:614, 1991

23. Almdal T, Feldt-Rasmussen B, Norgaard K, Deckert T: The predictive value of microalbuminuria in IDDM. Diabetes Care 17:120, 1994

24. Parving H-H, Oxenboll B, Svendsen PAA et al: Early detection of patients at risk of developing diabetic nephropathy: a longitudinal study of urinary albumin excretion. Acta Endocrinol (Copenh) 100:550, 1982

25. Viberti GC, Hill RD, Jarrett RJ et al: Microalbuminuria as a predictor of clinical nephropathy in insulin-dependent diabetes mellitus. Lancet 1:1430, 1982

26. Mogensen CE, Christensen CK: Predicting diabetic nephropathy in insulin-dependent patients. N Engl J Med 311:89, 1984

27. Mathiesen ER, Oxenboll B, Johansen K et al: Incipient nephropathy in type 1 (insulin-dependent) diabetes. Diabetologia 26:406, 1984

28. Deckert T, Andersen AR, Christiansen JS, Andersen JK: Course of diabetic nephropathy. Factors related to development. Acta Endocrinol (Copenh), suppl. 242, 97:14, 1981

29. Andersen AR, Christiansen JS, Andersen JK et al: Diabetic nephropathy in type 1 (insulin-dependent) diabetes mellitus. Diabetologia 28:590, 1985

30. Kofoed-Enevoldsen A, Borch-Johnsen K, Kreiner S et al: Declining incidence of persistent proteinuria in type I (insulin-dependent) diabetic patients in Denmark. Diabetes 36:205, 1987

31. Krolewski AS, Warram JH, Christlieb AR et al: The changing natural history of nephropathy in type I diabetes. Am J Med 78:785, 1985

32. Bojestig M, Arnqvist HJ, Hermansson G et al: Declining incidence of nephropathy in insulin-dependent diabetes mellitus. N Engl J Med 330:15, 1994

33. Gall MA, Rossing P, Skott P et al: Prevalence of micro- and macroalbuminuria, arterial hypertension, retinopathy and large vessel disease in European type 2 (non-insulin-dependent) diabetic patients. Diabetologia 34:655, 1991

34. Schmitz A: Renal function changes in middle-aged and elderly Caucasian type 2 (non-insulin-dependent) diabetic patients—review. Diabetologia 36:985, 1993

35. Gall MA, Nielsen FS, Smidt UM, Parving HH: The course of the kidney function in type 2 (non-insulin-dependent) diabetic patients with diabetic nephropathy. Diabetologia 36:1071, 1993

36. Seaquist ER, Goetz FC, Rich S, Barbosa J: Familial clustering of diabetic kidney disease—evidence for genetic susceptibility to diabetic nephropathy. N Engl J Med 320:1161, 1989

37. Doria A, Warram JH, Krolewski AS: Genetic predisposition to diabetic nephropathy—evidence for a role of the angiotensin I-converting enzyme gene. Diabetes 43:690, 1994

38. Viberti GC, Keen H, Wiseman MJ: Raised arterial pressure in parents of proteinuric insulin dependent diabetics. BMJ 295:515, 1987

39. Krolewski AS, Canessa M, Warram JH et al: Predisposition to hypertension and susceptibility to renal disease in insulin-dependent diabetes mellitus. N Engl J Med 318:140, 1988

40. Mangili R, Bending JJ, Scott G et al: Increased sodium-lithium countertransport activity in red cells of patients with insulin-dependent diabetes and nephropathy. N Engl J Med 318:146, 1988

41. Jensen JS, Mathiesen ER, Norgaard K et al: Increased blood pressure and erythrocyte sodium/lithium countertransport activity are not inherited in diabetic nephropathy. Diabetologia 33:619, 1990

42. Walker JD, Tariqu T, Viberti GC: Sodium-lithium countertransport activity in red cells of patients with insulin dependent diabetes and nephropathy and their parents. BMJ 301:635, 1990

43. Elving LD, Wetzels JFM, de Nobel E, Berder JHM: Erythrocyte sodium-lithium countertransport is not different in type 1 (insulin-dependent) diabetic patients with and without diabetic nephropathy. Diabetologia 34:126, 1994

44. Deckert T, Feldt-Rasmussen B, Borch-Johnsen K et al: Albuminuria reflects widespread vascular damage—the Steno hypothesis. Diabetologia 32:219, 1989

45. Kanwar YS, Liu ZZ, Kashihara N, Wallner EI: Current status of the structural and functional basis of glomerular filtration and proteinuria. Semin Nephrol 11:390, 1991

46. Abuelo JG: Renal Pathophysiology—The Essentials. Williams & Wilkins, Baltimore, 1989

47. Gellman DD, Pirani CC, Soothill JF: Diabetic nephropathy: a clinical and pathologic study based on renal biopsies. Medicine (Baltimore) 38:321, 1959

48. Arieff AI, Myers BD: Diabetic nephropathy. p. 1906. In Brenner BM, Rector FC Jr (eds): The Kidney. WB Saunders, Philadephia, 1981

49. Kimmelstiel P, Wilson C: Intercapillary lesions in glomeruli of kidney. Am J Pathol 12:83, 1936

50. Steffes MW, Osterby R, Chavers B, Mauer M: Mesangial expansion as a central mechanism for loss of kidney function in diabetic patients. Diabetes 38:1077, 1989

51. Mogensen CE: The effect of blood pressure intervention on renal function in insulin-dependent diabetes. Diabete Metab 15:343, 1989

52. Hirsch IB: Current concepts in diabetic nephropathy. Clin Diabetes 12:8, 1994

53. Christiansen JS, Gammelgaard J, Tronier B: Kidney function and size in diabetics before and during initial insulin treatment. Kidney Int 21:683, 1982

54. Mogensen CE: Glomerular filtration rate and renal plasma flow in short-term juvenile diabetes mellitus. Scand J Clin Lab Invest 28:91, 1971

55. Hirose K, Tsuchida H, Osterby R, Gundersen HJG: A strong correlation between glomerular filtration rate and filtration surface in diabetic kidney hyperfunction. Lab Invest 43:434, 1980

56. Mogensen CE, Christensen CK, Vittinghus E: The stages in diabetic renal disease, with emphasis on the stage of incipient diabetic nephropathy. Diabetes, suppl. 2, 32:64, 1983

57. Viberti GC, Bilous RW, Mackintosh D, Keen H: Monitoring glomerular function in diabetic nephropathy: a prospective study. Am J Med 74:256, 1983

58. Mogensen CE, Osterby R, Gundersen HJG: Early functional and morphologic vascular renal consequences of the diabetic state. Diabetologia 17:71, 1979

59. Brochner-Mortensen J, Ditzel J: Glomerular filtration rate and extracellular fluid volume in insulin-dependent patients with diabetes mellitus. Kidney Int 21:696, 1982

60. Ellis EN, Steffes MW, Goetz FC et al: Glomerular filtration surface in type I diabetes mellitus. Kidney Int 29:889, 1986

61. Osterby R, Parving HH, Nyberg G et al: A strong correlation between glomerular filtration rate and filtration surface in diabetic nephropathy. Diabetologia 31:265, 1988

62. Osterby R, Gundersen HJG: Glomerular size and structure in diabetes mellitus. I. Early abnormalities. Diabetologia 11:225, 1975

63. Osterby R, Gundersen HJG, Nyberg G, Aurell M: Advanced diabetic glomerulopathy: quantitative structural characterization of non-occluded glomeruli. Diabetes 36:612, 1987

64. Chavers BM, Bilous FW, Ellis EN et al: Glomerular lesions and urinary albumin excretion in type I diabetes without overt proteinuria. N Engl J Med 320:966, 1989

65. Diabetes Control and Complications Trial Research Group: The effect of intensive treatment of diabetes on the development and progression of long-term complications in insulin-dependent diabetes mellitus. N Engl J Med 329:977, 1993

66. Silverstein JH, Fennell R, Donnelly W: Correlates of biopsy-studied nephropathy in young patients with insulin-dependent diabetes mellitus. J Pediatr 106:196, 1985

67. Osterby R, Gundersen HJG, Horlyck A et al: Diabetic glomerulopathy. Structural characteristics of the early and advanced stages, Diabetes, suppl. 2, 32:79, 1983

68. Bilous RW, Mauer SM, Sutherland DER, Steffes MW: Mean glomerular volume and rate of development of diabetic nephropathy. Diabetes 38:1142, 1989

69. Nakamura Y, Myers BD: Charge selectivity of proteinuria in diabetic glomerulopathy. Diabetes 37:1202, 1988

70. Viberti G, Mackintosh D, Keen H: Determinants of the penetration of proteins through the glomerular barrier in insulin-dependent diabetes mellitus. Diabetes, suppl. 2, 32:92, 1983

71. Kreisberg JI, Venkatachalam M, Troyer D: Contractile properties of cultured mesangial cells. Am J Physiol 249: F457, 1985

72. Eisenbach GM, VanLiew JB, Boylen JW: Effect of angiotensin on the filtration of protein in the rat kidney: a micropuncture study. Kidney Int 8:80, 1975

73. Myers BD, Vinetz JA, Chui F, Michaels AS: Mechanisms of proteinuria in diabetic nephropathy: a study of glomerular barrier function. Kidney Int 21:633, 1982

74. Deckert T, Feldt-Rasmussen B, Djurup R, Deckert M: Glomerular size and charge selectivity in insulin dependent diabetes mellitus. Kidney Int 33:100, 1988

75. Makino H, Yamasaki Y, Haramoto T et al: Ultrastructural changes of extracellular matrices in diabetic nephropathy revealed by high resolution scanning and immunoelectron microscopy. Lab Invest 68:45, 1993

76. Chigguri GM, Candiano G, Delfino G et al: Glycosyl albumin and diabetic microalbuminuria: demonstration of altered renal handling. Kidney Int 25:565, 1984

77. Cohen M, Sharma K, Jin Y, Ziyadeh F: Abrogating effects of glycated albumin in vivo ameliorates diabetic nephropathy. Diabetes, suppl. 1, 43:105A, 1994

78. Friedman EA: Diabetic nephropathy: strategies in prevention and management. Kidney Int 21:780, 1982

79. Cagliero E, Roth T, Roy S, Lorenzi M: Characteristics and mechanisms of high-glucose-induced overexpression of basement membrane components in cultured human endothelial cells. Diabetes 40:102, 1991

80. Haneda M, Kikkawa R, Horide N et al: Glucose enhances type IV collagen production in cultured rat glomerular mesangial cells. Diabetologia 34:198, 1991
81. Pugliese G, Pricci F, Pugliese F et al: Mechanisms of glucose-enhanced extracellular matrix accumulation in rat glomerular mesangial cells. Diabetes 43:478, 1994
82. Vernier RL, Steffes MW, Sisson-Ross S, Mauer SM: Heparan sulfate proteoglycan in the glomerular basement membrane in type 1 diabetes mellitus. Kidney Int 41: 1070, 1992
83. Falk RJ, Scheinman JI, Mauer SM, Michael AF: Polyantigenic expansion of basement membrane constituents in diabetic nephropathy. Diabetes, suppl. 22, 32:34, 1983
84. Shimomura H, Spiro RG: Studies on macromolecular components of human glomerular basement membrane and alterations in diabetes—decreased levels of heparan sulfate proteoglycan and laminin. Diabetes 36: 374, 1987
85. Tamsma JT, Van Den Born J, Bruin JA et al: Expression of glomerular extracellular matrix components in human diabetic nephropathy: decrease of heparan sulphate in the glomerular basement membrane. Diabetologia 37: 313, 1994
86. Rohrbach DH, Wagner CW, Star VL et al: Reduced synthesis of basement membrane heparan sulphate proteoglycan in streptozotocin-induced diabetic mice. J Biol Chem 258:11672, 1983
87. Wu VY, Wilson B, Cohen MP: Disturbances in glomerular basement membrane glycosaminoglycans in experimental diabetes. Diabetes 36:679, 1987
88. Groggel GC, Marindes GN, Hovingh P et al: Inhibition of rat mesangial cell growth by heparan sulfate. Am J Physiol 258:F259, 1990
89. Cohen MP, Klepser H, Wu VY: Undersulfation of glomerular basement membrane heparan sulfate in experimental diabetes and lack of correction with aldose reductase inhibition. Diabetes 37:1324, 1988
90. Kofoed-Enevoldsen A: Inhibition of glomerular glucosaminyl N-deacetylase in diabetic rats. Kidney Int 41: 763, 1992
91. Unger E, Pettersson I, Eriksson UJ et al: Decreased activity of the heparin sulfate modifying enzyme glucosaminyl N-deacetylase in hepatocytes from streptozotocin-diabetic rats. J Biol Chem 266:8671, 1991
92. Tarsio FJ, Reger LA, Furcht LT: Molecular mechanisms in basement membrane complications of diabetes—alterations in heparin, laminin and type IV collagen association. Diabetes 37:532, 1988
93. Brownlee M, Cerami A, Vlasser H: Advanced glycosylation end products in tissue and the biochemical basis of diabetic complications. N Engl J Med 318:1315, 1988
94. Brownlee M: Glycation and diabetic complications. Diabetes 43:836, 1994
95. Vlassara H, Bucala R, Striker L: Pathogenic effects of advanced glycosylation: biochemical, biologic, and clinical implications for diabetes and aging. Lab Invest 70: 138, 1994
96. Skolnik EY, Yang Z, Makita Z et al: Human and rat mesangial cell receptors for glucose-modified proteins: potential role in kidney tissue remodelling and diabetic nephropathy. J Exp Med 174:515, 1994
97. Doi T, Vlassara H, Kirstein M et al: Receptor specific increase in extracellular matrix production in mouse mesangial cells by advanced glycosylation end products is mediated via platelet derived growth factor. Proc Natl Acad Sci USA 89:2873, 1992
98. Striker LJ, Peten EP, Elliot SJ et al: Mesangial cell turnover: effect of heparin and peptide growth factors. Lab Invest 64:446, 1991
99. Esposito C, Gerlach H, Brett J et al: Endothelial receptor-mediated binding of glucose-modified albumin is associated with increased monolayer permeability and modulation of cell surface coagulant properties. J Exp Med 170:1387, 1989
100. Edelstein D, Brownlee M: Aminoguanidine ameliorates albuminuria in diabetic hypertensive rats. Diabetologia 35:96, 1992
101. Ellis EN, Good BH: Prevention of glomerular basement membrane thickening by aminoguanidine in experimental diabetes mellitus. Metabolism 40:1016, 1991
102. Shah SV: Role of reactive oxygen metabolites in experimental glomerular disease. Kidney Int 35:1093, 1989
103. Wolff SP, Dean RT: Glucose autoxidation and protein modification: the potential role of autoxidative glycosylation in diabetes. Biochem J 245:243, 1987
104. Packer L: The role of anti-oxidative treatment in diabetes mellitus. Diabetologia 36:1212, 1993
105. Tada H, Kuboki K, Ishii H et al: Impaired degradation of hydrogen peroxide in isolated glomeruli of streptozocin-induced diabetes. Diabetes, suppl. 1, 43:105A, 1994
106. Mullarkey CJ, Edelstein D, Brownlee M: Free radical generation by early glycation products: a mechanism for accelerated atherogenesis in diabetes. Biochem Biophys Res Commun 173:932, 1990
107. King GL, Shiba T, Oliver J et al: Cellular and molecular abnormalities in the vascular endothelium of diabetes mellitus. Annu Rev Med 45:179, 1994
108. Greene DA, Lattimer SA, Sima AAF: Sorbitol, phosphoinositides, and sodium-potassium-ATPase in the pathogenesis of diabetic complications. N Engl J Med 316: 599, 1987
109. Chang WP, Dimitriadis E, Allen T et al: The effect of

aldose reductase inhibitors on glomerular prostaglandin production and urinary albumin excretion in experimental diabetes mellitus. Diabetologia 34:225, 1991

110. Kern T, Engerman R: Effect of aldose reductase inhibition on renal disease in diabetic dogs. Diabetes, suppl. 1, 43:105A, 1994

111. Derubertis FR, Craven PA: Activation of protein kinase C in glomerular cells in diabetes. Diabetes 43:1, 1994

112. Craven PA, DeRubertis FR: Protein kinase C is activated in glomeruli from streptozotocin diabetic rats: possible mediation by glucose. J Clin Invest 83:1667, 1989

113. Ayo SH, Radnik R, Garoni J et al: High glucose increases diacylglycerol mass and activates protein kinase C in mesangial cell cultures. Am J Physiol 260:F185, 1990

114. Craven PA, Davidson CM, DeRubertis FR: Increase in diacylglycerol mass in isolated glomeruli by glucose from de novo synthesis of glycerolipids. Diabetes 39:667, 1990

115. Spurney RF, Onorato JJ, Alberts FJ, Cofman TM: Thromboxane binding and signal transduction in rat glomerular mesangial cells. Am J Physiol 264:F292, 1993

116. Williams B, Schrier RW: Glucose-induced protein kinase C activity regulates arachidonic acid release and prostaglandin production by cultured rat glomerular mesangial cells. J Am Soc Nephrol 2:302, 1991

117. Oliver JA: Adenylate cyclase and protein kinase C mediate opposite reactions on endothelial junctions. J Cell Physiol 145:536, 1990

118. Lynch JJ, Ferro TJ, Blumenstock FA et al: Increased endothelial albumin permeability mediated by protein kinase C activation. J Clin Invest 85:1991, 1990

119. Studer RK, Craven PA, DeRubertis FR: Activation of protein kinase C reduces thromboxane receptors in glomeruli and mesangial cells. Kidney Int 44:58, 1993

120. Studer RK, Craven PA, DeRubertis FR: Thromboxane stimulation of mesangial cell fibronectin synthesis is signaled by activation of protein kinase C and is modulated by cGMP. J Am Soc Nephrol 4:458, 1993

121. Brenner BM: Hemodynamically mediated glomerular injury and the progressive nature of kidney disease. Kidney Int 23:647, 1983

122. Parving H-H, Viberti GC, Keen H et al: Hemodynamic factors in genesis of diabetic microangiopathy. Metabolism 32:943, 1983

123. Hostetter TH: Diabetic nephropathy. N Engl J Med 312:642, 1985

124. Wiseman M, Viberti GC: Kidney size and glomerular filtration rate in type I (insulin-dependent) diabetes mellitus revisited. Diabetologia 25:530, 1983

125. Ellis EN, Steffes MW, Goetz FC et al: Relationship of renal size to nephropathy in type I (insulin-dependent) diabetes. Diabetologia 28:12, 1985

126. Wiseman MJ, Saunders AJ, Keen H, Viberti G: Effect of blood glucose control on increased glomerular filtration rate and kidney size in insulin-dependent diabetes. N Engl J Med 3112:617, 1985

127. Hostetter TH, Renneke HG, Brenner BM: The case for intrarenal hypertension in the initiation and progression of diabetic and other glomerulopathies. Am J Med 72:375, 1982

128. Steffes MW, Brown DM, Mauer SM: Diabetic glomerulopathy following unilateral nephrectomy in the rat. Diabetes 27:35, 1978

129. Christiansen JS, Frandsen M, Parving H-H: Effect of intravenous glucose infusion on renal function in normal man and insulin-dependent diabetics. Diabetologia 21:368, 1981

130. Ditzel J, Brochner-Mortensen J: Tubular reabsorption rates as related to elevated glomerular filtration in diabetic children. Diabetes, suppl. 2, 32:28, 1983

131. Körner A, Eklöf A-C, Celsi G, Aperia A: Increased renal metabolism in diabetes: mechanism and functional implications. Diabetes 43:629, 1994

132. Bank N: Mechanisms of diabetic hyperfiltration. Kidney Int 40:792, 1991

133. Brosius FC III: Molecular and cellular aspects of diabetes mellitus: applications to diabetic nephropathy. Semin Nephrol 12:554, 1994

134. Kasiske BL, O'Donnell MP, Keane WF: Glucose-induced increases in renal hemodynamic function. Possible modulation by renal prostaglandins. Diabetes 34:360, 1985

135. Bank N, Aynedjian JS: Role of EDRF (nitric oxide) in diabetic renal hyperfiltration. Kidney Int 43:1306, 1993

136. Kreisberg JI, Ayo SH: The glomerular mesangium in diabetes mellitus. Kidney Int 43:109, 1993

137. Feldt-Rasmussen B: Increased transcapillary escape rate of albumin in type 1 (insulin-dependent) diabetic patients with microalbuminuria. Diabetologia 29:282, 1986

138. Jensen T: Increased plasma concentration of von Willebrand factor in insulin dependent diabetics with incipient nephropathy. BMJ 298:27, 1989

139. Valdorf-Hansen F, Jensen T, Borch-Johnsen K, Deckert T: Cardiovascular risk factors in type I (insulin-dependent) diabetic patients with and without proteinuria. J Intern Med 222:439, 1987

140. Deckert T, Jensen T, Feldt-Rasmussen B et al: Albuminuria, a risk marker of atherosclerosis in insulin-dependent diabetes mellitus. Cardiovasc Risk Factors 1:347, 1991

141. Feldt-Rasmussen B, Norgaard K, Jensen T et al: The role of hypertension in the development of nephropathy in type 1 (insulin-dependent) diabetes mellitus. Acta Diabetol 27:173, 1990

142. Mogensen CE, Hansen KW, Osterby R, Damsgaard EM: Blood pressure elevation versus abnormal albuminuria in the genesis and prediction of renal disease in diabetes. Diabetes Care 15:1192, 1992

143. Chase HP, Garg SK, Harris A et al: High-normal blood pressure and early diabetic nephropathy. Arch Intern Med 150:639, 1990

144. Kasiske BL, Kalil RSN, Ma JZ et al: Effect of antihypertensive therapy on the kidney in patients with diabetes: a meta-regression analysis. Ann Intern Med 118:129, 1993

145. Heeg JE, de Jong PE, Van der Hem GK, de Zeuuw D: Efficacy and variability of the antiproteinuric effect of ACE inhibitors by lisinopril. Kidney Int 36:272, 1989

146. Slataper R, Vicknair N, Sadler R, Bakris L: Comparative effects of different antihypertensive treatments on progression of diabetic renal disease. Arch Intern Med 153:973, 1993

147. Viberti B, Mogensen CE, Groop LC et al: Effect of captopril on progression to clinical proteinuria in patients with insulin-dependent diabetes mellitus and microalbuminuria. JAMA 271:275, 1994

148. Lewis EJ, Hunsicker LG, Bain RP et al: The effect of angiotensin-converting-enzyme inhibition on diabetic nephropathy. N Engl J Med 329:1456, 1993

149. Hanssens M, Keirse MJNC, Vankelecom F, Assche FAV: Fetal and neonatal effects of treatment with angiotensin-converting enzyme inhibitors in pregnancy. Obstet Gynecol 78:128, 1991

150. Consensus Statement. Diabetic nephropathy. Am J Kidney Dis 13:2, 1989

151. Mogensen CE, Hansen KW, Pederson MM, Christensen CK: Renal factors influencing blood pressure threshold and choice of treatment for hypertension in IDDM. Diabetes Care, suppl. 4, 14:13, 1991

152. Consensus Statement. Treatment of hypertension in diabetes. Diabetes Care 16:1394, 1993

153. Fairlie FM, Sibai BM: Hypertensive diseases in pregnancy. p. 938. In Reece EA, Hobbins JC, Mahoney MJ, Petrie RH (eds): Medicine of the Fetus and Mother. JB Lippincott, Philadelphia, 1992

154. Cockburn J, Ounsted M, Moar VA, Redman CWG: Final report of study on hypertension during pregnancy: the effects of specific treatment on the growth and development of the children. Lancet 1:647, 1982

155. Bakris GL: The effects of calcium antagonists on renal hemodynamics, urinary protein excretion and glomerular morphology in diabetic states. J Am Soc Nephrol, suppl. I, 2:21, 1991

156. Bakris GL, Barnhill BW, Sadler R: Treatment of arterial hypertension in diabetic man: importance of therapeutic selection. Kidney Int 41:898, 1992

157. Demarie B, Barkris GL: Effects of different calcium antagonists on proteinuria associated with diabetes mellitus. Ann Intern Med 113:987, 1990

158. Jerums G, Cooper ME, Seeman E et al: Comparison of early renal dysfunction in type I and type II diabets: differing associations with blood pressure and glycaemic control. Diabetes Res Clin Pract 4:133, 1988

159. McNally PG, Burden AC, Swift PGF et al: The prevalence and risk factors assocaited with the onset of diabetic nephropathy in juvenile-onset (insulin-dependent) diabetics diagnosed under the age of 17 years in Leicestershire 1930–1985. Q J Med 76:831, 1990

160. Kalk WJ, Osler C, Taylor D, Panz VR: Prior long term glycaemic control and insulin therapy in insulin-dependent diabetic adolescents with microalbuminuria. Diabetes Res Clin Pract 9:83, 1990

161. Watts F, Harris R, Shaw KM: The determinants of early nephropathy in insulin-dependent diabetes mellitus: a prospective study based on the urinary excretion of albumin. Q J Med 79:365, 1991

162. McCance DR, Hadden DR, Atkinson AB et al: The relationship between long-term glycaemic control and diabetic nephropathy. Q J Med 82:53, 1992

163. Feldt-Rasmussen B, Mathiesen ER, Hegedus L, Deckert T: Kidney function during 12 months of strict metabolic control in insulin-dependent diabetic patients with incipient nephropathy. N Engl J Med 314:665, 1986

164. Tuttle KR, Bruton JL, Perusek MC et al: Effect of strict glycemic control on renal hemodynamic response to amino acids and renal enlargement in insulin-dependent diabetes mellitus. N Engl J Med 324:1626, 1991

165. Tuttle KR, DeFronzo RA, Stein JH: Treatment of diabetic nephropathy: a rational approach based on its pathophysiology. Semin Nephrol 11:220, 1991

166. Feldt-Rasmussen B, Mathiesen ER, Jensen T et al: Effect of improved metabolic control on loss of kidney function in type 1 (insulin-dependent) diabetic patients: an update of the Steno studies. Diabetologia 34:164, 1991

167. Reichard P, Rosenqvist U: Nephropathy is delayed by intensified insulin treatment in patients with insulin-dependent diabetes mellitus and retinopathy. J Intern Med 226:81, 1989

168. Reichard P, Nilsson B-Y, Rosenqvist U: The effect of long-term insulin treatment on the development of microvascular complication of diabetes mellitus. N Engl J Med 329:304, 1993

169. Viberti GC, Bilous RW, Mackintosh D: Long-term correction of hyperglycemia and progression of renal failure in insulin-dependent diabetes. BMJ 286:598, 1983

170. Cataland S, O'Dorisio TM: Diabetic nephropathy. JAMA 249:2059, 1983

171. Tamborlane WV, Pukoin JE, Bergman M et al: Long-term improvement of metabolic control with the insulin

pump does not reverse microangiopathy. Diabetes Care, suppl. 1, 5:58, 1982

172. Brenner BM, Meyer TW, Hostetter TH: Dietary protein intake and the progressive nature of kidney disease: the role of hemodynamically mediated glomerular injury in the pathogenesis of progressive glomerular sclerosis in aging, renal ablation, and intrinsic renal disease. N Engl J Med 307:652, 1982

173. Zatz R, Meyer TW, Rennke HG et al: Predominance of hemodynamic rather than metabolic factors in the pathogenesis of diabetic glomerulopathy. Proc Natl Acad Sci USA 82:5963, 1985

174. Barsotti G, Ciardella F, Morelli E et al: Nutritional treatment of renal failure in type 1 diabetic nephropathy. Clin Nephrol 29:280, 1988

175. Evanoff G, Thompson C, Brown J, Weinman E: Prolonged dietary protein restriction in diabetic nephropathy. Arch Intern Med 149:1129, 1989

176. Walker JD, Dodds RA, Murrells TJ et al: Restriction of dietary protein and progression of renal failure in diabetic nephropathy. Lancet 2:1411, 1989

177. Dodds RA, Keen H: Low protein diet and conservation of renal function in diabetic nephropathy. Diabete Metab 16:464, 1990

178. Zeller K, Whittaker E, Sullivan L et al: Effect of restricting dietary protein on the progression of renal failure in patients with insulin-dependent diabetes mellitus. N Engl J Med 324:78, 1991

179. Brodsky IG, Robbins DC, Hiser E et al: Effects of low-protein diets on protein metabolism in insulin-dependent diabetes mellitus patients with early nephropathy. J Clin Endocrinol Metab 75:351, 1992

180. Levine SE, D'Elia JA, Bistrian B et al: Protein-restricted diets in diabetic nephropathy. Nephron 52:55, 1989

181. Schichiri M, Hishio Y, Ogura M, Marumo F: Effect of low-protein, very-low-phosphorus diet on diabetic renal insufficiency with proteinuria. Am J Kidney Dis 18:26, 1991

182. Sawicki PT, Didjurget U, Muhlhauser I et al: Smoking is associated with progression of diabetic nephropathy. Diabetes Care 17:126, 1994

183. Fuhrmann K, Reiher H, Semmler K, Glockner E: The effect of intensified conventional insulin therapy before and during pregnancy on the malformation rate in offspring of diabetic mothers. Exp Clin Endocrinol 83:173, 1984

184. Steel JM, Johnstone FD, Hepburn DA, Smith A: Can pre-pregnancy care of diabetic women reduce the risk of abnormal babies? BMJ 301:1070, 1990

185. Kitzmiller JL, Gavin LA, Gin GD et al: Preconception care of diabetes: glycemic control prevents congenital anomalies. JAMA 265:731, 1991

186. Combs CS, Kitzmiller JL: Spontaneous abortion and congenital malformations in diabetes. Baillieres Clin Obstet Gynaecol 5:315, 1991

187. Damm P, Molsted-Pedersen L: Significant decrease in congenital malformations in newborn infants of an unselected population of diabetic women. Am J Obstet Gynecol 161:1163, 1989

188. Combs CA, Wheeler BC, Kitzmiller JL: Urinary protein/creatinine ratio before and during pregnancy in women with diabetes mellitus. Am J Obstet Gynecol 165:920, 1991

189. Manske CL, Thomas W, Wang Y, Wilson RF: Screening diabetic transplant candidates for coronary artery disease: identification of a low risk subgroup. Kidney Int 44:617, 1993

190. Kitzmiller JL, Brown ER, Phillippe M et al: Diabetic nephropathy and perinatal outcome. Am J Obstet Gynecol 141:741, 1981

191. Reece EA, Coustan DR, Hayslett JP et al: Diabetic nephropathy: pregnancy performance and fetomaternal outcome. Am J Obstet Gynecol 159:56, 1988

192. Jovanovic R, Jovanovic L: Obstetric management when normoglycemia is maintained in diabetic pregnant women with vascular compromise. Am J Obstet Gynecol 149:617, 1984

193. Grenfell A, Brudenell JM, Doddridge MC et al: Pregnancy in diabetic women who have proteinuria. Q J Med 59:379, 1986

194. Combs CA, Rosenn B, Kitzmiller JL et al: Early-pregnancy proteinuria in diabetes related to preeclampsia. Obstet Gynecol 82:802, 1993

195. Kimmerle R, Zass R-P, Cupisti S et al: Pregnancies in women with diabetic nephropathy: longterm outcome for mother and child. Diabetologia 38:227, 1995

196. Winocour PH, Taylor RJ, Steel JM: Early alterations of renal function in insulin-dependent diabetic pregnancies and their importance in predicting pre-eclamptic toxaemia. Lancet 2:975, 1984

197. Ogburn PL Jr, Kitzmiller JL, Hare JW et al: Pregnancy following renal transplantation in class T diabetes mellitus. JAMA 255:911, 1986

198. Greene MF, Hare JW, Krache M et al: Prematurity among insulin-requiring diabetic gravid women. Am J Obstet Gynecol 161:106, 1989

199. Yankowitz J, Piraino B, Laifer A et al: Use of erythropoietin in pregnancies complicated by severe anemia of renal failure. Obstet Gynecol 80:485, 1992

200. Kitzmiller JL: Sweet success with diabetes. The development of insulin therapy and glycemic control for pregnancy. Diabetes Care, suppl. 3, 16:107, 1993

201. Landon MD, Langer O, Gabbe SG et al: Fetal surveillance in pregnancies complicated by insulin-dependent diabetes mellitus. Am J Obstet Gynecol 167:617, 1992

202. Salvesen DR, Higueras MT, Brudenell JM et al: Doppler

velocimetry and fetal heart rate studies in nephropathy diabetics. Am J Obstet Gynecol 167:1297, 1992

203. Biesenbach G, Stoger H, Zazgornik J: Influence of pregnancy on progression of diabetic nephropathy and subsequent requirement of renal replacement therapy in female type I diabetic patients with impaired renal function. Nephrol Dial Transplant 7:105, 1992

204. Reece EA, Winn HN, Hayslett JY et al: Does pregnancy alter the rate of progression of diabetic nephropathy? Am J Perinatol 7:193, 1990

205. Hare JW: Diabetic neuropathy and coronary heart disease. p. 515. In Reece EA, Coustan DR (eds): Diabetes Mellitus in Pregnancy: Principles and Practice. 1st Ed. Churchill Livingstone, New York, 1988

21
Diabetic Neuropathy and Coronary Heart Disease

FLORENCE M. BROWN
JOHN W. HARE

NEUROPATHY AS A COMPLICATION OF DIABETIC PREGNANCY

Neuropathic complications of both type I and type II diabetes are remarkably common. Pregnancy in women with diabetes is also a common event and receives a great deal of attention, both in the literature and in professional societies. Nevertheless, only a few scientific articles report on neuropathy as a complication of pregnancy, and these focus on the topic of autonomic neuropathy. It is unclear whether, and to what extent, pregnancy influences the short- and long-term complications of neuropathy. Given the beneficial effect of improved diabetes control on peripheral neuropathy, as demonstrated by the Diabetes Control and Complications Trial,[1] one might expect that the improved metabolic parameters that are mandated during a diabetic pregnancy would lead to short-term improvement in measures of nerve function. By contrast, because compression neuropathies are more common with pregnancy and with diabetes independently, one would expect an even higher incidence of these during the diabetic pregnancy. The purpose of this section of the chapter is to discuss the serious potential impact of autonomic neuropathy on the diabetic pregnancy and to review other forms of neuropathy so that the reader will be able to recognize them, should they become manifested during pregnancy.

Autonomic Neuropathy

Autonomic neuropathy refers to dysfunction of the nerves that innervate the heart and blood vessels, bladder, bowel, stomach, and sweat glands. Orthostatic hy-

potension, one manifestation of autonomic neuropathy, is defined by a fall of 20 to 30 mm Hg in systolic blood pressure or fall of 10 to 15 mm Hg in diastolic blood pressure, when changing from a supine to standing position, and it may cause patients to have symptoms of lightheadedness or near syncope. Failure of the heart rate to increase with standing distinguishes orthostatic hypotension from hypovolemia. Orthostatic hypotension appears to be an infrequent complicating factor in diabetic pregnancies. Interestingly, in one case report, symptoms of severe orthostatic hypotension were ameliorated by pregnancy, possibly as a result of the volume expansion of the pregnant state.[2] Signs and symptoms of bladder neuropathy include incomplete bladder emptying, which predisposes to urinary tract infections. Severe symptoms of bladder dysfunction, such as overflow incontinence and urinary retention, which requires intermittent self-catheterization, have not been reported during the pregnancies of women with insulin-dependent diabetes mellitus (IDDM). Routine screening of urine for culture and antibiotic sensitivities should be performed on a monthly basis. Positive urine cultures should be treated with appropriate antibiotics. Lower bowel neuropathy may result in the embarrassing symptoms of nocturnal diarrhea and fecal incontinence alternating with constipation. Symptoms of diarrhea are safely treated with loperamide (Food and Drug Administration pregnancy category B) during pregnancy,[3] after other causes of diarrhea such as viral, bacterial (including *Clostridium difficile*), and parasitic infections have been ruled out. Constipation, when it occurs in the setting of autonomic neuropathy, without the characteristic diarrhea, may be difficult to distinguish from constipation that is common to pregnancy. However, treatment for both situations is similar and includes increasing oral water intake and the use of sugar-free bulking agents.

Severe gastroparesis may result in significant maternal and fetal morbidity and mortality rates. Symptoms of early satiety, nausea, and postprandial vomiting that occur in the nonpregnant state may be exacerbated by the "morning sickness" that is normal to early pregnancy. Late in pregnancy, mechanical compression of the stomach by an enlarging uterus may also aggravate symptoms of gastroparesis. In the worst cases, intractable vomiting has resulted in maternal and fetal malnutrition and dehydration with the requirement of hyperalimentation during the pregnancy. In one case report, aspiration of vomitus resulted in a maternal anoxic cardiac arrest and a fetal demise.[4] In another case, intractable nausea and vomiting in a patient with nephrotic-range proteinuria resulted in severe hypoalbuminemia. Repeated episodes of pulmonary edema occurred during the pregnancy, and a stillborn fetus was delivered.[5]

In less severe cases, gastroparesis may result in erratic blood sugar control with an increase in the already significant risk of severe maternal hypoglycemia because of the delayed absorption of food. Conversely, profound hyperglycemia may result when food is finally absorbed and there is inadequate insulin available to metabolize the glucose. The potential benefit of greater metabolic stability with metoclopromide probably outweighs the theoretical risks of this Food and Drug Administration pregnancy category B drug,[3] which may be instituted when symptoms of gastroparesis are present.

Prospective controlled studies from Finland have demonstrated that patients with IDDM and asymptomatic autonomic neuropathy, as defined by an abnormality of either the expiratory/inspiratory ratio or heart rate response to standing (30:15 ratio), have double the risk of aggregated pregnancy-related complications compared with those who have normal autonomic function tests. Data comparing the risk of specific complications between the two groups, such as spontaneous abortion, perinatal mortality rate, congenital malformations, respiratory distress syndrome, preeclampsia, maternal ketoacidosis, and severe maternal hypoglycemia, were not significant, possibly because the study group was too small to evaluate these low-frequency complications independently.[6] Cross-sectional studies from Finland also demonstrated that increasing parity was not associated with a higher incidence of abnormal autonomic function tests, suggesting that pregnancy itself does not lead to deterioration of autonomic neuropathy.[7]

The screening of asymptomatic women with IDDM for autonomic neuropathy has not been performed routinely because management decisions, generally, have not been altered with this information. Women with symptoms of gastroparesis before pregnancy should be aware that exacerbations are likely to occur during pregnancy and that there is a potential for significant maternal or fetal morbidity. Women in whom symptoms of gastroparesis develop during pregnancy should be treated with metoclopromide to improve comfort level, nutritional status, and blood sugar control. Total parenteral nutrition should be instituted early, in cases of severe gastroparesis, when malnutrition threatens the pregnancy.

Peripheral Neuropathy

Involvement of the peripheral nerves is the most common nerve disorder in diabetes. The longest nerves are the most commonly affected, so that the feet, hands, and anterior thoracoabdominal region (intercostal nerves) are most commonly affected. The usual clinical picture is a sensory disorder characterized by paresthesia, which may be variously described as painful, burning, tingling, numb, or a feeling that the extremity is asleep.

The physical examination may be normal in mild cases but, more typically, includes some findings of sensory loss. In the very common distal neuropathy of the lower extremity, the anterior part of the foot is involved, particularly the toes and the ball of the foot. Both the symptoms and the findings may extend retrograde to the knee, but rarely about it. For this reason, knee jerk reflexes are present, and ankle jerk reflexes are typically absent. Examination of the foot often reveals loss of pin prick, light touch, proprioception, vibration, and temperature sensations. The foot is particularly vulnerable to injury, with resulting ulceration and potentially severe infection. It is also likely that there is some neural alteration in the integrity of the skin, making the foot vulnerable to damage. Ulceration of the toes and the feet, which are so common in the middle-aged diabetic population, are fortunately rare in the younger childbearing group. Hare has seen only a few neuropathic ulcerations of the feet in 20 years' experience with pregnant diabetic women. One of these resulted in the amputation of a toe while the patient was under anesthesia for a cesarean section. It is not the ulcerated lesion itself, which necessitates an amputation, but the development of infection in the bone or joint that is a problem.

Similar findings of peripheral neuropathy may be present in the hands but need to be distinguished from carpal tunnel syndrome. In the latter, there is a distinct change in the nerve conduction velocity across the wrist; in peripheral neuropathy, the changes in conduction velocity are more gradual. Ulnar entrapment syndrome causes changes in nerve function at the level of the elbow and below. Although pregnancy may aggravate these two compression neuropathies, surgical intervention during pregnancy may be unnecessary, since these conditions usually improve postpartum.

Intercostal neuropathy is distinctly uncommon in pregnancy. However, the clinical nature of this syndrome should be kept in mind to distinguish it from other discomforts of pregnancy, particularly the round ligament syndrome or rib cage distention. Symptomatic patients complain of discomfort, which may be unilateral or bilateral, usually along the distribution of one or two intercostal nerves. Pain and dysesthesia are common symptoms. Physical findings may be extremely difficult to elicit.

Cranial Neuropathy

The third, sixth, and seventh (Bell's palsy) cranial nerves may be involved in diabetes. Anecdoctal reports indicate that Bell's palsy is more common both in pregnancy and in diabetes. Cranial neuropathies usually have an abrupt onset, are typically (but not invariably) painless, and have a clinical presentation that is predominantly motor (diploplia or facial droop), although some patients with Bell's palsy may complain of dysesthesia in the distribution of the peripheral facial nerve. The course is self-limited over a period of weeks to months, and complete recovery is expected. The diagnostic dilemma presented by such patients is the concern that the sudden onset of painless cranial nerve palsy may reflect a vascular event or a tumor. When cranial neuropathies occur in diabetes, they are unilateral, isolated events. If a cerebral vascular accident has occurred or a tumor is present, cranial neuropathies are usually not neurologically isolated. Therefore, if one finds no other neurologic deficit at the time of onset, one can be on safe clinical ground in assuming that this is only a cranial neuropathy. Radiographic investigation such as a computed tomographic scan of the head is not necessary.

Neuropathic Fractures

Patients with diabetes may have difficulty with spontaneous and often painless fractures of the bones in the foot (Charcot fractures); peripheral neuropathy is almost always clinically evident in these patients. Because the fractures are usually painless, they go unnoticed initially and further damage occurs. Altered neural function and input to the bone is involved in the pathogenesis. The foot may be red and swollen, suggesting the presence of infection, which can be virtually excluded by the absence of ulceration of the skin. This point is particularly important because the radiographic appearance suggests osteomyelitis. Since the treatment of osteomyelitis is amputation, it is obviously critical not to make this diagnosis erroneously. The treatment for a Charcot foot is primarily lack of weight bearing to allow healing of the fractures. Casting may be required. Healing is often slow and may take several months. Assiduous avoidance of weight bearing is important to prevent compounding the damage and increasing the degree of deformity. Unfortunately, such patients often do have a residual deformity of the foot. Because they have a neuropathic foot, they are also prone to neuropathic ulceration and additional fractures. The most common deformity results from fractures of the metatarsal bones and distortion of the arch, leading to a rocker bottom deformity.

Because this complication may occur in young women, it may occur in pregnancy. A report of nine women who became pregnant after prior renal transplantation included two with neuropathic fractures of the foot.[8] In this special situation, the use of corticosteroid therapy plus alterations in vitamin D and calcium metabolism in renal failure may have contributed to the propensity for bony dissolution.

CORONARY ARTERY DISEASE AS A COMPLICATION OF DIABETIC PREGNANCY

Myocardial infarction is infrequent in women of childbearing age, occurring with an estimated incidence of 1 in 10,000 pregnancies, in the general population.[9,10] One can understand the rarity of myocardial infarction during pregnancy by examining data from the Framingham Heart study. A low cumulative mortality rate of 4 percent has been shown for women up to the age of 55, which is approximately one-half the risk of men of similar age.[11–13] The incidence of death from coronary artery disease in 35- to 45-year-old women, in the general population, is extremely low at 0.2 per 1,000 per year. Before age 35 years, the risk of death from coronary artery disease is negligible.[11]

Data from patients with IDDM from the Joslin Clinic provides an interesting contrast to the Framingham Heart study.[13] Cohorts of patients with IDDM were identified based on the year of their first visit to the clinic (1939, 1949, and 1959). The subjects were younger than 21 years of age and had IDDM of less than 1-years duration. In 1981, surviving subjects were evaluated for the presence of coronary artery disease, based on questionnaires, review of medical records, and exercise tolerance testing. Mortality information

was based on autopsy reports, medical records, and death certificates. Premenopausal women with IDDM had the same incidence of coronary artery disease as did men with IDDM of similar ages. By the age of 55 years, 35 percent of all men and women with IDDM had died from coronary artery disease (Fig. 21-1). Compared with their nondiabetic counterparts, women and men with IDDM had, respectively, eight and four times the risk of coronary artery disease, indicating that the protective effect of female gender is eliminated in IDDM.

For women aged 25 to 35 years with IDDM, the yearly incidence of death from coronary artery disease is 1 per 1,000 for those without nephropathy and 3 to 4 per 1,000 for those with nephropathy.[13] The yearly incidence of death from coronary artery disease is considerably higher in women aged 35 to 45, occurring at a rate of 7 per 1,000 for those without diabetic nephropathy and 30 per 1,000 for those with nephropathy[13] (Fig. 21-2).; Thus, nephropathy is a powerful risk factor for women with IDDM. The risk of coronary artery disease in women with IDDM may be modified, to a greater or lesser extent,[14] by the other established risk factors for the general population, such as smoking, hyperlipidemia, hypertension, and a history of toxemia of pregnancy.[15] Past oral contraceptive use does not appear to increase the risk of coronary artery dis-

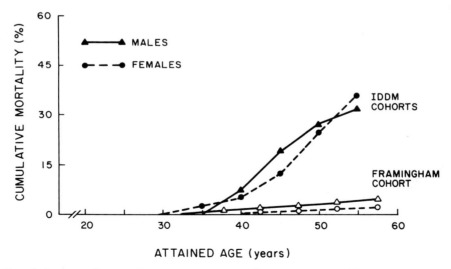

Fig. 21-1. Cumulative mortality rate from coronary artery disease up to age 55 years in patients with insulin-dependent diabetes mellitus (IDDM) and in the population of the Framingham Heart Study. (From Krolewski et al,[13] with permission.)

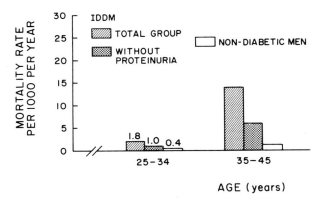

Fig. 21-2. Mortality rate from coronary artery disease (CAD) in the total study group and the estimated CAD mortality rate that would be expected if diabetic nephropathy were not present, and, for comparison, the CAD mortality rate in non-diabetic men in the Framingham Heart Study. The presence of diabetic nephropathy increases the incidence of death from CAD, to 3 to 4 in 1,000 person-years for ages 25 to 34 and 30 in 1,000 person-years for ages 35 to 45. (Data not shown. J. Warram, personal communication). (Adapted from Krolewski et al,[13] with permission.)

ease.[16,17] Of note, deaths from coronary artery disease, in both the IDDM and Framingham cohorts, do not seem to occur before the latter part of the third decade.[13] For women with IDDM who delay their childbearing until the fourth and sometimes fifth decades, there is an associated increased risk of coronary artery disease just on the basis of age.

There have been no more than 15 scattered case reports of coronary artery disease occurring during the pregnancies of woman with IDDM.[5,18-26] The incidence of coronary artery disease in pregnancies of women with IDDM has not been reported. Between the years 1978 through 1993, approximately 1,400 pregnancies complicated by IDDM were followed at the Joslin Diabetes Center. During these years, four pregnancies were complicated by coronary artery disease (class H diabetes), an incidence of 1 per 350 pregnancies. Two of these patients were reported in the previous edition of this textbook,[5] and the third was reported subsequently.[26] Since then, a fourth patient, 36 years old, with toxemia of pregnancy complicating both her pregnancies, had an anterior wall myocardial infarction 1 week after delivery of her second infant. She developed chest pain while visiting her infant in the neonatal intensive care unit and went into cardiogenic shock but was successfully resuscitated.

Table 21-1 provides clinical information on each of these four patients. Two women (SOE and MAM) had myocardial infarctions during pregnancy or immediately postpartum. There was one death (SOE), occurring at 10 weeks' gestation. One patient (VJ) survived 28 weeks of pregnancy, in spite of angina and congestive heart failure, but died 5 years postpartum. Interestingly, three of the four women were older than age 35 years at the time of their pregnancies. All women had IDDM of greater than 20 years' duration. Anatomic information was available in three of the four women, and in each of these, single-vessel left anterior descending coronary artery disease was present. In addition to IDDM, all of the women had at least one other risk factor for coronary artery disease such as smoking, hypertension, and family history. All four also had diabetic renal involvement. One had microalbuminuria noted before her pregnancy, and three had overt diabetic nephropathy (class F diabetes).

In light of these findings, it seems prudent to provide an assessment of coronary artery disease risk when preconception counseling is given to women with IDDM. Diabetic nephropathy is a substantial risk factor for coronary artery disease in women with IDDM, increasing the risk two- to fourfold, compared with women without nephropathy. Women older than 30 to 35 years, who have other risk factors for coronary artery disease, including diabetic nephropathy, might be advised to undergo exercise tolerance testing before pregnancy. Women with documented coronary artery disease should be advised against pregnancy because of the high associated mortality rate of symptomatic coronary artery disease during pregnancy. Specific guidelines require consensus from the many centers that follow women with IDDM throughout their pregnancies.

In summary, the presence of either coronary artery disease or gastroparesis may lead to increased morbidity and mortality risks for pregnant women with IDDM. Women who have risk factors for coronary artery disease, especially advanced maternal age and diabetic nephropathy, should be screened for coronary artery disease before pregnancy, if possible. Women with gastroparesis that is symptomatic before pregnancy should be advised that their symptoms may worsen during pregnancy.

Table 21-1. Coronary Artery Disease in Pregnancy, 1978 to 1993, at the Joslin Diabetes Center

Patient	Year of Event	Outcome	Lesion	Risk Factors	Age (years)	Duration of IDDM (years)	Timing of Event Relative to Pregnancy
MAM	1992	Survived anterior wall MI with cardiogenic shock	100% LAD	IDDM, smoking hypertension, pre-eclampsia in both pregnancies, microalbuminuria	36	23	1 week postpartum
SOE	1986	Died	90% LAD, porcine aortic valve replacement at age 22; multifocal subendocardial MIs at autopsy	IDDM, hypertension diabetic nephropathy	27	25	10 weeks gestation
MC	1982	Asymptomatic during pregnancy; termination at 19 weeks due to congenital malformation	Coronary artery bypass graft of LAD	IDDM, diabetic nephropathy, family history (+): mother died MI age 50, father survived MI age 40+	37	26	1 month before pregnancy
VJ	1978	Survived; baby died after delivery at 28 weeks	Unknown	IDDM, smoking, hypertension, diabetic nephropathy; (+) Family history; brother had MI at age 42	38	24	Angina before and during pregnancy. Congestive heart failure 22–28 weeks.

Abbreviation: LAD, left anterior descending artery; IDDM, insulin-dependent diabetes mellitus; MI, myocardial infarction.

REFERENCES

1. The DCCT Research Group: The effect of intensive treatment of diabetes on the development and progression of long-term complications in insulin-dependent diabetes mellitus. N Engl J Med 329:977, 1993
2. Scott AR, Tattersall RB, McPherson M: Improvement of postural hypotension and severe diabetic autonomic neuropathy during pregnancy. Diabetes Care 11:369, 1988
3. Briggs GG, Freeman RK, Yaffe SJ: Drugs in Pregnancy and Lactation. Williams & Wilkins, Baltimore, 1994
4. Macleod AF, Smith SA, Sonksen PH, Lowy C: The problem of autonomic neuropathy in diabetic pregnancy. Diabetic Med 7:80, 1990
5. Hare JW: Diabetic neuropathy and coronary heart disease. p. 515. In Reece EA, Coustan DR (eds): Diabetes Mellitus in Pregnancy: Principles and Practice. Churchill Livingstone, New York, 1989
6. Airaksinen KEJ, Anttila LM, Linnaluoto MK et al: Autonomic influence on pregnancy outcome in IDDM. Diabetes Care 13:756, 1990
7. Airaksinen KEJ, Salmela PI: Pregnancy is not a risk factor for a deterioration of autonomic nervous function in diabetic women. Diabetic Med 10:540, 1993
8. Ogburn PL, Kitzmiller JL, Hare JW et al: Pregnancy following renal transplantation in class T diabetes mellitus. JAMA 255:911, 1986
9. Fletcher E, Knox EW, Morton P: Acute myocardial infarction in pregnancy. BMJ 3:586, 1967
10. Sullivan JM, Ramanathan KB: Management of medical problems in pregnancy—severe cardiac disease. N Engl J Med 313:304, 1985
11. Lerner DJ, Kannel WB: Patterns of coronary heart disease morbidity and mortality in the sexes: a 26 year follow-up of the Framingham population. Am Heart J 111:383, 1986
12. Sorlie P: The Framingham Study section 32; cardiovascular disease and death following myocardial infarction and angina pectoris—20 year follow-up. Publication no. (NIH) 77-1247. Department of Health and Human Services, 1977
13. Krolewski AS, Kosinski EJ, Warram JH et al: Magnitude and determinants of coronary artery disease in juvenile-

onset, insulin-dependent diabetes mellitus. Am J Cardiol 59:750, 1987

14. Warram JH, Laffel LMB, Ganda OP, Christlieb AR: Coronary artery disease is the major determinant of excess mortality in patients with insulin-dependent diabetes mellitus and persistent proteinuria. J Am Soc Nephrol 3: s104, 1992

15. Croft P, Hannaford PC: Risk factors for acute myocardial infarction in women: evidence form the Royal College of General Practitioners' oral contraception study. BMJ 298:165, 1989

16. Stamfer MJ, Willett WC, Colditz GA et al: Past use of oral contraceptives and cardiovascular disease: a meta-analysis in the context of the Nurse's Health Study. Am J Obstet Gynecol 163:285, 1990

17. Stampfer MJ, Willett WC, Colditz GA et al: A prospective study of past use of oral contraceptive agents and risk of cardiovascular diseases. N Engl J Med 319:1313, 1988

18. Brock HJ, Russel NG, Randall CL: Myocardial infarction in pregnancy: report of a case with normal spontaneous vaginal delivery seven months later. JAMA 152:1030, 1953

19. Siegler AM, Hoffman J, Bloom O: Myocardial infarction complicating pregnancy. Obstet Gynecol 7:306, 1956

20. Delaney JJ, Ptacek J: Three decades of experience with diabetic pregnancies. Am J Obstet Gynecol 106:550, 1970

21. White P: Life cycle of diabetes in youth. J Am Med Women Assoc 27:293, 1972

22. Hibbard LT: Maternal mortality due to cardiac disease. Clin Obstet Gynecol 18:27, 1975

23. Hare JW, White P: Pregnancy in diabetes complicated by vascular disease. Diabetes 26:953, 1977

24. Silfen SL, Wapner RJ, Gabbe SG: Maternal outcome in class H diabetes mellitus. Obstet Gynecol 55:749, 1980

25. Reece EA, Egan JFX, Coustan DR et al: Am J Obstet Gynecol 154:150, 1986

26. Hare JW: Complicated diabetes complicating pregnancy. Ballieres Clin Obstet Gynaecol 5:349, 1991

22
Delivery: Timing, Mode, and Management

DONALD R. COUSTAN

One of the most critical and controversial aspects of perinatal medicine is the precise timing of the delivery. Furthermore, once a decision has been made to accomplish delivery, the clinician is confronted with a choice between abdominal or vaginal routes. In the woman with diabetes, the management of glucose metabolism during cesarean section or labor appears to be an important determinant of at least some types of neonatal morbidity. As recently as 1966, *Williams Obstetrics*[1] contained the following statement:

> Because of the increase in fetal death as term approaches there is widespread belief that pregnancy should be terminated either by the induction of labor or by cesarean section about three weeks prior to term. The choice between cesarean section and induction of labor depends upon the level of the presenting part and the condition of the cervix.

As to the management of diabetes during labor, the above textbook recommends that "it is well to give the equivalent of 10 g of glucose approximately every hour."[1]

A great many changes have occurred in the approach to these issues during the past 30 years, and this chapter outlines current recommendations.

TIMING

With the improvements in management of the pregnancy complicated by diabetes discussed in earlier chapters, the necessity for early intervention to deliver such pregnancies has diminished remarkably. In the past, the high intrauterine fetal death rate after 36 to 37 weeks of gestation more than outweighed the risks of respiratory distress occurring in infants of diabetic mothers (IDMs) delivered after this gestational age. However, the convergence of both advancing perinatal technology and improved understanding of the relationship between meticulous maternal diabetic control and the prevention of perinatal death, has enabled the clinician to individualize decision making, allowing most diabetic women to proceed to term or near term before planned delivery.

The development of neonatal intensive care units has improved the survival chances for infants born prematurely, particularly those who have respiratory distress syndrome (RDS). Furthermore, the development and utilization of tests of fetoplacental function, which include antepartum fetal monitoring, biophysical profiles, and fetal movement quantitation, have allowed the evolution of a strategy that combines identification of those pregnancies at lowest risk of fetal deterioration, thereby avoiding the neonatal and maternal risks of untimely intervention.

In addition to identification of those pregnancies in which the fetus is compromised, it has also become possible to measure the likelihood of a particular fetus to develop RDS if delivered at a given point in time. The measurement of surfactant components in amniotic fluid has become a standard method of assessing fetal pulmonic maturity, critical for timing the elective delivery of a patient with diabetes. This technology allows the avoidance of iatrogenic RDS when delivery can be safely postponed. It is particularly helpful when antepartum biochemical or biophysical assessment of fetal well-being is equivocal or when other indications for delivery are present but not absolute.

In parallel with the above mentioned advances in fetal assessment has come the elucidation of the relationship between the achievement of maternal euglycemia and a marked reduction in perinatal mortality rates. It is thus clear that the approach to timing delivery can be two pronged: (1) we can prevent the necessity for intentional early delivery in most cases by strict metabolic control of maternal diabetes and (2) we can identify those few fetuses still at high risk of perinatal death with antepartum testing. What remains is the vast majority of diabetic pregnancies in which there is no specific indication for delivery at a given time. The principle that should guide our determination of the optimal date for intervention in these individuals is one that is familiar to every doctor and medical student: primum non nocere. As discussed in the next section of this chapter, vaginal delivery is preferable to cesarean section if all other factors are equal. Therefore, a management scheme that will optimize the chances for a normal vaginal delivery without increasing perinatal mortality and morbidity rates is desirable. On the other hand, perinatal risk increases when pregnancies in general go much beyond term, and most clinicians are reluctant to allow women with diabetes to continue pregnancies beyond the estimated date of confinement. Although in the well-controlled and otherwise uncomplicated diabetic pregnancy this position may be emotional rather than data based, it is unlikely to change in the near future, particularly with medicolegal concerns lurking in the conscious or subconscious of every practicing obstetrician. Therefore, the following approach has evolved in our diabetes center:

1. Delivery is accomplished even without documented lung maturity if maternal or fetal compromise places the life of either mother or fetus at significant risk, for example, proven severe fetal compromise at a time when fetal survival after delivery is considered possible, currently 24–25 weeks at our center. Maternal eclampsia or severe pre-eclampsia is present, in which maternal well-being is compromised by continuing the pregnancy, and little improvement in fetal outcome is anticipated. In such situations, the likelihood of extrauterine survival must be weighed against the severity of fetal or maternal compromise.

2. Delivery is recommended as soon as lung maturity can be documented when there is a significant maternal or fetal problem, but neither poses an immediate risk. For example, when there is poor (mean plasma glucose >120 mg/dl) or undocumented maternal metabolic control, maternal hypertensive disorder of pregnancy or worsening pre-existing hypertension, intrauterine growth retardation, strongly suspected fetal macrosomia (as outlined in the next portion of this chapter), previous classic cesarean section, or equivocal antepartum assessment of fetal condition.

3. In patients who do not fulfill any of the above criteria, elective delivery is *considered* at 38 weeks of gestation to decrease the expense and anxiety associated with continuing the pregnancy, if the cervix is clinically "ripe" and fetal lung maturity is documented by studies on amniotic fluid. If the cervix is unfavorable, amniocentesis is not attempted because fetal pulmonic maturity would not lead to induction of labor under these circumstances. After 38 weeks, if oligohydramnios precludes successful amniocentesis, this is taken as an indication to proceed with delivery without amniotic fluid studies. Repeat cesarean sections are performed at 38 weeks if lung maturity is documented.

Although an earlier chapter (see Ch. 7) is devoted to discussing neonatal respiratory problems in IDMs, it is worthwhile to reiterate that there is not total agreement on the need for chemical documentation of fetal pulmonic maturity before elective delivery at term. The above approach was supported by data in the 1970s that showed (1) a greater likelihood of RDS among IDMs, even when they were delivered at term and (2) a greater likelihood of false-positive lecithin/sphingomyclin ratios in diabetic pregnancies, leading to the use of the more accurate phosphatidylglycerol (PG) measurement. Data published since the previous edition of this book confirm the absence of PG in amniotic fluid samples of approximately 20 percent of patients with gestational diabetes at 38 weeks' gestation and a similar proportion of patients with pre-existing diabetes at 38 weeks' gestation.[2] Because the patients were not delivered when PG was absent, no data are available concerning RDS in the offspring. A number of other studies have suggested that RDS is no more common in the IDMs whose glucose metabolism has been well controlled during pregnancy than among normal controls[3,4] and that false-positive test results at term are no more likely in IDMs than in normal pregnancies. These data would suggest that, if fetal hyperinsulinemia can be avoided by meticulous control of maternal blood glucose levels, RDS in near-term IDMs is not likely. The study of Piper and Langer[5] that showed a greater prevalence of immature lung profiles in poorly controlled than in well-controlled diabetic pregnancies would tend to confirm this. It is almost certainly true that, in diabetic pregnancies, as in other pregnancies, the single most important determinant of pulmonic maturity is gestational age. In some centers, amniocentesis for lung maturity before elective delivery at term is forgone if maternal diabetes has been documented to be in good control and reliable early dating places the pregnancy at 38 weeks or beyond.

It should be apparent that, in this scheme, the White class of the maternal diabetes does not enter into clinical decision making as to timing of delivery. Although it is undoubtedly true that women with vascular disease are more likely to have adverse outcomes such as perinatal death, this increased risk is most likely associated with problems such as hypertension and intrauterine growth retardation, which would themselves prompt early delivery. Conversely, if a particular woman whose diabetes has been in excellent metabolic control, has normal blood pressure, and has an appropriately growing fetus with normal antenatal monitoring parameters, it would be unreasonable to induce labor, possibly increasing the likelihood of a cesarean section, at a predetermined number of weeks before term merely because she has had diabetes for 20 years rather than 19 years.

The otherwise uncomplicated diabetic pregnancy that reaches 40 weeks of gestation with a cervix unfavorable for induction can present a dilemma. The options include continuing the pregnancy while awaiting cervical change, using methods such as prostaglandin E gel or laminaria to effect cervical ripening, or proceeding with a primary cesarean section. Except in the presence of macrosomia (discussed in the next section of this chapter), we almost never choose the last of the options. The performance of a cesarean section without labor seems extreme. Although the efficacy of cervical ripening among diabetic pregnancies at 40

weeks or more has not been unequivocally demonstrated, this option is often chosen to alleviate the anxiety of both patient and obstetrician when a diabetic pregnancy has exceeded 40 weeks. The above approach to the timing of delivery should allow most patients to deliver at or beyond the 38 weeks, generally accepted as "term."

MODE

There has been considerable controversy concerning the appropriate mode of delivery for diabetic pregnancies over the past 50 years. During the first 70 years of the present century, some experts advocated almost routine cesarean section for such pregnancies and reported cesarean section rates of 65 percent or more[6-9] at a time when overall cesarean section rates in most hospitals were below 5 percent. Other experts disagreed and reported cesarean section rates of approximately 16 percent.[7,10-12]

During the 1970s, overall cesarean section rates in the United States increased for reasons outside the scope of this chapter. At the same time, the advances in management discussed earlier enabled clinicians to feel more and more comfortable in allowing pregnancies to proceed closer to term in women with diabetes. These two trends would be expected to have opposing effects on cesarean section rates for diabetic pregnancies. In a nonexhaustive review of 17 series of overt diabetic pregnancies published between 1975 and 1985, cesarean section rates varied between 19 and 83 percent.[13-29] When all results were combined, 995 of 2,138 (47 percent) deliveries were performed by cesarean section. It was not possible to distinguish the characteristics of diabetes management that predisposed to higher or lower cesarean rates. However, in the two series with cesarean section rates of 19 and 25 percent, most patients were managed without induction and were allowed to go into spontaneous labor.[22,29] Cesarean section rates have not changed drastically since the publication of the previous edition of this book. The cesarean section rate for diabetic pregnancy at the National Maternity Hospital in Ireland has increased from 19[29] to 28 percent.[30] A prospective nationwide study in Sweden found the overall cesarean section rate for diabetic pregnancies to be 45 percent versus

12 percent for nondiabetic pregnancies,[31] and a multicenter prospective survey in France reported a 60 percent cesarean section rate for women with pre-existing diabetes.[32] A notable exception came from the State of Hesse in Germany, where only 13 percent of 446 diabetic pregnancies were delivered by cesarean section, compared with 5.4 percent in the general population.[33] In a survey of 273 American subspecialists in maternal-fetal medicine, only 31 percent reported cesarean rates for insulin-dependent diabetic women to be 25 percent or less; 58 percent estimated that their rates were between 26 and 50 percent; and 10 percent reported rates above 50 percent.[34]

Cesarean section may be considered as an adverse outcome for the mother, given the greater incidence of infectious morbidity among diabetic pregnancies compared with that in the general population[35,36] and the increased maternal mortality rates ascribed to cesarean section. In addition, the total cost of cesarean section exceeds that of vaginal delivery, and maternal discomfort is arguably greater. From the fetal-neonatal point of view, there is a clear increase in the incidence of RDS when delivery is by cesarean.[37,38] Thus, all other things being equal, vaginal delivery is preferable to cesarean section.

Certain complications that are more likely to occur in diabetic pregnancy may necessitate cesarean delivery, making the higher than usual cesarean section rates likely to continue. Among these are the association of hypertensive disorders of pregnancy with maternal diabetes, which may make early intervention necessary at a time when cervical ripening has not occurred and the uterus is not as likely to respond to oxytocin stimulation. Likewise, the greater likelihood of fetal compromise in the diabetic woman whose glucose metabolism is suboptimally controlled may necessitate early intervention and cesarean section.

The increased incidence of fetal macrosomia, with the accompanying risk of shoulder dystocia, prompts many clinicians to opt for cesarean section when the estimated fetal weight exceeds certain limits. This is understandable, particularly in view of the fact that the macrosomic infant of a diabetic mother is likely to have a body that is disproportionately large in relation to its head size, thus predisposing to shoulder dystocia at any given birthweight.[39,40] Shoulder dystocia has been reported to occur in 3[41] to 12 percent[42] of deliveries that result in neonates weighing 4,000 g or more and in 8.4[42] to 14.6 percent[43] of those weighing more than

4,500 g. In one study, 31 percent of diabetic women who had babies weighing 4,000 g or more experienced shoulder dystocia.[42] In another study, 21 percent of infants weighing more than 4,000 g and undergoing midpelvic vaginal delivery after a prolonged second stage had shoulder dystocia.[41] Thus, diabetes, macrosomia, midpelvic delivery, and a prolonged second stage all appear to be risk factors for shoulder dystocia. Shoulder dystocia is of greatest concern because of the possibility that Erb's palsy may result. Erb's palsy was found in the offspring of 10 in 1,000 diabetic pregnancies compared with 0.6 in 1,000 normal controls.[44] This has prompted many obstetricians to resort to elective cesarean section when infants of diabetic mothers are estimated to weigh 4,000 g or more or 4,500 g or more. Problems associated with this type of plan include the poor predictive value of clinical estimates of fetal weight when macrosomia is present[45,46] and the lack of agreement as to the accuracy of ultrasound measurements for such predictions. In babies who weigh 4,000 to 4,500 g, the usually acceptable 10 percent error in ultrasound fetal weight estimation may lead to under- or overestimation by 400 to 450 g. This problem has prompted a number of proposals for predicting shoulder dystocia, including ultrasonic measurement of anthropometric data[39] such as abdominal circumference,[47] the difference between chest diameter and biparietal diameter,[48] the rate of abdominal growth,[49] magnetic resonance imaging of fetal fat,[50] and ultrasound imaging[51] or computed tomographic scanning[52] of shoulder soft tissue width. No such system has been tested thoroughly enough in a prospective manner at this time to allow evaluation of its function as a screening test for shoulder dystocia. Therefore, ultrasound estimation of fetal weight is currently the most accurate available method and continues to be relied on for clinical decision making. It should be noted that the use of a relatively inaccurate method to diagnose macrosomia has drawbacks as well as benefits and that overdiagnosis may increase morbidity by prompting unnecessary interventions.[53] In our center, we continue to use arbitrary ultrasound-generated estimated fetal weight criteria to guide our decision, as described below.

Given the risks of macrosomia, a reasonable option might be to induce labor before the appearance of fetal overgrowth in the hope of preventing morbidity. A retrospective study found that elective induction of labor in fetuses estimated to be above the 90th percentile for weight increased the cesarean section rate without preventing shoulder dystocia.[54] However, a randomized prospective clinical trial of induction when diabetic pregnancies reached 38 weeks demonstrated a reduction in macrosomia and shoulder dystocia without an increase in cesarean sections.[55]

Decision making as to the mode of delivery in a pregnancy complicated by overt diabetes is guided by the following principles:

1. Diabetes is not an a priori indication for cesarean section, although its complications may necessitate this route of delivery.
2. The closer to term a pregnancy is allowed to continue, the greater is the likelihood of a vaginal delivery.
3. The decision for cesarean section is made on obstetric indications.
4. To minimize the risk of shoulder dystocia, the fetal weight should be estimated with as much accuracy as possible before a decision is made as to the mode of delivery. We consider the following to be indications for cesarean section without a trial of labor: Estimated fetal weight more than 4,500 g, in most instances or estimated fetal weight of 4,000 to 4,500 g, depending on history, clinical assessment of the pelvis, and progress of labor. Midforceps deliveries in such patients should be avoided, if possible, particularly after a long second stage. A history of shoulder dystocia, unless the estimated fetal weight is significantly lower than the birthweight of the previous baby, would also indicate cesarean delivery.
5. The history of a previous transverse lower uterine segment cesarean section does not preclude attempted vaginal delivery.

MANAGEMENT OF DIABETES DURING LABOR AND DELIVERY

The principle guiding management of maternal diabetes during labor and delivery is the maintenance of maternal euglycemia. Animal studies have demonstrated that maternal-fetal hyperglycemia may be associated with increasing fetal lactate levels and oxygen consumption, with subsequent acidosis and occasional fetal death.[56,57] It has also been suggested that the combination of hyperglycemia and hypoxia in primates may predispose to brain damage.[58] In human studies,

the infusion of large amounts of glucose into normal[59,60] and diabetic[61] women about to undergo cesarean section has been associated with fetal and neonatal acidemia.

One of the more common neonatal morbidities in IDMs is neonatal hypoglycemia. This is caused by fetal and neonatal hyperinsulinemia. Although the pancreas of the fetus of the diabetic mother may be more responsive to hyperglycemia, even the normal fetus responds to maternal hyperglycemia with an outpouring of insulin.[62] The administration of intravenous glucose solutions during labor, leading to maternal hyperglycemia, has been associated with neonatal hypoglycemia in both diabetic[63-65] and normal[66] pregnancies. Thus, the continued meticulous control of maternal glycemia during labor is necessary to avoid neonatal hypoglycemia.

In the past, it was customary to administer subcutaneous short-acting insulin to diabetic women undergoing labor, using a lower dose than the daily prepregnancy amount. Given that even short-acting insulin does not reach a peak of absorption for a few hours, it is no wonder that glycemia was difficult to control during labor. In 1977, West and Lowy[67] described the use of a constant intravenous infusion of glucose and low-dose (1 to 2 U/h) insulin as a means to control glycemia during labor. Soon thereafter, numerous centers reported satisfactory results with this system, although neonatal hypoglycemia was not entirely eliminated.[68-70] In the first study, glucose was infused at a rate of 8.3 g/h, and all 15 patients required at least 1.4 U/h of insulin throughout the labor.[67] In the later studies, lower rates of glucose infusion were used (5 to 6 g/h), and lower infusion rates of insulin were necessary. In fact, some patients required no insulin.

In 1978, Nattrass et al[71] reported the use of the artificial pancreas during labor in three laboring insulin-dependent diabetic women. The average infusion rates to maintain normoglycemia were 0.7 to 6.7 U/h of insulin and 3.0 to 6.4 g/h of glucose. By contrast, Jovanovic and Peterson[72] reported that 12 pregnant women with insulin-dependent diabetes managed with an artificial pancreas required no insulin during active first-stage labor despite glucose infusion rates of approximately 10 g/h. Golde et al[73] used glucose infusion rates of 6 g/h in 33 women with insulin-dependent diabetes during oxytocin induction of labor. One-half of the patients required no insulin to maintain euglycemia; the other half required insulin infusions of 0.6 to 1.2 U/h or more. It is thus apparent that at least some women with diabetes require no insulin during active labor; others may need more intensive treatment. It is most important to monitor circulating glucose levels frequently during this dynamic period of labor and to be prepared to add insulin if hyperglycemia occurs.

Our current approach to the metabolic management of diabetes during labor is based on the goal of maternal euglycemia at delivery and acknowledges the caloric requirements attributable to the work of labor and that laboring women should not be allowed to ingest food because of the potential hazard of aspiration if anesthesia is required:

1. On the day before induction of labor when the patient has been in satisfactory metabolic control, the existing insulin and meal regimen is followed to ensure that euglycemia will be present on the morning of induction.
2. On the morning of induction, withhold insulin and breakfast.
3. Start an intravenous infusion of 5 percent dextrose in half-normal saline, at a rate of 125 ml/h, using an infusion pump.
4. Measure the glucose level at the bedside every 1 to 2 hours, maintaining a glucose concentration between 70 and 120 mg/dl.
5. If the glucose level exceeds 120 mg/dl, add 10 U of regular insulin to 1,000 ml of dextrose 5 percent in half-normal saline and continue the infusion rate of 125 mg/h. This yields an insulin dose of approximately 1.25 U/h.
6. Further adjustments in insulin dosage are made by doubling or halving the insulin concentration but keeping the infusion rate constant.
7. Another option is to use a separate infusion line for insulin, in a nonglucose-containing solution, and to piggyback this into the glucose infusion. Such an approach requires three infusion pumps: one for glucose, one for insulin, and a third for oxytocin.
8. If spontaneous labor occurs, the procedure is the same. However, the patient may be less likely to require insulin, since she may have taken some intermediate-acting insulin before the onset of labor.

When elective cesarean section is planned, the procedure is simpler. The patient is instructed to follow her usual meal and insulin regimen on the day and evening before surgery. If it is assumed that the patient has been in good metabolic control, she should awaken on the morning of cesarean section with a normal blood glucose level. An intravenous line is inserted, and normal saline, without glucose, is infused. The diabetic patient's cesarean section should be the first one on the morning schedule, commencing at an early hour so that no perturbations in glucose metabolism have yet occurred. Once the baby has been delivered, glucose with or without insulin can be infused as needed.

With the approach outlined above, it is possible to maintain normal or near-normal glucose levels in most laboring diabetic women and prevent the sudden surge of fetal insulin release at the time of delivery that might increase the risk of neonatal hypoglycemia. Occasionally, this meticulous control of circulating glucose levels during labor can be abruptly negated by the infusion of a large quantity of glucose-containing solution just before the initiation of conduction anesthesia to prevent maternal hypotension. It is thus important that the entire health care team, including nurses and anesthesiologists, be aware of the importance of maintaining maternal euglycemia. Because it is usually necessary to expand the mother's intravascular volume before an epidural or spinal anesthetic is administered, nonglucose-containing solutions should be used.

REFERENCES

1. Eastman NJ, Hellman LM: Williams Obstetrics. 13th Ed. Appleton & Lange, New York, 1966
2. Ojomo EO, Coustan DR: Absence of evidence of pulmonary maturity at amniocentesis in term infants of diabetic mothers. Am J Obstet Gynecol 163:954, 1990
3. Mimouni F, Miodovnik M, Whitsett JA et al: Respiratory distress syndrome in infants of diabetic mothers in the 1980s: no direct adverse effect of maternal diabetes with modern management. Obstet Gynecol 69:191, 1987
4. Kjos SL, Walther FJ, Montoro M et al: Prevalence and etiology of respiratory distress in infants of diabetic mothers: predictive value of fetal lung maturation tests. Am J Obstet Gynecol 163:898, 1990
5. Piper JM, Langer O: Does maternal diabetes delay fetal pulmonary maturity? Am J Obstet Gynecol 168:783, 1993
6. White P: Pregnancy complicating diabetes. Am J Med 6: 609, 1949

7. Pedowitz P, Shlevin EL: Review of management of pregnancy complicated by diabetes and altered carbohydrate metabolism. Obstet Gynecol 23:716, 1964

8. Harley JMG, Montgomery DAD: Management of pregnancy complicated by diabetes. BMJ 1:14, 1965

9. Schwartz RH, Kyle GC: Timing of delivery in the pregnant diabetic patient. Obstet Gynecol 34:787, 1969

10. Jones WS: Diabetes in pregnancy. Am J Obstet Gynecol 66:322, 1953

11. Hall RE, Tillman AJB: Diabetes in pregnancy. Am J Obstet Gynecol 61:1107, 1951

12. Delaney JJ, Ptacek J: Three decades of experience with diabetic pregnancies. Am J Obstet Gynecol 106:550, 1970

13. Brearley BF: The management of pregnancy in diabetes mellitus. Practitioner 215:644, 1975

14. Ayromlooi J, Mann LI, Weiss RR et al: Modern management of the diabetic pregnancy. Obstet Gynecol 49:137, 1977

15. Boehm FH, Graber AL, Hicks MML: Coordinated metabolic and obstetric management of diabetic pregnancy. South Med J 71:37, 1978

16. Cassar J, Gordon H, Dixon HG et al: Simplified management of pregnancy complicated by diabetes. Br J Gynaecol 85:585, 1978

17. Gabbe SG, Lowensohn RI, Wu PYK, Guerra G: Current patterns of neonatal morbidity and mortality in infants of diabetic mothers. Diabetes Care 1:335, 1978

18. Goldstein AI, Cronk DA, Garite T, Amlie RN: Perinatal outcome in the diabetic pregnancy: a retrospective analysis. J Reprod Med 20:61, 1978

19. Kitzmiller JL, Cloherty JP, Younger MD et al: Diabetic pregnancy and perinatal morbidity. Am J Obstet Gynecol 131:560, 1978

20. Jervell J, Moe N, Skjaeraasen J et al: Diabetes mellitus and pregnancy—management and results at Rikshospitalet, Oslo, 1970–1977. Diabetologia 16:151, 1979

21. Martin TR, Allen AC, Stinson D: Overt diabetes in pregnancy. Am J Obstet Gynecol 133:275, 1979

22. Roversi GD, Gargiulo M, Nicolini U et al: A new approach to the treatment of diabetic pregnant women: report of 479 cases seen from 1963 to 1975. Am J Obstet Gynecol 135:567, 1979

23. Coustan DR, Berkowitz RL, Hobbins JC: Tight metabolic control of overt diabetes in pregnancy. Am J Med 68:845, 1980

24. Haukkamaa M, Nilsson CG, Luukkainen T: Screening, management, and outcome of pregnancy in diabetic mothers. Obstet Gynecol 55:596, 1980

25. Tevaarwerk GJM, Harding PGR, Milne KJ et al: Pregnancy in diabetic women: outcome with a program aimed at normoglycemia before meals. Can Med Assoc J 125:435, 1981

26. Fadel HE, Hammond SD: Diabetes mellitus in pregnancy: management and results. J Reprod Med 27:56, 1982

27. Traub AI, Harley JMG, Montgomery DAD, Hadden DR: Pregnancy and diabetes—the improving prognosis. Ulster Med J 52:118, 1983

28. Piras G, Cherchi PL, Delfino F et al: Diabetes in pregnancy: an epidemiologic study by Department of Obstetrics and Gynecology of Sassari University from 1974 to 1983. Clin Exp Obstet Gynecol 12:26, 1985

29. Drury MI, Stronge JM, Foley ME, MacDonald DW: Pregnancy in the diabetic patient: timing and mode of delivery. Obstet Gynecol 62:279, 1983

30. Rasmussen MJ, Firth R, Foley M, Stronge JM: The timing of delivery in diabetic pregnancy: a 10-year review. Aust NZ J Obstet Gynaecol 32:313, 1992

31. Hanson U, Persson B: Outcome of pregnancies complicated by type 1 insulin-dependent diabetes in Sweden: acute pregnancy complications, neonatal mortality and morbidity. Am J Perinatol 10:330, 1993

32. Gestation and Diabetes in France Study Group: Multicenter survey of diabetic pregnancy in France. Diabetes Care 14:994, 1991

33. Lang U, Künzel W: Diabetes mellitus in pregnancy. Eur J Obstet Gynecol Reprod Biol 33:115, 1989

34. Landon MB, Gabbe SG, Sachs L: Management of diabetes mellitus and pregnancy: a survey of obstetricians and maternal-fetal specialists. Obstet Gynecol 75:635, 1990

35. Diamond MP, Entman SS, Salyer SI et al: Increased risk of endometritis and wound infection after cesarean section in insulin-dependent women. Am J Obstet Gynecol 155:297, 1986

36. Stamler EF, Cruz ML, Mimouni F et al: High infectious morbidity in pregnant women with insulin-dependent diabetes: an understated complication. Am J Obstet Gynecol 163:1217, 1990

37. Usher RH, Allen AC, McLean FH: Risk of respiratory distress syndrome related to gestational age, route of delivery, and maternal diabetes. Am J Obstet Gynecol 111:826, 1971

38. Robert MF, Neff RK, Hubbell JP et al: Association between maternal diabetes and the respiratory distress syndrome in the newborn. N Engl J Med 294:357, 1976

39. Modanlou HD, Komatsu G, Dorchester W et al: Large-for-gestational-age neonates: anthropometric reasons for shoulder dystocia. Obstet Gynecol 60:417, 1982

40. Langer O, Berkus M, Huff RW, Samueloff A: Shoulder dystocia: should the fetus weighing ≥4000 grams be delivered by cesarean section? Am J Obstet Gynecol 165:831, 1991

41. Benedetti TJ, Gabbe SG: Shoulder dystocia: a complication of fetal macrosomia and prolonged second stage of labor with midpelvic delivery. Obstet Gynecol 52:526, 1978

42. Acker DB, Sachs BP, Friedman EA: Risk factors for shoulder dystocia. Obstet Gynecol 60:417, 1982

43. Spellacy WN, Miller S, Winegar A, Peterson PQ: Macrosomia: maternal characteristics and infant complications. Obstet Gynecol 66:762, 1985

44. Acker DB, Gregory KD, Sachs BP, Friedman EA: Risk factors for Erb-Duchenne palsy. Obstet Gynecol 71:389, 1988

45. Benson CB, Doubilet PM, Saltzman DH: Sonographic determination of fetal weights in diabetic pregnancies. Am J Obstet Gynecol 156:441, 1987

46. Miller JM, Brown HL, Khawli OF et al: Fetal weight estimates in diabetic gravid women. J Clin Ultrasound 16:569, 1988

47. Ogata ES, Sabbagha RE, Metzger BE et al: Serial ultrasonography to assess evolving fetal macrosomia: studies in 23 pregnant diabetic women. JAMA 243:2405, 1980

48. Elliott JP, Garite TJ, Freeman RK et al: Ultrasonic prediction of fetal macrosomia in diabetic patients. Obstet Gynecol 60:159, 1982

49. Landon MB, Mintz MC, Gabbe SG: Sonographic evaluation of fetal abdominal growth: predictor of the large-for-gestational-age infant in pregnancies complicated by diabetes mellitus. Am J Obstet Gynecol 160:115, 1989

50. Jovanovic-Peterson L, Crues J, Durak E, Peterson CM: Magnetic resonance imaging in pregnancies complicated by gestational diabetes predicts infant birth weight ratio and neonatal morbidity. Am J Perinatol 10:432, 1993

51. Mintz MC, Landon MB, Gabbe SG et al: Shoulder soft tissue width as a predictor of macrosomia in diabetic pregnancies. Am J Perinatol 6:240, 1989

52. Kitzmiller JL, Mall JC, Gin GD et al: Measurement of fetal shoulder width with computed tomography in diabetic women. Obstet Gynecol 70:941, 1987

53. Levine AB, Lockwood CJ, Brown B et al: Sonographic diagnosis of the large for gestational age fetus at term: does it make a difference? Obstet Gynecol 79:55, 1992

54. Combs CA, Singh NB, Khoury JC: Elective induction versus spontaneous labor after sonographic diagnosis of fetal macrosomia. Obstet Gynecol 81:492, 1993

55. Kjos SL, Henry OA, Montoro et al: Insulin-requiring diabetes in pregnancy: a randomized trial of active induction of labor and expectant management. Am J Obstet Gynecol 169:611, 1993

56. Robillard JE, Sessions C, Kennedy RI, Smith FG Jr: Metabolic effects of constant hypertonic glucose infusion in well-oxygenated fetuses. Am J Obstet Gynecol 130:199, 1978

57. Phillips AF, Rosenkrantz TS, Raye J: Consequences of perturbations of fetal fuels in ovine pregnancy. Diabetes, suppl. 2, 34:32, 1985

58. Myers RE: Brain damage due to asphyxia: mechanism of causation. J Perinat Med 9:78, 1981

59. Kenepp NB, Shelley WC, Gabbe SG et al: Fetal and neonatal hazards of maternal hydration with 5% dextrose before cesarean section. Lancet 1:1150, 1982

60. Philipson EH, Kalhan SC, Riha MM, Pimentel R: Effects of maternal glucose infusion on fetal acid-base status in human pregnancy. Am J Obstet Gynecol 157:866, 1987

61. Datta S, Kitzmiller JL, Naulty JS et al: Acid-base status in diabetic mothers and their infants following spinal anesthesia for cesarean section. Anesth Analg 61:662, 1982

62. Cordero L Jr, Grunt JA, Anderson GG: Hypertonic glucose infusion in labor. Am J Obstet Gynecol 107:560, 1970

63. Light IJ, Keenan WJ, Sutherland JM: Maternal intravenous glucose administration as a cause of hypoglycemia in the infant of the diabetic mother. Am J Obstet Gynecol 113:345, 1972

64. Anderson O, Hertel J, Schmolker L, Kühl C: Influence of the maternal plasma glucose concentration at delivery on the risk of hypoglycaemia in infants of insulin-dependent diabetic mothers. Acta Paediatr Scand 74:268, 1985

65. Soler NG, Soler SM, Malins JM: Neonatal morbidity among infants of diabetic mothers. Diabetes Care 1:340, 1978

66. Grylack LJ, Chu SS, Scanlon JW: Use of intravenous fluids before cesarean section: effects of perinatal glucose, insulin, and sodium homeostasis. Obstet Gynecol 63:654, 1984

67. West TET, Lowy C: Control of blood glucose during labour in diabetic women with combined glucose and low-dose insulin infusion. BMJ 1:1252, 1977

68. Yeast JD, Porreco RP, Ginsberg HN: The use of continuous insulin infusion for the peripartum management of pregnant diabetic women. Am J Obstet Gynecol 131:861, 1978

69. Caplan RH, Pagliara AS, Beguin EA et al: Constant intravenous insulin infusion during labor and delivery in diabetes mellitus. Diabetes Care 5:6, 1982

70. Bowen DJ, Daykin AP, Nacekievill ML, Normal J: Insulin dependent diabetic patients during surgery and labour: use of continuous intravenous insulin-glucose-potassium infusions. Anaesthesia 39:407, 1984

71. Nattrass M, Alberti KGMM, Dennis KJ, Gillibrand PN: A glucose-controlled insulin infusion system for diabetic women during labour. BMJ 2:599, 1978

72. Jovanovic JL, Peterson CM: Insulin and glucose requirements during the first stage of labor in insulin-dependent diabetic women. Am J Med 75:607, 1983

73. Golde SH, Good-Anderson B, Montoro M, Artal R: Insulin requirements during labor: a reappraisal. Am J Obstet Gynecol 144:556, 1982

23

Perinatal Mortality and Morbidity

DONALD R. COUSTAN

The pathogenesis of many of the perinatal morbidities associated with maternal diabetes, including fetal macrosomia, respiratory distress syndrome, and congenital anomalies, are discussed in earlier chapters of this book. Neonatal morbidities are discussed in Chapter 24. The pathogenesis of perinatal death in pregnancies complicated by diabetes is therefore the primary concern of this chapter. In addition, suggestions are made for the prevention of both morbidity and death in these pregnancies.

PERINATAL MORTALITY

Before the discovery of insulin in 1922, those few reported pregnancies among diabetic individuals yielded a perinatal mortality rate of approximately 65 percent.[1] However, maternal mortality rates were in the range of 30 percent, so that fetal considerations were secondary at that time. Once insulin was available, maternal mortality rates plummeted; currently, it is reasonable to conclude that the maternal mortality risk for diabetic pregnancy is approximately equal to that of the general pregnant population plus the risk associated with having diabetes over a 9-month period. Exceptions would include those diabetic individuals with coronary artery disease.[2] In addition, there have been reports of maternal mortality related to severe insulin reactions.[3] Denominator figures are not available, and it cannot presently be determined whether the hypoglycemia-related death rate during pregnancy exceeds the risk to nonpregnant diabetic women.

Although maternal death rates diminished rapidly with the availability of insulin treatment for diabetes, fetal and neonatal losses were much more difficult to eliminate. Unexplained sudden fetal death was a common way for such losses to occur. In the 1930s and 1940s, approximately 20 percent of diabetic pregnancies ended in this manner.[4–6] In the 1950s and 1960s, fetal death rates had fallen to approximately 12 percent,[7] and by the 1970s, most centers were reporting fetal mortality rates below 3 percent and perinatal mortality rates below 5 percent.[8–16] The reasons for this decline is perinatal mortality rate are not entirely clear. During the seven decades since the discovery of insulin, technological advances such as blood transfusions, safer anesthesia techniques, neonatal intensive care units, fetal monitoring, amniocentesis, biochemical and biophysical antepartum testing, and ultrasound may all have contributed to the improvement. However, an increased understanding of the effects of perturbations in maternal metabolism on the unborn fetus and techniques that allow the achievement of better metabolic control during diabetic pregnancy may have had even greater significance.

The groundbreaking publications of Harley and Montgomery[17] in 1965 and Karlsson and Kjellmer[18] in 1972 demonstrated an inverse relationship between mean maternal ambient glucose levels during the third trimester and perinatal mortality rates (Table 23-1). At the time of Karlsson and Kjellmer's publication, many centers in the United States were attempting to maintain glucose levels at around 150 mg/dl in diabetic pregnant women in the belief that maternal hypoglycemia was equally disadvantageous for the fetus as was hyperglycemia, although there was little evidence to support that view. When the pregnancies of 237 dia-

Table 23-1. Perinatal Mortality Rates in Diabetic Pregnancies as a Function of Third Trimester Maternal Inpatient Glucose Control

	Average Blood Glucose (mg/dl)		
	<100	100–150	>150
N	52	77	38
Perinatal mortality rate (%)	2 (3.4)[a]	12 (16)	9 (24)

[a] P < .05.
(Modified from Karlsson and Kjellmer,[18] with permission.)

betic women among the 50,000 pregnancies in the Collaborative Study of Cerebral Palsy were analyzed, no effect of maternal "insulin shock" on mental or motor performance at 8 months or 4 years of age in the offspring could be demonstrated.[19] Furthermore, Roversi et al[20] maintained diabetic pregnant women at the brink of symptomatic hypoglycemia with increasing insulin doses and reported a perinatal mortality rate of 3.6 percent.

Jovanovic and Peterson[21] reviewed the literature in 1980, citing those studies that reported both perinatal mortality rates and mean maternal circulating glucose levels. A scatterplot of these two variables was constructed, and the line of best fit (Fig. 23-1) suggests that the optimal perinatal survival is associated with a mean plasma glucose level of approximately 84 mg/dl. At about the same time that these data were being published and accepted, a number of centers began to explore the normal range of maternal glycemia during the third trimester (Fig. 23-2). These studies determined that normal, nondiabetic pregnant women manifest fasting plasma glucose levels averaging 74 to 88 mg/dl and postprandial values that rarely exceed 130 mg/dl at 1 hour or 120 mg/dl at 2 hours.[22–24]

Although the above evidence is indirect and the appropriate randomized controlled trial of intensive metabolic management in diabetic pregnancy has not been performed to date, the weight of these data strongly suggests that maternal hyperglycemia is associated with increased perinatal mortality rates in diabetic pregnancy and that normalization of glucose levels can reduce the incidence of perinatal loss.

Because the initiation of attempts to normalize maternal glucose metabolism was coincident with the development of methods to assess fetal condition, it is possible that the above improvements in perinatal outcome were related to timely identification and delivery of fetuses in jeopardy, rather than to the prevention of fetal compromise. Such an explanation seems unlikely

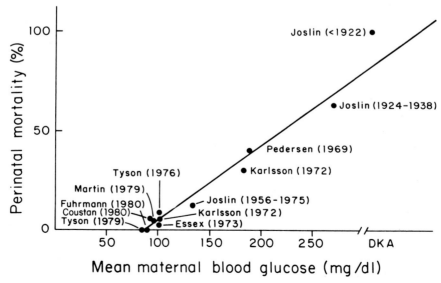

Fig. 23-1. Perinatal mortality rate in diabetic pregnancies as a function of mean maternal blood glucose level in third trimester. (Adapted from Jovanovic and Peterson,[21] with permission.)

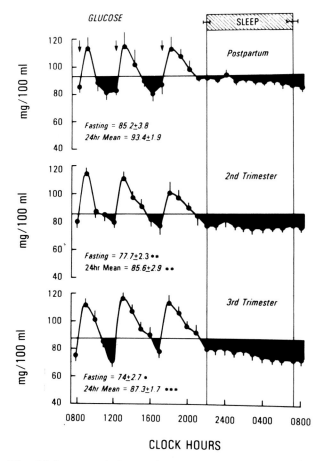

GLUCOSE

SLEEP

Postpartum

Fasting = 85.2±3.8
24hr Mean = 93.4±1.9

2nd Trimester

Fasting = 77.7±2.3 **
24hr Mean = 85.6±2.9 **

3rd Trimester

Fasting = 74±2.7 *
24hr Mean = 87.3±1.7 ***

CLOCK HOURS

Fig. 23-2. Diurnal glucose level excursions in six normal pregnant women during the second and third trimesters and 6 weeks postpartum. (From Cousins et al,[24] with permission.)

in light of the fact that the Karlsson and Kjellmer[18] series did not use antepartum fetal assessment. Furthermore, if advances in antepartum fetal monitoring (e.g., estriol measurement and nonstress and stress testing) were responsible for the noted improvements, it would be expected that approximately 10 to 20 percent of surviving newborns would have to be delivered expeditiously because of evidence of deteriorating fetoplacental function. In one series, in which 77 percent of diabetic women had mean plasma glucose levels below 120 mg/dl in the third trimester, only 2.8 percent of babies were delivered because of falling estriol levels or abnormal stress test results.[15] In another series of 52 very tightly controlled diabetic pregnancies, none

of 52 infants were delivered because of deteriorating fetal or placental function.[16]

Because sudden intrauterine fetal death occurs rarely, if at all, during intensive efforts at metabolic normalization in diabetic pregnancy, this phenomenon is difficult to study. In the past, hypotheses to explain the losses included unnoticed hypoglycemia and undiagnosed ketoacidosis. However, episodes of profound maternal hypoglycemia have generally been associated with fetal survival, and it is unlikely that episodes so mild as to go unnoticed would lead to fetal death. Diabetic ketoacidosis, on the other hand, has been associated with perinatal mortality rates of 50 to 90 percent.[25,26] It is impossible to document whether this was the mechanism for the fetal deaths reported in the past, but an alternative explanation is plausible. Myers[27] demonstrated that monkeys do not tolerate periods of hypoxia as well if they are hyperglycemic compared with euglycemic or even hypoglycemic. He found that hypoxia in the hyperglycemic rhesus monkey led to large accumulations of lactic acid in the central nervous system, which resulted in more severe brain damage. In studies in which sheep and rhesus monkey fetuses were made hyperinsulinemic by the direct infusion of glucose[28] or insulin,[29] the high fetal insulin levels led to increased glucose and oxygen uptake across the umbilical cord, hypoxia, acidosis, and fetal death. Similarly, when large amounts of glucose were infused into normal[30–33] and diabetic[34] pregnant humans in labor, neonatal hypoxemia or acidemia (or both) occurred with increased frequency. Bradley et al[35] obtained fetal blood by cordocentesis from diabetic pregnancies in the second and third trimesters. Although there was no difference from normal during the second trimester, the fetuses of type 1 diabetic mothers at term manifested higher lactate levels and lower pH, even before labor and delivery. Given these data, it appears likely that at least some intrauterine fetal deaths in diabetic pregnancies were caused by maternal hyperglycemia, which leads to fetal hyperinsulinemia and results in hypoxia and acidosis. Given lesser degrees of insult, it is possible that perinatal compromise in diabetic pregnancies may result from the same mechanism.

In summary, stillbirth occurs with increased frequency among pregnancies in diabetic mothers. There is an association between the rate of stillbirth and maternal hyperglycemia, and the incidence of this outcome has decreased steadily with improvements in diabetic control during pregnancy. The mechanism may be that of fetal hyperinsulinemia, but this has not been clearly proved. Currently, the appropriate strategy for prevention of perinatal loss is to attempt normalization of maternal glycemia, particularly during the third trimester.

PATHOPHYSIOLOGY OF PERINATAL MORBIDITY

As mentioned at the beginning of this chapter, the various types of perinatal morbidity seen in diabetic pregnancies are covered in other portions of this book. This section presents a unifying theme as to the pathophysiology of these types of morbidity, followed in the next by a plan for their prevention.

The "Pedersen[36] hypothesis" suggests that, in pregnant women with diabetes, maternal hyperglycemia is rapidly translated into fetal hyperglycemia. The fetal pancreas responds to this glycemic stimulus with islet cell hypertrophy and hyperplasia, and fetal hyperinsulinemia results. It is this fetal hyperinsulinemia that results in the diabetic fetopathy or perinatal morbidities seen in such pregnancies. The Pedersen hypothesis has been modified to allow for the possibility that nonglucose secretogogues for fetal pancreatic insulin may also be important[37] (Fig. 23-3).

As noted in Chapter 6, fetal hyperinsulinemia can induce macrosomia in rhesus monkeys. Similarly, macrosomic human infants of diabetic mothers demonstrate elevated cord blood[38] and amniotic fluid[39–41] insulin levels. There is also evidence that some macrosomic infants of nondiabetic mothers may manifest high cord blood insulin levels, which suggests that the pancreas of some fetuses may be particularly responsive to seemingly normal glucose levels.[42] Neonatal hypoglycemia is related to high fetal insulin levels in an obvious way. Neonatal polycythemia and hyperbilirubinemia, likewise, may be the result of fetal hyperinsulinemia, which leads to chronic hypoxia, as noted above, with a resultant increase in fetal erythropoietin.[43,44] The possible influence of fetal hyperinsulinemia on respiratory distress syndrome has been thoroughly covered elsewhere (see Ch. 7). Although it has been suggested that the hydramnios seen in diabetic pregnancy is related to fetal hyperglycemia with os-

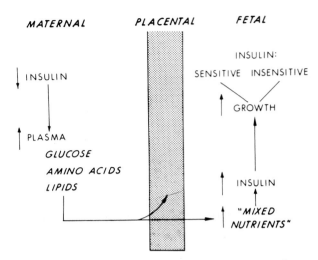

Fig. 23-3. Genesis of fetal hyperinsulinemia according to the "modified Pedersen hypothesis." (From Freinkel,[37] with permission.)

motic diuresis, this has not been documented to date. The increased incidence of hypertensive disorders of pregnancy among diabetic individuals may be related to diabetic vasculopathy rather than hyperglycemia, but an increasingly likely pathophysiologic explanation is the association between insulin resistance, hyperinsulinemia, and hypertension.[45,46]

STRATEGIES FOR PREVENTION

Because most complications in diabetic pregnancy are related, directly or indirectly, to maternal hyperglycemia-fetal hyperinsulinemia, it is apparent that therapeutic strategies should be directed toward normalization of maternal circulating glucose levels. As illustrated earlier, when this is done, both perinatal mortality and morbidity are reduced. They are not reduced to levels comparable to those observed in the nondiabetic general population, suggesting that either absolute euglycemia has not been achieved or that other fetal pancreatic secretogogues must be likewise normalized. The answer to this question remains for future research to uncover.

The appropriate use of dietary prescriptions and various insulin delivery systems and schemes are discussed earlier in this book. A third, and extremely important, strategy toward maintenance of euglycemia is the team concept of perinatal care. It is critical that pregnant women with diabetes are cared for in centers where such patients are frequently encountered. A critical mass of personnel, programs, and facilities are necessary to offer the diabetic gravid woman the optimal chance for a good outcome The obstetrician or internist who cares for the occasional diabetic pregnant woman simply does not have the time or the familiarity with problems specific to this group of patients to do a thorough job.

The team caring for diabetic pregnancies might consist of (1) an obstetrician who specializes in high-risk pregnancy (perinatologist) and/or (2) a diabetologist, internist, or obstetrician who is thoroughly familiar with modern concepts of diabetes care; (3) an ophthalmologist who is expert in detecting and treating diabetic retinopathy; (4) a nurse who devotes a significant proportion of time to patients with diabetes; (5) a dietitian; (6) a social worker; and (7) appropriate laboratory backup, including ultrasound. A neonatologist should be part of the team, and a highly competent neonatal unit should be available in the facility where delivery is planned. In most circumstances, the major interface of the team with the patient is the diabetes nurse specialist, who is in frequent telephone contact with each patient, often daily, and serves as the "anchor," that is, the one who is easily available when problems arise. Consistency in obtaining the daily blood glucose results is the most important means of preventing hyperglycemia in these individuals. An immediate response to aberrations in metabolic control tends to limit these to minor problems rather than major ones such as episodes of ketoacidosis, which may result when unacceptably high glucose values are ignored.

In some centers, the patient herself is made responsible for day-to-day adjustments in insulin dosage, with results being reported to the center at weekly or greater intervals. It has been our experience that, for many patients, this system is less than optimal. There is a tendency to assume that glucose values outside the intended range are the result of factors that are nonrecurrent and thus to put off adjustments in insulin because the glucose was high "for a reason." Although this assessment is sometimes accurate, we try to instill in our patients a sense that "fault" is not the issue and that the fetus does not "care" *why* its blood glucose

concentration is high only *that* it is elevated. Thus, having another person to report to, one who is not "emotionally involved" with the stresses and strains of the patient's daily life, tends to keep the patient on track toward the stated goal.

This frequent one-on-one contact (usually by telephone) has the added advantage of serving as an "early warning system" for complications. When the diabetic pregnant woman talks to the nurse and mentions that she has a "cold" coming on, the nurse takes the opportunity to review sick day management with the patient and to reinforce the need to step up surveillance of circulating glucose levels. If the patient mentions that she has, for example, "a little fluid coming out of her vagina," the nurse instructs her to come in for evaluation and not to wait for her next appointment. Thus, this contact is helpful not only for diabetic control but also for maintenance of the patient's overall obstetric state.

Thus, with the use of frequent home glucose monitoring, diet, insulin, and a team approach, it is possible to achieve euglycemia in most diabetic pregnancies and, in this way, to prevent much of the perinatal morbidity and mortality seen in former times.

REFERENCES

1. Williams JW: The clinical significance of glycosuria in pregnant women. Am J Med Sci 137:1, 1909
2. Silfen SL, Wapner RJ, Gabge SG: Maternal outcome in class H diabetes mellitus. Obstet Gynecol 55:749, 1980
3. Gabbe SG, Mestman JH, Hibbard LT: Maternal mortality in diabetes mellitus: an 18-year survey. Obstet Gynecol 48:549, 1976
4. Miller HC, Hurwitz D, Kuder K: Fetal and neonatal mortality in pregnancies complicated by diabetes mellitus. JAMA 124:271, 1944
5. White P: Pregnancy complicating diabetes. Am J Med 7: 609, 1949
6. Hall RE, Tillman AJB: Diabetes in pregnancy. Am J Obstet Gynecol 61:117, 1951
7. North AF, Mazumdar S, Logrillo VM: Birth weight, gestational age, and perinatal deaths in 5,471 infants of diabetic mothers. J Pediatr 90:444, 1977
8. Cassar J, Gordon H, Dixon HG et al: Simplified management of pregnancy complicated by diabetes. Br J Obstet Gynaecol 85:585, 1978
9. Jervell J, Moe N, Skjaerassen J et al: Diabetes mellitus and

pregnancy—management and results in Rikshospitalet, Oslo, 1970–1977. Diabetologia 16:151, 1979

10. Lemons JA, Vargas P, Delaney JJ: Infant of the diabetic mother: review of 225 cases. Obstet Gynecol 57:187, 1981

11. Soler NG, Soler SM, Malins JM: Neonatal morbidity among infants of diabetic mothers. Diabetes Care 1:340, 1978

12. Tevaarwerk GJM, Harding PGR, Milne KJ et al: Pregnancy in diabetic women: outcome with a program aimed at normoglycemia before meals. Can Med Assoc J 125:435, 1981

13. Gabbe SG, Mestman JH, Freeman RK et al: Management and outcome of pregnancy in diabetes mellitus, classes B to R. Am J Obstet Gynecol 129:723, 1977

14. Kitzmiller JL, Cloherty JP, Younger MD et al: Diabetic pregnancy and perinatal morbidity. Am J Obstet Gynecol 131:560, 1978

15. Coustan DR, Berkowitz RL, Hobbins JC: Tight metabolic control of overt diabetes in pregnancy. Am J Med 68:845, 1980

16. Jovanovic L, Druzin M, Peterson CM: Effect of euglycemia on the outcome of pregnancy in insulin-dependent diabetic women as compared with normal control subjects. Am J Med 71:921, 1981

17. Harley JMG, Montgomery DAD: Management of pregnancy complicated by diabetes. BMJ 1:14, 1965

18. Karlsson K, Kjellmer I: The outcome of diabetic pregnancies in relation to the mother's blood sugar level. Am J Obstet Gynecol 112:213, 1972

19. Churchill JA, Berendes HW, Nemore J: Neuropsychological deficits in children of diabetic mothers: a report from the collaborative study of Cerebral Palsy. Am J Obstet Gynecol 105:257, 1969

20. Roversi GD, Gargiulo M, Nicolini U et al: A new approach to the treatment of diabetic pregnant women. Am J Obstet Gynecol 135:567, 1979

21. Jovanovic L, Peterson CM: Management of the pregnant, insulin-dependent diabetic woman. Diabetes Care 3:63, 1980

22. Lewis SB, Wallin JD, Kuzuya H et al: Circadian variation of serum glucose, C-peptide imunoreactivity and free insulin in normal and insulin-treated diabetic pregnant subjects. Diabetologia 12:343, 1976

23. Gilmer MDG, Beard RW, Brooke F, Oakley NW: Carbohydrate metabolism in pregnancy. I. Diurnal plasma glucose profile in normal and diabetic women. BMJ 3:399, 1975

24. Cousins L, Rigg L, Hollingsworth D et al: The 24-hour excursion and diurnal rhythm of glucose, insulin, and C-peptide in normal pregnancy. Am J Obstet Gynecol 136:483, 1980

25. Drury MI, Greene AT, Stronge JM: Pregnancy compli-

cated by clinical diabetes mellitus: a study of 600 pregnancies. Obstet Gynecol 49:519, 1977

26. White P: Pregnancy and diabetes. p. 583. In Marble A, White P, Bradley R, Krall L (eds): Joslin's Diabetes Mellitus. 11th Ed. Lea & Febiger, Philadelphia, 1971

27. Myers RE: Brain damage due to asphyxia: mechanism of causation. J Perinat Med 9:78, 1981

28. Phillips AF, Dubin JW, Matty PJ, Raye JR: Arterial hypoxemia and hyperinsulinemia in the chronically hyperglycemic fetal lamb. Pediatr Res 16:653, 1982

29. Susa JB, Groppuso PA, Widness JA et al: Chronic hyperinsulinemia in the fetal rhesus monkey: effects of physiologic hyperinsulinemia on fetal substrates, hormones and hepatic enzymes. Am J Obstet Gynecol 150:415, 1984

30. Mauad-Filho F, deMorais EN, Parente JV et al: Effect of glucose infusion on the maternal and fetal acid-base equilibrium during labor. J Perinat Med 10:99, 1982

31. Kenepp NB, Shelley WC, Gabbe SG et al: Fetal and neonatal hazards of maternal hydration with 5% dextrose before cesarean section. Lancet 1:1150, 1982

32. Lawrence GF, Brown VA, Parsons RJ, Cooke ID: Fetomaternal consequences of high-dose glucose infusion during labour. Br J Obstet Gynaecol 89:27, 1982

33. Philipson EH, Kalhan SC, Riha MM, Pimentel R: Effects of maternal glucose infusion on fetal acid-base status in human pregnancy. Am J Obstet Gynecol 157:866, 1987

34. Datta S, Brown WU: Acid-base status in diabetic mothers and their infants following general or spinal anesthesia for cesarean section. Anesthesiology 47:272, 1977

35. Bradley RJ, Brudenell JM, Nicolaides KH: Fetal acidosis and hyperlacticaemia diagnosed by cordocentesis in pregnancies complicated by maternal diabetes mellitus. Diabetes Med 8:464, 1991

36. Pedersen JL: The Pregnant Diabetic and Her Newborn. Williams & Wilkins, Baltimore, 1967

37. Freinkel N: Banting lecture 1980: of pregnancy and progeny. Diabetes 19:1023, 1980

38. Weiss PAM, Hofmann H, Purstner P et al: Fetal insulin balance: gestational diabetes and postpartal screening. Obstet Gynecol 64:65, 1984

39. Lin CC, River P, Mosawad AH et al: Prenatal assessment of fetal outcome by amniotic fluid C-peptide levels in pregnant diabetic women. Am J Obstet Gynecol 141:671, 1981

40. Stangenberg M, Persson B, Vaclavinkova V: Amniotic fluid volumes and concentrations of C-peptide in diabetic pregnancies. Br J Obstet Gynaecol 89:536, 1982

41. Weiss PAM, Hofmann H, Winter et al: Gestational diabetes and screening during pregnancy. Obstet Gynecol 63:776, 1984

42. Hoegsberg B, Gruppuso PA, Coustan DR: Hyperinsulinemia in macrosomic infants of nondiabetic mothers. Diabetes Care 16:32, 1993

43. Widness JA, Sousa JB, Garcia JF et al: Increased erythropoiesis and elevated erythropoietin in infants born to diabetic mothers and in hyperinsulinemic rhesus fetuses. J Clin Invest 67:637, 1981
44. Phillips AF, Widness JA, Garcia JF et al: Erythropoietin elevation in the chronically hyperglycemic fetal lamb. Proc Soc Exp Biol Med 170:42, 1982
45. Bauman WA, Maimen M, Langer O: An association between hyperinsulinemia and hypertension during the third trimester of pregnancy. Am J Obstet Gynecol 159:446, 1988
46. Moller DE, Flier JS: Insulin resistance—mechanisms, syndromes and implications. N Engl J Med 325:938, 1991

24
Neonatal Outcome and Care

WILLIAM OH

Basic research and clinical investigations have generated new information during the past 2 to 3 decades that enhanced our understanding of morbidities encountered in infants of diabetic mothers (IDMs). Although optimal medical and obstetric management can indeed reduce the incidence and severity of the perinatal complications, it is very clear that, because of a multitude of factors, including lack of patient compliance, such an ideal situation is difficult to achieve. Therefore, it is important to understand clearly the pathophysiology, diagnosis, and management of the various neonatal complications.

As shown in Figure 24-1, one can postulate that, when maternal diabetes goes undetected or if good control of diabetes is not achieved, maternal episodic hyperglycemia leads to fetal episodic hyperglycemia, possible enhanced placental transfer of amino acids, and increased availability of fatty acids to the fetus. The epidodic fetal hyperglycemia is due to the direct relationship between the maternal and fetal blood glucose concentrations.[1] In mammalian species, the fetus derives most of its caloric and metabolic needs from glucose, transported from the mother across the placenta by facilitated diffusion.[2-4] Fetal hyperglycemia is associated with fetal hyperinsulinism with hypertrophy and hyperplasia of the β-cells of the fetal pancreas. There is strong evidence suggesting that insulin serves as the primary growth factor for the fetus.[5,6] Therefore, in the presence of an abundant supply of substrate, the hyperinsulinemic state accelerates fetal growth, leading to macrosomia. The presence of fetal macrosomia, in turn, sets the stage for the possibility of dystocia and an increased risk for birth injury and asphyxia during delivery. It has been shown that, in the nonhuman primate, chronic fetal hyperinsulinemia is associated with fetal macrosomia and selective organomegaly.[7] In spite

of increasing understanding of the pathophysiology and the management of diabetes during pregnancy, the incidence of macrosomia in IDMs appears to be unchanged.[8] Cardiomyopathy has been observed, and the morphologic cardiac abnormality has been correlated with functional changes. Using the echocardiographic technique, Walther et al[9] demonstrated an indirect correlation between the thickness of the atrioventricular septum and cardiac output in IDMs. The functional aberration is transient and is resolved at the end of the first week of life.

Another important clinical aspect of fetal macrosomia in IDMs is its relationship to obesity in later childhood. Vohr et al[10] demonstrated a direct correlation between neonatal macrosomia and obesity during the adolescent period. A similar relationship has been shown in an animal model in which neonatal macrosomia, a result of mild maternal hyperglycemia, was associated with obesity in young adult rats.[11-13] Furthermore, the obesity was also associated with glucose intolerance,[14] which raised the intriguing association between maternal diabetes, fetal macrosomia, adolescent obesity, and the development of glucose intolerance in young obese adult subjects.

Fetal hyperinsulinemia appears to be an important factor in the pathogenesis of the respiratory distress syndrome (RDS), which occurs more frequently in IDMs than it does in the offspring of nondiabetic mothers at similar gestational ages.[15,16] Several studies have shown the inhibitory effect of insulin on surfactant production, which provides an experimental rationale for the increased risk of RDS.[17-20] Furthermore, fetal hyperinsulinemia is also the mechanism involved in the increased risk of neonatal hypoglycemia in these infants.[21]

The mechanism for the increased risks of polycythe-

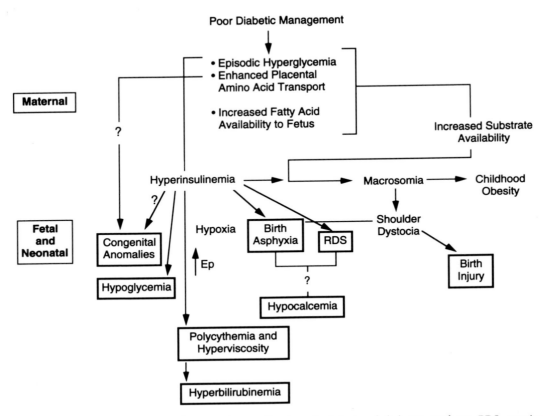

Fig. 24-1. Proposed pathogenesis of neonatal complications in infants of diabetic mothers. RDS, respiratory distress syndrome. Ep, erythropoietin.

mia and hyperviscosity in IDMs is less well defined. It has been shown that fetal hypoxia stimulates fetal erythropoietin production,[22] resulting in an increase in erythropoiesis. Such an association has been documented in infants of diabetic mothers (Fig. 24-2), although the precise relationship to polycythemia and hyperviscosity was not shown in this report.[22] Using the chronic sheep preparation an an animal model, Stonestreet et al[23] showed that fetal hypersinsulinemia is associated with increased fetal blood volume. Furthermore, the increased blood volume may also be explained on the basis of acute fetal distress and asphyxia. It has been shown previously that, in the presence of an intact umbilical circulation, fetal distress or birth asphyxia is associated with "intrauterine placental transfusion," that is, with an increase in fetal blood volume derived from the placenta.[24–26] After the acute

expansion of blood volume at birth, a process of adjustment between circulating blood volume and circulatory capacity occurs that results in hemoconcentration. Under these circumstances, some infants may have polycythemia and hyperviscosity on the basis of high hematocrit and blood viscosity.[27]

The precise mechanism for the increased incidence of neonatal hypocalcemia in IDMs is unknown. In IDMs, there are other complicating factors such as prematurity, birth asphyxia, and respiratory distress with acidosis that may adversely influence calcium and phosphate homeostasis during the first few days of life.

The higher incidence of hyperbilirubinemia in the offspring of diabetic mothers probably stems from the higher red blood cell volumes and an increased amount of "physiologic hemolysis" during the first days of life. There is currently no other mechanism

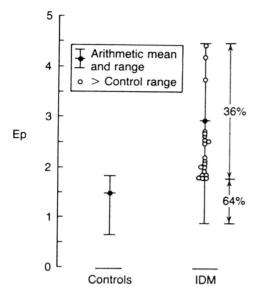

Fig. 24-2. Erythropoietin (Ep) levels in cord blood of infants of diabetic mothers (IDM). (From Widness et al,[22] with permission.)

that accounts for this common neonatal complication in IDMs. Other neonatal conditions for which the pathogenesis remains to be elucidated in the offspring of diabetic women include the increased incidence of congenital malformations. However, it has been suggested that good control of diabetes during preconception and during the first trimester of pregnancy significantly reduces the incidence of congenital anomalies in infants.[28]

It is clear from this overview that, if obstetric and medical management of diabetes is optimal during pregnancy and if the maternal blood glucose level is controlled throughout the period of gestation, the opportunity exists to reduce these various forms of perinatal morbidity and to improve survival for IDMs. The decreased perinatal mortality rate that has been achieved in association with careful maternal metabolic control is clear evidence that maternal management and diabetic status play an important role in the neonatal outcome.[29–31]

It is useful to bear in mind that the clinical abnormalities seen in IDMs usually occur in a predictable temporal sequence. There is a typical age of onset and duration for each of the common complications. As shown in Figure 24-3, neonatal depression, birth injury, and most congenital malformations are readily detectable at the time of birth by a careful assessment and physical examination of the infant in the delivery room. Respiratory distress, irrespective of cause, usually occurs soon after birth and characteristically persists for 3 to 5 days unless complications such as pneumothorax or pneumonitis prolong its course. Hypoglycemia usually develops during the first 3 hours of life, with a peak incidence at 1.5 hours after birth..In most instances, the hypoglycemia is transient in nature, and the blood glucose concentration returns to normal by 3 to 5 days of age. Because hemoconcentration occurs maximally at 3 to 6 hours of life, polycythemia and hyperviscosity usually present at this age. Therefore, a capillary hematocrit should be performed at that time as a screen of these complications. With treatment (by partial exchange transfusion), polycythemia and hyperviscosity generally occurs around 24 hours and re-

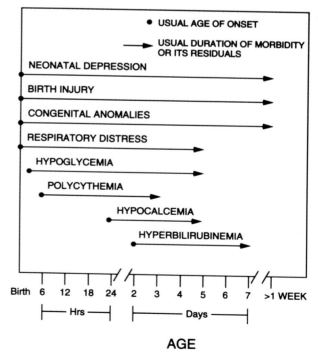

Fig. 24-3. Usual age of onset and duration of neonatal complications in infants of diabetic mothers.

solves at 3 to 5 days of age. Hyperbilirubinemia generally occurs around the second or third day and lasts through the first week of life.

NEONATAL MACROSOMIA

Neonatal macrosomia is a situation in which the birthweight exceeds standard deviations of the mean at a certain gestational age. The condition can be identified at birth and, with the aid of fetal ultrasonography, is often identified before birth. The recognition of fetal macrosomia is important because it is often associated with a number of perinatal morbidities, including birth injury, neonatal depression, respiratory distress, hypoglycemia, and hyperbilirubinemia. The relationship between neonatal macrosomia and obesity in later childhood has been discussed presviously. However, there are inadequate data to allow for more definitive anticipatory guidance in regard to the role of the dietary and nutritional management of the infants to prevent the development of childhood obesity.

NEONATAL DEPRESSION

Depression at birth is a common problem in IDMs if the control of diabetes during pregnancy is not optimal. As indicated in the previous discussion, fetal hyperinsulinemia is asssociated with fetal hypoxemia, probably on the basis of increased metabolic demand. Fetal status should be monitored, and if fetal distress is present, apropriate timing and mode of delivery are critical to avoid fetal demise or significant fetal distress that eventually may lead to neonatal depression. If fetal macrosomia is present, there is an increased likelihood that dystocia and difficulty during delivery may contribute to the occurrence of neonatal depression. Thus, with a history of inappropriate control of the diabetic condition, evidence of compromise in fetal status and fetal macrosomia, the possibility of neonatal depression should be strongly suspected and anticipated. Facilities, equipment, and personnel for neonatal resuscitation should be available during delivery of this infant for the prompt management of neonatal depression. Management consists of maneuvers to prevent cold injury, maintain airway, and establish cardiopulmonary function. After vaginal delivery, the umbilical cord is best clamped at 15 to 30 seconds after the delivery of the fetal body to avoid excessive placental transfusion.

BIRTH INJURY

The presence of an excessive-sized fetus in a mother with a small to normal-sized pelvis may result in prolonged labor, dystocia, or birth injury, particularly when a vaginal delivery is attempted. Some of the more common birth injuries in the macrosomic IDM include Erb's palsy, fractured clavicle, facial paralysis, phrenic nerve injury, and intracranial hemorrhage in the form of intracerebral bleeding or subdural hematomas.

The symptoms and signs of these various types of birth injury are well known to most clinicians. An awareness of such potential complications makes them readily identifiable soon after birth. For instance, facial palsies and Erb's paralysis can be detected by physical examination; phrenic nerve injuries are recognizable by the presence of respiratory distress together with asymmetric excursions of the hemidiaphragms during respiration. A fractured clavicle can be suspected by a lack of movement in the upper extremity on the side of injury and confirmed by radiologic examination. The diagnosis of intracranial hemorrhage is sometimes more difficult to make. A history of a difficult delivery in a macrosomic infant with birth depression in whom marked hypo- or hypertonia later develops associated with seizures should alert the clinician to the potential for intracranial pathologic conditions, including intracranial hemorrhage. When intracranial hemorrhage is suspected, cranial ultrasonography may be useful in arriving at this diagnosis. Computed tomographic scan can also identify other forms of intracranial hemorrhage. The medical management of these birth injuries is largely supportive because many of the injuries resolve over time. However, it should be pointed out that bleeding disorders in the intracranial areas may have longer lasting effects and sequelae.

CONGENITAL MALFORMATIONS

The incidence of congenital malformations in infants of diabetic mothers is significantly higher than in the normal newborn population. The precise reason for this increased risk of congenital anomalies is unknown, but it has been theorized that a "disturbed homeostatic state" during embryonic development, resulting from poor maternal metabolic control, may serve as a contributing factor.[32–34] The two most common groups of malformations encountered are those that involve the cardiovascular and skeletal systems, especially of the neural axis. Among the cardiovascular anomalies, transposition of the great vessels, atrial and ventricular septal defects, endocardial cushion defects, and coarctation of the aorta are most common. Caudal regression syndrome (sacral agenesis), although rare, is commonly associated with IDMs. Clinicians attending the IDM immediately after birth must be alert to these possibilities, and careful physical examination is essential for prompt detection. In cases in which strong possibilities for congenital malformations are present, diagnostic studies, including chest radiography, ultrasonography with echocardiography, and electrocardiography, should be done.

RESPIRATORY DISTRESS

Respiratory distress is also a common neonatal morbidity in the IDM. Causes of respiratory distress are not limited to RDS or hyaline membrane disease. "Retained lung fluid" secondary to cesarean birth,[35] transient tachypnea of the newborn,[36] hypoglycemia, and polycythemia and hyperviscosity[37] are some of the other known etiologic factors for respiratory difficulties in the newborn period. However, these metabolic and transitional causes of respiratory distress are usually benign and transient in nature and most often resolve by the second or third day of life. RDS, on the other hand, can be more severe, particularly for those infants who are born at a gestational age of less than 33 or 34 weeks. In the prenatal assessment of fetal lung maturity in the diabetic pregnancy, the conventional value of a mature lecithin/sphingomyelin (L/S) ratio (2:1) may often be misleading. In IDMs, an amniotic fluid L/S ratio of 2.0 may not necessarily indicate lung maturity because many of these fetus lack phosphatidyl glycerol (PG), one of the phospholipids in the lung that serves an important role in maintaining alveolar stability.[38] In normal pregnancy, fetal lung maturation is associated with a parallel increase in the various specific phospholipids (e.g., lecithin, PG, phosphatidyl-

inositol, and phosphatidylserine). In IDMs, for yet unknown reasons, there is delay in maturation of the PG synthesis system so that one may have a relatively normal L/S ratio with lack of PG, which leads to the development of RDS. Some investigators recommend using an L/S ratio of greater than 3.0 as an indicator of lung maturity for the IDM.[38,39] The most direct method to assess the level of lung maturity is to analyze both L/S ratio and PG. In many perinatal centers, the latter is routinely done in the clinical laboratory.

The management of IDMs with respiratory distress is supportive and is similar to the management on an infant with respiratory difficulty who is not an IDM. Recently, the use of surfactant replacement therapy has been shown to be effective in the treatment of infants with RDS.[40] However, its efficacy has not been shown specifically in IDMs. Nevertheless, because the pathophysiology of RDS is similar in IDMs and non-IDMs, there is no reason to suspect that surfactant replacement therapy will not be equally effective in the treatment of RDS in IDMs. Thus, in the presence of prematurity, evidence of fetal lung immaturity, and classic clinical signs of RDS (tachypnea, chest retraction, and typical radiologic findings of homogeneous granular infiltrate and air bronchogram), the use of surfactant therapy in IDMs is appropriate.

NEONATAL HYPOGLYCEMIA

This is the most common and well-defined metabolic complication in IDMs. The major contributing factor to the hypoglycemia is hyperinsulinemia at birth. The hyperinsulinemia leads to suppressed endogenous glucose production[41] by decreased gluconeogenesis and glycogenolysis, which occurs despite an abundance of glycogen stores in the liver and myocardium.[42] Hyperinsulinemia also leads to increased peripheral glucose utilization.

The peak age of onset for hypoglycemia is at 1 to 1.5 hours of life, and the frequency of this complication is greater in infants born to insulin-dependent mothers,[43] in infants whose mother's diabetic status is poor during pregnancy, and in those whose mothers receive large doses of intravenous glucose during labor or at the time of delivery.[30] Many IDMs with hypoglycemia may be asymptomatic; in those who are symptomatic, the manifestations may be nonspecific in nature. These manifestations include jitteriness, twitching of the extremities, apnea, tachypnea, and in extreme cases, seizures. The condition is confirmed by a determination of the plasma glucose level, and hypoglycemia is diagnosed when the plasma glucose concentration is less than 35 mg/dl in a term infant or less than 25 mg/dl in a preterm infant. All IDMs should have semiquantitative examinations of blood for glucose level (Dextrostix) at hourly intervals during the first 3 hours of life. If the Dextrostix findings suggest blood glucose level below 40 mg/dl, a plasma sample for glucose determination by the clinical laboratory should be obtained. The infant may be given an intravenous glucose infusion at a dose of 5 to 6 mg/kg/min, preferably through a peripheral vein. If the plasma glucose concentration confirms the diagnosis of hypoglycemia, the glucose infusion can be continued. If the plasma glucose value is normal and a repeat determination at 6 to 12 hours of age reveals normal results, the intravenous glucose can be discontinued if the infant's condition is stable and oral feeding is feasible. Otherwise, the intravenous glucose infusion can be continued and gradually tapered as the infant's ability to feed orally increases.

Early initiation of oral feeding (4 to 6 hours of age) is useful for earlier establishment of glucose and calcium homeostasis. However, it should not be done if the infant's cardiopulmonary status is unstable. The risk of aspiration is real and should be avoided.

The use of bolus hypertonic glucose infusion should be avoided because the hyperinsulinemia induced by a rise in plasma glucose level may lead to rebound hypoglycemia.[44] In infants with symptomatic hypoglycemia, a bolus dose of 200 mg/kg of 10 percent glucose may be given intravenously over a 5- to 10-minute period followed by continuous infusion with a dose that is indicated above. It has been shown that this method of glucose therapy provides a prompt increase in serum glucose concentration with no risk of a rebound hypoglycemia.[45] The use of glucagon during the first 6 hours of life has been proposed at a dosage of 300 μg/kg body weight.[46] However, there appears to be no real advantage to glucagon infusion. Glucagon administration may produce a brisk rise in blood glucose concentration so that the risk of rebound hypoglycemia is present and may constitute a potential disadvantage for this therapeutic regimen. Epinephrine has also been used in the treatment of neonatal hypoglycemia on the basis of its glycogenolytic property. However,

it has the disadvantages of producing untoward cardiovascular side effects and lactic acidosis in an infant who may already have cardiopulmonary difficulties.[47]

In most instances, neonatal hypoglycemia in the IDM is a transient condition. However, occasionally, the hypoglycemia may persist beyond the second or third day of life and may require the use of additional therapeutic agents, such as glucocorticoids. If hypoglycemia still persists despite adequate therapy, other underlying causes, such as β-cell hyperplasia (nesidioblastosis) or islet cell tumor, should be entertained. The prognosis for IDMs with hypoglycemia is usually favorable, and when the problem is treated promptly, neurologic sequelae are minimal.

POLYCYTHEMIA AND HYPERVISCOSITY

The precise incidence of polycythemia complicating the newborn period in IDMs has not been well documented. However, it is accepted by most clinicians that this morbidity is fairly common. The mechanism is based on a hypoxia-induced increase in erythropoietin and subsequent enhanced erythropoiesis. If fetal hypoxia occurs during labor, there is an increased possibility of placental transfusion and hypervolemia. In the presence of hypervolemia and subsequent hemoconcentration, a rise in hematocrit ensues. Those infants with a venous hematocrit value that exceeds two standard deviations (65 percent) are considered to be polycythemic.

Clinically, infants with polycythemia appear plethoric, and the condition is often initially suspected on the basis of the newborn's appearance and is confirmed by hematocrit determination. In this respect, it is important to consider the site of blood sampling because it is well known that capillary blood generally yields higher hemoglobin and hematocrit values than venous blood.[47,48] Figure 24-4 shows the correlation between capillary and venous hematocrits in term newborn infants during the first 24 hours of life. It may be used as a guide for estimating the venous hematocrit when a capillary blood measurement is used for screening purposes. It should be emphasized, however, that to establish the diagnosis of polycythemia definitively, a venous blood hematocrit is required.

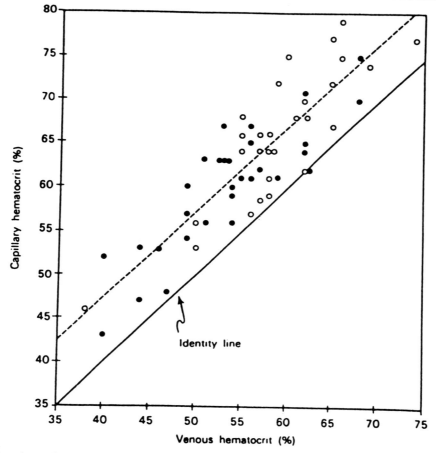

Fig. 24-4. Correlation between capillary and venous hematocrit in normal newborn infants during first 6 hours of life. (Modified from Oh and Lind,[48] with permission.)

It has been shown that the venous blood hematocrit and the blood viscosity are directly related.[49] When the hematocrit value exceeds 65 percent, the viscosity of the blood exceeds two standard deviations above the normal range, hence constituting a state of hyperviscoity.[49] Although it is ideal to diagnose hyperviscosity by actual measurement of blood viscosity,[50] many clinical laboratories may not have this service available. Thus, it is often assumed that an infant who evidences polycythemia also has hyperviscosity. It should be emphasized that this is not an entirely valid assumption.

The clinical manifestations of polycythemia are nonspecific in nature, mainly because the symptom complex may be attributed to one or more of the following four factors.

1. *Effects of perinatal asphyxia:* because perinatal asphyxia is often the primary event that leads to polycythemia and hyperviscosity, many polycythemic infants may have signs and symptoms relating to perinatal asphyxia
2. *Effects of transudation of fluid from intravascular into extravascular (interstitial) space of various organs:* the clearest evidence for this is the association of less efficient respiratory functions in infants with large placental transfusions. In the presence of acute expansion of blood volume, the newborn compensates by hemoconcentration, resulting in transvascular movement of fluid into interstitial tissue, including that of the lung.[51] The latter gives rise to low lung compliance and tachypnea

3. *Effect of increased erythrocyte mass* (e.g., increased incidence of hyperbilirubinemia in polycythemic infants because of "physiologic hemolysis")
4. *Effect of hyperviscosity itself,* which may impede the velocity of blood flow in various microcirculatory beds

The treatment of polycythemia or hyperviscosity consists of a partial exchange transfusion during which blood is removed and replaced by an equal quantity of a volume expander such as plasma, plasmanate, or salt-poor albumin. The formula used is as follows:

Blood volume to be exchanged (ml)

$$= \frac{\text{observed hematocrit} - \text{desired hematocrit (55\%)}}{\text{observed hematocrit}} \times \text{blood volume (90 ml)} \times \text{body weight (kg)}$$

Three to four hours after the procedure is done, it is prudent to re-examine the neonate's venous blood hematocrit and viscosity; if both parameters are still abnormally high, a repeat partial exchange transfusion may be indicated.

NEONATAL HYPOCALCEMIA

Neonatal hypocalcemia is the other major metabolic problem encountered in IDMs. The mechanism of hypocalcemia in this group of infants remains under investigation, but it has been suggested that a state of relative maternal hyperparathyroidism plays a role.[52] Although it has been shown that an elevated immunoreactive parathyrin level exists in normal pregnant women,[53] the precise parathyroid status in the diabetic mother has not been well defined. Other predisposing factors that could contribute to the increased incidence of hypocalcemia in IDMs include the greater frequency of respiratory distress with acidosis. It has been shown that, during a state of acidosis, calcium ions may diffuse from the intracellular into the extracellular fluid, including the intravascular compartment, hence producing an apparently normal serum calcium level. When acidosis is corrected either by treatment or through spontaneous recovery from the respiratory difficulties, the calcium ion re-equilibrates into the intracellular fluid compartment, resulting in an abrupt fall in the serum calcium concentration.[54] This may account for the fact that the peak age of onset of hypocalcemia is in the second or third day of life, coinciding with the usual recovery phase from respiratory distress. Hypoglucagonemia has also been implicated as another possible contributing factor to the hypocalcemia in IDMs.[55] However, this hypothesis is yet to be confirmed. Although IDMs with hypocalcemia may be asymptomatic, their hypocalcemia is usually treated with calcium supplementation administered either intravenously or orally. There are no follow-up data established in regard to the potential harmful or innocuous nature of asymptomatic hypocalcemia during the neonatal period.

HYPERBILIRUBINEMIA

It is well established that hyperbilirubinemia is a common problem in IDMs. It was previously believed that this was due mainly to prematurity because, in the past, most IDMs were delivered before term. It has been shown, however, that, even when matched for gestational age, the IDM has a higher risk of hyperbilirubinemia than does the normal infant.[56] The reason for this increased risk of jaundice is not known, but polycythemia with an associated increase in the breakdown of red blood cells is considered to be a contributing factor. In spite of this higher incidence of jaundice, the risk of kernicterus in IDMs does not appear to be unusually high. One hypothesis invoked to explain this observation in IDMs makes use of their suppressed lipolytic response to adrenergic-provoking stimuli such as hypothermia, hypoglycemia, stress, and so forth.[43] It has been speculated that the increased risk of kernicterus in infants with hyperbilirubinemia, under situations of stress, results from a reduction of bilirubin-binding capacity secondary to epinephrine-induced elevations in free fatty acids.[57,58] Therefore, reducing the lipolytic response to stress in IDMs may provide a degree of protection from kernicterus because the bilirubin-binding capacity will not be altered even in the presence of stress. More recently, there is increasing evidence that the risk of kernicterus in full-term infants with nonhemolytic jaundice is extremely low.[59] This observation is applicable in IDMs because most of these infants are full term and the hyperbilirubinemia is due to causes other than hemolysis. The management of hyperbilirubinemia in IDMs is similar to that in other infants. The main goal is to prevent kernicterus by keeping the serum bilirubin levels within the range of safety by phototherapy and, if needed, by exchange transfusion.

REFERENCES

1. Spellacy WN, Goetz FC, Greenberg BZ et al: The human placental gradient for plasma insulin and blood glucose. Am J Obstet Gynecol 90:753, 1964
2. Widdas WF: Transport mechanisms in the foetus. Br Med Bull 17:107, 1961
3. Karvonen MJ, Raiha N: Permeability of placenta of the guinea pig to glucose and fructose. Acta Physiol Scand 31:194, 1954
4. Battaglia FC, Hellegers AE, Heller CG et al: Glucose concentration gradients across the maternal surface, the placenta, and the amnion of the rhesus monkey (Macaca mulatta). Am J Obstet Gynecol 88:22, 1964
5. Hill DE: Effect of insulin on fetal growth. Semin Perinatol 2:319, 1978
6. Picon L: Effect of insulin on growth and biochemical composition of the rat fetus. Endocrinology 81:1419, 1967
7. Susa JB, Schwartz R: Effects of hyperinsulinemia in the primate fetus. Diabetes 34:36, 1985
8. Hod M, Merlob P, Friedman S et al: Gestational diabetes mellitus. A survey of perinatal complications in the 1980s. Diabetes, Suppl. 2, 40:74, 1991
9. Walther FJ, Siassi B, King J, Wu PY-K: Cardiac output in infants to insulin-dependent diabetic mothers. J Pediatr 107:109, 1985
10. Vohr BR, Lipsitt LP, Oh W: Somatic growth of children of diabetic mothers with reference to birth size. J Pediatr 97:196, 1980
11. Gelardi NL, Cha C-J, Oh W: Evaluation of insulin sensitivity in obese offspring of diabetic rats by hyperinsulinemic-euglycemic clamp. Pediatr Res 30:40, 1991
12. Cha C-JM, Gelardi NL, Oh W: Accelerated growth and abnormal glucose tolerance in young female rats exposed to fetal hyperinsulinemia. Pediatr Res 21:83, 1987
13. Gelardi NL, Cha C-JM, Oh W: Glucose metabolism in adipocytes of obese offsprings of mild hyperglycemic rats. Pediatr Res 28:641, 1990
14. Oh W, Cha C-JM, Gelardi NL: The cross generation effect of neonatal macrosomia in rat pups of streptozotocin induced diabetes. Pediatr Res 29:606, 1991
15. Vileisis RA, Oh W: Enhanced fatty acid synthesis in hyperinsulinemic rat fetuses. J Nutr 113:246, 1983
16. Robert MF, Neff RK, Hubbel JP et al: Association between diabetes and the respiratory distress syndrome in the newborn. N Engl J Med 294:357, 1976
17. Smith BT, Giroud LJP, Robert MF et al: Insulin antagonism of cortisol action on lecithin synthesis by cultured fetal lung cells. J Pediatr 87:953, 1975
18. Neufeld ND, Servanian A, Barrett CT, Kaplan SA: Inhibition of surfactant production by insulin in fetal rabbit lung slices. Pediatr Res 13:752, 1979
19. Epstein MF, Farrell PM, Chez RA: Fetal lung lecithin metabolism in the glucose-intolerant rhesus monkey pregnancy. Pediatrics 57:722, 1976
20. Morishige WK, Uetake CA, Greenwood FC, Akaka J: Pulmonary insulin responsivity: in vivo effects of insulin binding to lung receptors in normal rats. Endocrinology 100:1710, 1977
21. Cornblath M, Schwartz R: Disorders of Carbohydrate Metabolism in Infancy. 2nd Ed. WB Saunders, Philadelphia, 1976
22. Widness JA, Susa JB, Garcia JF et al: Increased erythropoiesis and elevated erythropoietin in infants born to diabetic mothers and in hyperinsulinemic rhesus fetuses. J Clin Invest 67:637, 1981
23. Stonestreet BS, Goldstein M, Oh W, Widness JA: Effects of prolonged hyperinsulinemia on erythropoiesis in fetal sheep. Am J Physiol 257:R1199, 1989
24. Oh W, Omori K, Emmanouilides GC, Phelps DL: Placenta to lamb fetus transfusion in utero during acute hypoxia. Am J Obstet Gynecol 122:316, 1975
25. Flod NE, Ackerman BD: Perinatal asphyxia and residual placental blood volume. Acta Paediatr Scand 60:433, 1971
26. Yao AC, Wist A, Lind J: The blood volume of the newborn infant delivered by caesarean section. Acta Paediatr Scand 56:585, 1967
27. Oh W: Neonatal polycythemia and hyperviscosity. Pediatr Clin North Am 33:523, 1986
28. Jovanovic L, Druzin M, Peterson CM: Effects of euglycemia on the outcome of pregnancy in insulin-dependent diabetic women as compared with normal control subjects. Am J Med 68:105, 1980
29. Gabbe SG, Mestman JH, Freeman RK et al: Management and outcome of pregnancy in diabetes mellitus, classes B to R. Am J Obstet Gynecol 129:723, 1977
30. Karlsson K, Kjellmer I: The outcome of diabetic pregnancies in relation to the mother's blood sugar level. Am J Obstet Gynecol 112:213, 1972
31. Coustan DR, Berkowitz RI, Hobbins JC: Tight metabolic control of overt diabetes in pregnancy. Am J Med 68:845, 1980
32. Cousins L: Congenital anomalies among infants of diabetic mothers. Am J Obstet Gynecol 147:333, 1983
33. Fuhrmann K, Reiher H, Semmler K, Glockner E: The

effect of intensified conventional insulin therapy before and during pregnancy on the malformation rate in off-spring of diabetic mothers. Exp Clin Endocrinol 83:173, 1984

34. Kylinen P, Stenman U-H, Kesaniemi-Kuokkanen T, Teramo K: Risk of minor and major fetal malformations in diabetics with high haemoglobin A_{1c} values in early pregnancy. BMJ 289:345, 1984

35. Milner AD, Saunders RA, Hopkin IE: Effects of delivery by caesarean section on lung mechanics and lung volume in the human neonate. Arch Dis Child 53:545, 1978

36. Avery ME, Gatewood OB, Brumley G: Transient tachypnea of the newborn: possible delayed resorption of fluid at birth. Am J Dis Child 1111:380, 1966

37. Richardson DW: Transient tachypnea of the newborn associated with hypervolemia. Can Med Assoc J 103:70, 1970

38. Meuller-Beubach E, Caritis SN, Edelstone DI et al: Lecithin/sphingomyelin ratio in amniotic fluid and its value for the prediction of neonatal respiratory distress syndrome in pregnant diabetic women. Am J Obstet Gynecol 130:28, 1978

39. Cunningham MD, Desai NS, Thompson SA et al: Amniotic fluid phosphatidylglycerol in diabetic pregnancies. Am J Obstet Gynecol 131:719, 1978

40. Mercier CE, Soll RF: Clinical trials of natural surfactant extract in respiratory distress syndrome. Clin Perinatol 20:711, 1993

41. Kalhan SC, Savin SM, Adam PAJ: Attenuated glucose production rate in newborn infants of insulin dependent diabetic mothers. N Engl J Med 296:375, 1977

42. Cardell BS: The infants of diabetic mothers. A morphological study. Br J Obstet Gynaecol 60:834, 1953

43. Chen CH, Adam PAJ, Laskowski DE et al: The plasma free fatty acid composition and blood glucose of normal and diabetic pregnant women and of their newborns. Pediatrics 36:843, 1965

44. Haworth JC, Dilling LA, Vidyasagar D: Hypoglycemia in infants of diabetic mothers. Effect of epinephrine therapy. J Pediatr 82:94, 1973

45. Lilien LD, Pildes RS, Sainivasan G et al: Treatment of neonatal hypoglycemia with minibolus and intravenous glucose infusion. J Pediatr 97:295, 1980

46. Wu PYK, Modanlou H, Karelitz M: Effect of glucagon on blood glucose homeostasis in infants of diabetic mothers. Acta Paediatr Scand 64:441, 1975

47. Oettinger L Jr, Mills WB: Simultaneous capillary and venous hemoglobin determinations in the newborn infant. J Pediatr 35:362, 1949

48. Oh W, Lind J: Venous and capillary hematocrit in newborn infants and placental transfusion. Acta Paediatr Scand 56:197, 1966

49. Gross GP, Hathaway EW, Boyle E: Hyperviscosity in the neonate. J Pediatr 82:2004, 1973

50. Wells RE, Denton R, Merrill EW: Measurement of viscosity of biologic fluids by cone-plate viscometer. J Lab Clin Med 57:646, 1961

51. Oh W, Wallgren G, Hanson JS, Lind J: The effects of placental transfusion on respiratory mechanics of normal term newborn infants. Pediatrics 40:6, 1967

52. Tsang RC, Kleinman LL, Sutherland JM et al: Hypocalcemia in infants of diabetic mothers. J Pediatr 80:384, 1972

53. Cushard WG Jr, Creditor MA, Canterbury JM et al: Physiologic hyperparathyroidism in pregnancy. J Clin Endocrinol Metab 34:767, 1972

54. Tsang RC, Oh W: Neonatal hypocalcemia in low birth weights infants. Pediatrics 45:773, 1970

55. Bergman L: Studies on early neonatal hypocalcemia. Acta Pediatr Scand Suppl 248:5, 1974

56. Taylor PM, Wofson JH, Bright NH et al: Hyperbilirubinemia in infants of diabetic mothers. Biol Neonate 5:289, 1963

57. Schiff D, Aranda JV, Chan G et al: Metabolic effects of exchange transfusions. I. Effect of citrated and heparinized blood on glucose, nonesterified fatty acids, 2-(4-hyporoxy-benzeneazo)benzoic acid binding, and insulin. J Pediatr 78:603, 1971

58. Brown AK: Variations in the management of neonatal hyperbilirubinemia. Impact of our understanding of fetal and neonatal physiology. Birth Defects 6:22, 1970

59. Newman TB, Maisels MJ: Evaluation and treatment of jaundice in the term newborn: a kinder, gentler approach. Pediatrics 89:809, 1992

25

Long-Term Outcome of Infants of Diabetic Mothers

DAVID J. PETTITT
PETER H. BENNETT

The infant of the diabetic mother eventually becomes the child, the adolescent, and the adult offspring of the diabetic mother. The legacy of the diabetic intrauterine environment, acquired during gestation, cannot be ignored. It is increasingly clear that the effects of the diabetic intrauterine environment extend beyond those that are readily apparent at birth. Anthropometric, neurologic, and metabolic differences are found between such offspring and those of normal pregnancies.[1]

The long-range anatomic and functional changes that result from development in a diabetic intrauterine environment can be divided into four areas:

1. *Growth:* growth rate, height, and development as they relate to obesity are excessive during the latter stages of gestation and are also excessive during childhood and early adulthood
2. *Glucose homeostasis:* because of genetic and environmental factors, glucose tolerance is more likely to be abnormal than that observed in offspring of nondiabetic women
3. *Neurologic and psychological development:* offspring of high-risk pregnancies often have neurologic defects, which are usually relatively minor, but which may be significant causes of morbidity
4. *Miscellaneous:* there are long-term sequelae of congenital structural abnormalities and residua of birth trauma, especially if the abnormalities are severe enough to be recognized during the newborn period

GROWTH

As is evident from standardized growth curves, there is great variation in height and weight among growing children, even within a family. For a given height, the heaviest "normal" individuals may weigh almost twice as much as the lightest. Consequently, factors that affect growth may need to exert a very large effect to cause an otherwise average child to meet some arbitrary definition for obesity, and a child genetically destined to be near the low end of the scale may end up well above the mean without appearing abnormal. Thus, individual children within the normal range for height and weight may be very different from what they would have been without an antecedent insult. Nevertheless, the offspring of diabetic women are, on average, heavier for their height than the offspring of nondiabetic women.

In 1953, White et al[2] at the Joslin Clinic reported "superiority of growth in stature and weight" in the offspring of women with diabetes. Subsequently, reports from many parts of the world have confirmed and documented excessive growth in the offspring of diabetic women after the first few years of life. Table 25-1 summarizes the results from such studies.[2–13] Several reports indicate that the offspring of diabetic women are slightly taller than those of nondiabetic women,[2,3,13] but in other reports, the offspring of diabetic women have, on average, been normal[4,5,7,12] or short.[5,6] Most investigators report overweight or obesity in these children. Most recently, using published growth curves for comparison, Silverman et al[12,13] re-

Table 25-1. Growth in the Offspring of Diabetic Women

Ages (y)	Stature[a]	Overweight	Comments	References
1–20	Tall	+		White et al[2]
6–16	Tall	+	"Gigantism"	White[3]
0.5–10	Normal	+		Farquhar[4]
≤18	Normal/short	+		Farquhar[5]
0.5–30	Short	+		Hagbard et al[6]
1–23	Normal	+		Breidahl[7]
6–14		+		Adler et al[8]
4.5–13.5		+		Cummins et al[9]
0.2–1		–	Strict diet	Enzi et al[10]
5–19		+		Pettitt et al[11]
20–29		–		Current chapter
6	Normal	+		Metzger et al[12]
8	Tall	+		Silverman et al[13]

[a] Blank if data on stature not presented.

Abbreviations: +, overweight or obesity present; –, overweight not found.

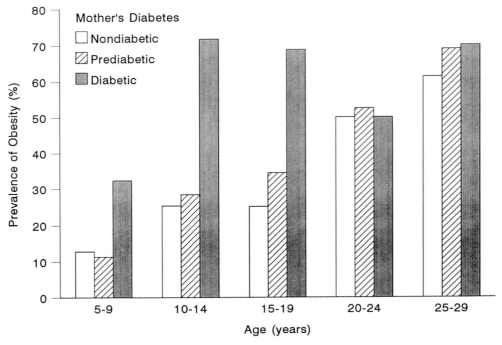

Fig. 25-1. Prevalence of obesity by age group in the offspring of nondiabetic, prediabetic (i.e., women who, during pregnancy, had documented normal glucose tolerance but who subsequently developed diabetes), and diabetic women. (Adapted from Pettitt et al,[11] with permission.)

ported that by age 8 years, the offspring of women with diabetes or gestational diabetes were slightly taller than expected. In addition, one-half of the children were at or above the 90th percentile for weight on these curves. A direct correlation was found between amniotic fluid insulin concentration and relative obesity at ages 6 and 8 years, suggesting a possible mechanism for the excessive growth.[12,13]

Among Pima Indian children of Arizona examined after the age of 5 years, the offspring of women who had diabetes during pregnancy were heavier for height, and more likely to be obese, than the offspring of either nondiabetic or prediabetic women (i.e., women who had normal glucose tolerance during pregnancy but in whom diabetes subsequently developed).[11] Even normal-birthweight offspring of diabetic women were larger by age 5 to 9 years than were those of nondiabetic women.[14] This association between diabetes in pregnancy and childhood obesity was not confounded by, and did not appear to be related to, maternal obesity. Figure 25-1 shows the prevalence of obesity according to age. Before the age of 20 years, the offspring of diabetic women were heavier for height than those of nondiabetic and prediabetic women,[11,15] which suggests an important influence of the diabetic intrauterine environment. However, after age 20 years, there was little difference in relative weight between offspring whose mothers were diabetic and those whose mothers did not have diabetes. By this age, the effects of the diabetic intrauterine environment on obesity, so important at younger ages, were apparently superseded by other determinants of obesity.

Evidence that excess growth is not due to genetic factors alone comes from three areas. First, obesity is no more common in the offspring of women in whom diabetes developed after delivery than in those of nondiabetic women.[6,11] Second, obesity in the offspring of diabetic women cannot be accounted for by maternal obesity.[11,14] Third, the excessive growth seen in the offspring of diabetic mothers was not found in those of diabetic fathers in either the Joslin Clinic[3] or the Pima Indians series.[16]

GLUCOSE HOMEOSTASIS

Standard methods for the diagnosis of diabetes and impaired glucose tolerance, which have been generally accepted since 1979, require the ingestion of a standard carbohydrate load in asymptomatic individuals.[17-19] Such tests have seldom been performed in clinical practice in children, even for those whose parents have diabetes. Surveys of populations and selected groups, however, have allowed an evaluation of glucose tolerance in children in relation to their mothers' glucose tolerance or diabetes status at the time of pregnancy.

Reports from several countries document high rates of diabetes in the offspring of diabetic parents or high rates of diabetes in the parents of children with diabetes. Some of these reports are summarized in Table 25-2.[2,3,20-29] Many studies of the familial occurrence of diabetes, however, have not distinguished between parental diabetes that developed before and after the pregnancy. Consequently, children who are the products of metabolically normal pregnancies but whose mothers eventually developed diabetes are often included along with those whose mothers had diabetes during pregnancy. Nevertheless, studies that look at the offspring of women with diabetes generally find higher rates of diabetes than in those of nondiabetic women.[2,3,20-23,26,29]

The rates of diabetes in the offspring of diabetic women range from 5 to 225 times the rates in the general population, and there are no reports of lower than expected rates of diabetes in the offspring of parents with diabetes. Although it is generally accepted that diabetes is familial, transmission does not follow simple mendelian patterns and appears to be influenced by both the environment and the genetic background.[30-32] Factors such as viral infection[33] are associated with insulin-dependent diabetes mellitus (IDDM), and diuretic use,[34,35] obesity,[36-40] and physical inactivity[41-43] play important roles in impairment of glucose tolerance and non-insulin-dependent diabetes mellitus (NIDDM). How much of the excess diabetes in the offspring of diabetic mothers can be attributed to heredity and how much can be attributed to the environment is not clear, but there is evidence that the intrauterine environment plays an important role. Inheritance of a "diabetes gene" or genes may be necessary in order for the environment to have an effect.

Only in longitudinal studies that follow women who have normal glucose tolerance during pregnancy but who subsequently develop diabetes, can women be identified, in retrospect, as prediabetic. Comparison of the offspring of prediabetic pregnancies with those of

Table 25-2. Glucose Tolerance in the Offspring of Diabetic Parents

Ages (y)	Diabetes Present[a] (%)	Relative Risk[b]	Other	Reference
1–20	10.5	255		White et al[2]
1–30	8		2% with diabetic fathers	White[3]
All	Boys			Simpson[20,21]
	1.4		Mother's age of onset <20 y	
	1.2		Mother's age of onset ≥20 y	
	Girls			
	1.1		Mother's age of onset <20 y	
	0.8		Mother's age of onset ≥20 y	
1.5–26	1	20–30		Yssing[22]
≤15	0.7	20		Bibergeil et al[23]
1–32	3.4		1.5% of offspring of women with type 1	Köbberling and Brüggeboes[24]
0–adult			High risk of type 1 in parents; more likely, the father	Wagener et al[25]
0.1–20	1.3	5	6.1% in offspring of diabetic fathers	Warram et al[26]
Adult			More diabetic parents; diabetic parents, especially mother, had early age of onset	Lee et al[27]
0–14			High risk of type 1 in parents, especially father, of diabetic children	Dahlquist et al[28]
10–24	7.4	12.3		Pettitt et al[29]

[a] Blank if rate not presented.
[b] Relative risk of diabetes in the offspring of diabetic children.

diabetic pregnancies identifies differences that are likely to be the effect of the diabetic intrauterine environment. High rates of diabetes have generally been found in the offspring of diabetic fathers, but it has been recognized for some time, as stated by White[3] in 1960, that the "... maternal environment, prenatal, natal and post natal, has a greater influence upon the second generation than did the diabetic paternal environment." The maternal environment has also been shown to have a much greater effect on the occurrence of diabetes in Pima Indians,[29] as described below.

A greater influence of the maternal environment is not always apparent. In contrast to the Pima studies, Warram et al[26] reported higher rates of IDDM among the offspring of diabetic men than of diabetic women with IDDM. They speculated that women with a diabetic susceptibility may experience selective intrauterine loss of fetuses that inherit this susceptibility. This would not occur if the parent with the diabetes susceptibility were the father and would lead to the survival of a larger percentage of infants in whom diabetes eventually develops from diabetic fathers than from diabetic mothers. The hypothesis is that the fetus who inherits the susceptibility to IDDM is less likely to sur-

vive the pregnancy if the mother also has this susceptibility. Other studies of the familial occurrence of IDDM in children have also found that a greater proportion had diabetic fathers than diabetic mothers, findings that are in accord with Warram et al's hypotheses.[25,27]

Among the Pima Indians, a population with a very high prevalence of NIDDM, the diabetic intrauterine environment appears to have a greater effect on glucose tolerance in the offspring than does paternal diabetes.[29] Figure 25-2 shows the prevalence of diabetes by age in the offspring of nondiabetic, prediabetic, and diabetic women. The high prevalence among the offspring of diabetic women persists through the older age group even though there is little difference in obesity by this age.

Pathogenesis

Data from laboratory animals and autopsies done on infants of diabetic women suggest possible mechanisms that may result in abnormal glucose tolerance in the child of the diabetic woman. From 34 weeks of gestation, the infants of diabetic women have histologic evidence of hyperplasia of the islet cells, a higher

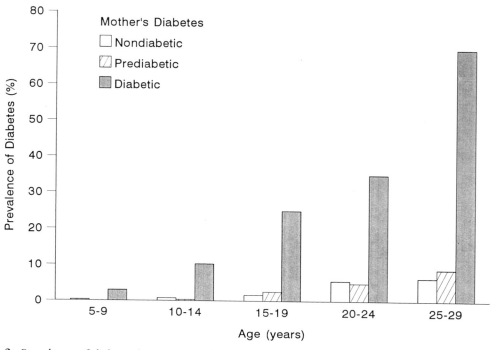

Fig. 25-2. Prevalence of diabetes by age group (see legend for Figure 25-1 for description of groups). (Adapted from Pettitt et al,[29] with permission.)

β-cell mass, and a greater pancreatic insulin content than do infants of nondiabetic mothers.[44–47] The serum insulin (and C-peptide) is elevated, sometimes resulting in hypoglycemia.[45,48–50] Hypoglycemia is transient, resolving within a few days of birth, but islet abnormalities persist. Naeye[51] found an increase in islet tissue in infants of diabetic women, regardless of birth weight, that was caused both by hypertrophy and hyperplasia of the islet cells. Hultquist and Olding[52] found pancreatic islet fibrosis at autopsy in infants of diabetic women who survived up to 5 months, and Nelson et al[53] found fibrosis in the infants of diabetic women who survived up to 14 months. Fibrosis of the fetal islets and hypertrophy and hyperplasia of the islets may persist throughout life in some offspring, thereby affecting glucose tolerance later. The presence of islet cell hyperplasia and hypertrophy suggests that such infants may be more susceptible to the later development of hyperinsulinemia and, perhaps secondarily, compensatory insulin resistance that could then lead to glucose intolerance. On the other hand, any process that causes pancreatic fibrosis could lead to a decrease in islet cell mass and potentially to insulin deficiency and then to diabetes. The critical investigations that would allow differentiation between these hypotheses remain to be performed.

NEUROLOGIC AND PSYCHOLOGICAL DEVELOPMENT

Past reports of neurologic problems of the children of diabetic women have included impaired visual motor function, low intelligence, Erb's palsy, seizure disorder, cerebral palsy, mental retardation, speech disturbances, reading difficulties, behavior disturbance, psychosis, and deafness.[9,22,54–69] Possible reasons for the infants of diabetic women to be at risk of neurologic impairment include more birth trauma, especially trauma to the head and neck because of large infant size, and shoulder dystocia,[54] which leads to structural damage and hypoxic necrosis; metabolic abnormalities during gestation, which may cause aberrations in neurologic development; neonatal hypoglycemia, which rarely may damage the central nervous system with potentially permanent deficits[58,59]; and neonatal hyperbilirubinemia, which leads to kernicterus.[60,61] In addition, even though the infant of the diabetic woman tends toward general macrosomia, the brain is underweight for gestational age.[48,62] Major cerebral dysfunction has been related to more severe diabetes in pregnancy.[22] In the newborn offspring of women with well-controlled diabetes, Rizzo et al[67] found a significant inverse correlation between maternal glycemia during pregnancy and newborn behavior.

At least two studies have found an association between acetonuria during pregnancy and lower intelligence quotients (IQ) in the offspring of diabetic mothers.[63,64] In one of these, birthweight was also predictive of IQ, with smaller infants at birth having lower IQ scores at age 5 years.[63] Rizzo et al,[68] although finding no correlation between maternal acetonuria and the child's IQ, found an inverse correlation between maternal second trimester β-hydroxybutyrate concentrations and the offspring's mental development index scores at age 2 years. The mothers of these children had well-controlled diabetes during pregnancy and only infrequently had acetonuria.

Although hypoglycemia can result in potentially permanent damage to the central nervous system, no relationship was found between neonatal hypoglycemia in the offspring of diabetic women and low IQ.[65] The offspring of diabetic women fared better on follow-up than did hypoglycemic infants whose mothers did not have diabetes.[58] It appears either that the underlying cause of the hypoglycemia in these other infants was different, or that early recognition and treatment of the infant of the diabetic mother was responsible for the difference (i.e., it may not be the hypoglycemia per se that causes the problem in most cases). Delivery of very large infants by cesarean section and control of blood glucose concentrations throughout gestation may prevent neurologic problems in the offspring of diabetic women.[59,61] Indeed, several studies have reported very good neurologic outcomes for the offspring of diabetic women, with normal IQ scores and no overall difference between these children and the offspring of nondiabetic women.[9,65,69]

MISCELLANEOUS

Congenital anomalies, by definition anomalies present at birth, are frequently induced during organogenesis by the diabetic intrauterine environment.[70] The outlook for those with nonfatal abnormalities depends on the nature of the specific anomaly, and a complete discussion of the long-term outlook for infants with various anomalies is beyond the scope of this chapter. There is no evidence that the offspring of diabetic women fare any better or worse than do others with similar anomalies. Likewise, trauma, most notably to the head and brachial plexus, but to a lesser extent to abdominal organs, occurs more frequently in the offspring of diabetic women because of the increased frequency of very large and premature infants and often leads to permanent disability. In addition, the pronounced decrease in the plasma calcium concentration after birth in the offspring of women with diabetes is thought to be responsible for enamel hypoplasia and structural abnormalities in deciduous teeth.[8,71–73]

Animal Studies

There is good evidence that, in addition to any genetic effects that may be present, the diabetic intrauterine environment has lasting effects on the offspring. Evidence in humans is supported by studies in which hyperglycemia was induced in animals not genetically predisposed to diabetes. These studies have clearly shown that the abnormal intrauterine environment alone is sufficient to have long-lasting effects on the offspring.[74–76] Streptozotocin-induced diabetes in rats was shown by Aerts and Van Assche[74] to result in abnormal pancreatic morphology in the offspring. As adults, both the second- and third-generation offspring had impaired glucose tolerance and gestational diabetes.[75] Gauguier et al[76] showed similar abnormalities in the offspring of rats kept hyperglycemic by glucose infusion during pregnancy.

PROJECTIONS FOR THE FUTURE

The effect of maternal diabetes on the child may be viewed as a vicious cycle.[77,78] Children whose mothers had NIDDM during pregnancy are at increased risk of becoming obese and having diabetes develop at young

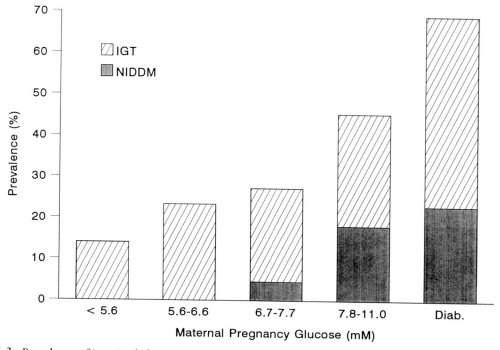

Fig. 25-3. Prevalence of impaired glucose tolerance (IGT) and non-insulin-dependent diabetes mellitus (NIDDM) at pregnancy in women aged 15 to 24 years by their mothers' 2-hour postload glucose test result during pregnancy.

ages. Many of these children already have diabetes or abnormal glucose tolerance by the time they reach their childbearing years, thereby perpetuating the cycle. As seen in Figure 25-3, higher rates of impaired glucose tolerance and diabetes were found in Pima Indian women by the time of pregnancy if their mothers had had diabetes during their own pregnancies.[79]

Although rigorous control of diabetes during pregnancy has been shown to decrease infant mortality, reduce the prevalence of macrosomia, and normalize the delivery and postpartum course for the mother,[80–83] there is little evidence that this leads to longer term benefits for the offspring. Indeed, even levels of abnormal glucose tolerance that are not diagnostic of diabetes in the nonpregnant state are associated with slightly higher glucose concentrations and more obesity in the offspring.[79,84] However, Dorner et al[85] speculated that treatment of diabetes and impaired glucose tolerance in pregnant women, along with the prevention of overnutrition in the newborn, by preventing hyperinsulinism in the fetus and newborn dur-

ing differentiation and maturation of the neuroendocrine system, may be responsible for the decrease in the prevalence of childhood diabetes seen in Berlin. Enzi et al[10] provided evidence that the excess obesity seen in the offspring of women with diabetes during the pregnancy may not be inevitable. They followed infants whose diabetic mothers had been receiving strict low-calorie diets during the pregnancy. Those of normal birthweight and who had been receiving carefully controlled diets to age 1 year were not obese by that time. They concluded that overnutrition in utero, such as occurs with maternal diabetes, does not have long-lasting effects on adiposity if the birthweight is normal and infant overfeeding is prevented.

In the past, high perinatal mortality claimed many offspring of diabetic women. These were those who had the greatest perinatal difficulties and whose mothers for the most part had poorly controlled diabetes. Long-term follow-up, therefore, was limited to the survivors who may not have been as severely affected as those who died in utero or in infancy. Today, infant survival is the norm, even for infants of women with severe diabetes that is difficult to control. The long-term effects in the offspring of diabetic women who are being born today, therefore, may differ from those reported previously. The long-term outcome in the future may be no better than in the past because children, who in former times would have died in utero, now survive. By contrast, because of better prenatal care and monitoring and better newborn care, adverse effects may be less than in former times. The challenge for the future is to see whether a degree of diabetic control can be achieved throughout pregnancy that would prevent the developing fetus from recognizing that its mother has diabetes, thus breaking the vicious cycle. If this is achievable, it will in turn probably reduce the prevalence of diabetes in the next generation of pregnancies and, therefore, be beneficial for future generations as well as the immediate offspring.

REFERENCES

1. Freinkel N: Banting lecture 1980: of pregnancy and progeny. Diabetes 29:1023, 1980
2. White P, Koshy P, Duckers J: The management of pregnancy complicating diabetes and of children of diabetic mothers. Med Clin North Am 39:1481, 1953
3. White P: Childhood diabetes: its course, and influence on the second and third generations. Diabetes 9:345, 1960
4. Farquhar JW: The child of the diabetic woman. Arch Dis Child 34:76, 1959
5. Farquhar JW: Prognosis for babies born to diabetic mothers in Edinburgh. Arch Dis Child 44:36, 1969
6. Hagbard IO, Reinard T: A follow-up study of 514 children of diabetic mothers. Acta Paediatr Scand 48:184, 1959
7. Breidahl HD: The growth and development of children born to mothers with diabetes. Med J Aust 1:268, 1966
8. Adler P, Fett KD, Bohatka L: The influence of maternal diabetes on dental development of the non-diabetic offspring in the stage of transitional dentition. Acta Paediatr Hung 18:181, 1977
9. Cummins M, Norrish M: Follow-up of children of diabetic mothers. Arch Dis Child 55:259, 1980
10. Enzi G, Inelmen EM, Rubaltelli FF et al: Postnatal development of adipose tissue in normal children on strictly controlled calorie intake. Metabolism 31:1029, 1982
11. Pettitt DJ, Baird HR, Aleck KA et al: Excessive obesity in offspring of Pima Indian women with diabetes during pregnancy. N Engl J Med 308:242, 1983
12. Metzger BE, Silverman BL, Freinkel N et al: Amniotic fluid insulin concentration as a predictor of obesity. Arch Dis Child 65:1050, 1990
13. Silverman BL, Rizzo T, Green OC et al: Long-term prospective evaluation of offspring of diabetic mothers. Diabetes, suppl. 2, 40:121, 1991
14. Pettitt DJ, Knowler WC, Bennett PH et al: Obesity in offspring of diabetic Pima Indian women despite normal birthweight. Diabetes Care 10:76, 1987
15. Pettitt DJ, Nelson RG, Saad MF et al: Diabetes and obesity in the offspring of Pima Indian women with diabetes during pregnancy. Diabetes Care, suppl. 1, 16:310, 1993
16. Pettitt DJ, Bennett PH: Long-term outcome of infants of diabetic mothers. p. 559. In Reece EA, Coustan D (eds): Diabetes Mellitus in Pregnancy: Principles and Practice. Churchill Livingstone, New York, 1988
17. National Diabetes Data Group: Classification and diagnosis of diabetes mellitus and other categories of glucose intolerance. Diabetes 28:1039, 1979
18. WHO Study Group: WHO Expert Committee on Diabetes Mellitus. 2nd Report. World Health Organization Technical Report Series 646. World Health Organization, Geneva, 1980
19. WHO Study Group: Diabetes Mellitus. World Health Organization Technical Report Series 727. World Health Organization, Geneva, 1985
20. Simpson NE: Diabetes in the families of diabetics. Can Med Assoc J 98:427, 1968
21. Simpson NE: Heritabilities of liability to diabetes when sex and age at onset are considered. Ann Hum Genet 32:283, 1969
22. Yssing M: Long-term prognosis of children born to mothers diabetic when pregnant. p. 575. In Camerini-Davalos RA, Cole HS (eds): Early Diabetes in Early Life. Academic Press, San Diego, 1975
23. Bibergeil H, Godel E, Amendt P: Diabetes and pregnancy: early and late prognosis of children of diabetic mothers. p. 427. In Camerini-Davalos RA, Cole HS (eds): Early Diabetes in Early Life. Academic Press, San Diego, 1975
24. Köbberling J, Brüggeboes B: Prevalence of diabetes among children of insulin-dependent diabetic mothers. Diabetologia 18:459, 1980
25. Wagener DK, Sacks JM, LaPoret RE, MacGregor JM: The Pittsburgh study of insulin-dependent diabetes mellitus. Diabetes 31:136, 1982
26. Warram JH, Krolewski AS, Gottlieb MS, Kahn CR: Differences in risk of insulin-dependent diabetes in offspring of diabetic mothers and diabetic fathers. N Engl J Med 311:149, 1984
27. Lee ET, Anderson PS Jr, Bryan J et al: Diabetes, parental diabetes and obesity in Oklahoma Indians. Diabetes Care 8:107, 1985
28. Dahlquist G, Blom L, Holmgren G et al: The epidemiol-

ogy of diabetes in Swedish children 0–14 years—a six-year prospective study. Diabetologia 28:802, 1985

29. Pettitt DJ, Aleck KA, Baird HR et al: Congenital susceptibility to NIDDM: role of intrauterine environment. Diabetes 37:622, 1988

30. Neel JV: Diabetes mellitus—a geneticist's nightmare. p. 1. In Creutzfeldt W, Köbberling J, Neel JV (eds): The Genetics of Diabetes Mellitus. Springer-Verlag, New York, 1976

31. Friedman JM, Fialkow PJ: The genetics of diabetes mellitus. p. 199. In Steinberg AG, Bearn AG, Motulsky AG, Childs B (eds): Progress in Medical Genetics. Vol. 4. WB Saunders, Philadelphia, 1980

32. Rotter JI, Rimoin DL: The genetics of the glucose intolerance disorders. Am J Med 70:116, 1981

33. Yoon J-W, Austin M, Onodera T, Notkins AL: Virus-induced diabetes mellitus: isolation of a virus from the pancreas of a child with diabetic ketoacidosis. N Engl J Med 300:1173, 1979

34. Amery A, Berthaux P, Bulpitt C et al: Glucose intolerance during diuretic therapy: results of trial by the European Working Party on Hypertension in the Elderly. Lancet 1:681, 1978

35. Ames RP, Hill P: Improvement of glucose tolerance and lowering of glycohemoglobin and serum lipid concentrations after discontinuation of antihypertensive drug therapy. Circulation 65:899, 1982

36. Knowler WC, Pettitt DJ, Savage PJ, Bennett PH: Diabetes incidence in Pima Indians: contributions of obesity and parental diabetes. Am J Epidemiol 113:144, 1981

37. Knowler WC, Savage PJ, Nagulesparan M et al: Obesity, insulin resistance and diabetes mellitus in the Pima Indians. p. 243. In Köbberling J, Tattersall R (eds): The Genetics of Diabetes Mellitus. Academic Press, San Diego, 1982

38. Haffner SM, Stern MP, Hazuda HP et al: Role of obesity and fat distribution in non-insulin-dependent diabetes mellitus in Mexican Americans and non-Hispanic whites. Diabetes Care 9:153, 1986

39. Everhart JE, Pettitt DJ, Bennett PH, Knowler WC: Duration of obesity increases the incidence of NIDDM. Diabetes 41:235, 1992

40. McCance DR, Pettitt DJ, Hanson RL et al: Glucose, insulin concentrations and obesity in childhood and adolescence as predictors of NIDDM. Diabetologia 37:617, 1994

41. Helmrich SP, Ragland DR, Leung RW, Paffenbarger RS: Physical activity and reduced occurrence of non-insulin-dependent diabetes mellitus. N Engl J Med 325:147, 1991

42. Manson JE, Rimm EB, Stampfer MJ et al: Physical activity and incidence of non-insulin-dependent diabetes mellitus in women. Lancet 2:774, 1991

43. Kriska AM, LaPorte RE, Pettitt DJ et al: The association of physical activity with obesity, fat distribution and glucose intolerance in Pima Indians. Diabetologia 36:863, 1993

44. Steinke J, Driscoll SG: The extractable insulin content of pancreas from fetuses and infants of diabetic and control mothers. Diabetes 14:573, 1965

45. Obenshain SS, Adam PAJ, King KC et al: Human fetal insulin response to sustained maternal hyperglycemia. N Engl J Med 283:566, 1970

46. Heding LG, Persson B, Stangenberg M: β-Cell function in newborn infants of diabetic mothers. Diabetologia 19:427, 1980

47. Reiher H, Fuhrmann K, Noack S et al: Age-dependent insulin secretion of the endocrine pancreas in vitro from fetuses of diabetic and nondiabetic patients. Diabetes Care 6:446, 1983

48. Hill DE: Effect of insulin on fetal growth. Semin Perinatol 2:319, 1978

49. Gerö L, Baranyi É, Békefi D: Investigation on serum C-peptide concentrations in pregnant diabetic women and in newborns of diabetic mothers. Horm Metab Res 14:516, 1982

50. Soltész G, Aynsley-Green A: Hyperinsulinism in infnacy and childhood. Ergeb Inn Med Kinderheilkd 51:151, 1984

51. Naeye RL: Infants of diabetic mothers: a quantitative, morphologic study. Pediatrics 35:980, 1965

52. Hultquist GT, Olding LB: Pancreatic-islet fibrosis in young infants of diabetic mothers. Lancet 2:1015, 1975

53. Nelson L, Turkel S, Shulman I, Gabbe S: Pancreatic-islet fibrosis in young infants of diabetic mothers. Lancet 2:362, 1977

54. Dor N, Mosberg H, Stern W et al: Complications in fetal macrosomia. N Y State J Med 84:302, 1984

55. Drorbaugh JE, Moore DM: The effect of maternal diabetes on development of central nervous system function in the child. p. 106. In Moghissi KS (ed): Birth Defects and Fetal Development: Endocrine and Metabolic Factors. Charles C Thomas, Springfield, IL, 1974

56. Pedersen J: Future years of surviving babies. p. 233. In Pedersen J (ed): The Pregnant Diabetic and Her Newborn. 2nd Ed. Munksgaard, Copenhagen, 1977

57. Sack RA: The large infant. Am J Obstet Gynecol 104:195, 1969

58. Knobloch H, Sotos JF, Sherard ES Jr et al: Prognostic and etiologic factors in hypoglycemia. Pediatrics 70:876, 1967

59. Pildes RS: Infants of diabetic mothers. N Engl J Med 289:902, 1973

60. Peevy KJ, Landaw SA, Gross SJ: Hyperbilirubinemia in infants of diabetic mothers. Pediatrics 66:417, 1980

61. Cowett RM, Schwartz R: The infant of the diabetic mother. Pediatr Clin North Am 29:1213, 1982

62. Driscoll SG, Benirschke K, Curtis GW: Neonatal deaths

among infants of diabetic mothers. Am J Dis Child 100:818, 1960

63. Stehbens JA, Baker GL, Kitchel M: Outcome at ages 1, 3, and 5 years of children born to diabetic women. Am J Obstet Gynecol 127:408, 1977

64. Churchill JA, Berendes HW, Newmore J: Neuropsychological deficits in children of diabetic mothers. Am J Obstet Gynecol 105:257, 1969

65. Persson B, Gentz J: Follow-up of children of insulin-dependent and gestational diabetic mothers. Acta Paediatr Scand 73:349, 1984

66. Naeye RL, Chez RA: Effects of maternal acetonuria and low pregnancy weight gain on children's psychomotor development. Am J Obstet Gynecol 139:189, 1981

67. Rizzo T, Freinkel N, Metzger BE et al: Correlations between antepartum maternal metabolism and newborn behavior. Am J Obstet Gynecol 163:1458, 1990

68. Rizzo T, Metzger BE, Burns WJ, Burns K: Correlations between antepartum maternal metabolism and intelligence of offspring. N Engl J Med 325:911, 1991

69. Hadden DR, Byrn E, Trotter I et al: Physical and psychological health of children of type 1 (insulin-dependent) diabetic mothers. Diabetologia 26:250, 1984

70. Mills JL, Baker L, Goldman AS: Malformations in infants of diabetic mothers occur before the seventh gestational week. Diabetes 28:292, 1979

71. Grahnen H, Edlune K: Maternal diabetes and changes in the hard tissues of primary teeth. Odontol Rev 18:157, 1967

72. Noren J, Grahnen H, Magnusson BO: Maternal diabetes and changes in the hard tissues of primary teeth. Acta Odontol Scand 36:127, 1978

73. Noren JG: Microscopic study of enamel defects in deciduous teeth of infants of diabetic mothers. Acta Odontol Scand 42:153, 1984

74. Aerts L, Van Assche FA: Is gestational diabetes an acquired condition? J Dev Physiol 1:219, 1979

75. Aerts L, Holemans K, Van Assche FA: Maternal diabetes during pregnancy: consequences for the offspring. Diabetes Metab Rev 6:147, 1990

76. Gauguier D, Bihoreau M-T, Ktorza A et al: Inheritance of diabetes mellitus as a consequence of gestational hyperglycemia in rats. Diabetes 39:734, 1990

77. Pettitt DJ, Knowler WC: Diabetes and obesity in the Pima Indians: a cross-generational vicious cycle. J Obesity Weight Regul 7:61, 1988

78. Knowler WC, Pettitt DJ, Saad MF, Bennett PH: Diabetes mellitus in the Pima Indians: incidence, risk factors and pathogenesis. Diabetes Metab Rev 6:1, 1990

79. Pettitt DJ, Bennett PH, Saad MF et al: Abnormal glucose tolerance during pregnancy in Pima Indian women: long-term effects on the offspring. Diabetes, suppl. 2, 40:126, 1991

80. Karlsson K, Kjellmer I: The outcome of diabetic pregnancies in relation to the mother's blood sugar level. Am J Obstet Gynecol 112:213, 1972

81. Gyves MT, Rodman HM, Little AB et al: A modern approach to management of pregnant diabetics: a two-year analysis of perinatal outcomes. Am J Obstet Gynecol 128:606, 1977

82. Coustan DR, Berkowtiz RL, Hobbins JC: Tight metabolic control of overt diabetes in pregnancy. Am J Med 68:845, 1980

83. Jovanovic L, Druzin M, Peterson CM: Effect of euglycemia on the outcome of pregnancy in insulin-dependent diabetic women as compared with normal control subjects. Am J Med 71:921, 1981

84. Pettitt DJ, Bennett PH, Knowler WC et al: Gestational diabetes mellitus and impaired glucose tolerance during pregnancy: long-term effects on obesity and glucose tolerance in the offspring. Diabetes 34:119, 1985

85. Dorner G, Steindel E, Thoelke H, Schliack V: Evidence for decreasing prevalence of diabetes mellitus in childhood apparently produced by prevention of hyperinsulinism in the foetus and newborn. Exp Clin Endocrinol 84:134, 1984

26

The Interaction Between Pregnancy, Diabetes, and Long-Term Maternal Outcome

JOHN B. O'SULLIVAN

Pregnancy can be evaluated both for its possible etiologic relationships to, and its predictive ability for, subsequent maternal diabetes mellitus. That parity may be related to the development of diabetes is a topic with etiologic implications. The predictive role of pregnancy, on the other hand, relates to asymptomatic hyperglycemia that can be precipitated temporarily during pregnancy or by the delivery of a macrosomic infant. The occurrence of an exaggerated response to glucose ingestion, confined to gestation, does indeed foretell diabetes for a substantial proportion of mothers with this manifestation. The predictive ability of the birth of a large baby, on the other hand, is less clear but does function as a prognosticator for women with gestational diabetes.

ETIOLOGIC ROLE: PARITY AND DIABETES

The hypothesis attributing an etiologic role to the recurrent metabolic stresses of pregnancy was first proposed over 50 years ago to explain the higher prevalence of diabetes among women.[1] Numerous studies supported the initial report. Pyke,[2] for example, showed that the excess of female diabetic patients was confined to women who had borne children and that the incidence increased with increasing parity. Also in favor of the hypothesis were the publications of Joslin et al,[3] Monroe et al,[4] Fitzgerald et al,[5] and others. These authors attributed the greater frequency of diabetes among women to the associated influences of obesity

and parity, although Pykes' data indicated that the excess incidence of diabetes was not accounted for by the greater tendency of multiparous women to become fat. There has not been unanimity on the role of parity and subsequent diabetes, however, and authors such as Steinberg[6] and Vincke et al[7] have questioned the relationship.

Parity data from two population studies were subjected to collaborative analyses.[8] One was the epidemiologic study of the town of Sudbury, Massachusetts. Seventy-seven percent of the adult population, aged 15 years and older, had medical examinations and blood tests, with a detailed verification process being used to document diabetes. The other study was the 1960 to 1962 Health Examination Survey (HES) of the National Center for Health Statistics based on a cross-sectional sample of the entire noninstitutionalized U.S. population.

The age-adjusted probability of diabetes for women was found to increase with parity in the HES survey (Fig. 26-1). Mean parity for diabetic women was higher than in nondiabetic women, and this difference was statistically significant, some inconsistencies among various age groups notwithstanding. Much smaller differences for diabetic and nondiabetic women were found in Sudbury, but the data were not inconsistent with the HES findings (Table 26-1). The absence of an association between family size and diabetes in fathers would have been supportive of a causal relationship for parity and diabetes in women. Data on family size for men in Sudbury were, however, equally inconclusive when age differences were controlled. The rela-

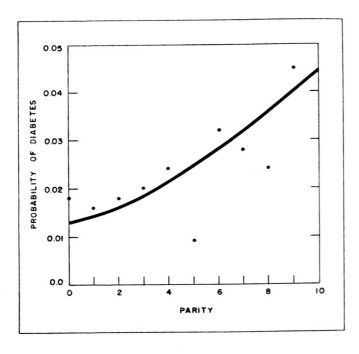

Fig. 26-1. Age-adjusted probability of having diabetes, by parity.

tionship between parity and diabetes has also been explored by cross-sectional studies based on single blood glucose values after a glucose challenge. Blood glucose levels 1 hour after ingestion of 50 g of glucose in the HES survey showed no clear parity/blood glucose relationships, the one possible exception being in women of parity nine or more. Another study examined a 10 percent sample of prenatal registrants.[9] The significant association between blood glucose levels (1 hour after ingestion of 50 g of glucose) and parity that emerged from a simple regression analysis was found not to be significant when considered in a multivariate context. Moreover, data from the 1976 to 1980 National Health and Nutrition Examination Survey of National Center for Health Statistics (HANES survey) was recently explored by O'Sullivan et al[10] with the conclu-

Table 26-1. Parity and Diabetes by Age and Sex: Sudbury, Massachusetts[a]

| | No. of Persons | | | | Mean No. of Children Ever Born | | | |
| | Men | | Women | | Men | | Women | |
Age (y)	Diabetic[a]	Nondiabetic	Diabetic[a]	Nondiabetic	Diabetic[a]	Nondiabetic	Diabetic[a]	Nondiabetic
All ages	53	2,154[b]	31	2,385[b]	2.7	2.1	2.6	2.3
15–24	—	371	—	391	—	0.1	—	0.3
25–34	5	526	2	706	2.4	2.2	1.5	2.6
35–44	8	741	2	701	2.6	2.8	4.0	3.0
45–54	18	305	4	298	2.9	2.6	2.0	2.5
55–64	6	130[c]	9	162	2.3	2.0	1.2	2.1
65–74	14	65	6	85	2.6	2.4	3.0	2.5
≤75	2	16[c]	8	42[c]	3.5	3.6	4.2	2.3

[a] Includes the stated, confirmed, and newly discovered diabetic patients in the Sudbury populations.
[b] Excludes two persons with number of children not stated.
[c] Excludes one person with number of children not stated.

sion that serum glucose levels, obtained 2 hours after the ingestion of 75 g of glucose, were not related to parity.

Epidemiologic studies, therefore, agree that there is no significant relationship between parity and blood glucose when single blood glucose levels are used for analyses. Agreement among studies of this nature contrasts with findings based on studies of persons with diabetes, the results of which cannot clearly exclude an opposite conclusion. By contrast, the higher prevalence of diabetes among women, responsible for introducing the original hypothesis, is now questioned by several studies, including the Sudbury study reported here (Table 26-1).

The question can best be resolved by prospective rather than cross-sectional data. Such data exist in the Boston Gestational Diabetes Study. Participants at risk of diabetes in that study were subjected to periodic tests of glucose tolerance over many years. Data from the 16-year follow-up interval formed the basis of an assessment of predictor variables present at the outset of the study.[11] Results indicated that parity, in a multivariate context, was not related to the later development of diabetes, whether diabetes was defined by the U.S. Public Health Service diagnostic criteria or by additional criteria designating further decompensation of carbohydrate control.

In summary, although cross-sectional data show no significant relationship between single blood glucose levels and parity, they do suggest that diabetic women have more children than their nondiabetic counterparts. The relationship is not sufficiently strong or consistent to confirm that it is etiologically related to the development of diabetes. Prospective data, however, show parity to have no predictive value for diabetes, and, consequently, this factor is unlikely to play an etiologic role. Alternative explanations for the higher parity of diabetic women, such as altered fertility rates or more subtle psychosocial causes, are possible. Whatever the explanation, current data indicate that there is no reason for women with a high risk of diabetes to be concerned about having a family.

PREDICTIVE ROLE: SUBSEQUENT MORBIDITY AND MORTALITY

The underlying basis for predicting long-term morbid events is related to the increased metabolic demands accompanying pregnancy that become particularly sig-

nificant in persons with a marginal capacity to respond. Aggravation of existing diabetes, unmasking of latent diabetes, and exaggeration of responses to a glucose challenge are among the well-recognized clinical manifestations that result. A notable study by Hagbard and Svanborg[12] revealed, in this context, that one-half of the women with the onset of symptomatic diabetes in pregnancy, including cases of diabetic coma, had a condition that was transitory, that is, all symptoms of diabetes disappeared after delivery and lactation, and normoglycemia returned. This study dramatizes the surprising magnitude of the gestational changes that can be considered transitory. Insufficient data are provided to consider the frequency of such extreme reactions in the general population, however.

More structured studies show that rates of subsequent maternal diabetes are related to the degree of glucose intolerance, albeit temporary, in pregnancy. For example, the difference between two diagnostic criteria for the glucose tolerance test, with one set of critical glucose levels set higher than the other, is that the test requiring higher values selects patients who go on, in the years subsequent to pregnancy, to develop diabetes both sooner and in greater numbers.[13] It is to be expected, then, that currently available studies, which have not used identical criteria, or have used the same criteria with different application rules, would have differing results.[13] Another manifestation of variations in diagnostic standards is the proportion of tests that reveal diabetes in the postpartum period. The study of Metzger et al[14] exemplifies this with high incidence rates for diabetes, ranging from 23 to 86 percent, depending on the gestational fasting glucose level, in the year after delivery. Such high rates probably reflect the presence of women with unrecognized diabetes before the index pregnancy. Table 26-2 shows the results from two studies, contrasting the diabetes incidence rates both with and without women diagnosed with diabetes in the postpartum period.[15,16] Both studies had low numbers of women who had test results diagnostic for diabetes postpartum (4 and 2.1 percent) and, consequently, a small impact on their long-term diabetes incidence rates. Although factors interfering with interstudy comparisons abound, all published studies show the same trend—an increased risk of later diabetes.[13]

Figure 26-2 shows the cumulative incidence of diabetes in women with a history of gestational diabetes,

Table 26-2. Follow-Up Studies of Women With Gestational Diabetes (A) and Results ExcludingWomen With Diabetes Diagnosed Postpartum (B)

Author	No.	Follow-Up (y)	Diabetic Patients	
			USPHS	WHO
Fuhrmann[16]				
A	50	8		46.0
B	46	8		43.7
O'Sullivan[15]				
A	615	22–28	49.9	36.4
B	612	22–28	48.8	35.2

Abbreviations: USPHS, United States Public Health Service criteria; WHO, World Health Organization criteria.

and the rate is contrasted with those from concurrently selected controls who had normal glucose tolerance test results in the index pregnancy.[17] Differences between the diabetes incidence rates in the two groups are shown to be substantial, projecting a 73 percent (± 2.8 percent) likelihood of women with gestational diabetes going on to have subsequent diabetes mellitus and impaired glucose tolerance, when followed a full 24 years. When alternative criteria (Decompensated Diabetes, National Diabetes Data Group, and World Health Organization criteria) are applied to the

same data, the major thrust of the results remain unaltered.[18] It is evident from these data, then, that incidence rates for subsequent diabetes are highly significant, that results are not affected by a variety of currently recommended standards for diagnosing subsequent diabetes, and that variations in incidence rates among studies probably reflect differences in diagnostic standards for gestational diabetes.

Figure 26-3 also uses analyses from the Boston Gestational Diabetes Study. It indicates that initial maternal body weight plays an important, statistically significant, role in determining the incidence rates for subsequent diabetes.[19] The effect of maternal body weight is subjected to further analyses in Table 26-3. Here, the predictive capabilities of various body weight subsets among the study patients are explored.[11] Individuals with persistent obesity are seen to be at greatest risk of later diabetes; subjects who remain in the desirable weight range have the lowest incidence of diabetes. Subjects who were normal weight initially but gained weight or those who were overweight initially and subsequently lost weight had intermediary incidence rates for diabetes that were significantly lower than those persons with persistent obesity. In fact, those who had achieved weight reduction had an incidence of diabetes close to the lower rate of the nonobese woman

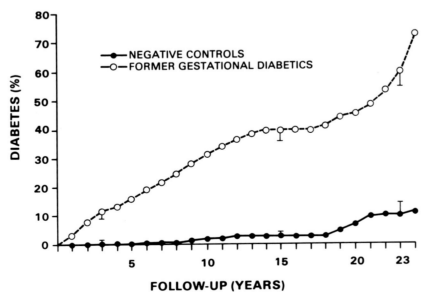

Fig. 26-2. Cumulative incidence of diabetes. Percentage ± SE. (From O'Sullivan,[17] with permission.)

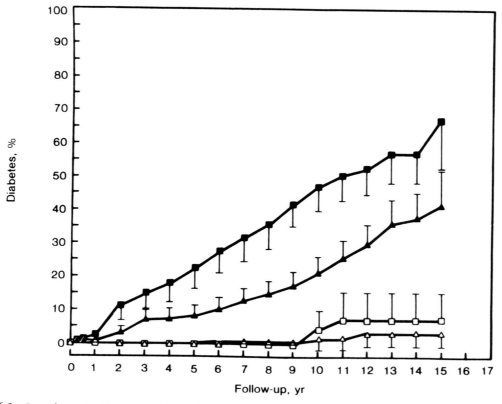

Fig. 26-3. Cumulative incidence of diabetes in overweight (black squares) and normal-weight (black triangles) women with gestational diabetes; overweight (white squares) and normal-weight (white triangles) controls. Percentage ± SE. (From O'Sullivan,[19] with permission.)

Table 26-3. Incidence of Diabetes (23-year) by Body Weight Subsets

Study Group	Weight Status[a]	Total No.	Diabetes Mellitus No.	%
GDM	Persistent obesity	205	125	61.0
	Weight increase	113	48	42.5
	Weight decrease	25	7	28.0
	Nonobese	235	63	26.8
Controls	Persistent obesity	54	4	7.4
	Weight increase	67	3	4.5
	Weight decrease	6	0	0.0
	Nonobese	170	5	2.9

Abbreviations: GDM, women with gestational diabetes.
[a] Status by 120% of desirable weight using initial and final weights.

with gestational diabetes. Although these data require further analyses to remove the possible effects of confounding variables, multivariate analysis confirms that the initial body weight is an independent predictor of diabetes.[19]

The most prominent obstetric outcome of gestational diabetes, now that the perinatal mortality rate has been brought under control, is the higher proportion of large baby births compared with that in normoglycemic women. The focus here is on the predictive capabilities of this event for the mother. A study of 120 gestational diabetic women found to have carbohydrate intolerance postpartum showed that macrosomia did not predict persistent carbohydrate intolerance.[20] Fitzgerald et al[21] studied the frequency of diabetes in a random sample of women 13 years after

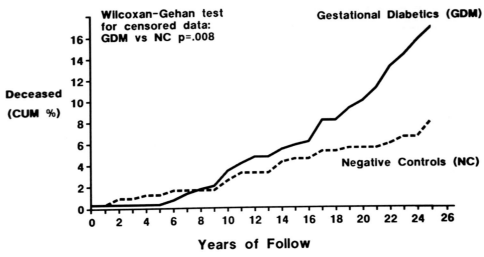

Fig. 26-4. Cumulative percentage of mortality rate for women with gestational diabetes and controls.

the birth of a 10.5-lb baby. Of the 61 women, 20 either definitely or probably had diabetes. The authors cautioned that firm conclusions concerning the predictive ability of the birth of a 10.5-lb baby could not be drawn because the effect of confounding variables had not been taken into account. The 16-year incidence of diabetes mellitus from 308 women with gestational diabetes who did not receive insulin treatment during pregnancy and from 328 concurrent random controls was unrelated to the birth of a 9-lb baby in either group. Further analyses of these data from the Boston Gestational Diabetes Study did show, however, that macrosomia was related to the severity of the subsequent diabetes and this finding was not explained by other factors such as age, weight, family history of diabetes, variations in observation periods, or the glucose level in the index pregnancy.[22]

Figure 26-4 presents the mortality status for the Boston Gestational Diabetes Study up to 24 years postpartum. This preliminary analysis indicates that women with gestational diabetes have a mortality rate that is significantly higher than that of controls. The total number of deaths are still too few to allow confirmatory analyses or a meaningful assessment of mortality by cause. Nevertheless, an indirect approach suggests a rationale for this mortality disparity. Because the major causes of death among women with diabetes are cardiovascular, analyses of cardiovascular risk factors were

undertaken. Women with gestational diabetes are found on follow-up to have more serum lipid abnormalities (total cholesterol, low-density lipoprotein-cholesterol, very low-density lipoprotein, and triglyceride levels) and higher mean systolic blood pressures than control patients who did not have elevated blood glucose values in their index pregnancies (Table 26-4). Women with gestational diabetes also show a significantly greater number of abnormalities in resting electrocardiograms than do negative control patients. Table 26-5 presents the results of a multifactor analysis with resting electrocardiograms as the dependent vari-

Table 26-4. Mean Values 17 to 23 Years Later for Women With Gestational Diabetes and Controls

Measurements	Former GDM	Negative Controls	P
Systolic BP (mm Hg)	130	122	<.01
Diastolic BP (mm Hg)	80	79	>.05
Total cholesterol	231	215	<.01
LDL-C	150	140	<.01
HDL-C	48	48	>.05
VLDL	33	28	<.01
Triglycerides	132	114	<.05

Abbreviations: GDM, women with gestational diabetes; BP, blood pressure; LDL-C, low-density lipoprotein-cholesterol; HDL-C, high-density lipoprotein-cholesterol; VLDL, very low-density lipoprotein.

Table 26-5. Logistic Regression on Resting Electrocardiogram

Variable	β	SE	P
Age	0.071	0.03	.01
Race	0.996	0.39	.01
Smoking	−0.148	0.38	.70
Weight	0.010	0.01	.11
Systolic BP	0.001	0.00	.47
Study category[a]	0.949	0.41	.02
TC/HDL	0.216	0.10	.03
Intercept	−7.837	0.10	

[a] Study. Category: Former Gestational Diabetics and Controls.
Abbreviations: TC/HDL, total cholesterol/high-density lipoprotein ratio; BP, blood pressure; SE, standard error.
(From O'Sullivan,[17] with permission.)

able. It shows that in the study category, that is, women with a history of gestational diabetes and negative controls, test findings were significantly different even when possible confounding cofactors were considered. In addition, the greater number of abnormal stress electrocardiograms among the women with gestational diabetes than among the controls remains statistically significant when subjected to a similar multifactor analysis. Coronary risk profiles consequently show women with gestational diabetes to be at greater risk of coronary artery disease. Moreover, clinical experence with the study subjects through this follow-up interval shows that there were some three to five times more cases of myocardial infarctions and angina pectoris among the women with gestational diabetes than among the control subjects.[17] Although these analyses need to be expanded in a multivariate context for confirmation, the trend is sufficiently evident to recommend counseling for women with gestational diabetes in the control of coronary risk factors as a particularly prudent approach to their health maintenance.

In summary, approximately three of four women with gestational diabetes can be expected to progress to diabetes or impaired glucose tolerance over a period of 24 years. The incidence rates for diabetes are greatly influenced by body weight, with the highest rates occurring in the persistently obese. Although the birth of a large baby may not, in general, predict diabetes for the mother, among women with a history of gestational diabetes, it has prognostic value in that, if

diabetes does occur, it is more likely to have progressed to a more advanced stage. Evidence of an increased mortality rate and more frequent cardiovascular disease among women with gestational diabetes, compared with controls in follow-up observations, is now beginning to emerge.

ETIOLOGIC AND PREDICTIVE ROLES: IMPLICATIONS FOR COUNSELING

An overview of the possible etiologic effects of parity and the long-term maternal outcome for the woman with gestational diabetes that has been presented here emphasizes several areas of importance to counseling programs and for the development of meaningful preventive medicine strategies. In the first place, reassurance can be provided to such patients that there is no evidence to show that multiple pregnancies will increase the risk of subsequent diabetes.

Whether or not further pregnancies are planned, the long-term risks associated with blood glucose responses in the index pregnancy of the woman with gestational diabetes should be explained to her, pointing out the very strong possibility of developing diabetes in the future, most particularly if she is overweight, and the added prognostic implications of the birth of a large baby. The growing evidence of an increased frequency of cardiovascular disease should be emphasized. Indeed, population-based information suggests that the relative sex advantage that women have for cardiovascular disease is obliterated by the development of diabetes.[23] The opportunities for delaying or preventing the development of diabetes and for minimizing the risks of cardiovascular disease should consequently be presented forcefully to the patient. The means of achieving this goal are deceptively simple. For the patient, nevertheless, it is often extremely difficult because life-style changes are involved. For the physician, the problem is also difficult because it takes both time and dedication—time to communicate effectively and dedication to motivate the patient successfully. Moreover, the patient will have many opportunities to rationalize noncompliance as the years pass without evidence of ill health. That the absence of diabetic or cardiovascular symptoms and signs provides no guide or reassurance must be underscored.

The following three-point plan of action can be presented:

1. *Periodic health assessment.* An annual health examination is recommended from age 40. In those younger than this age, the periodicity of the examination can be lengthened provided that the patient is without health problems, is maintaining an appropriate body weight, and is dedicated to a healthy life-style. The periodic health assessment, which invariably includes a detailed medical history, weight and blood pressure measurements, and blood glucose and serum cholesterol assays, should be expanded to include a lipid profile and, if necessary, a glucose tolerance test.

2. *Weight control.* Given the predilection of the woman with gestational diabetes for overt diabetes, she should be told that she can moderate the risk of this disease through weight control. Measures that incorporate weight control as an integral part of her life-style need to be outlined in detail. Maintaining a normal weight is a keystone in any problem of preventive medicine for women with gestational diabetes. The presence of obesity in such patients can be considered one of the categories of high-risk obesity, and it should be clear to the patient that its treatment is not cosmetic but is specifically therapeutic.

3. *Cardiovascular risk factor control.* The higher mortality rate and the greater cardiovascular risks for the woman with gestational diabetes indicate a trend that requires particular attention to be paid to risk modification. A prudent approach requires weight control, an exercise program, a diet that favors both fish and low saturated fat and cholesterol foods over those that are cholesterol rich, and when appropriate, blood pressure control and smoking cessation. Each component of the risk profile should be reviewed and used to motivate compliance. Obesity is designated as high-risk obesity here also if it is associated with hypertension of any degree or lipid abnormalities. The key role of weight reduction in both the prevention and treatment of these abnormalities should be repeatedly emphasized, and its beneficial effects on each of the individual components of the lipid profile should be explained to the patient. In addition, a more focused approach must be adopted when the patient shows evidence of alterations among the components of the lipid profile. Appropriate diets should be prescribed. For example, a diet is designed that lowers cholesterol for those patients with elevated low-density lipoprotein-cholesterol levels, one is prescribed that restricts carbohydrate foods for persons with elevated triglyceride levels, and aerobic exercise and smoking cessation are used for those exhibiting low high-density lipoprotein-cholesterol levels. Thyroid disorders and other causes of secondary hyperlipoproteinemias should be excluded before more specific therapy is instituted in the patient whose early changes do not respond to the outlined measures. Regarding exercise, the minimum standards for cardiovascular fitness by the American Heart Association require exercise for at least 20 minutes three times a week and of sufficient intensity to raise the heart rate.

In conclusion, women with gestational diabetes provide an outstanding opportunity for practicing prevention. Their pregnancies expose them to more regular medical care than others at comparable ages. Health education, with specific risk factor reduction instructions, can thus be given with an increased likelihood of success. Periodic reinforcement of the long-term commitment to diet, weight control, and exercise are necessary even for the most dedicated patient. Such surveillance demands from the physician a willingness to make time for the frequently unrewarding task of follow-up on the patient's regimen. The long-term results, however, make such mutual efforts rewarding.

REFERENCES

1. Mosenthal HO, Boldan C: Diabetes mellitus—problems of present day treatment. Am J Med Sci 186:605, 1933
2. Pyke DA: Parity and the incidence of diabetes. Lancet 1: 818, 1956
3. Joslin EP, Dublin LI, Marks HH: Studies in diabetes mellitus. IV. Etiology. Part I. Am J Med Sci 191:759, 1936
4. Monroe HN, Eaton JC, Glenn A: Survey of a Scottish diabetic clinic. J Clin Endocrinol 9:48, 1949
5. Fitzgerald M, Malins J, O'Sullivan D, Wall M: The effect of sex and parity on the incidence of diabetes mellitus. Q J Med 117:57, 1961
6. Steinberg AG: Heredity and diabetes. Diabetes 7:244, 1958
7. Vincke B, Nagelsmit WF, van Buchem FSP, Smid LJ: Some

statistical investigations in diabetes mellitus. Diabetes 8: 100, 1959

8. O'Sullivan JB, Gordon T: Childbearing and Diabetes Mellitus. Public Health Service Publication No. 1000, Series 11, Number 21. U.S. Government Printing Office, Washington, DC, 1966

9. O'Sullivan JB, Gellis SS, Tenney BO: Gestational blood glucose levels in normal and potentially diabetic women related to the birth weight of their infants. Diabetes 15: 466, 1966

10. O'Sullivan JB, Harris ML, Mills JL: Maternal diabetes in pregnancy. p. XX-12. In Harris MI, Hamman RF (eds): Diabetes in America. U.S. Dept. Health and Human Services, Public Health Service, NIH Publication No. 85-1468. U.S. Government Printing Office, Washington, DC, 1985

11. O'Sullivan JB: Gestational diabetes: factors influencing rates of subsequent diabetes. p. 429. In Sutherland HW, Stowers JM (eds): Carbohydrate metabolism in pregnancy and the newborn. Springer-Verlag, New York, 1978

12. Hagbard L, Svanborg A: Prognosis of diabetes mellitus with onset during pregnancy. Diabetes 9:296, 1960

13. O'Sullivan JB: Diabetes mellitus after gestational diabetes. Diabetes 40:131, 1991

14. Metzger BE, Bybee DE, Freinkel N et al: Gestational diabetes mellitus: correlations between the phenotypic and genotypic characteristics of the mother and abnormal glucose tolerance during the first year postpartum. Diabetes 34:111, 1985

15. O'Sullivan JB: The Boston Gestational Diabetes Studies: review and perspectives. p. 292. In Sutherland HW, Stowers JM, Pearson DWM (eds): Carbohydrate Metabolism in Pregnancy and the Newborn. Springer-Verlag, New York, 1989

16. Fuhrman K: Targets in oral glucose tolerance testing. p. 227. In Sutherland HW, Stowers JM, Pearson DWM (eds): Carbohydrate Metabolism in Pregnancy and the Newborn. Springer-Verlag, New York, 1989

17. O'Sullivan JB: Subsequent morbidity among gestational diabetic women. p. 174. In Sutherland HW, Stowers JM (eds): Carbohydrate Metabolism in Pregnancy and the Newborn. Churchill Livingstone, Edinburgh, 1984

18. O'Sullivan JB: Quarter century of glucose intolerance: incidence of diabetes mellitus by USPHS, NIH, and WHO criteria. p. 126. In Eschwege E (ed): Advances in Diabetes Epidemiology. Elsevier Biomedical Press, Amsterdam, 1982

19. O'Sullivan JB: Body weight and subsequent diabetes mellitus. JAMA 248:949, 1982

20. Lam KS, Li DS, Lauder IJ et al: Prediction of persistent carbohydrate intolerance in patients with gestational diabetes. Diabetes Res Clin Pract 12:181, 1991

21. Fitzgerald MG, Malins JM, O'Sullivan DJ: Prevalence of diabetes thirteen years after bearing a big baby. Lancet 1:1250, 1961

22. O'Sullivan JB, Mahan CM: Diabetes subsequent to the birth of a large baby: a sixteen year prospective study. J Chronic Dis 33:37, 1980

23. Garcia MJ, McNamara PM, Gordon T, Kannell WB: Morbidity and mortality in the Framingham population. Diabetes 23:105, 1974

27

Genetic Counseling and Family Planning

E. ALBERT REECE
SUSAN KOCH

Significant advances in the understanding of genetic factors in diabetes mellitus, particularly the insulin-dependent form, have been achieved in the past 25 years.[1] Diabetes mellitus is not one single disease but a group of disorders that share glucose intolerance in common. These disorders are also genetically heterogeneous. In an attempt to classify the different forms of diabetes, the National Diabetes Data Group[2] introduced a classification in 1979, which Hollingsworth and Resnik[3] subsequently modified (Table 27-1). Generally, diabetes can be categorized into four groups: (1) insulin-dependent diabetes mellitus (IDDM; type I); (2) non-insulin-dependent diabetes mellitus (NIDDM; type II); (3) gestational diabetes mellitus (GDM; type III); and (4) diabetes associated with other conditions or genetic syndromes (secondary diabetes; type IV).

Since the early 1970s, it has been known that IDDM is a human leukocyte antigen (HLA)-linked disorder, whereas NIDDM is not, supporting the genetic distinctions between these two clinically separate classifications. The magnitude of the differences in genetic factors that lead to either type I or type II diabetes was demonstrated by twin studies.[4,5] When one member of a monozygotic twin pair has IDDM, the probability that the second twin will develop the disease is between 20 and 50 percent, suggesting that genetic factors are required but not sufficient. By contrast, the risk of developing NIDDM is almost 100 percent in monozygotic co-twins of NIDDM patients[6,7] (Table 27-2).

Besides twin studies, classic familial pedigree and population studies have also been used to study the genetics of diabetes. Recently, a variety of newer physiologic, serologic, and molecular approaches has also been applied. It is clear from these works that a variety of etiologic and pathophysiologic mechanisms is involved in each of the different forms of IDDM and NIDDM. The distinction between the different types of diabetes is crucial for genetic counseling, even though this differentiation is not always clinically feasible.

This chapter reviews what is known regarding the various genetic factors that predispose an individual to glucose intolerance. Although great progress has been achieved in unraveling the genetic basis of diabetes, the exact mechanisms of inheritance remain unclear. Nonetheless, it will not be too long before expansion of our knowledge will allow the physician to prevent, treat, and perhaps, cure these disorders effectively.

HLA AND DISEASE SUSCEPTIBILITY

The major genetic susceptibility to IDDM is provided by genes near or within the HLA region.[8] The HLA region, otherwise known as the major histocompatibility complex (MHC), is a family of closely linked genes located on the short arm of chromosome 6 (Fig. 27-1). This single genetic region occupies about 1/3,000th of the human genome and controls antigens that are the primary targets of cell-mediated and antibody-mediated reactions to transplanted tissues.[9] The MHC

Table 27-1. Classification of Glucose Intolerance

Nomenclature	Old Names
Type I: Insulin-dependent diabetes mellitus	Juvenile diabetes Juvenile-onset diabetes Ketosis-prone diabetes
Type II: Non-insulin-dependent diabetes mellitus nonobese, obese	Adult-onset diabetes Maturity-onset diabetes Ketosis-resistant diabetes Stable diabetes, maturity-onset diabetes of youth
Type III: Gestational or carbohydrate intolerance, nonobese, obese	Gestational diabetes mellitus
Type IV: Secondary diabetes	Conditions and syndromes associated with impaired glucose tolerance

(Modified from Hollingsworth and Resnick,[3] with permission.)

Table 27-2. Predominant Characteristics of IDDM and NIDDM

Characteristics	IDDM	NIDDM
revalence	0.1–0.5%	5–10%[a]
Weight at onset	Nonobese	Often obese
Age at onset	Usually young, <30 years	Usually older, >40 years
Seronal variations	Yes	No
Insulin level	Low or absent	Variable
Ketosis	Most often	Unusual
Major histocompatibility complex gene associations	HLA-DR4, HLA-DR3, HLA-DQ	None
Twin studies	30–50% concordance	80–100% concordance
Anti-islet cell antibodies	Positive in 70% of new IDDM or prediabetic IDDM	None

[a] Prevalence in Western countries.
(From Hagay et al.,[108] with permission.)

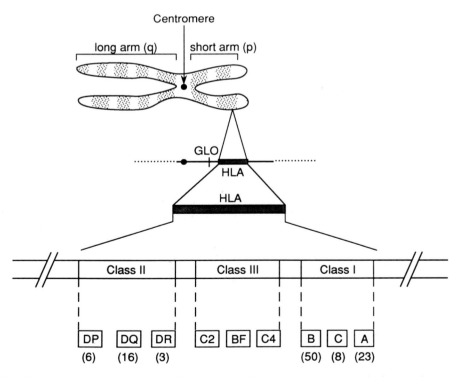

Fig. 27-1. The HLA gene complex located on the short arm of human chromosome 6. The numbers in parentheses indicate the minimum number of alleles per locus. (From Hagay et al,[108] with permission.)

plays a critical role in immune functions, regulating immune cooperation between monocytes and lymphocytes. Furthermore, it is believed that MHC molecules play a significant role in susceptibility to certain diverse diseases, possibly via an immunoregulatory role.[10,11]

The HLA complex is composed of several closely linked loci (i.e., selected chromosomal regions), the best known of which are the HLA-A, -B, -C, and -D/DR loci. Each of these loci is composed of several different alleles, which code for various antigens that can be distinguished serologically or by mixed lymphocyte culture.[9] An important feature of the HLA system is linkage disequilibrium, which occurs when the association of two alleles from different regions is observed at a much higher frequency than predicted by the individual allele frequencies in that population[9,12] (Fig. 27-2).

Three major classes of HLA gene products have been described[11,13,14] (Fig. 27-1). Class I gene products are surface antigens controlled by the HLA-A, -B, and -C genes. These surface antigens are found on all nucleated cells and platelets. Each of these class I genes is highly polymorphic, meaning many separate alleles have been identified in humans at each of these loci. At least 23 alleles for HLA-A, 50 for HLA-B, and 8 for HLA-C have been described.

Control of class II gene products occurs within the HLA-D region. These molecules are expressed primarily on the surface of antigen presenting cells such as B lymphocytes, macrophages, and activated T lymphocytes. Biochemical and DNA molecular studies have indicated the presence of at least three distinct loci within the HLA-D region, referred to as DP, DQ, and DR. Each of these regions is further divided into α- and β-subunits, encoded by the respective A and B

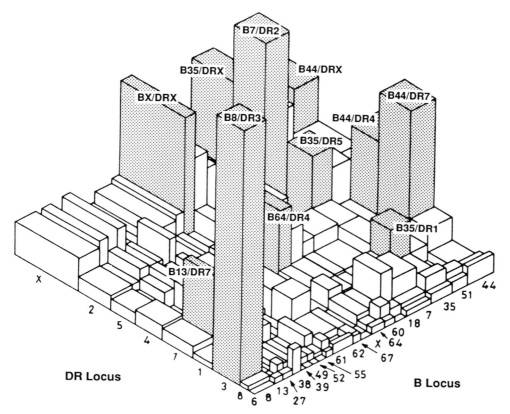

Fig. 27-2. Schematic presentation of linkage disequilibrium between the alleles of HLA-DR and HLA-B loci. (Modified from Tiwari and Terasaki,[110] with permission.)

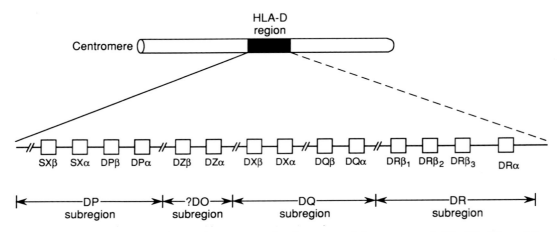

Fig. 27-3. The HLA-D region with its subregions on the short arm of chromosome 6. (Modified from Hitman,[1] with permission.)

genes. For the class II HLA-DR subregion, the allelic products defined by serology were given numbers from DR1 to DRW14. Many alleles from the DP and DQ loci have been cloned and sequenced.[15,16] The genomic organization of the currently identified class II loci is presented in Figure 27-3. The primary biologic significance of both class I and class II gene products probably relates to their role as receptor elements in antigen recognition and immune response. Class I epitopes contribute to the immune system by presenting foreign (or self) antigens to cytotoxic T lymphocytes, whereas class II gene products present antigens to T-helper cells (Table 27-3).

Between classes I and II are the genes encoding class III molecules, which are not directly involved with the immune reaction.

In 1964, Lilly et al[17] observed that the MHC of mice (the H2 system) controls the genetic susceptibility to viral leukemogenesis. In 1972, an association between certain HLA factors and disease states was observed in humans: HLA-B8 and celiac disease[18] and HLA-B13, B17, and psoriasis.[19,20] During the following years, several additional associations between HLA loci and disease associations were described (Table 27-4). A significant association with disease suggests either a causative role for the gene polymorphism or linkage between the marker allele and a disease susceptibility allele. It is now clear that certain HLA antigens are associated with disease susceptibility to a greater extent than any other known genetic marker in humans.[21]

In Table 27-4, an individual's chances of acquiring a specified disease, if the indicated antigen is inherited, is expressed as the "relative risk." For example, those who have inherited the HLA-B27 allele have an 87 times

Table 27-3. Three Distinct Types of Major Histocompatibility Complex Antigens

	Class I Antigen	Class II Antigen	Class III Antigen
Genetic control	HLA-A, -B, and -C	HLA-DR, -DP and -DQ	HLA-C2, -C4, and -BF
Tissue distribution	All nucleated cells and platelets	B cells, activated T cells, monocytes/ macrophages, some have marrow-precursor cells	Plasma protein
Function	Important in tissue transplantation and presentation of antigen to cytotoxic T cells	Associated with activation of immune system and present antigen to T-helper cells	Perform several biologic functions related to the mechanism of defense against infection (i.e., enhances phagocytosis)

(From Reece et al,[109] with permission.)

Table 27-4. Association Between HLA and Selected Diseases

Disease	HLA	Frequency of Antigen (%)		Relative Risk
		In Patients	In Controls	
Congenital adrenal hyperplasia	B47	9	0.6	15.4
Ankylosing spondylitis	B27	90	9.4	87.4
Insulin-dependent diabetes	DR3 and DR4	91	57.3	7.9
Systemic lupus erythematosus	DR3	70	28.2	5.8
Multiple sclerosis	DR2	59	25.8	4.1
Hasimoto's thyroiditis	DR5	19	6.9	3.2

(Modified from Svejgaard et al,[21] with permission.)

greater chance of developing ankylosing spondylitis than those who have not inherited this gene. It should be stressed that for each disease, only the antigen with the strongest association is recorded in Table 27-4.

The association of HLA and disease may have important implications for diagnosis, prognosis, and possible pharmacologic prophylaxis. In many cases, this association helped to clarify disease heterogeneity; however, the areas that have so far profited most markedly from the discovery of these associations are probably the "genetically inherited" diseases, especially IDDM.[21] In IDDM, the disease is not inherited per se; it is the susceptibility to the disease that is inherited, and the development of the disease is dependent on other genetic factors and possibly environmental factors as well (Table 27-5).

GENETIC FACTORS INVOLVED IN INSULIN-DEPENDENT DIABETES MELLITUS

HLA Association with IDDM

Singal and Blajchman[8] were the first to report an association between IDDM and class I antigens, specifically B15 in Canadian patients. This was corroborated 1 year later both in Denmark and Britain, where studies showed a significant increase of HLA-B15 and HLA-B8 in IDDM, whereas HLA-B7 showed a negative association.[22,23] The association of these class I antigens and IDDM is now known to be due to linkage disequilibrium between class I and class II alleles. Thus, significant linkage disequilibrium was found between HLA-B7 and HLA-DR2, B8 and DR3, and B15 with DR4 (Fig.

Table 27-5. Proposed Six Stages in the Pathogenesis of IDDM

Stage and Occurrence	Comments
Stage I: Genetic susceptibility	Most likely polygenic
	HLA association with IDDM (chromosome 6); 95% of whites with IDDM express HLA-DR3 or -DR4, or both
	Non-HLA association with IDDM; immunoglobulin loci (encoded on chromosomes 2, 14); polymorphic region 5' of the insulin gene (chromosome 11); T-cell receptor (chromosome 7, 14)
Stage II: Triggering factors	Environmental factors: toxic chemicals (?), viruses such as Coxsackie B, rubella, mumps (?), stress (?)
Stage III: Active autoimmunity	Many immunologic abnormalities may precede overt diabetes mellitus (DM) by >9 years; anti-islet cell antibodies may be present in up to 70% of pre-DM patients
Stage IV: Progressive loss of glucose-stimulated insulin secretion	Reduction in β-cell mass, evident from abnormal intravenous glucose tolerance test in ≥50% of first-degree relatives (IDDM) with islet-cell antibodies
Stage V: Early onset of overt DM	≥10% of β-cells remain
	Trials of immunotherapy (such as steroids and cyclosporine) have been attempted
Stage VI: Overt DM with complete β-cell destruction	Several years may elapse between stages V and VI

(From Hagay and Reece,[108] with permission.)

27-2). Studies of the DR region (class II antigens) have shown stronger association with IDDM than the B locus; although approximately 60 percent of IDDM patients possess HLA-B8 or -B15, more than 90 percent possess DR3 and/or DR4.[24] The higher frequency of certain HLA-DR molecules in IDDM compared with the HLA-B locus indicates that the DR subregion of class II is more closely linked to IDDM than the class I loci.[25] The relative risk of developing IDDM is increased to about 15-fold in individuals who co-inherit both DR3 and DR4 alleles, in contrast to the lower risk associated with individuals homozygous for either of these two alleles.[25–28] Conversely, the estimated relative risk of developing IDDM was increased only about threefold in HLA-B8 and -B15-positive individuals.[8,23] It is possible to calculate the absolute risk for inheriting IDDM according to various HLA haplotypes.[29] For example, individuals with DR2 have a lower absolute risk for IDDM (1:2,500) than the risk in the general population (1:500). However, individuals with DR3/DR4 have the highest risk (1:42) of developing IDDM[29] (Table 27-6). However, this association with the HLA-D region is not pathognomonic for IDDM, because DR3 and/or DR4 are also found in approximately 50 percent of healthy individuals.[24] Many investigators concur that DR3 and DR4 (as defined by conventional serology) are not themselves the only susceptibility alleles, and it has been suggested that perhaps susceptibility is due to certain subsets of DR3 and DR4 molecules or is influenced by more than one locus in the HLA region.

The rapid evolution of recombinant DNA technology and the development of genetic probes for the HLA region have initiated a new approach to the study of the genetics of IDDM.[30] Studies using monoclonal antibodies directed against distinct allelic products have

indicated that HLA-DQ may actually be more closely linked to the disease susceptibility locus than HLA-DR.[31] Sheehy et al[32] reported that a DR4 haplotype carries a higher risk for IDDM if it encodes a particular DQ subtype, DQW3.2 (now classified as DQB1*0302[33]). Furthermore, sequence analysis of the HLA-DQ3 gene product suggested that a single amino acid (aspartic acid) at position 57 is uniquely important for determining susceptibility or resistance to IDDM.[32,33] These groups of investigators have shown that among IDDM patients, the DQ β-alleles do not have aspartic acid at position 57. They suggest that the DQB allelic polymorphisms, particularly at position 57, determine the susceptibility or the lack thereof for IDDM. Moreover, these investigators suggested that an individual carrying one aspartic acid 57-negative and one aspartic acid 57-positive allele (DQB1*0302 and DQB1*0301), a so-called heterozygote state, has a much lower risk of developing IDDM. However, individuals homozygous for aspartic acid 57-negative had a high prevalence of IDDM. In this study of 39 IDDM patients, 35 were aspartic acid-negative homozygous. They concluded that full HLA susceptibility is dependent on the individual having two aspartic acid 57-negative DQ β-alleles, especially if they are from the DR4 and/or DR3 haplotypes. Although a similar finding was found in DR4-positive Northern Indian Asians,[36] this association was not confirmed transracially,[37,38] and DQB1*0302 is, therefore, unlikely to be a primary disease susceptibility determinant.

Because the structure, function, and expression of the α- and β-chains of the class II molecule are interdependent, a possible candidate for a gene product that can modify the function of the DQ β-chain is the α-chain. Transracial studies have implicated DQA1*0301 as the primary allele associated with IDDM in Japanese,[39] black Americans,[40] Northern Indians,[41] and whites.[42,43] In whites, this allele encodes arginine at position 52, and it has been postulated that disease susceptibility correlates with expression of a DQ molecule bearing Arg 52 on the α-chain and lacking Asp 57 on the β-chain.[42] This finding has not been confirmed in other races.[37,39]

In summary, the association between specific HLA regions and IDDM susceptibility is now defined more precisely. The "susceptibility" area is located within the D region and specifically in or close to DR3 and/or DR4 and/or DQ α- or β-alleles. However, it is still

Table 27-6. Absolute Risks for IDDM for Whites of Various HLA Genotypes[a]

HLA Genotype	Absolute Risk
DR3/DR3	1:125
DR3/DRX[b]	1:500
DR4/DR4	1:147
DR4/DRX	1:476
DR3/DR4	1:42
DRX/DRX	1:5565

[a] Based on IDDM prevalence rate of 1 in 500.
[b] X, non-DR3; non-DR4 antigen.
(Modified from Maclaren and Henson,[29] with permission.)

not known whether the DR and/or DQA or DQB antigens themselves predispose to IDDM or if the susceptibility is due to as-yet-undefined diabetes susceptibility genes located close to and inherited with these antigens.

HLA Susceptibility and β-Cell Destruction in IDDM

The development of IDDM can be divided into six stages conceptually, beginning with genetic susceptibility and ending with complete β-cell destruction. It now seems clear that genetic predisposition (i.e., HLA-linked susceptibility) when combined with other factors (i.e., environmental) leads to clinical diabetes. The aforementioned data indicate that IDDM may be due to immune disease of the pancreatic β-cells. Insulitis is regarded as a process in which insulin-secreting cells are gradually destroyed. Most theories attempting to explain autoimmunity either implicate primary dysfunction within the immune system as the cause or suggest primary islet cell anatomy damage, which may lead to secondary autoimmune destruction. Stage I represents genetic susceptibility inherent in some subjects in whom environmental factors (stage II) such as stress and viral infections occur. These insults trigger the development of β-cell immunity (stage III) in which immunologic abnormalities can precede the development of overt IDDM. In fact, immunologic abnormalities that can precede type I diabetes include anticytoplasmic islet cell antibodies, anti-insulin antibodies, and lymphocyte inhibition of insulin secretion.[44-46] Initially, individuals with immunologic abnormalities have normal insulin secretion. In stage IV, glucose-stimulated insulin secretion is progressively lost, although overt diabetes does not immediately occur.[47] This selective loss of response to glucose may reflect a reduction of β-cell mass. In stage V, overt diabetes is first recognized while some residual insulin secretion remains but eventually results in complete β-cell destruction (stage VI).

The immune response to foreign organisms depends on the responsiveness of the MHC to a given stimulus. The fundamental role of MHC genes is in the identification and distinction of foreign from self. T cells of the immune system can recognize and respond to an antigen only if they are presented in combination with an HLA molecule on the surface of antigen-pre-

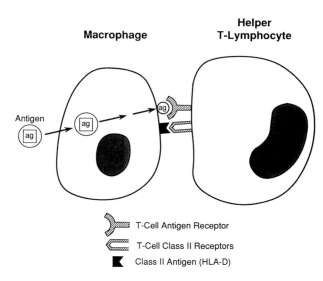

Fig. 27-4. Schematic illustration of the interaction between the macrophage and the helper T lymphocyte. The latter recognizes and responds to antigens if it sees both the foreign antigen and DR antigen on the surface of macrophages. (From Reece et al,[109] with permission.)

senting cells[48-50] (Fig. 27-4). The mechanism by which genes within the MHC of humans influence autoimmune processes is not clear. One recent suggestion by Todd[51] is that there is an impairment in the tolerance of the immune system so that self is recognized as foreign. Tolerance may, however, be maintained by a third class of T lymphocytes called suppressor T cells. These cells are able to suppress the proliferation of T-helper cells but may require HLA-DQ for their suppression. This suggests that IDDM patients with aspartic 57-negative DQ molecules have abnormal tolerance, perhaps leading to self-destruction of pancreatic β-cells.

Another theory regarding the pathogenesis of IDDM involves aberrant expression of HLA-D region gene products on the surface of cells outside the immune system. For example, the aberrant expression of these gene products on pancreatic β-cells may result in cell destruction. Class II antigens are normally limited to macrophages, B lymphocytes, and activated T lymphocytes. It has been suggested that under pathologic conditions, other cell types may become class II-positive, such as in Hashimoto's thyroiditis and Grave's disease. Bottazzo et al[52] have demonstrated DR expression on β-cells of the pancreatic islets of a young girl with IDDM in the very early stages of the disease. However, endocrine cells in the islets of a control pancreas were invariably DR-negative. Thus, expression of class II antigens on the surface of antigen-presenting cells capable of attracting T-helper cells specific for these antigens, resulted in the autoimmune destruction of the β-cells.

Non-HLA Associations with IDDM

There is ample evidence to support the idea that type I diabetes is a genetically programmed autoimmune disease, and its association with HLA has provided new ways to explore certain aspects of the mode of disease inheritance. Nonetheless, although HLA association is strong, it does not explain or account for all the genetic predisposition to IDDM. For instance, many individuals with both DR3 and DR4 do not develop IDDM, whereas many diabetic individuals possess neither of these antigens.[15] Another interesting example is the finding of higher incidences of IDDM among black Americans compared with African blacks with similar HLA antigenic frequencies.[53] It has been estimated that loci in the HLA region account for from 30 percent to as much as 70 percent of the genetic predisposition. This suggests that genetic factors other than HLA contribute to IDDM susceptibility.[53,54] The search for non-HLA susceptibility genes has focused predominantly on the following three areas:

1. Immunoglobulin heavy chain (Gm) and light chain (Km) regions encoded on chromosomes 14 and 2, respectively
2. The insulin gene (INS), located on the short arm of chromosome 11; particularly the polymorphic 5' region
3. The T-cell receptor β-chain region on chromosome 7 and α-chain region on chromosome 14

Field et al[55] and Rich et al[56] reported an association between the DR type, particular genes in the immunoglobulin heavy chain (Gm) region and IDDM susceptibility. Field et al proposed that genes encoding Gm allotypes (or genes in linkage disequilibrium with them) may contribute to susceptibility to IDDM through interaction with HLA.[55] This finding was not corroborated subsequently in a fairly large sample of affected families. However, a significant association was observed between 5' insulin-region alleles and IDDM, although the significance of this relationship is not clear.

Because the autoimmune process leading to type I diabetes is specific to the β-cells of the pancreas that produce insulin, abnormalities of insulin secretion or processing are possible etiologic factors. Thus, the insulin (INS) gene remains a candidate for susceptibility to type I diabetes. The major polymorphism in the INS gene region is located 5' to the start of the transcription region of the INS gene on the short arm of chromosome 11 (11p15.5).[57] In whites, the size of this variable number tandem repeat falls into two main classes: small alleles of approximately 40 repeats (class I alleles) and large alleles of approximately 170 repeats (class II).[58] Many population association studies have shown an increase in the frequency of the class I allele in patients with IDDM compared with controls.[43] However, linkage analyses in multiplex families have failed to confirm this finding.[59] Julier et al[60] were able to detect linkage by considering only parents heterozygous for the common disease-associated alleles. In that study, the parental origin of the INS gene appeared to be important in imparting disease susceptibility, suggesting a role for genomic imprinting.

Other candidate genes for IDDM susceptibility include those coding for T-cell receptors, because type I diabetes appears to be T-cell-mediated. T-cell receptors are surface molecules composed of both an α- and β-chain, each with constant and variable regions. These receptors mediate antigen recognition by T lymphocytes.

There are only limited numbers of studies analyzing polymorphisms of both α- and β-subunit genes of the T-cell receptors.[8] Both association and linkage analyses of polymorphisms of the genes coding for the α-subunit and IDDM susceptibility have been negative.[61] An early association study of polymorphisms within the T-cell receptor β-chain gene suggested a higher frequency of heterozygosity among diabetic individuals compared with controls.[62] Later studies using larger populations and linkage analysis, however, failed to confirm this observation.[63] There is no convincing evidence that genes in the T-cell receptor β-chain or α-chain regions influence predisposition to IDDM, either directly or indirectly through interaction with HLA region genes. However, Field[64] showed that diabetic individuals who are positive for the IgG_2 allotype G2m(23) have significantly different frequencies of a T-cell receptor β-chain restriction fragment length polymorphism than those who are negative for the allotype, suggesting an interaction between T-cell receptor β-genes and immunoglobulin heavy chain genes.

In summary, other candidate genes related to susceptibility to IDDM are characterized by the relative inconsistencies of the findings compared with those for HLA. However, it seems that all three genes: the immunoglobulin, the T-cell receptor, and the insulin gene play a certain role in the immunopathogenesis of IDDM. It seems likely that as the approaches and tools for mapping such susceptibility genes become more clearly defined, the identification of further susceptibility determinants will be accomplished in the near future.[65]

GENETIC COUNSELING

Insulin-Dependent Diabetes Mellitus

Although great progress has been made in the understanding of the genetics of IDDM, the exact mode of inheritance of the disease remains controversial. It is possible that manifestations of IDDM require the interaction of at least five different genes (on chromosomes 2, 6, 7, 11, and 14) along with environmental factors. Hence, it is clear why genetic counseling in IDDM is not simple.

Because the exact mechanism of inheritance of IDDM is not known, genetic counseling is based on empirical risk. For example, the estimated overall risk of siblings of IDDM proband developing the disease ranges from 4.6 to 6.6 percent.[66,67] HLA typing of the entire family permits more precise estimates, because the risk of a sibling is related to the number of haplotypes that the sibling shares with the diabetic proband.

If disease occurs independently of HLA, then the expected frequency of affected sibling pairs sharing one, two, or no haplotypes will be 50, 25, and 25 percent, respectively. However, the expected frequencies assuming linkage of susceptible genes to HLA should be increased for sibling pairs sharing two haplotypes and decreased if only one or no haplotype was shared. In fact, this is precisely what has been found in family studies of IDDM: observed frequencies among affected sibling pairs are 58.5 percent being HLA identical, 37.3

Table 27-7. Distribution of the Number of HLA Haplotypes Shared among IDDM Subpairs According to the Observed vs. Expected Proportions

Siblings	Number of Haplotypes Shared (%) with Proband		
	0	1	2
Expected percentage of IDDM in siblings if disease is independent of HLA	25	50	25
Observed percentage in IDDM siblings	4.2	37.3	58.5

(From Reece et al,[109] with permission.)

percent sharing one haplotype, and 4.2 percent for HLA nonidentical. Table 27-7 displays the distribution of the number of HLA haplotypes shared among IDDM sibling pairs according to observed frequency versus the expected proportions if disease was independent of HLA.

Thompson et al,[68] in an extensive international multicenter study involving 1,792 white probands with IDDM, calculated the risk to siblings on the basis of DR type of the proband and haplotype sharing of the sibling and probands (Table 27-8). It is apparent that for an HLA-identical sibling, the risk is 13.1 percent; but if only one haplotype is shared, the risk is 4.6 percent. The risk for siblings sharing no haplotype with the proband and therefore not depending on the DR genotype of the proband is 1.8 percent. This risk is greater than the prevalence of the disease (0.4 percent) in the general population and may indicate that additional factors are involved in the disease predisposi-

Table 27-8. Estimates of Risks to Siblings of IDDM Probands on the Basis of DR Type of Proband and Haplotype Sharing

Proband DR Type	Risk to Siblings According to Number of Haplotypes Shared (%)		
	2	1	0
DR3/DR4	19.2	3.7	1.3
DR4/DR4	7.4	3.5	1.0
DR4/X	11.1	6.8	1.6
DR3/DR3	14.1	3.9	2.4
DR3/X	11.2	4.9	2.8
X/X[a]	5.7	3.3	3.8
Overall risk	13.1	4.6	1.8

[a] X, non-DR3; non-DR4 antigen.
(From Reece et al,[109] with permission.)

tion. It is also evident from Table 27-8 that siblings who share two haplotypes with a DR3/DR4 proband have the highest risk (19.2 percent) of developing IDDM. This is in agreement with other studies that showed increased risk of IDDM for DR3/DR4 heterozygotes in comparison to either DR3/DR3 or DR4/DR4 homozygotes.[1,25,27]

What is the risk of offspring developing the disease if a parent has IDDM? The most common answer until recently was that the cumulative risk of IDDM by age 20 to 30 years is in the range of 16 percent.[69,70] However, Warram et al[71] studied the incidence of IDDM in offspring of patients with the disease. They found that by the age of 20 years, 6.1 percent of the offspring of the diabetic fathers had diabetes. By contrast, only 1.3 percent of the offspring of the diabetic mothers had the disease by the age of 20 years. Hence, IDDM is transmitted less frequently to the offspring of diabetic mothers than to those of diabetic fathers. The mechanism responsible for this preferential transmission is not clear. A possible explanation offered is the lower frequency of recombination between linked loci during gametogenesis in men than in women.[72] Another possible mechanism is one that depends on the intimate relation between the mother and fetus, as evidenced by increased pregnancy loss rate in mothers with IDDM.[71]

Non-Insulin-Dependent Diabetes Mellitus

There are clear genetic and immunologic differences between IDDM and NIDDM. The latter is not linked with HLA, and no specific genetic markers have been found. Furthermore, NIDDM does not seem to be an autoimmune or endocrine disease. Current available information indicates that NIDDM is due to both impaired insulin secretion and insulin resistance.[73] Although the genetic markers for NIDDM are not yet defined, it is evident from family and twin studies that the genetic component of NIDDM is much stronger. As mentioned previously, monozygotic twins have a much higher rate of concordance for type II diabetes (almost 100 percent) than for type I diabetes (20 to 50 percent).[6,7] Based on twin studies, one may expect that there is a consistent pattern of inheritance in NIDDM; unfortunately, this is not the case. Environmental factors also play an important role in the etiology of

NIDDM, as reflected in the rapid changes in frequency in NIDDM seen in migrant populations and the major effect of obesity on its frequency and clinical course.

It is likely that there is genetic heterogeneity in NIDDM, and the modes of inheritance, for the most part, are poorly defined. However, there is a special subgroup of NIDDM in which the disease develops not in midlife but much earlier, in adolescence or young adulthood.[74,75] This subgroup is referred to as maturity-onset diabetes of the young. This disease is transmitted as an autosomal dominant trait, with as many as 50 percent of offspring inheriting the disease or manifesting glucose intolerance.[75,76] Another example of genetic heterogeneity in NIDDM is found in differences in familial aggregations (i.e., among nonobese diabetic individuals, 15 percent of first-degree relatives [siblings, parent, or offspring] are also affected compared with 7.3 percent of first-degree relatives of obese diabetic individuals) (Table 27-9).[77]

The empirical risk of NIDDM relatives developing the disease is thus much higher than that of IDDM relatives. The transmission of the disease to first-degree relatives of NIDDM probands is almost 15 percent, and as many as 30 percent will have impaired glucose tolerance. When both parents have type II diabetes, the chance of developing the disease is much higher and reaches 60 to 75 percent.[78] Given the magnitude of these risks, periodic screening of first-degree

Table 27-9. Empirical Risk for Offspring of IDDM and NIDDM Developing Diabetes

Affected Parents	Empirical Risk Estimates of Offspring
IDDM	
Diabetic mother	1%
Diabetic father	6%
Parents unaffected but previous sibling affected	Overall, 5–6%; No. haplotypes shared with proband:
	1 haplotype = 5%
	2 haplotype = 13%
	No haplotypes = 2%
Both parents affected	33%
NIDDM	
Maturity-onset diabetes of the young	50%
Obese	7%
Nonobese	15%
First-degree relatives	15–30%
Both parents affected	60–75%

(From Hagay and Reece,[108] with permission.)

relatives with oral glucose tolerance tests is not unreasonable. Those found to have impaired glucose tolerance should be advised to attain ideal body weight. Obesity is certainly a risk factor among this group that should be avoided.

Gestational Diabetes Mellitus

Carbohydrate intolerance of variable severity discovered or presumably arising during pregnancy is defined as GDM. Glycemic control is often achieved by diet or insulin therapy, or both.[2,79] GDM patients are usually identified by means of an oral glucose tolerance test. Fifteen percent or more of those patients will require insulin treatment in the pregnancy, either because of fasting or postprandial hyperglycemia.[79] These differences demonstrate that the severity of metabolic disturbances can vary between patients with GDM. This raises the question of whether this group of patients consists of a single homogeneous entity. Until recently, GDM was believed to be a variant of NIDDM. Available data, however, support the concept that GDM is a heterogeneous disorder representing, at least in part, patients who are destined to develop diabetes in later life, either IDDM or NIDDM.[79–82] The exact percentage difference of each subgroup is unknown, but it seems that most of the cases represent a preclinical state of NIDDM.

Long-term follow-up of patients who had GDM showed an increased incidence of acquiring diabetes during middle age or later (30 to 50 percent).[83] However, this risk can be modified by weight reduction in later years. The possibility that GDM may represent some patients who are destined to develop IDDM later in life was raised by the following: first, IDDM may occur in the age group of pregnancy (hence, the disease may arise as a result of the stress of pregnancy); second, it has become clear that autoimmunity plays a key role in IDDM, and the disease process is believed to be a slow destructive process of β-cells in the pancreas (Table 27-5).[82,84] Immunologic studies have shown that as many as 30 percent of GDM patients may have circulating islet cell antibodies,[82,85] and anti-islet cell antibodies have been found in high proportions of patients with pre-IDDM.[86–90] Recently, Tarn and coworkers[89] reported that up to 54 percent of first-degree relatives of IDDM who were found to be positive for complement-fixing islet cell antibodies (ICAs) on three or more occasions developed IDDM within a maximum of 8 years of follow-up. Furthermore, they showed that GDM patients who were ICA-positive had a higher prevalence of HLA-DR3 or DR4 than those who were ICA-negative, and more than half of them developed IDDM 11 years after the diagnosis of GDM.[89] In a recent study of Pima Indians[91] (a group in whom the incidence of NIDDM is high), there was a higher prevalence of diabetes in the offspring of women who had NIDDM during pregnancy than in the offspring of women who developed diabetes only after the pregnancy (45 versus 8.6 percent at age 20 to 24 years). The authors suggested that the intrauterine environment is an important determinant of the development of diabetes and its effect is additive to genetic factors.

The previously mentioned data support the concept that GDM is clearly heterogeneous and composed of patients who are prone to develop either IDDM or NIDDM later in life. Further studies are needed to clarify this heterogeneity.

FAMILY PLANNING

Effective contraception, pregnancy planning, and preconception care are all important components of a comprehensive reproductive care program for women with diabetes. Every physician visit offers an excellent opportunity for regular discussions of the need for preconception glucose control and for development of a care plan for future pregnancies.

Prepregnancy Planning

Preconception planning is important to prevent undesired pregnancies and to allow conception to occur only after the achievement of stringent metabolic control. The incidence of congenital anomalies among children of diabetic women is four to ten times higher than among their nondiabetic counterparts. Current evidence suggests that normalization of blood glucose in the preconceptional period and the maintenance of normal glycemic control throughout the critical phase of organogenesis results in a reduced incidence of anomalies. The other advantages of prepregnancy glycemic control include improved cooperation among those involved in the care of these patients, an increased proportion of planned pregnancies, earlier antenatal care, and identification of infertility.

Maternal Complications

Women with diabetes are living longer and hence more women with vascular complications are becoming pregnant. The major cause of maternal death has shifted from diabetic ketoacidosis to cardiorenal complications. In the past, diabetic women with vasculopathy were counseled to avoid pregnancy or terminate pregnancy if it occurred. New data, however, suggest that with the possible exception of coronary artery disease, women with vasculopathy may be counseled toward more favorable outcomes.[92]

The chronic complications of diabetes, however, may in fact be affected by pregnancy. Evidence suggests that pregnancy per se is an independent risk factor that accelerates diabetic retinopathy.[93] Furthermore, both hyperglycemia and hypertension have been shown to potentiate this acceleration.[94,95] This information serves to underscore the importance of women with proliferative retinopathy seeking preconception care and achieving euglycemia before pregnancy. A recently published study by Reece and colleagues[96] in 20 women with advanced diabetic retinopathy demonstrates that with appropriate contemporary management satisfactory retinal and perinatal outcomes are possible. None of their patients experienced progressive visual changes that were not amenable to photocoagulation therapy, and successful perinatal outcomes were reported in 94 percent of their sample.

The effect of pregnancy on diabetic nephropathy is less clear but is believed not to accelerate the rate of progression to end-stage renal disease.[97–99] However, nephropathy has important implications during pregnancy because of its association with an increased risk of pre-eclampsia, accelerated hypertension, fetal growth retardation, fetal distress, preterm delivery, and perinatal death. At least in women with mild-to-moderate renal insufficiency, successful perinatal outcomes are possible with meticulous attention to blood glucose and blood pressure control as well as fetal surveillance.[96,98] Diabetic women with vascular disease need sensitive but explicit counseling to make informed decisions regarding their reproductive futures. Because the risk for vascular complications increases with duration of the disease, women with pregestational diabetes may not be well advised to delay childbearing until their later years.

Contraceptive Choices

When considering the potential risks of contraception in women with diabetes mellitus, the clinician must also consider the other major alternative, which is a possibly undesired pregnancy. Despite advances in obstetric care and diabetes management, the risks of morbidity and mortality are increased for the woman with diabetes and her offspring. Today, there are many contraceptive options for women with diabetes that do not increase the risk for the vascular complications of diabetes.

The vast majority of the more than 30 formulations of oral contraceptives available on the American market contain various doses of synthetic estrogen and progestin. Most of the preparations are considered to be low dose, containing less than 0.05 mg of ethinyl estradiol or mestranol. The major metabolic side effects of progestins include decreased glucose tolerance as the result of increased peripheral insulin resistance. Also, progestins decrease high-density lipoprotein cholesterol and increase low-density lipoprotein cholesterol. Estrogens, however, increase insulin sensitivity in muscle and adipose cells and favorably alter lipid levels. Therefore, the combinations of estrogen and progesterone in most preparations are thought to balance the metabolic effects of each other.[100] Studies in nondiabetic women have demonstrated that low-dose oral contraceptives have little effect on glucose tolerance or serum insulin an glucagon levels.[101] Both human[102,103] and animal[104] studies have failed to demonstrate accelerated atherosclerosis with oral contraceptive use or increased risk of myocardial infarction in former oral contraceptive users.

Low-dose oral contraceptives can be selectively used in women with pregestational diabetes as well as in women with a history of gestational diabetes. Most recent studies of low-dose oral contraceptives in women with diabetes have demonstrated little if any change in glucose tolerance or insulin requirements. Little data are available to evaluate the effect of oral contraceptive use on diabetic complications. However, a recent cross-sectional study[105] of 384 women with IDDM found no association among vasculopathy and prior history or years of oral contraceptive use.

Diabetic women placed on oral contraceptive therapy should be evaluated after the first cycle of oral contraceptive use and every 3 to 4 months thereafter. Evaluations should include monitoring of weight, blood pressure, lipid levels, postprandial glucose levels, and HbA_{1c}.[100,101]

Long-acting progestins are currently available on the U.S. market and offer another alternative for the woman with diabetes. Depo Provera is administered as an intramuscular injection every 3 months. Studies in nondiabetic women have demonstrated a statistically significant but not clinically significant deterioration in glucose tolerance. Norplant, which is a subdermal implant, provides 5 years of contraceptive protection. Increases in glucose and insulin levels have been seen in nondiabetic women with this therapy. Therefore, close medical surveillance is indicated when used in women with diabetes.

In the past, intrauterine devices have not been recommended for use in women with diabetes because the potential increased risk for infection was considered unacceptable. Two recent prospective trials[106,107] in women with IDDM have failed to support this belief. Therefore, women with diabetes who are at very low risk of sexually transmitted disease may consider this additional option. Women should receive antibiotic prophylaxis at the time of insertion and be followed closely to ensure the detection and early treatment of infection.[100]

Other options include barrier methods such as the diaphragm, condom, spermicidal jelly or foam, contraceptive sponges, and cervical caps. Because these methods produce no metabolic alterations, they can be safely used in women with diabetes. However, these methods are user-dependent and have a much higher failure rate than the previously discussed options. Last, permanent sterilization is a reasonable option for women who have completed their childbearing and desire no more children.

CONCLUSION

Meticulous care and strict metabolic control of the diabetic woman during pregnancy have dramatically improved both maternal and fetal outcomes. However, unintended pregnancies and an increased risk for congenital anomalies in the offspring of women with diabetes remain major obstacles yet to be overcome. A systematic approach to family planning and repeated encouragement by providers of the importance of preconception care must be included as essential components of comprehensive diabetes care.

SUMMARY

In the past decade, the genetics and immunology of IDDM have received considerable attention. With the advent of recombinant DNA techniques, significant advances have been made in identifying the genetic factors involved in IDDM. It is clear that genes within the HLA region contribute to the development of IDDM. It seems that 60 percent of the genetic basis of IDDM is related to the HLA gene locus on chromosome 6 and another 40 percent is non-HLA-associated (i.e., chromosomes 2, 7, 11, and 14). Nevertheless, the mode of inheritance of IDDM remains controversial. New data have emerged in the past few years regarding the risk estimates of transmitting the disease that permit genetic counseling of diabetic patients.

Our current knowledge thus far has led us to understand that diabetes mellitus is not a single disease. Therefore, its inheritance pattern will be influenced by its heterogeneity as well as its multifactorial origin. Twin study data demonstrate that NIDDM is transmitted at a higher rate to twins than observed in IDDM, suggesting a greater genetic contribution in NIDDM. However, the genetic factors involved in this latter group are largely unknown; whereas in IDDM, more is known about the genetic factors associated with this disease. Genetic counseling for most patients and families is still limited to a discussion of the empirical risks, followed by recommendations of a lifestyle that will avoid high-risk factors. This is especially true for patients who have had GDM, as weight reduction has been shown to be associated with a lower relative risk for the onset of diabetes in later years. As more information accrues and permits differentiation between the subgroups of diabetes, the impact on therapy, prognosis, and genetic counseling will be realized.

REFERENCES

1. Hitman GA: Progress with the genetics of insulin-dependent diabetes mellitus. Clin Endocrinol 25:463, 1986
2. National Diabetes Data Group: Classification and diagnosis of diabetes mellitus and other categories of glucose intolerance. Diabetes 28:1039, 1979
3. Hollingsworth DR, Resnik R (eds): Medical Counseling Before Pregnancy. Churchill Livingstone, New York, 1988

4. Gottlieb MS, Root HF: Diabetes mellitus in twins. Diabetes 17:693, 1968

5. Tattersall RB, Pyke DA: Diabetes in identical twins. Lancet 2:1120, 1972

6. Pyke DA: Diabetes: the genetic connections. Diabetologia 17:333, 1979

7. Barnett AH, Eff C, Leslie RDG, Pyke DA: Diabetes in identical twins. Diabetologia 20:87, 1981

8. Singal DP, Blajchman MA: Histocompatibility (L-A) antigens, lymphocytotoxic antibodies and tissue antibodies in patients with diabetes mellitus. Diabetes 22:429, 1973

9. Sachs D: The majority histocompatibility complex. p. 303. In Paul WE (ed): Fundamental Immunology. Raven Press, New York, 1984

10. Zinkernagel RM: Associations between major histocompatibility antigens and susceptibility to disease. Annu Rev Microbiol 33:201, 1979

11. Sondel PM: Immunogenetics: the major histocompatibility complex. p. 89. In Graziano FM, Lemanske RF (eds): Williams and Wilkins, Baltimore, 1989

12. Benacerraf B: Role of MHC gene products in immune regulation. Science 212:1229, 1980

13. Gjerset GF, Slichter SJ, Hansen JA: HLA, blood transfusion and the immune system. Clin Immunol Allergy 4:503, 1984

14. Scott DW, Dawson JR: Key Facts in Immunology. Churchill Livingstone, New York, 1985

15. Kaufman JF, Auffray B, Korman AJ et al: The class II molecules of the human and murine major histocompatibility complex. Cell 36:1, 1984

16. Bach FH, Sachs DH: Current concepts: immunology transplantation. N Engl J Med 317:489, 1987

17. Lilly T, Boyse EA, Old LJ: Genetic basis of susceptibility to viral leukemogenesis. Lancet 2:1207, 1964

18. Falchuk ZM, Rogentine GN, Strober W: Predominance of histocompatibility antigen HLA8 in patients with gluten-sensitive enteropathy. J Clin Invest 51:1602, 1972

19. Svejgaard A, Nielsen LS, Svejgaard E et al: HLA in psoriasis vulgaris and in pustular psoriasis—population and family studies. Br J Dermatol 91:145, 1974

20. White SH, Newcomer VC, Mickey MR et al: Disturbance of HLA antigen frequency in psoriasis. N Engl J Med 287:740, 1972

21. Svejgaard A, Platz P, Ryder LP: HLA and disease 1982: a survey. Immunol Rev 70:10, 1983

22. Nerup J, Platz P, Anderson OO et al: HLA-antigens and diabetes mellitus. Lancet 2:864, 1974

23. Cudworth AG, Woodrow JC: HLA system and diabetes mellitus. Diabetes 24:245, 1975

24. Wolf E, Spencer KM, Cudworth AG: The genetic susceptibility to type I (insulin-dependent) diabetes: analysis of the HLA-DR association. Diabetologia 24:224, 1983

25. Sachs JA, Cudworth AG, Jaruquemada D et al: Type I diabetes and the HLA D locus. Diabetologia 418:41, 1980

26. Thompson G: Handbook of Experimental Immunology. Vol. 10. Blackwell Scientific Publications, Oxford, 1986

27. Svejgaard A, Platz P, Ryder LP: Insulin-dependent diabetes mellitus. p. 638. In Terasaki PI (ed): Histocompatibility Testing. UCLA, Tissue Typing Laboratory, Los Angeles, 1980

28. Thompson G: HLA-DR antigens and susceptibility to insulin-dependent diabetes mellitus. Am J Hum Genet 36:1309, 1984

29. Maclaren NK, Henson V: The genetics of insulin-dependent diabetes. Growth Genet Horm 2:1, 1986

30. Todd JA: Genetic analysis of susceptibility to type I diabetes. Springer Semin Immunopathol 14:33, 1992

31. Kim SJ, Holbeck SL, Nisperos B et al: Identification of a polymorphic variant associated with HLA-BQW3 and characterized by specific restriction sites within the DQ beta-chain gene. Proc Natl Acad Sci USA 82:8139, 1985

32. Sheehy J, Rowe JR, Nepom BS: Defining the IDDM-susceptible genotype. Diabetes 37:91A, 1988

33. Bodner JG, Marsh SGE, Parham P et al: Nomenclature for factors of the HLA system. Hum Immunol 28:326, 1989

34. Todd JA, Bell JI, McDevitt HO: HLA-DQB gene contributes to susceptibility and resistance to insulin-dependent diabetes mellitus. Nature 329:599, 1987

35. Todd JA, Bell JI, McDevitt HO: A molecular basis for genetic susceptibility to insulin-dependent diabetes mellitus. Trends Genet 4:129, 1988

36. Fletcher J, Odugbesan O, Mijovic C et al: Class II HLA DNA polymorphisms in type I (insulin-dependent) diabetic patients of North Indian origin. Diabetologia 31:343, 1988

37. Penny M, Jenkins D, Mijovic CH et al: Susceptibility to IDDM in a Chinese population: role of HLA class II alleles. Diabetes 41(8):914, 1992

38. Jacobs KH, Jenkins D, Mijovic CH et al: An investigation of Japanese subjects maps susceptibility to type I (insulin-dependent) diabetes mellitus close to the DQA1 gene. Hum Immunol 33:53, 1992

39. Todd JA, Fukui Y, Kitagawa T et al: The A3 allele of the HLA-DQA1 locus is associated with susceptibility to type I diabetes in Japanese. Proc Natl Acad Sci 87:1094, 1990

40. Mijovic CH, Jenkins D, Jacobs KH et al: HLA-DQA1 and DQ3, alleles associated with genetic susceptibility to IDDM in a black population. Diabetes 40:748, 1991

41. Jenkins D, Mijovic C, Jacobs KH et al: Allele-specific gene probing supports the DQ molecule as a determinant of inherited susceptibility to type I (insulin-dependent) diabetes mellitus. Diabetologia 34:109, 1991

42. Khalil I, d'Auriol L, Gobet M et al: A combination of HLA-DQβ Asp57-negative and HLA-DQα Arg52 confers susceptibility to insulin-dependent diabetes mellitus. J Clin Invest 85:1315, 1990

43. Kockum I, Wassmuth R, Holmberg E et al: HLA-DQ primarily confers protection and HLA-DR susceptibility in type I (insulin-dependent) diabetes studied in population-based affected families and controls. Am J Hum Genet 53:150, 1993

44. MacCuish AC, Barnes EW: Pancreatic islet cell in insulin-dependent disease. Lancet 2:1529, 1974

45. Palmer JP, Asplin CM, Clemons P et al: Insulin antibodies in insulin-dependent diabetics before insulin treatment. Science 222:1337, 1983

46. Dobersen MJ, Scharff JE, Ginsberg-Fellner F et al: Cytotoxic autoantibodies to beta cells in the serum of patients with insulin-dependent diabetes mellitus. N Engl J Med 303:1493, 1980

47. Srikanta S, Ganda OP, Rabizadeh A et al: First-degree relatives of patients with type I diabetes: islet-cell antibodies and abnormal insulin secretion. N Engl J Med 313:461, 1985

48. Schwartz RH: T-lymphocyte recognition of antigen in association with gene products of the major histocompatibility complex. Annu Rev Immunol 3:237, 1985

49. Sette A, Buus S, Colon S et al: Structural characteristics of an antigen required for its interaction with 1a and recognition by T cells. Nature 328:395, 1987

50. Marrack P, Kappler I: The antigen specific major histocompatibility complex-restricted receptor on T cells. Adv Immunol 38:1, 1986

51. Todd JA: Genetic control of autoimmunity in type I diabetes. Immunol Today 11:112, 1990

52. Bottazzo GF, Dean BM, McNally JM et al: In situ characterization of autoimmune phenomena and expression of HLA molecules in the pancreas in diabetic insulitis. N Engl J Med 313:353, 1985

53. Risch N: Assessing the role of HLA-linked and unlinked determinants of disease. Am J Hum Genet 40:1, 1987

54. Rotter JI, Landau EM: Measuring the genetic contribution of a single locus to multilocus disease. Clin Genet 26:529, 1984

55. Field LL, Anderson CE, Neiswanger K et al: Interaction of HLA and immunoglobulin antigens in type I (insulin-dependent) diabetes. Diabetologia 27:504, 1984

56. Rich SS, Weitkamp LR, Guttormsen S, Barbosa J: Gm, Km and HLA in insulin-dependent diabetes mellitus: a log-linear analysis of association. Diabetes 35:927, 1986

57. Bell GI, Horita S, Karam JH: A highly polymorphic locus near the human insulin gene is associated with insulin-dependent diabetes mellitus. Diabetes 33:176, 1984

58. Hitman GA, Tarn AC, Winter RM et al: Type I (insulin-dependent) diabetes and a highly variable locus close to the insulin gene on chromosome 11. Diabetologia 28:218, 1985

59. Tuomilehto-Wolf E, Tuomilehto J, Cepaitis Z et al: New susceptibility haplotype for type I diabetes. Lancet 2:299, 1989

60. Julier C, Hyer RN, Davies J et al: Insulin-IGF2 region on chromosome 11p encodes a gene implicated in HLA-DR4 dependent diabetes susceptibility. Nature 354:155, 1991

61. Concannon P, Wright JA, Wright LG et al: T cell receptor genes and insulin dependent diabetes mellitus (IDDM): no evidence for linkage from affected sib-pairs. Am J Hum Genet 47:45, 1990

62. Millward BA, Leslie RDG, Welsh HI et al: T-cell receptor beta chain gene polymorphisms are associated with insulin-dependent diabetes in identical twins. Clin Exp Immunol 70:152, 1987

63. Field LL, Anderson CE, Neiswanger K et al: Interaction of HLA and immunoglobulin antigens in type I (insulin-dependent) diabetes. Diabetologia 27:504, 1984

64. Field LL: Non-HLA region genes in insulin-dependent diabetes mellitus. Baillieres Clin Endocrinol Metab 5:413, 1991

65. Bell JI: Polygenic disease. Curr Opin Genet Dev 3:466, 1993

66. Chern MM, Anderson VE, Barbosa J: Empirical risk for insulin-dependent diabetes (IDDM) in sibs: further definition of genetic heterogeneity. Diabetes 31:1115, 1982

67. Tillil H, Kobberling J: Age-corrected empirical genetic risk estimates for first-degree relatives of IDDM patients. Diabetes 36:93, 1987

68. Thompson G, Robinson WP, Kuhner MK et al: Genetic heterogeneity, modes of inheritance, and risk estimates for a joint study of Caucasians with insulin-dependent diabetes mellitus. Hum Genet 43:799, 1988

69. Wagener DK, Sacks JM, Laporte RE et al: The Pittsburgh study of insulin-dependent diabetes mellitus: risk for diabetes among relatives of IDDM. Diabetes 31:136, 1982

70. Kobberling J, Bruggeboes B: Prevalence of diabetes among children of insulin-dependent diabetic mothers. Diabetologia 18:459, 1980

71. Warram JH, Krolewski AS, Gottlieb MS et al: Differences in risk of insulin-dependent diabetes in offspring of diabetic mothers and diabetic fathers. N Engl J Med 311:149, 1984

72. Vadheim CM, Rotter JI, MacLaren NH et al: Preferential transmission of diabetic alleles within the HLA gene complex. N Engl J Med 315:1314, 1986

73. Cahill GF Jr: Heterogeneity in type II diabetes (editorial). West J Med 142:240, 1985

74. Tattersall RB, Fajans SS: A difference between the inheritance of classical juvenile-onset and maturity-onset diabetes of young people. Diabetes 24:44, 1975

75. O'Rahilly S, Spivey RS, Holman RR et al: Type II diabetes of early onset: a distinct clinical and genetic syndrome? BMJ 294:923, 1987

76. Heiervang E, Folling I, Sovik D et al: Maturity-onset diabetes of the young. Studies in a Norwegian family. Acta Paediatr Scand 78:74, 1989

77. Permutt MA, Andreone T, Chirgwin J et al: The genetics of type I and type II diabetes: analysis by recombinant DNA methodology. Adv Exp Med Biol 189:89, 1985

78. Zimmet P, Taft P: The high prevalence of diabetes mellitus in Nauru, a central Pacific island. Adv Metab Disord 9:225, 1978

79. Freinkel N, Josimovich J, Conference Planning Committee: American Diabetes Association workshop conference on gestational diabetes: summary and recommendations. Diabetes Care 3:499, 1980

80. Ober C, Wason CJ, Andrew K, Dooley S: Restriction fragment length polymorphisms of the insulin gene hypervariable in gestational onset diabetes mellitus. Am J Obstet Gynecol 157:1364, 1987

81. Freinkel N, Metzger BE, Phelps RL et al: Gestational diabetes mellitus. Heterogeneity of maternal age, weight, insulin secretion, HLA antigens, and islet cell antibodies and the impact of maternal metabolism on pancreatic B-cell and somatic development in the offspring. Diabetes 34:1, 1985

82. Ginsberg-Fellner F, Mark EM, Nechemias C et al: Islet cell antibodies in gestational diabetics. Lancet 2:362, 1980

83. O'Sullivan JB: Subsequent morbidity among gestational diabetic women. p. 174. In Sutherland HW, Stowers JM (eds): Carbohydrate Metabolism in Pregnancy and the Newborn. Churchill Livingstone, Edinburgh, 1984

84. Freinkel N, Metzger BE: Gestational diabetes: problems in classification and implications for long-range prognosis. p. 47. In Vranic M, Hollenberg CH, Steiner G (eds): Comparison of Type I and Type II Diabetes. Similarities and Dissimilarities in Etiology, Pathogenesis, and Complications. Plenum Press, New York, 1985

85. Stowers JM, Sutherland HW, Kerridege DR: Long-range implications for the mother: the Aberdeen experience. Diabetes 34:106, 1985

86. Powers AC, Eisenbarth GS: Autoimmunity to islet cells in diabetes mellitus. Annu Rev Med 36:31, 1985

87. Vardi P, Dib SA, Tuttlemen M et al: Competitive insulin autoantibody assay. Prospective evaluation of subjects at high risk for development of type I diabetes mellitus. Diabetes 36:1286, 1987

88. Ginsberg-Fellner F, Witt ME, Franklin BH et al: Triad of markers for identifying children at high risk of developing insulin-dependent diabetes mellitus. JAMA 254:1469, 1985

89. Tarn AC, Thomas JM, Dean BM et al: Predicting insulin-dependent diabetes. Lancet 1:845, 1980

90. Srikanta S, Ricker AT, McCulloch DK et al: Autoimmunity to insulin, beta cell dysfunction, and development of insulin-dependent diabetes mellitus. Diabetes 35:139, 1986

91. Pettit DJ, Aleck KA, Baird HR et al: Congenital susceptibility to NIDDM. Role of intrauterine environment. Diabetes 37:622, 1988

92. Reece EA, Homko CJ: Diabetes-related complication of pregnancy. J Natl Med Assoc 85:537, 1993

93. Klein BE, Moses SE, Klein R: Effect of pregnancy on progression of diabetic retinopathy. Diabetes Care 13:34, 1990

94. Jovanovic-Peterson L, Peterson CM: Diabetic retinopathy. Clin Obstet Gynecol 34:516, 1991

95. Rosenn B, Midovnik M, Kranias G et al: Progression of diabetic retinopathy in pregnancy: association with hypertension in pregnancy. Am J Obstet Gynecol 166:1214, 1992

96. Reece EA, Lockwood CJ, Tuck S et al: Retinal and pregnancy outcomes in the presence of diabetic proliferative retinopathy. J Reprod Med 39:799, 1994

97. Hayslett JP, Reece EA: Managing diabetic patients with nephropathy and other vascular complications. Baillieres Clin Obstet Gynaecol 1:939, 1987 (The updated version of this paper was done as a chapter for a book, Renal Disease in Pregnancy (2nd Ed.).

98. Reece EA, Winn HN, Hayslett JP et al: Does pregnancy alter the rate of progression of diabetic nephropathy? Am J Perinat 7:193, 1990

99. Reece EA, Coustan DR, Hayslett JP et al: Diabetic nephropathy: pregnancy performance and fetomaternal outcome. Am J Obstet Gynecol 159:56, 1988

100. Kjos SL: Contraception in women with diabetes mellitus. Diabetes Spectrum 6:80, 1993

101. Kjos SL: Contraception in diabetic women. Clin Perinat 20:649, 1993

102. Porter JB, Hunter JR, Jick H, Stergochis A: Oral contraceptives and nonfatal vascular disease. Obstet Gynecol 66:1, 1985

103. Rosenberg L, Palmer JR, Lesko SM, Shapiro S: Oral contraceptive use and the risk of myocardial infarction. Am J Epidemiol 131:1009, 1990

104. Clarkson TB, Shively CA, Morgan TM et al: Oral contraceptives and coronary artery atherosclerosis of cynomolgus monkeys. Obstet Gynecol 75:217, 1990

105. Klein BEK, Moss SE, Klein R: Oral contraceptives in women with diabetes. Diabetes Care 13:895, 1990

106. Wiese J: Intrauterine contraception in diabetic women. Fertil Steril 28:422, 1977

107. Skouby SO, Molsted-Pedersen L, Kosonen A: Consequences of intrauterine contraception in diabetic women. Fertil Steril 42:568, 1984

108. Hagay Z, Reece EA, Hobbins JC: Diabetes mellitus in pregnancy and periconceptional genetic counseling. Am J Perinat 9:88, 1992

109. Reece EA, Hagay Z, Hobbins J: Insulin-dependent diabetes mellitus and immunogenetics: maternal and fetal considerations. Obstet Gynecol Surv 46:257, 1991

110. Tiwari JL, Terasaki PI: Endocrinology. p. 1. In: HLA and Disease Associations. Springer-Verlag, New York, 1985

28
Preconception, Conception, and Contraception

JUDITH M. STEEL

PREPREGNANCY COUNSELING

Excellent antenatal care has improved the outlook for the infant of the diabetic mother. There are, however, several important problems that can only be influenced by counseling women before conception. These include congenital abnormalities, problem patients, and patients with micro- and macrovascular angiopathy.

Congenital Abnormalities

The high incidence of severe abnormalities in infants of diabetic mothers has been recognized for many years,[1,2] and it is known that the abnormalities arise as maldevelopments before the seventh week of gestational life.[3] Work on rats shows that both in vitro and in vivo hyperglycemia is associated with a high incidence of developmental abnormalities (see Ch. 9). Measurement of glycosylated hemoglobin (HbA$_1$) enables us to look retrospectively at blood glucose control over the previous 6 to 8 weeks. Many workers have shown an association between high HbA$_1$ levels in early pregnancy and congenital abnormalities.[4–6] The title of the article by the National Institute of Child Health and Human Development throws some doubt on the subject,[7] but the study itself supports the view that hyperglycemia in early pregnancy is associated with a high incidence of malformations.[8] If we are to prevent these abnormalities, it is clear that it is necessary to initiate strict glucose level control before conception.

Problem Patients

Patients who are unreliable and those who have unplanned pregnancies are particularly at risk of delivering an infant with an anamoly because they tend to present late in pregnancy, may be unsure of their dates, and often are poorly controlled.

Patients with Micro- and Macrovascular Angiopathy

Retinopathy is no longer a contraindication to pregnancy but should be treated, if necessary, before conception. Women with severe renal disease, especially if it is associated with hypertension, have a reduced chance of delivering a live baby, and in the case of ischemic heart disease, the mother's life may also be at risk.[9]

It is clear that the only way to make any impact on these problems is to see and advise women before conception.

AIMS AND PRACTICES OF PREPREGNANCY CARE

We started our prepregnancy clinic in Edinburgh in 1976. The aims of the clinic were published in 1980[10] and details of the practice in 1982.[11] There have been no major changes over the years since then.

In view of the importance of planned pregnancies and of good control in early pregnancy, pregnancy should be discussed with all young women with diabetes, and contraceptive advice should be offered to all women of childbearing age. This could be described as pre-prepregnancy care.

When a couple decide that they would like to have a baby, they are seen by a diabetologist and an obstetrician at a formal visit. The aims of this visit are

1. *To assess the woman's fitness for pregnancy.* A full medical, obstetric, and gynecologic, and medication history is taken. Fundi are examined, blood pressure measured, and renal function assessed, and in those with long-standing diabetes, an exercise electrocardiogram and autonomic nerve function tests are carried out. Any necessary treatment is given for hypertension, avoiding the use of angiotension-converting enzyme inhibitors.

2. *To obtain maximum cooperation from patients and their partners.* The importance of good control over the time of conception and during pregnancy is explained, and the program for antenatal care is discussed. Couples are encouraged to ask questions, and written information is provided.

3. *To optimize control.* Control is assessed by frequent blood glucose monitoring and by HbA_1 measurement. Patients are usually on "pen" regimens with multiple injections of short-acting insulin and intermediate-acting insulin before bed. Sometimes, twice-daily injections of short- and intermediate-acting insulin are given, often increasing to three injections by giving the evening intermediate-acting insulin before bed. Ideally, HbA_1 levels should be in the normal nondiabetic range before conception (6 to 8 percent in our laboratory), but it may be difficult for some women with long-standing diabetes to achieve this. It is important that women are not made to feel guilty or to have too frequent or severe episodes of hypoglycemia. The aim is, therefore, to individualize treatment and obtain the best possible HbA_1 level without undue risk of hypoglycemia. Control is optimized on an outpatient basis. Dietary advice is given to ensure accuracy with the prescribed diet and to ensure that it is adequate in all essential nutrients, particularly folic acid. Women are given folic acid supplements. The partner, friends, and family are taught how to recognize and treat hypoglycemia, and the partner is taught how to administer glucagon. The importance of testing the urine for ketones if the blood glucose level is

high, at the time of illness and particularly if vomiting occurs, is stressed.

4. *To ensure good general health.* Rubella antibodies and thyroid function are measured. Advice is given regarding the risks of obesity and smoking if necessary.

5. *To discuss the inheritance of diabetes.*

6. *To identify the time of conception.* After the second formal visit, when the results are discussed and further questions are answered, women whose diabetes is well controlled and who have no complications of diabetes stop contraception. Other women may require treatment for complications, and some may take more time to optimize their level of diabetic control. After stopping contraception, women are asked to keep a log of their menstrual periods. Some are given ovulation kits, and all are instructed to send off a pregnancy test if it has been 5 weeks since their last menstrual period. If the pregnancy test result is negative, they are asked to repeat the test weekly until the result is positive or they begin menstruating. They are asked to schedule for antenatal care as soon as the test finding is positive. Women are always told that it is normal to take some time to conceive and are encouraged to maintain good control if there is a delay.

7. *To identify and treat infertility early.* As the risks of diabetes and pregnancy are related to the presence of complications, women are evaluated, if they wish, after 1 year of infertility.

Experience of the Edinburgh Prepregnancy Clinic

Over the 18 years from 1976 to 1993, we have seen 294 couples. Twenty-six have been advised against pregnancy, 9 have decided not to become pregnant, 39 have been evaluated for infertility, 11 have moved away, 5 have left their partners, and several are currently pregnant or trying to conceive. There have been 196 pregnancies (excluding spontaneous abortions).

Patients Advised Against Pregnancy

In 1976, one woman was advised against pregnancy because of proliferative retinopathy; however, since that time, laser therapy has been available, and retinopathy is no longer a contraindication to pregnancy.

Three patients had severe ischemic heart disease, and 11 had multiple medical, obstetric, and psychological problems.

The most common single reason for advising against pregnancy was renal disease with hypertension. There were 11 patients in this group, 5 of them have since died, and 2 are undergoing dialysis. The situation is changing, and over the past few years, no women have been advised against pregnancy. This is because the outlook has improved as a result of better treatments, including renal transplants, and advances in the management of premature babies.[12] There are still risks in this type of situation, and the woman's life expectancy may be limited. However, the couples are helped to make an informed decision.

Retinopathy

Seven patients with previously untreated retinopathy received laser treatment during pregnancy, three of these with proliferative retinopathy were referred from other centers, two were our own patients who had not attended the prepregnancy clinic, and two had only mild background retinopathy before pregnancy, which deteriorated during pregnancy. Nineteen patients with proliferative retinopathy and four with preproliferative retinopathy were treated with laser therapy before pregnancy, and only one required further treatment during pregnancy. Four patients had both laser treatment and vitrectomies before pregnancy, and none showed any deterioration during pregnancy. No pregnancies were terminated because of retinopathy.

Attendance at the Prepregnancy Clinic

It was 1977 before the first patients coming through the clinic were delivered; by 1979, the clinic was running well. Over the 15 years from 1979 to 1993, we have had 277 pregnancies in insulin-dependent diabetic women; 188 (68 percent) of these patients have come through the clinic. Of the 89 patients not from our own general clinic, 36 have come to us from other centers who were already pregnant. If these women are excluded, 78 percent of our patients have come through the clinic. We are able to see a large proportion of women at the clinic because

1. Our clinic is run by the British National Health Service, and there is virtually no private practice, so all young insulin-dependent diabetic women attend our general diabetes clinic.
2. We have diabetes nurse specialists who discuss pregnancy with all young women and can counsel and follow poorly controlled and noncompliant women.
3. I have worked for 24 years in the same department doing five diabetes clinics a week, including a children's and an adolescent clinic and thus have been in an ideal position to get to know personally nearly all the women of child-bearing age.

Control in Patients Coming Through the Clinic

During the early years of the clinic, I compared the HbA_1 levels in those coming through the prepregnancy clinic with those who had not on an annual basis. Although the patients coming through the clinic were self-selected, initially, their control was only slightly better than that in those who had not attended. Motivation toward pregnancy was not necessarily associated with good control. Those coming through the clinic achieved good control before conception and presented earlier for antenatal care. The other group presented later but also improved so that, by the end of pregnancy, the two groups were equally well controlled. The important difference between the two groups was of course that the prepregnancy group were well controlled throughout pregnancy while the others were only well controlled in the latter half of pregnancy.[13,14] Over the years, the two groups have become more and more similar because of a marked improvement in those not coming through the clinic. When 50 of our own patients who had not attended the prepregnancy clinic were interviewed in detail, it became clear that they had nearly all been told (usually repeatedly) about the importance of good control in early pregnancy and the importance of early antenatal care. There were only three truly unplanned pregnancies in this group. All the other women (many unmarried) had carefully planned their pregnancies. They had not told me nor, in many cases, their partners, but most of them had improved their control and come early for antenatal care. This raises the question as to whether it is necessary to run a formal prepregnancy clinic, and this is discussed later in this chapter. We did have six women who did not chose to take the advice they were given; two of these women each had two children with congenital anomalies. Despite the efforts of all our staff to target them, this small group remains a problem.

First Pregnancy Visit

The time of first attendance for antenatal care has fallen dramatically in both groups, and it is now unusual to see anyone later than 6 weeks of gestation. It is usually necessary to delay the early scan to assess gestation until the second visit.

Congenital Malformations

Over all the years of our clinic (1976–1993), we have had 14 abnormalities in 117 pregnancies in which the mothers have not come through the prepregnancy clinic (12.0 percent) compared with three (1.5 percent) in the 196 women who have come through the prepregnancy clinic. This gives an overall incidence of 5.4 percent. The difference between the two groups was statistically significant ($P < .001$). Details of the abnormalities are shown in Table 28-1, which demonstrates that all the mothers who had babies with congenital anomalies were poorly controlled. Some of the earlier patients came too late to have HbA$_1$ levels measured in the first trimester, but several of them admitted to omitting their insulin completely on several occasions during early pregnancy. Two of the patients attending the prepregnancy clinic who gave birth to anomalous infants were well controlled, as judged by HbA$_1$ levels. It is unrealistic to expect to eliminate all congenital abnormalities because the background level is around 1 percent. Greene et al[15] showed that there is a broad range over which risks are not substantially elevated but that it is possible that swings in blood glucose levels or those of other metabolites are also important. The one poorly controlled patient in the prepregnancy group conceived by accident as a result of failed contraception at a time of social and metabolic turmoil. It is important to note that only 3 of the 17 abnormalities were perinatal deaths. Several pregnancies were aborted; this is becoming and will continue to become more common as ultrasound detection improves. Some babies died after the perinatal period, and some survived with handicaps. We have followed 96 percent of our babies. If we had defined congenital abnormalities as those detected before or at birth, four

Table 28-1. Major Congenital Abnormalities (1976–1993)

No.	HbA$_1$ Level First Trimester (%)	Defect	Outcome
Nonattenders at prepregnancy clinic
1	Before assay	Encephalocele	Major surgery, survived retarded
2	Too late Omitted insulin	Anencephaly	Aborted
3	Too late Omitted insulin	Sacral hypoplasia	Urinary incontinence
4	Too late	Microcephaly	Survived, retarded
5	13.4	Sirenomelia, renal agenesis	Died
6	11.6	Kyphoscoliosis, deafness	Major surgery, survived
7	11.4	Monomelia, renal agenesis	Died
8	13.8	Kyphoscoliosis, deafness	Major surgery, survived
9	13.7	Single ventricle, mitral atresia	Died
10	14.9	Fallot's tetralogy	Shunt, for surgery
11	12.2	Encephalocele	Aborted
12	Too late Omitted insulin	Anencephaly	Aborted
13	12.9	Sacral agenesis	Severely handicapped
14	11.7	Situs inversus, atrial and ventricular septal defects	For surgery
Attenders at prepregnancy clinic
15	8.8	Anencephaly	Aborted
16	9.5	Transposition of great vessels	Diagnosed at 6 weeks Died during surgery at 8 weeks
17	12.0	Pulmonary atresia, left atrial isomerism	Intrauterine death at 14 weeks

of the abnormalities (numbers 3,6,8, and 10 in Table 28-1) would have been missed. This demonstrates that the impressive perinatal mortality figures from some "centers of excellence" grossly underestimate the serious problems that affect the infants of diabetic mothers.

A few years ago, we became concerned that work on rat models demonstrated that rat embryos, exposed to a period of hypoglycemia at a stage equivalent to days 32 to 38 of human pregnancy, developed abnormalities (see Ch. 9). Our retrospective data[16] agreed with Pedersen's[17] observation in his book *The Pregnant Diabetic and Her Newborn* published in 1967 in which he stated that "the occurrence of hypoglycemia reactions and insulin coma during the first trimester was low in mothers with malformed infants indicating a poor compensation of diabetes at that time." (When we started our prepregnancy clinic, the relationship between high blood glucose levels and congenital abnormalities had not yet been described, and this statement of Pedersen was one of the reasons we thought good control in early pregnancy might be important.) Looking prospectively at days 28 to 42 in our last 101 consecutive pregnancies, we found that 48 women had clinical hypoglycemia during that period. Forty-six had mild episodes, 16 had severe episodes (defined as requiring help from someone), and 12 required glucagon. One patient required 10 vials of glucagon over that period. All these women had normal babies. There were six women who had babies with congenital malformation, and none of them had had any hypoglycemic reactions over the period studied. I do not think that there is any evidence that hypoglycemia in early pregnancy causes abnormalities in humans.

Infertility

It is difficult to know whether infertility is any more common in women with diabetes. Some patients who were identified as infertile were successfully treated.[16]

Experience of Other Prepregnancy Clinics

The first articles that suggested that improving control in early pregnancy can reduce the abnormality rate in infants of diabetic mothers were from Fuhrmann et al[18,19] in East Germany. They had only two malforma-

tions in 185 insulin-dependent women who attended their prepregnancy clinic (1.1 percent) compared with 31 in 473 patients who did not attend (6.6 percent). The patients were admitted to hospital every 3 months before conception and were admitted again as soon as their basal body temperature had been raised for more than 16 days. Numerous blood glucose measurements were made, but HbA_1 levels were not measured. In a small study of 44 patients who received prepregnancy care compared with 31 who did not, Goldman et al[20] found a reduced incidence of congenital malformations. The Copenhagen group[21] showed a reduction in congenital malformations over the period from 1982 to 1986 compared with the period from 1967 to 1981. They did not have HbA_1 results for all the patients studied, but it seems likely that the reduction reflected the fact that 75 percent of pregnancies during the second time period were planned after preconception advice. In a smaller study of 28 women who had attended a prepregnancy program compared with 71 enrolled after conception, Rosenn et al[22] reported a decreased rate of early pregnancy loss. He had a high dropout rate from his prepregnancy group possibly because his criteria for tight control were too strict and women did not receive enough encouragement. In a larger study, Kitzmiller et al[23] reported an abnormality rate of 1.2 percent in 84 women recruited before conception compared with 12 of 110 (10.9 percent) in those first seen postconception. These findings are similar to our own.[24] It has also been shown that women with diabetes who have elevated HbA_1 levels in the first trimester have a significantly increased risk of having a spontaneous abortion.[25] Reports from the United States have shown that prepregnancy care is cost effective.[26]

Is Formal Prepregnancy Care Necessary?

Gregory and Tattersall[27] maintain that a formal clinic is not necessary and that all the work can be done by nurses as part of their normal counseling and education. I agree that nurse specialists are invaluable in discussing pregnancy and particularly in focusing on patients who default from general diabetic clinics and are particularly at risk. They should be encouraged, as many are, to take on this role. Everyone would agree that there is always the problem that, in any type of preventative medicine, those needing it most are least likely to come and the whole team puts a lot of energy into attempting to improve the control and motivation of a few more difficult patients.

There is considerable confusion over the use of the term *clinic*. Some people see couples by appointment at a mutually convenient time, as I do; others see couples on a special day at a prepregnancy clinic; some see patients during a routine diabetes clinic visit; and others see couples at an antenatal or gynecology clinic. I continue to use the word "clinic" to distinguish those who declare a wish to become pregnant and come through the formal system system described from women who are simply told about the importance of pregnancy during a routine diabetes visit. In an ideal world where all women know a great deal about both diabetes and pregnancy and where diabetes in all women is perfectly controlled, it will not be necessary to offer formal preconception planning. However, we have not yet reached that stage, and women do appreciate being told in detail about what to expect by the people who will be caring for them during their pregnancy. In my experience, women who have attended a prepregnancy clinic are much easier to look after antenatally. Although many of the things done at the formal clinic may have already been done at a good diabetic clinic, the formality ensures that nothing is missed and that there are no misunderstandings. In the case of patients with complications of diabetes, those who are difficult to control, those who are taking medications, and those with previous obstetric or gynecologic problems, I believe that prepregnancy care is essential.

Prepregnancy Care in Women with Non-Insulin-Dependent Diabetes Mellitus and Previous Gestational Diabetes

Women with non-insulin-dependent diabetes mellitus also require prepregnancy care.[28] If they are overweight, they should be encouraged to lose weight before conception. Those who are inadequately controlled on diet alone and those who take oral agents should be converted to insulin therapy before pregnancy.

Appropriate advice should also be given to women with a previous history of gestational diabetes.[29]

Conclusion

There is reasonable evidence that prepregnancy counseling can improve the cooperation of couples during pregnancy, optimize the outcome for mother and fetus in those with complications of diabetes, increase the proportion of planned pregnancies, reduce the incidence of spontaneous abortions, help patients to present early for antenatal care, improve control in early pregnancy, and reduce the incidence of major congenital malformations. It can also enable us to identify infertility early and is a very interesting and rewarding experience.

IDENTIFICATION OF THE DATE OF CONCEPTION AND THE "EARLY GROWTH DELAY" HYPOTHESIS

One important consequence of establishing a prepregnancy clinic is the opportunity afforded to study the physiology of early gestation in this group of patients. Pedersen and Molsted-Pedersen[30,31] reported that early growth retardation occurs in 30 percent of diabetic pregnancies and that a fetus showing early growth delay is more likely to be abnormal. They claim that a similar delay is also seen in placental development.[32] By the age of 4 to 5 years, children with a history of growth delay in early pregnancy had lower scores on the Denver developmental screening test for personal-social development and gross motor development and statistically significantly lesser scores in language and speech development compared with infants of diabetic mothers who did not show a delay.[33] If correct, these findings have serious implications. Although they included only patients with "previous regular cycles," menstrual irregularities are even more common in diabetic than in nondiabetic women.[34] All their data depended on predicting ovulation from menstrual dates apart from a very small series of 10 women who measured basal body temperature. These 10 pregnancies did show a slight delay compared with nondiabetic pregnancies, but only 1 woman with a discrepancy of 6 days fulfilled their criteria of a delay of more than 5 days.[35] It is possible that the appearance of growth retardation in their series was in fact due to delayed ovulation.

Nondiabetic Women

We found that only 197 (10.5 percent) of 1,873 nondiabetic women fulfilled Pedersen and Molsted-Pedersen's criteria for unequivocal menstrual data and that 32 of these women had ultrasound estimates of gestation greater than 5 days behind the menstrual age, which suggested to us that there is tendency for ovulation to be delayed, even in these women.[36]

Diabetic Women

We identified the time of ovulation using salivary progesterone levels in 12 insulin-dependent diabetic women compared with the gestation day from ultrasound scan and found no evidence of early growth delay.[37] More recently, in collaboration with Drs. S. G. Hillier and Vicky Sweeting in the Reproductive Endocrinology Unit, Edinburgh University, we identified ovulation by the use of home ovulation kits (an enzyme-linked immunosorbent assay method of measuring luteinizing hormone levels in urine) in an additional 20 women and by measuring urinary luteinizing hormone levels in the laboratory by immunoassay in 17 of them.[37a] The results of the two methods were almost identical, and there was no evidence of growth delay, although when dating was based on menstrual data, six fetuses showed apparent growth delay.

In addition, we have seen two patients who had ovulation induced and recorded on ultrasound on a known day; neither of these pregnancies showed evidence of growth delay. We have, therefore, accurately identified the time of ovulation in 34 pregnant women with insulin-dependent diabetes and seen no evidence of growth delay.

Other Studies

Whittaker et al[38] measured human placental lactogen levels in 13 diabetic women and were unable to detect early growth delay. Hieta-Heikurainen and Teramo[39] monitored basal body temperature in 24 insulin-dependent diabetic women and found that conception occurred, on average, on the 18th day of the cycle. They found no evidence of early growth delay. Cousins et al[40] repeatedly measured early fetal growth in a group of 20 diabetic pregnancies, which included two abnormal fetuses, and found that early fetal growth was similar to that in control fetuses.

Possible Effect of Control

Women with poorly controlled diabetes are more likely to have abnormal fetuses, and Pedersen and Molsted-Pedersen[35] suggested that a similar mechanism may cause altered somatic growth. This view is supported by the fact that the incidence of growth delay in their series decreased as control in early pregnancy improved. Our patients' diabetes was not all well controlled. The average HbA_1 level was high in both Hieta-Heikurainen and Teramo's[39] and Cousins et al[40] series. Women with poorly controlled diabetes are more likely to have irregular cycles; therefore, there is more likely to be an error in estimating ovulation from menstrual dates in these women.[41]

Conclusion

Although early growth delay has been described in animals and has been shown to occur in diabetic rats,[42,43] there are no unequivocal reports in humans. On the contrary, ultrasonic fetal measurement in humans in early pregnancy has been shown to predict the onset of spontaneous labor, resulting in the delivery of a mature fetus even more precisely than an impeccable menstrual history. Experience has shown that, when a fetal measurement falls below the normal range for gestational age because of intrauterine growth retardation, it usually remains below normal.[44] It seems likely that "early growth delay" in diabetic pregnancy does not exist and that the concept has resulted from incorrect estimations of conception from menstrual histories and therefore carries no sinister implications.

CONTRACEPTION FOR INSULIN-DEPENDENT DIABETIC WOMEN

When deciding on the best form of contraception for an insulin-dependent diabetic patient, in addition to the usual factors that are important for all women, there are several other important considerations:

1. The importance of periconceptual diabetic control (described above)
2. The constraints imposed by diabetes in pregnancy

3. The problems of patients with complications of diabetes
4. The reduction in life expectancy of women with insulin-dependent diabetes

All forms of contraception carry some risks. Every couple must be considered individually, and their relative risks and preferences must be discussed to find the method most suited to them.

Combined Oral Contraceptives

The combined oral contraceptive has obvious attractions because of its reliability.

There have been many studies that look at the metabolic effects of contraceptive steroids on glucose metabolism,[45] but in practice, the currently used low-dose preparations rarely cause any change in insulin requirements.

The original high-dose estrogen preparations were shown to increase the risk of vascular disease in the general population. Because young women with diabetes are already at high risk and may have some adverse changes in blood lipid and coagulation factor levels, there was understandably concern about the safety of the combined oral contraceptive in such patients. Evidence that there might be a problem was largely ancedotal,[46] and fortunately, before large studies were done, the dose of estrogen was greatly reduced, and the type and dose of progestin was changed in combined oral contraceptives. Skouby et al[47] studied the metabolic effects of four oral contraceptives in women with insulin-dependent diabetes mellitus, monophasic combination of a nonalkylated estrogen with 500 µg of norethindrone, a monophasic low-dose estrogen (35 µg ethinyl estradiol with 500 µg norethindrone), a progestin-only pill (300 µg norethindrone), and a low-dose triphasic preparation. No differences were found in insulin requirements, HbA_1 levels, nonesterified fatty acids, or low-density/high-density lipoprotein-cholesterol ratios between the treatment groups. However, the low-dose combined preparation produced significant increases in plasma triglyceride and very low-density lipoprotein-cholesterol levels. Every preparation has slightly different metabolic effects, but fortunately, the low-dose preparations in current use have very small effects. Diabetic and nondiabetic subjects may react differently to the same preparation. It is reassuring that Radberg and Gustafson,[48] using a preparation of ethinyl estradiol 50 µg and lynestrenol 2.5 mg, found less deleterious effects on lipids in insulin-dependent diabetic than in nondiabetic women.

Most specialists in the field believe that the low-dose modern combined oral contraceptives can be safely recommended for most women with diabetes. Some, including myself, have reservations about their use in those with serious complications of diabetes and other risk factors for vascular disease.

Progestin-Only Contraceptives

The progestin-only oral contraceptive has many advantages. There is no epidemiologic evidence associating this medication with vascular side effects, and there are no detrimental effects on lipid or clotting factor levels because of the small dose of progestin involved. The progestin-only oral contraceptive is usually criticized on two accounts. First, that it is not as reliable as the combined oral contraceptive and, second, that it may cause irregular cycles. Our experience with norethindrone in more than 200 patients has been satisfactory. The few patients who became pregnant had "forgotten" to take it for several days, and only two stopped because of irregular bleeding. There were no ectopic pregnancies; no changes in blood pressure, retinopathy, or lipid levels; and no other side effects. It seems likely that the high failure rates sometimes reported are due to patient failure; for once, the woman with diabetes has an advantage in that she takes her insulin every evening. Our patients keep their oral contraceptives with their insulin and are thus reminded to take one with each evening injection. Minor intermenstrual bleeding usually improves spontaneously, and more severe cases usually respond to doubling the dose for a few cycles or changing the preparation. It is difficult to understand why doctors sometimes change contraception when patients have amenorrhea. Most of these patients are very happy when it is explained to them that the absence of bleeding has no harmful consequences. It is important to arrange a pregnancy test in a patient with amenorrhea, but if the results are negative, the preparation is inhibiting ovulation and is particularly effective as a contraceptive. The injectable progestin preparations may have a place for the occasional patient with a difficult problem. Levonorgestrel rod implants (Norplant) may prove to be very useful.

Intrauterine Contraceptive Device

The intrauterine contraceptive device has the advantage of being unlikely to cause any detrimental metabolic effects, and its success does not depend on patient compliance.

The most worrisome problem, which immediately comes to the mind of a diabetologist, is the risk of infection. These devices have been found to increase the incidence of salpingitis, and diabetic women are particularly susceptible to all forms of bacterial infection.[49] Infection can lead in turn to infertility or ectopic gestation. Despite this theoretical problem, Scouby et al[50] reported no increase in infection rates in 105 women with insulin-dependent diabetes.

In 1974, Weise[51] in Copenhagen reported five pregnancies in 44 diabetic patients with intrauterine devices in situ, and we had 11 pregnancies in 30 women.[52] Differences in the deposits on the coils suggested a difference in endometrial metabolism in women with diabetes.[53] Another group reported decreased fibrinolytic activity in endometrial biopsies from diabetic patients,[54] and there is evidence that the enhancement of endometrial fibrinolytic activity prevents implantation.[55] However, in the large Danish series of 105 women with insulin-dependent diabetes, the authors only reported one accidental pregnancy and one infection; nine coils were removed for reasons other than pregnancy, which was similar to their experience in 119 nondiabetic controls.[50] They also found no difference in corrosion of copper devices between diabetic and nondiabetic subjects. Kimmerle et al[56] reported only two accidental pregnancies and eight other medical removals in 59 women with insulin-dependent diabetes, which was similar to the rates in a control group. It should, however, be noted that 37 percent of their diabetic patients were already using an intrauterine device when they were recruited into the study and so were preselected as successful with regard to that form of contraception. It is difficult to explain the different experiences, but in the early reports, patients were selected for an intrauterine device because they were unreliable and often poorly controlled. The devices were also different. There is still some dispute about the suitability of such devices, especially for nulliparous women with diabetes.[57] However, experience in large numbers of women with modern devices supports the view that they are a suitable form of contraception for women with diabetes.

Mechanical Contraception

Barrier methods of contraception are still popular and have been widely promoted since acquired immunodeficiency syndrome became a problem. The high failure rate is largely because they tend to be used incorrectly or not at all. However, there is also a failure rate for the methods themselves, and they are not recommended if it is essential to avoid pregnancy. They have no metabolic consequences and are usually free from local side effects, although a slightly raised incidence of urinary tract infections has been reported in women using a diaphragm.[58] Some couples do wish to use this method, and highly motivated couples taught to use the diaphragm and sheath correctly may find this an effective and acceptable form of contraception, especially if combined with the use of a spermicidal cream or gel.

Natural Family Planning

Natural family planning depends on identifying ovulation by examining cervical mucus.[59] It is only suitable for highly motivated couples who will accept the self-discipline required during the interval of abstinence. It is likely to be less successful in diabetic women because of their tendency to have irregular cycles.

Sterilization

Sterilization is requested by most mothers with diabetes when they have completed their family. Regretfully, it is occasionally necessary to advise sterilization because pregnancy would represent a serious risk to a woman's life. For some couples, vasectomy may be appropriate, but it is important to bear in mind the reduced life expectancy of those with long-standing diabetes when making this decision.

Conclusion

It is important to individualize therapy because there are advantages and disadvantages for all forms of contraception. Many diabetic women can reasonably chose between a low-dose combined oral contraceptive preparation, a progestin-only preparation, or an intrauterine device. Many chose sterilization when their family is complete.

REFERENCES

1. Molsted-Pedersen L, Tygstrup I, Pedersen J: Congenital malformations in newborn infants of diabetic women. Lancet 1:1124, 1964

2. Soler NJ, Walsh CH, Malins JM: Congenital malformations in infants of diabetic mothers. Q J Med 178:303, 1976

3. Mills JL, Baker L, Goldman AS: Malformations in infants of diabetic mothers occur before the seventh gestational week: implications for treatment. Diabetes 28:292, 1979

4. Leslie RDJ, John PN, Pyke DA, White JM: Haemoglobin A₁ in diabetic pregnancy. Lancet 2:958, 1978

5. Miller E, Hare JW, Cloherty JP et al: Elevated maternal hemoglobin A₁c in early pregnancy and major congenital anomalies in infants of diabetic mothers. N Engl J Med 304:1331, 1981

6. Ylinen K, Raivo K, Termao K: Haemoglobin A₁c predicts the perinatal outcome in insulin-dependent diabetic pregnancies. Br J Obstet Gynaecol 88:961, 1977

7. Mills JL, Knopp RH, Simpson JL et al: Lack of relation of increased malformation rates in infants of diabetic mothers to glycemic control during organogenesis. N Engl J Med 318:671, 1988

8. Anonymous: Congenital abnormalities in infants of diabetic mothers, editorial. Lancet 1:1313, 1988

9. Reece EA, Egan JFX, Coustan DR et al: Coronary artery disease in diabetic pregnancy. Am J Obstet Gynecol 154:150, 1986

10. Steel JM, Parboosingh J, Cole RA, Duncan LJP: Pre-pregnancy counseling—a logical prelude to the management of the pregnant diabetic. Diabetes Care 3:371, 1980

11. Steel JM, Johnstone FD, Smith AF, Duncan LJP: Five years experience of a pre-pregnancy clinic for insulin dependent diabetics. BMJ 285:353, 1982

12. Reece AR, Coustan DR, Haylett JP et al: Diabetic nephropathy: pregnancy performance and fetomaternal outcome. Am J Obstet Gynecol 159:56, 1988

13. Steel JM, Johnstone FD, Smith AP, Duncan LJP: The pre-pregnancy approach. p. 75. In Sutherland H, Stowers JM (eds): Third International Symposium on Carbohydrate Metabolism in Pregnancy. Churchill Livingstone, New York, 1984

14. Steel JM: Pre-pregnancy counseling and contraception in the insulin dependent diabetic patient. Clin Obstet Gynecol 28:3, 1985

15. Greene MF, Hare JW, Clocherty JP et al: First-trimester hemoglobin A₁ and risk for major malformation and spontaneous abortion in diabetic pregnancy. Teratology 39:225, 1989

16. Steel JM, Johnstone FD, Smith AF: Prepregnancy preparation. p. 129. In Sutherland H, Stowers JM, Pearson DWM (eds): Fourth International Symposium on Carbohydrate Metabolism in Pregnancy. Springer-Verlag, New York, 1989

17. Pedersen J: The Pregnant Diabetic and Her Newborn. Munksguaard, Copenhagen, 1967

18. Fuhrmann K, Reiher H, Semmler K et al: Prevention of congenital malformations in infants of insulin dependent diabetic mothers. Diabetes Care 6:219, 1983

19. Fuhrmann K, Reiher H, Semmler K, Glockner E: The effect of intensified conventional insulin therapy before and during pregnancy on the malformation rate in offspring of diabetic mothers. Exp Clin Endocrinol 83:173, 1984

20. Goldman JA, Dicker D, Feldberg D et al: Pregnancy outcome in patients with insulin-dependent diabetes mellitus with preconceptional diabetic control: a comparative study. Am J Obstet Gynecol 155:293, 1986

21. Damm P, Molsted-Pedersen L: Significant decrease in congenital malformations in infants of an unselected population of diabetic women. Am J Obstet Gynecol 161:1163, 1989

22. Rosenn B, Miodovnik M, Combs CA et al: Pre-conception management of insulin-dependent diabetes: improvement of pregnancy outcome. Obstet Gynecol 77:846, 1991

23. Kitzmiller JL, Gavin LA, Gin GD et al: Preconception care of diabetes—glycemic control prevents congenital anomalies. JAMA 265:1163, 1991

24. Steel JM, Johnstone FD, Hepburn DA, Smith AF: Can pre-pregnancy care of diabetic women reduce the risk of abnormal babies? BMJ 301:1070, 1990

25. Mills JL, Simpson JL, Driscoll SG et al: Incidence of spontaneous abortion among normal women and insulin-dependent diabetic women whose pregnancies were identified within 21 days of conception. N Engl J Med 319:1617, 1988

26. Scheffler RM, Feuchtbaum LB, Ciaran S: Prevention: the cost-effectiveness of the California Diabetes and Pregnancy Program. Am J Public Health 82:168, 1992

27. Gregory R, Tattersall RB: Are pre-pregnancy clinics worthwhile? Lancet 340:371, 1992

28. Rowe BR, Rowbotham CJF, Barnet AH: Pre-conception counselling, birth weight and congenital abnormalities in established and gestational diabetic pregnancy. Diabetes Res 6:33, 1987

29. Molsted-Pedersen L, Skouby SO, Damm P: Pre-conception counseling and contraception after gestational diabetes. Diabetes, suppl. 2, 40:147, 1991

30. Pedersen JF, Molsted-Pedersen L: Early growth retardation in diabetic pregnancy. BMJ 278:18, 1979

31. Pedersen JF, Molsted-Pedersen L: Early fetal growth delay detected by ultrasound marks increased risk of congenital malformation in diabetic pregnancy. BMJ 283:269, 1981

32. Pedersen JF, Molsted-Pedersen L, Lebech P: Is the early growth delay in the diabetic pregnancy accompanied by a delay in placental development? Acta Obstet Gynecol Scand 65:675, 1986

33. Petersen M, Pedersen S, Greisen G, et al: Early growth delay in diabetic pregnancy: relation to psychomotor development at age four. BMJ 296:598, 1988

34. Bergquist N: The gonadal function in female diabetics. Acta Endocrinol (Copenh), suppl., 19:3, 1953

35. Pedersen FJ, Molsted-Pedersen L: Early growth delay in diabetic pregnancy. p. 121. In Jovanovic L, Pederson CM, Fuhrmann K (eds): Diabetes and Pregnancy, Teratology, Toxicity and Treatment. Praeger, New York, 1986

36. Steel JM: Preconception, conception and contraception. p. 601. In Reece EA, Coustan DR (eds): Diabetes Mellitus in Pregnancy: Principles and Practice. Churchill Livingstone, New York, 1988

37. Steel JM, Johnstone FD, Corrie J: Early assessment of gestation in diabetics. Lancet 2:975, 1984

37a. Steel JM, Wu PS, Johnstone FD et al: Does early growth delay occur in diabetic pregnancy? Brit J Obstet Gynaecol (in press)

38. Whittaker P, Aspilla M, Lind T: Accurate assessment of early gestational age in normal and diabetic women by serum human placental lactogen concentration. Lancet 2:304, 1983

39. Hieta-Heikurainen H, Teramo K: Comparison of menstrual history and basal body temperature with early fetal growth by ultrasound in diabetic pregnancy. Acta Obstet Gynecol Scand 68:457, 1989

40. Cousins L, Key TC, Schorzman L, Moore TR: Ultrasound assessment of early fetal growth in insulin-treated diabetic pregnancies. Am J Obstet Gynecol 159:1186, 1988

41. Adcock CJ, Perry LA, Lindsell et al: Menstrual irregularities are more common in adolescents with type I diabetes and are associated with poor glycaemic control and weight gain. Diabetic Med 11:463, 1994

42. Eriksson UL, Dahlstrom E, Larsson S, Hellerstrom C: Increased incidence of congenital malformations in the offspring of diabetic rats and their prevention by maternal insulin therapy. Diabetes 31:1, 1982

43. Reece E, Pinter E, Leranth C et al: Malformations of the neural tube induced by in vitro hyperglycemia: an ultrastructural analysis. Teratology 32:363, 1985

44. Little DJ, Stubbs SM, Brudnell M, Campbell S: Early growth retardation in diabetic pregnancy. BMJ 278:488, 1979

45. Spellacy WM: Metabolic effects of oral contraceptives. Clin Obstet Gynecol 17:53, 1974

46. Steel JM, Duncan LJP: Serious complications of oral contraception in insulin-dependent diabetics. Contraception 17:291, 1978

47. Skouby SO, Molsted-Pedersen L, Kuhl C, Bennett P: Oral contraceptives in diabetic women: metabolic effects of four compounds with different estrogen/progestogen profiles. Fertil Steril 46:858, 1986

48. Radberg T, Gustafson A: Oral contraception in diabetic women: a cross over study on serum and high density lipoproteins (HDL) lipids and diabetes control during progestogen and combined oestrogen/progestgen contraception. Horm Metab Res 14:61, 1982

49. Westrom L, Bengtsson P, Mardh PA: The risk of pelvic inflammatory disease in women using intrauterine contraceptive devices compared to non-users. Lancet 2:221, 1976

50. Skouby SO, Molsted-Pedersen L, Kosonen A: Consequences of intrauterine contraception in diabetic women. Fertil Steril 42:568, 1984

51. Weise J: Contraception in diabetic patients. Acta Endocrinol (Copenh), suppl., 182:87, 1974

52. Steel JM, Duncan LJP: Contraception for the insulin-dependent diabetic. Diabetes Care 3:557, 1980

53. Gosden C, Steel JM, Ross A, Springbett A: Intrauterine contraceptive devices in diabetic women. Lancet 1:530, 1982

54. Larsson B, Karlsson K, Liedholm P et al: Fibrinolytic activity of the endometrium in diabetic women using Cu-IUD's. Contraception 15:711, 1977

55. Liedholm P, Asted B: Fibrinolytic activity of the rat ovum, appearance during tubal passage and disappearance at implantation. Int J Fertil 20:24, 1975

56. Kimmerle R, Weiss R, Berger M, Kurz K: Effectiveness, safety, and acceptability of a copper intrauterine device (Cu Safe 300) in type 1 diabetic women. Diabetes Care 16: 1227, 1993

57. Kjaer K, Hagen C, Sando SH, Eshoj O: Contraception in women with IDDM: an epidemiological study. Diabetes Care 15:1585, 1992

58. Vessey MP: Urinary tract infection and the diaphragm. Br J Fam Plan 2:81, 1988

59. Flynn AM, Lynch SS: Cervical mucus and identification of the fertile phase of the menstrual cycle. Br J Obstet Gynaecol 83:656, 1976

29

Postpartum Management and Lactation

ANN M. FERRIS
E. ALBERT REECE

POSTPARTUM MANAGEMENT

There is fairly unanimous agreement that improved control of maternal blood glucose is associated with decreased perinatal mortality and morbidity. Programs designed to care for pregnant diabetic women emphasize optimal glucose control as a major goal in antepartum management. However, too little attention is given to the postpartum period. In this chapter, we review the current data on postpartum care and lactation and make recommendations for management.

Insulin Requirements

After delivery, insulin requirements among women with diabetes decrease precipitiously. In the first half of the pregnancy, maternal glucose is transferred to the fetus, and food intake is ordinarily decreased because of the nausea and vomiting of pregnancy, leading to lower insulin requirements in diabetic women. Later on in the pregnancy, the increased need for insulin results from the antagonistic action to insulin by placental hormones. These "contrainsulin" hormones, which are lost after delivery, include estrogen,[1,2] human growth hormone,[3,4] human placental lactogen,[5,6] and two distinct insulin-degrading enzymes within the placenta.[7] All these changes are reversed postpartum after the expulsion of the placenta. The sensitivity to insulin increases, and so the postpartum period becomes another critical period for careful glycemic control to prevent multiple episodes of hypoglycemia.

Most diabetic patients require little or no insulin for 48 to 96 hours postpartum. Jovanovic and Peterson[8,9] recommend the resumption of insulin therapy when a 1-hour postprandial glucose value exceeds 160 mg/dl or a fasting glucose determination is above 100 mg/dl. They also recommend using a dose of 0.6 U/kg/24 h based on postpartum weight and administered in divided quantities. The caloric requirement postpartum is also less than that required during pregnancy. This is generally 25 kcal/kg/d. Breast-feeding women require about 30 kcal/kg/d.[10]

As stated previously, the sensitivity to insulin increases markedly postpartum. However, there is no general agreement on the insulin dosage or the method of insulin administration during this period. Many investigators have suggested short-acting insulin because of concerns regarding prolonged hypoglycemia if large doses of intermediate- or long-acting insulin are given.

Metabolic Control

Tyson and Hock[11] claimed that one of the most important times for precise metabolic management is postpartum. Insulin has a half-life of 15 to 17 minutes and, therefore, is active at the cellular membrane receptor for 10 to 15 minutes.[12] In that light, Tyson and Hock[11] used intravenous insulin and glucose to maintain maternal glucose homeostasis. They recommended insulin administration at a rate of 1 to 2 U/h, and blood samples for glucose determination were done periodically. In the first hour postpartum, glucose determinations were performed every 30 minutes and then hourly for up to 12 hours postpartum. They suggest close metabolic surveillance is important because hypoglycemic episodes can be anticipated at 5 and 7 hours postpartum. Furthermore, the total insulin requirement during the first 24 hours is usually less than 30 U.

Yeast et al[13] also used a continuous insulin infusion system. They studied 16 pregnant diabetic patients who received insulin infusions starting during labor and continuing through the first postpartum day or until oral intake was tolerated. Then their insulin was changed to subcutaneous longer-acting insulin. Blood glucose levels remained in the range of 75 to 150 mg/dl, with insulin infusion rates between 0.25 and 2.00 U/h. There was no apparent correlation between the severity of diabetes, or preinfusion insulin requirements, and the dose of insulin and glucose required for stabilization. In addition, the ease with which these patients' blood glucose values were maintained antepartum did not predict whether infusion would proceed smoothly postpartum. No patients exhibited hypoglycemia postpartum while receiving continuous insulin infusions, and none required any change in the insulin dose from delivery. Hence, the postpartum dose was easily calculated.

An alternative approach was used by Hanson et al[14] in a study of 55 diabetic subjects. Rather than a continuous insulin infusion, they used a reduced dosage of subcutaneous insulin. On the day of delivery, and on the first 2 postpartum days, their patients were treated with one daily injection of intermediate-acting insulin. The amount of insulin given was one-third of the total dose given on the day before delivery. Blood glucose values were determined every 4 hours for 48 hours and remained within normal limits for this period, without any evidence of hypoglycemia.

Although different approaches were used in the above studies, similar results were obtained. It should be noted, however, that both approaches (continuous intravenous insulin infusions or intermittent insulin injections) used a significantly reduced amount of insulin for postpartum management while monitoring blood glucose levels frequently, particularly for the first 24 to 48 hours postpartum.

Like Hanson et al,[14] the method of Cohen and Gabbe[15] also involved subcutaneous insulin. However, recommendations for therapy depend on the route of delivery. Patients who were delivered vaginally and could immediately tolerate oral intake could be given one-half of the pregnancy dose of insulin as NPH insulin on the first postpartum day. No additional insulin was necessary if glucosuria was absent. However, if glucosuria was present at 2+ or greater and a blood glucose value of 250 mg/dl was measured, additional insulin was given the following day. The patient who has undergone a cesarean section usually requires no additional insulin the day of delivery but might require one-third of her prepregnancy dosage of insulin as NPH insulin a few days later when her diet is being adjusted.

The above discussion describes different methods that have been used by various investigators to achieve euglycemia during the immediate postpartum period. Because the mother is prone to hypoglycemia during this period, it is important that blood glucose evaluations continue irrespective of the method of glucose control used.

The postpartum period is also one in which patients should receive counseling regarding long-term diabetic complications. If the patient had gestational diabetes, her risk of recurrence in a subsequent pregnancy and the likelihood of her developing diabetes in the future should be discussed. Much of this information is covered in the chapters on gestational diabetes and diabetic complications. A few important facts are restated below.

Gestational Diabetes

Gestational diabetes can persist postpartum. Estimates have ranged from 3 to 20 percent, with the remainder of patients reverting to normal shortly after delivery.[16–18] In a recent study, Kjos et al[19] examined the prevalence of abnormal carbohydrate metabolism in the early postpartum period (5 to 8 weeks) in 246 women with gestational diabetes mellitus. They found that 19 percent of patients had an abnormal oral glucose tolerance test result in the early puerperium. The prevalence of postpartum diabetes mellitus increased in parallel with the degree of maternal metabolic control during pregnancy, and diagnosis before 24 weeks was an additional risk factor for postpartum glucose intolerance. Their findings support the need for glucose tolerance testing at the 6-week postpartum visit, especially for women with elevated fasting serum glucose levels during pregnancy. O'Sullivan[16] found a much lower rate of persistence. It may be a matter of the demographics of the population or the adequacy of medical care before pregnancy.

A glucose tolerance test should be performed 6 weeks postpartum or when breast feeding is terminated, and those patients with persistent glucose intolerance should receive continued diabetes care. In a subsequent pregnancy, the probability of recurrence of gestational diabetes is about 60 percent. Therefore, such patients ought to be screened at their first visit. If diabetes is not diagnosed at that time, they should receive repeat screening at 26 to 28 weeks. Diabetes may also develop in patients several years after a pregnancy complicated by gestational diabetes. It has been estimated that diabetes develops in 60 percent of gestational diabetic patients within 16 years postpartum.[16] In addition, overweight patients and those in whom the initial 3-hour glucose tolerance test result was very abnormal (greater than three standard deviations above the mean) have about a 60 percent chance of manifesting diabetes in 20 years.[16,17]

More recently, Coustan et al[20] tested the hypothesis that the development of abnormal glucose tolerance after gestational diabetes could be predicted by clinical variables. They found the risk of subsequent glucose abnormality among women with a history of gestational diabetes to be quantifiable based on prepregnant body mass index and fasting plasma glucose levels during gestation.

LACTATION

Special Management Problems During Lactation

The normalization of maternal blood glucose levels (60 to 120 mg/dl) has been associated with a greater prevalence of full-term deliveries and improved fetal outcomes.[21] The impact of improved metabolic control on lactation is unknown. A variety of factors and events, including medical practices, metabolic control, infection rates, and hormonal changes, influence the initiation of lactation and the composition and volume of milk produced (Table 29-1).

Women with diabetes have more difficulty establishing and maintaining lactation.[22–25] Ferris et al[22] fol-

Table 29-1. Maternal and Infant Characteristics in Insulin-Dependent Diabetes Mellitus

Maternal characteristics
  Altered metabolism
  Difficulty maintaining glycemic control
  Increased infection rate
  Increased dehydration
  Scheduled lifestyle
Infant characteristics
  Increased birth weight
  Poor suckling ability
  Increased possibility of prematurity and related problems
    Hypoglycemia
    Hypocalcemia
    Hyperbilirubinemia
Hospital protocol
  Increased mother/infant separation
  Increased cesarean section rate

lowed 30 mothers with insulin-dependent diabetes mellitus (IDDM) from birth to 6 weeks postpartum. As many women with IDDM (53 percent) as without intended to breast feed. However, early maternal-infant separation delayed the first breast feeding until 3 days postpartum and increased the change to formula supplements more rapidly than in the general hospital population. Miyake et al[25] in Japan and Ferris et al[23] in the United States noted a significant increase in mixed breast and bottle feeding among women with IDDM (Table 29-2). In the American study, women with

Table 29-2. Frequency (%) of Breast Feeding in Women with Diabetes

	No.	Breast Feeding	Breast and Formula	Formula Only
New England[a]				
Day 14				
Women with diabetes	33	56.7	33.3	10.0
Controls	33	88.5	11.5	0
Day 42				
Women with diabetes	33	30.0	40.0	30.0
Controls	33	37	52	11
Japan[b]				
Day 30				
Women with diabetes	40	37.5	52.5	10.0
Controls	40	55.5	39.5	5.0

[a] Data from Ferris et al.[23]
[b] Data from Mikaye et al.[25] The number of women with insulin-dependent and non-insulin-dependent diabetes was not specified.

IDDM used more formula supplementation soon after delivery than the comparison group. Postpartum separation of neonates from mothers with IDDM caused this early use of formula. The continued use of formula may impair the ability of the mother to nurse adequately or the responsiveness of the neonate to breast feeding.

Medical Practices

Prenatal care of the pregnant mother with diabetes is necessarily intensive. The mother with diabetes may have neither the time nor the financial resources to attend classes that prepare her for nursing.[26] Thus, the high-risk obstetrician significantly influences the patient's decision of whether or not to breast feed. Postnatal care of the infant often involves procedures that interfere with the initiation of lactation.[27,28] The condition of the infant of a mother with diabetes often requires that the baby be separated for a minimum of 6 hours. Early and frequent suckling is considered necessary for optimal lactation,[29–31] although the importance of this early feeding is still controversial.[32,33] Early feeding of colostrum may also help prevent the higher incidence of neonatal hyperbilirubinemia.[34] If the mother cannot nurse during the observation period, then the initial advantage of early suckling may be lost. The use of scheduled feeds every 3 to 4 hours to help regulate the energy and insulin needs of the mother may adversely affect the process of lactation.[35] Furthermore, the discomfort and medications that accompany the reported 40 percent cesarean section rate add to the initial lactation difficulties for the mother with diabetes.[36]

The fetal condition may also indirectly affect lactation. Ferris et al[23] reported that at 7 and 14 days postpartum, respectively, more women with diabetes (44 and 33 percent) perceived that their infants have feeding problems than did controls (6 and 6 percent). Mothers with IDDM cite infant sleepiness as the most common infant feeding problem.

Glycemic Control

Lactating women with IDDM can have erratic insulin patterns that may cause multiple periods of hypoglycemia,[37] especially in the first week postpartum[23] and immediately after nursing.[38] Lawrence[38] cautions clini-cians that, although nursing depresses blood glucose levels, it also causes the spilling of lactose in the urine. Clinicians may misdiagnose the lactosuria as glucosuria and give additional insulin, further aggravating hypoglycemia. Murtaugh[39] found evidence of possible hypoglycemia through repeated nursing episodes. A high prevalence of hyperglycemia, as measured by fasting and postprandial blood glucose levels, was accompanied by periodic drops in blood glucose levels (Fig. 29-1).

Clinicians should maintain intensive monitoring of blood glucose concentrations at least until the sixth week postpartum and adjust insulin as needed. Women who maintain tight glycemic control during pregnancy find it more difficult to do so during lactation.[39,40] Dietary intakes below recommended levels did not improve the control.[39] Women who continue having difficulty maintaining normoglycemia should be assessed carefully for eating disorders, as these women use insulin withdrawal to increase weight loss.[41]

Fluctuations in metabolic control could also affect the composition of the milk. Hypoglycemia causes an increase in epinephrine concentrations that could decrease blood flow to the mammary gland[42] and decrease lactose secretion.[43] Although nursing decreases blood glucose levels, adequate insulin must be prescribed to prevent ketoacidosis.[38] Hyperglycemia in poorly controlled diabetic individuals can cause dehydration secondary to induced diuresis. This state of mild or moderate dehydration may lead to electrolyte imbalance. Decreased lactose and potassium concentrations and increased sodium and chloride levels have been found in milk from mildly dehydrated women.[44] Thus, good metabolic control is essential for optimal lactation in women with diabetes.

Lactation may aid in the control of diabetes by decreasing blood glucose. To ensure continued fat mobilization and prevent ketoacidosis, current data favor increasing calories while maintaining prepregnancy insulin levels. Both Tyson[45] and Lawrence[38] suggest that the additional calories be added as approximately 100 g of carbohydrate and 20 g of protein to account for the additional 500 kcal recommended in 1989 by the Food and Nutrition Board of the National Research Council.[46] Usual or recommended intakes to support lactation are approximately 2,300 to 2,700 kcal[47] or 37 kcal/kg.[48] Reducing energy intake below 1,800 kcal is not recommended.[47] Intakes of 1,500 kcal, often seen

Fig. 29-1. Postprandial glucose in lactating women (mean ± standard error). IDDM, insulin-dependent diabetes mellitus.

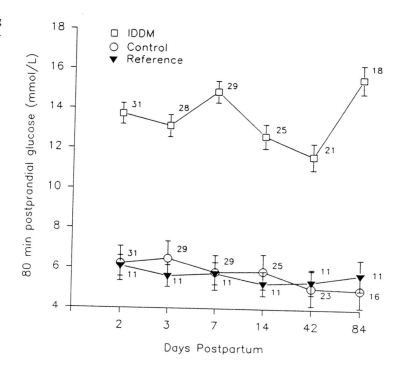

in women with IDDM, represent an approximate reduction of 30 to 40 percent in needed intake and could compromise lactation. Roberts et al[49] suggest in their work with baboons that in animals well nourished during pregnancy, lactation performance is not affected until food intake is limited by 40 percent. Intakes reduced by 20 percent are compatible with adequate lactation. Adequate lactation has been documented in women with IDDM who consumed diets of 31 kcal/kg/d.[22] However, women who stopped nursing by 42 days postpartum consumed an average of 25 kcal/kg/d. Thus, a clinician should not return mothers to prepregnancy diets but rather should prescribe diets of approximately 35 kcal/kg/d balanced with adequate insulin to ensure lactation.

No clinical data are available on the effect of daily distribution of calories or the portion of calories from each macronutrient on metabolic control during lactation. The demands of lactation, however, mandate that the mother distribute energy as snacks before nursing and eat enough to ensure lactation success.

Using breast milk lactose as a marker, Arthur et al[50] found that the onset of copious milk secretion was delayed significantly in women with IDDM; breast milk

lactose levels reached a plateau by 4 days postpartum in women with and without IDDM. An increase in milk lactose concentration parallels the decrease in milk protein and sodium[51] and precedes the increase in milk volume.[52] Neubauer et al[24] were able to measure both lactose and total nitrogen levels in a group of 33 women with IDDM. They compared their findings with those in 33 women without diabetes with comparable gestational age, delivery method, infant sex, and lactation experience. Both groups were compared with a group of 11 very healthy women who delivered vaginally and had no medical complications or difficulties with lactation. The point of the intersection of the levels of nitrogen and lactose (an indicator of lactogenesis) was significantly later in the women with IDDM (Fig. 29-2). The extent of the delay in lactogenesis correlated with maternal glycemic control. Women with poor metabolic control were more likely to experience a delay.

Delayed lactogenesis was coupled with reduced infant breast milk intake. Infants of women with IDDM consumed significantly less milk (in grams per day) than did comparison infants. At 7 days postpartum, the infants of women with IDDM consumed 310 ± 32

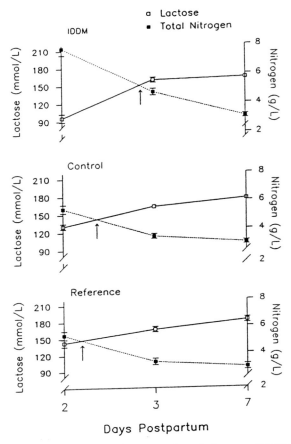

Fig. 29-2. Breast milk lactose and total nitrogen concentrations for women with insulin-dependent diabetes mellitus (IDDM) compared with control and reference women. Least squares means ± SEM, except when the SEM was smaller than the diameter of the symbol. SEM, standard error of the mean.

g/d; the controls; 455 ± 30 g/d; and the reference; 519 ± 38 g/d. For the infants of mothers with IDDM, the addition of formula increased the infant's intake at day 7 to 330 ± 28 g/d.[24] For the group with IDDM, these data are remarkably close to the intake of 376 ± 41 g/d of breast milk obtained in Japan at 6 days postpartum.[25] The breast milk intake of the reference group is comparable to that in other studies in which healthy mothers and babies were selected using similar criteria.[33] Infants of women with IDDM received more formula throughout the study.[24]

One cannot decide whether the infants in either of these studies needed a formula supplement. Perhaps if their mothers had not offered formula, the infants' demand would have stimulated increased breast milk production to a level that would have satisfied their appetites. Alternatively, without the formula, the reduced energy intake would have compromised their nutrition.

Milk Composition

In established human lactation, the breast milk of women with IDDM does not differ from that of nondiabetic controls in lactose,[53] protein,[54] lipid,[54,55] or calcium concentrations but may contain higher levels of glucose and sodium[54] and lower concentrations of low chain polyunsaturated fatty acids[55] (lipid and calcium data from Ostrom KM, Ferris AM: unpublished observation). The differences in the quality of the milk may not be clinically significant. However, the reduced maternal output may ultimately affect the growth of the infant. Coupling specific nutrient data with milk volume data provides further basis for concern. Neonatal hypocalcemia[56,57] and defective dental mineralization[58] have been documented in infants of mothers with diabetes. Phosphorus and calcitonin levels are normal. The hypocalcemia, thus, may be due to functional hypoparathyroidism.[59] Ionized and total calcium levels in umbilical venous blood of infants of patients with diabetes did not differ significantly from controls at delivery.[57] However, if the calcium concentration of the milk is not higher, despite the addition of formula, infants of mothers with IDDM may have significantly lower intake of milk and, thus, calcium.[57]

The lower energy intakes by infants born to mothers with IDDM may place them at nutritional risk, especially during lactation initiation. However, the energy needs of infants of women with IDDM may be lower. If the infants are more lethargic and sleep more, they might expend less energy and, consequently, have smaller appetites and energy needs. In addition, infants of women with IDDM may be born with higher fat stores,[60] which could explain their lower energy intakes. No data exist on comparative growth statistics beyond 3 months for breast-fed versus bottle-fed infants of women with IDDM.

Maternal Infections

Women with diabetes are prone to mastitis and monilial infections (*Candida albicans*),[38,61] especially if their disease is in poor control.[45] Changes in breast milk composition that result from mastitis can also affect the palatability of the milk for the infant if milk sodium concentrations increase to unacceptable levels.[62] Human mastitis results in significant decreases in milk production and milk lactose, glucose, potassium, and total protein concentrations and increases in sodium levels.[62] Large-scale clinical studies need to document the prevalence of these infections, including subclinical mastitis, not only in mothers with diabetes but also in the nondiabetic population.

Hormonal Changes

Both decreased[63–65] and normal[66] prolactin levels have been reported in diabetic pregnancy, and this has been related to blood glucose control.[34,63] Prolactin changes in pregnancy and lactation influence the quantity and quality of breast milk. Therefore, diabetic women with low prolactin levels may have difficulty initiating lactation. Prolactin is important for milk synthesis.[67] A deficiency of this hormone in lactating rats decreases fat synthesis in the mammary gland.[68] During mild synthesis in the mammary gland, prolactin may also influence insulin binding.[69] The mammary gland preferentially uses substrate as opposed to the liver of adipose tissue.[70,71] Ostrom and Ferris[72] found that circulating levels of serum prolactin declined temporally and were not different between women with and without diabetes. However, during the first week postpartum, milk immunoreactive prolactin levels were lower for women with IDDM. No data are available on oxytocin levels and diabetes.

CONCLUSION

Lactation in the mother with diabetes seems to be comparable to that in the mother without diabetes as long as good metabolic control is maintained. Therefore, women with diabetes should not be discouraged from breast feeding if they choose to do so. Breast feeding has been reported to enhance mother-infant bonding. To compensate for the energy demands of lactation,

physicians must prescribe adequate caloric intake. Relying on energy from adipose tissue does not appear sufficient. In the first 6 weeks postpartum, the mother with diabetes should be monitored frequently for glycemic control, and energy requirements should be adjusted or redistributed to include late night snacks if needed. Mothers with diabetes also need to be prepared for the behavior of their infants. Special help may be necessary for nursing if the baby suckles poorly or is fretful. If feeding is delayed, the mother's breast should be pumped using an electric pump on a consistent schedule. The resultant colostrum or milk, if any, may be fed to the infant. Clinicians should explain the symptoms of mastitis and encourage patients to call as soon as such symptoms occur.

The extra energy needs of lactation must be recognized, and the energy intake and the insulin dose must be adjusted to meet the maternal needs. Maintenance of metabolic control during lactation is associated with earlier lactogenesis and increased maternal milk production. Thus, to ensure adequate infant nutrition, mothers with IDDM should receive lactation counseling and continue with intensive metabolic control.

REFERENCES

1. Frantz AG, Rabkin MT: Effects of estrogen and sex differences on secretion of human growth hormone. J Clin Endocrinol Metab 25:1470, 1965
2. Beck P, Hoff DL: Oestrial modification and the effects of progesterone and human chorionic somatomammotropin on glucose tolerance and plasma insulin in rhesus monkeys. Diabetes 20:271, 1971
3. Parekh MC, Benjamin F, Gastillo N: The influence of maternal human growth hormone secretion of the weight of the newborn infant. Am J Obstet Gynecol 115:197, 1973
4. Catt KJ: Growth hormone. Lancet 1:933, 1970
5. Burt RL: Observations bearing on placental lactogenic hormone (HPL) function in pregnancy. p. 215. In Pecile A, Finzi C (eds): The Foeto-Placental Unit. Excerpta Medica, New York, 1969
6. Spellacy WN, Cohn JE: Human placental lactogen levels and daily insulin requirements in patients with diabetes mellitus complicating pregnancy. Obstet Gynecol 42:330, 1973
7. Posner BI: Insulin metabolizing enzyme activities in human placental tissue. Diabetes 22:552, 1973

8. Jovanovic L, Peterson CM: Management of the pregnant insulin-dependent diabetic woman. Diabetes Care 3:63, 1980

9. Jovanovic L, Peterson CM: Insulin and glucose requirements during the first stage of labor in insulin-dependent diabetic women. Am J Med 75:607, 1983

10. Jovanovic L, Braun SB, Druzin ML et al: Protocols for Managing Diabetes in Pregnancy. Biodynamics, Indianapolis, 1982

11. Tyson JE, Hock RA: Gestational and pregestational diabetes. An approach to therapy. Am J Obstet Gynecol 125:1009, 1976

12. Williams RH: Etiologic, pathophysiologic and clinical interrelationships in diabetes. Johns Hopkins Med J 136:25, 1975

13. Yeast JD, Porreco RP, Ginsberg HN: The use of continuous insulin infusion for the peripartum management of pregnant diabetic women. Am J Obstet Gynecol 131:861, 1978

14. Hanson U, Moberg P, Efendic S: Dosage of insulin during delivery and the immediate post-partum period in pregnant diabetics. Acta Obstet Gynecol Scand 60:183, 1981

15. Cohen AW, Gabbe SG: Intrapartum management of the diabetic patient. Clin Perinatol 8:165, 1981

16. O'Sullivan JB: Establishing criteria for gestational diabetes. Diabetes Care 3:437, 1980

17. Jovanovic L, Peterson C: Modern management of diabetes in pregnancy. p. 291. In Jovanovic L, Peterson CM, Fuhrmann K (eds): Diabetes and Pregnancy Teratology, Toxicity and Treatment. Praeger Publishers, New York, 1986

18. Coustan DR, Lewis SB: Insulin therapy for gestational diabetes. Obstet Gynecol 51:306, 1978

19. Kjos SL, Buchanan TA, Greenspoon JS et al: Gestational diabetes mellitus: the prevalence of glucose intolerance and diabetes mellitus in the first two months post partum. Am J Obstet Gynecol 163:93, 1990

20. Coustan DR, Carpenter MW, O'Sullivan PS, Carr SR: Gestational diabetes: predictors of subsequent disordered glucose metabolism. Am J Obstet Gynecol 168:1139, 1993

21. Jovanovic L, Peterson CM: Management of the pregnant insulin-dependent diabetic woman. Diabetes Care 3:63, 1980

22. Ferris AM, Dalidowitz C, Ingardia CJ et al: Lactation outcome in insulin-dependent diabetic women. J Am Diet Assoc 88:317, 1988

23. Ferris AM, Neubauaer SH, Bendel RB et al: Perinatal lactation protocol and outcome in mothers with and without insulin-dependent diabetes. Am J Clin Nutr 58:43, 1993

24. Neubauer SH, Ferris AM, Chase CG et al: Delayed lactogenesis in women with insulin-dependent diabetes. Am J Clin Nutr 58:54, 1993

25. Miyake A, Tahara M, Koike K, Tanizawa O: Decrease in neonatal suckled milk volume in diabetic women. Eur J Obstet Gynecol Reprod Biol 33:49, 1989

26. Dalidowitz C: Lactation in the Diabetic. Unpublished master's thesis. University of Connecticut, Storrs, CT, 1986

27. Hally MR, Bond J, Crawley J et al: What influences a mother's choice of infant feeding method? Nurs Times 80:65, 1984

28. Salariya EM, Eason PM, Cater JI: Duration of breast-feeding after early initiation and frequent feeding. Lancet 2:1141, 1978

29. Elander G, Lindberg T: Short mother-infant separation during the first week of life influences the duration of breastfeeding. Acta Pediatr Scand 73:237, 1984

30. Slaven S, Harvey D: Unlimited suckling time improves breastfeeding. Lancet 1:392, 1981

31. Ferris AM, McCabe LT, Allen LH et al: Biological and sociocultural determinants of successful lactation among women in eastern Connecticut. J Am Diet Assoc 87:316, 1987

32. Woolridge MW, Greasley V, Silpisornkosol S: The initiation of lactation: the effect of early versus delayed contact for suckling on milk intake in the first week postpartum. A study in Chiang Mia, northern Thailand. Early Hum Dev 12:260, 1985

33. Allen LH, Ferris AM, Pelto GH: Maternal factors affecting lactation. p. 51. In Hamosh M, Goldman AS (eds): Human Lactation 2. Maternal and Environmental Factors. Plenum Press, New York, 1986

34. Good J: The Diabetic Mother and Breastfeeding. Information Sheet No. 17. La Leche League International, Inc., Franklin Park, IL, 1983

35. Felig P, Coustan D: Diabetes mellitus. In Burrow GN, Ferris TF (eds): Medical Complications During Pregnancy. WB Saunders, Philadelphia, 1982

36. Gabbe SG, Quilligan EJ: General obstetric management of the diabetic pregnancy. Clin Obstet Gynecol 24:91, 1981

37. Jovanovic L, Peterson CM: Insulin and glucose requirements during the first state of labor in insulin-dependent diabetic women. Am J Med 75:607, 1983

38. Lawrence R: Breastfeeding, a Guide for the Medical Profession. 2nd Ed. CV Mosby, St. Louis, 1985

39. Murtaugh M: Factors Leading to Euglycemia in Lactating Women with Insulin-Dependent Diabetes Mellitus (IDD) in the First 12 Weeks Postpartum. Unpublished doctoral dissertation. University of Connecticut, Storrs, CT, 1991

40. Gagne M, Leff EW, Jefferies SC: The breast-feeding experience of women with type I diabetes. Health Care Women Int 13:249, 1992

41. Rodin GM, Daneman D, Johnson LE et al: Anorexia nervosa and bulimia in female adolescents with insulin-de-

pendent diabetes: a systemic study. J Psychiatr Res 19: 381, 1985

42. Rosenfeld C, Barton M, Meschia G: Effects of epinephrine on distribution of blood flow in the pregnant ewe. Am J Obstet Gynecol 124:15, 1976

43. Hove K: Maintenance of lactose secretion during acute insulin deficiency in lactating goats. Acta Pediatr Scand 103:173, 1978

44. Prentice A, Lamb W, Prentice A et al: The effect of water abstention on milk synthesis in lactating women. Clin Sci 66:291, 1984

45. Tyson JE: The diabetic nursing mother. Keeping Abreast J 1:106, 1976

46. National Research Council: Recommended Dietary Allowances. 10th Ed. Report of the Subcommittee of the Tenth Edition of the RDAs, Food and Nutrition Board, Commission on Life Sciences. National Academy press, Washington, DC, 1989

47. Food and Nutrition Board: Nutrition During Lactation. Report of Committee on Nutritional Status During Pregnancy and Lactation, Institute of Medicine. National Academy Press, Washington, DC, 1991

48. Butte NF, Garza C, Stuff JE et al: Effect of maternal diet and body composition on lactational performance. Am J Clin Nutr 39:396, 1984

49. Roberts SB, Cole TJ, Coward WA: Lactational performance in relation to energy intake in the baboon. Am J Clin Nutr 41:1270, 1985

50. Arthur PG, Smith M, Hartmann PE: Milk lactose, citrate, and glucose as markers of lactogenesis in normal and diabetic women. J Pediatr Gastroenterol Nutr 9:488, 1989

51. Kulski JK, Hartmann PE: Changes in human milk composition during the initiation of lactation. Aust J Exp Biol Med Sci 59:101, 1981

52. Neville MC, Allen JC, Archer PC et al: Studies in human lactations: milk volume and nutrient composition during weaning and lactogenesis. Am J Clin Nutr 54:81, 1991

53. Tolstoi E: The relationship of blood glucose to the concentration of lactose in the milk of lactating diabetic women. J Clin Invest 14:863, 1935

54. Butte NF, Garza C, Burr R et al: Milk composition of insulin-dependent diabetic women. J Pediatr Gastroenterol Nutr 6:936, 1987

55. Jackson MB, Lammi-Keefe CJ, Jensen RG et al: Total lipid and fatty acid composition of milk in women with and without insulin-dependent diabetes mellitus. Am J Clin Nutr (in press)

56. Salle B, David L, Glorieus F et al: Hypocalcemia in infants of diabetic mothers. Acta Paediatr Scand 71:573, 1982

57. Cruikshank D, Pitkin R, Varner M et al: Calcium metabolism in diabetic mother, fetus, and newborn infant. Am J Obstet Gynecol 145:1010, 1983

58. Noren JG: Microscopic study of enamel defects in deciduous teeth of infants of diabetic mothers. Acta Odontol Scand 42:153, 1984

59. Nogushi A, Eren M, Tsang RC: Parathyroid hormone in hypocalcemic and normocalcemic infants of diabetic mothers. J Pediatr 97:112, 1980

60. Pederson J: The Pregnant Diabetic and Her Newborn. 2nd Ed. Williams & Wilkins, Baltimore, 1977

61. Miller D: Birth and long-term unsupplemented breastfeeding in 17 insulin-dependent diabetic mothers. Birth Fam J 4:65, 1977

62. Ramadan M, Salah M, Eid S: Effect of breast infection on the composition of human milk. Int J Biochem 3:543, 1972

63. Larinkari J, Laatikainen L, Rants T et al: Metabolic control and serum hormone levels in relation to retinopathy in diabetic pregnancy. Diabetologia 22:327, 1982

64. Sadovsky E, Weinstein D, Ben-David M et al: Serum prolactin in normal and pathologic pregnancy. Obstet Gynecol 50:559, 1977

65. Botta RM, Donatelli M, Bucalo ML et al: Placental lactogen, progestrone, total estriol and prolactin plasma levels in pregnant women with insulin-dependent diabetes mellitus. Eur J Obstet Gynecol Reprod Biol 16:393, 1984

66. Jovanovic L, Peterson C, Dawood Y et al: The effect of normalization of blood glucose on the hromonal profile of insulin-dependent pregnant women. Diabetes, suppl. 2, 28:348, 1979

67. Hytten F: The physiology of lactation. J Hum Nutr 30:225, 1976

68. Agius L, Robinson A, Girard J et al: Alterations in the rate of lipogenesis in vovo in maternal liver and adipose tissue on premature weaning of lactating rats. Biochem J 180:689, 1979

69. Flint D: Regulation of insulin receptors by prolactin in lactating rat mammary gland. J Endocrinol 923:279, 1982

70. Roibinson A, Williamson D: Comparison of glucose metabolism in the lactating mammary gland of the rat liver in vitro. Biochem J 164:153, 1977

71. Ostrom KM, Ferris AM: Prolactin concentrations in serum and milk of mothers with and without insulin dependent diabetes mellitus. Am J Clin Nutr 58:49, 1993

Index

Page numbers followed by *f* represent figures; those followed by *t* represent tables.

A

Abdominal circumference measurements, fetal, 222, 223f
  compared to biparietal diameter, 224
  in macrosomia, 224–225, 225t
Abortion, spontaneous, 6, 114
Abstinence, in natural family planning, 425
Acesulfame-K, 194
Acetonuria, maternal, and intelligence quotient in offspring, 384
N-Acetylcholinesterase determination in spina bifida, 230
Acidemia, fetal, 256
Acrania, 121
Acylcarnitine transferase, hepatic, 48
Adenomatosis, islet, 87, 88, 89t
Adenosine deaminase gene, 18
Adipocytes, glucose uptake by, 60, 60t
Adipose tissue
  fetal, in hyperinsulinemia, 84, 84f
  in infants of diabetic mothers, in macrosomia, 107
  metabolic actions of insulin on, 37, 37t
Adrenal glands, hypoxic injury of, 108, 109
Aerobic exercise, 202–203
Age
  fetal, dating of, 219–222, 255, 355, 423
  in gestational diabetes, 266
  and incidence of diabetes, 12, 383f
    and parity, 390f, 390t
  in insulin-dependent diabetes, 12
  in non-insulin-dependent diabetes, 12
Agenesis, renal, 240, 241f, 242
Alanine
  in fasting, 39
    in pregnancy, 63–64
  in postabsorptive state, 38–39, 39f, 46, 47
  in pregnancy, 159
    compared to nonpregnant women, 63f
    and fasting, 63–64
  transfer to fetus, 156

Albumin
  glycated
    in gestational diabetes, 270
    glomerular handling of, 325
  urinary, 323–325
    in course of nephropathy, 320f, 320–323, 323f
    in definition of nephropathy, 315–316
    in exercise, 320
    in insulin-dependent diabetes, 315–316, 322, 323f, 324t
    in insulin therapy, 330
    and macrovascular disease, 328
    in microalbuminuria, 316, 322, 323f, 324t, 325
    preconception evaluation of, 331
Aldose reductase pathway, 326f
Alloxan-induced diabetes, 126
  fetal lung maturation in, 98, 99
Amino acid metabolism, 67
  in fasting, 39–40
    in pregnancy, 63–64
  in fetal hyperinsulinemia, 84
  gender-related differences in, 44
  ingestion of protein affecting, 43f, 43–44, 49
  in insulin-dependent diabetes, 46–47, 47f, 49
  in insulin therapy, 53
  in non-insulin-dependent diabetes, 47–48, 49
  in postabsorptive state, 38–39, 46–47, 47f
  in pregnancy, 65, 159
    compared to nonpregnant women, 62–63, 63f
    and fasting, 63–64
  and transfer to fetus, 156
Amniotic fluid
  in gestational diabetes, 270–271, 281
  indicators of fetal lung maturity in, 253, 254, 354, 373
  diabetic pregnancy affecting, 102
  predicting risk for respiratory distress syndrome, 96

in nephropathy, 335
  in respiratory distress syndrome, 96, 109–110, 253–254, 373
  volume of, 256, 257–258
    in hydramnios, 243–244, 293–294.
    See also Hydramnios
Amputation, in peripheral neuropathy, 347
Anabolism, 62
Anemia, in nephropathy, 333t, 334
Anencephaly, 121, 228, 229f
Angiotensin-converting enzyme, 316
  inhibitors of, 329
    contraindication in pregnancy, 329, 332
Animal models
  on congenital malformations, 125, 126–128
    and prevention of dysmorphogenesis, 139–145
  on exercise, 205, 207
  on fetal growth and development, 88, 88f
    compared to human studies, 88, 88f, 88t
    in hyperinsulinemia, 81–85, 88
    insulin-like growth factor levels in, 86
    lung maturation in, 98, 99
    in macrosomia, 88, 89t
    maternal glucose blood levels in, 185
    neural tube and yolk sac in, 133–139
    and prevention of malformations, 139–145
  on infants of diabetic mothers, 384
Antenatal care, 417–423
  in deviant fetal growth and congenital malformations, 219–244, 420–421
Antibodies
  glutamic acid decarboxylase, 16, 29
  insulin, 175–177
    in gestational diabetes, 279
    and macrosomia, 176–177
    in pathogenesis of insulin-dependent diabetes, 16, 29, 405
    placental transport of, 176
  islet cell
    cytoplasmic, 29, 405

439